# Nanozymes

# Nanozymes

## Advances and Applications

**Edited by**

*Sundaram Gunasekaran*

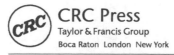

CRC Press
Taylor & Francis Group
Boca Raton London New York

CRC Press is an imprint of the
Taylor & Francis Group, an **informa** business

First edition published 2022
by CRC Press
2 Park Square, Milton Park, Abingdon, Oxon, OX14 4RN

and by CRC Press
6000 Broken Sound Parkway NW, Suite 300, Boca Raton, FL 33487-2742

*British Library Cataloguing-in-Publication Data*
A catalog record for this book is available from the British Library

---

### Library of Congress Cataloging-in-Publication Data

---

Names: Gunasekaran, Sundaram, 1957- editor.
Title: Nanozymes : advances and applications / edited by Sundaram Gunasekaran.
Description: First edition. | Boca Raton : CRC Press, [2022] | Includes bibliographical references and index. | Summary: "This book presents an up-to-date account of the emerging field of nanozymes. These nanomaterials function as enzymes to provide novel functionalities and rival that of traditional enzymes. The book focus on issues relating to the preparation and use of nanozymes and their attendant issues and the paths to overcome"– Provided by publisher.
Identifiers: LCCN 2021025842 (print) | LCCN 2021025843 (ebook) | ISBN 9780367623883 (pbk.) | ISBN 9780367619084 (hbk.) | ISBN 9781003109228 (ebk.)
Subjects: LCSH: Enzymes–Biotechnology. | Enzymes–Industrial applications. | Enzymes–Synthesis. | Nanotechnology. | Biomedical materials.
Classification: LCC TP248.65.E59 N36 2022 (print) | LCC TP248.65.E59 (ebook) | DDC 620/.5–dc23
LC record available at https://lccn.loc.gov/2021025842
LC ebook record available at https://lccn.loc.gov/2021025843

---

ISBN: 978-0-367-61908-4 (hbk)
ISBN: 978-0-367-62388-3 (pbk)
ISBN: 978-1-003-10922-8 (ebk)

DOI: 10.1201/9781003109228

Typeset in Times
by KnowledgeWorks Global Ltd.

# Contents

# Preface

Enzymes catalyze various important biochemical reactions that are essential to sustain life and for a myriad of industrial products and processes. As is the case with many biological entities, enzymes have evolved over the years to catalyze various compounds to different extents. Despite their extraordinary specificity, activity, and yield, enzymes are limited in many ways. Most enzymes work well only under a narrow range of physiological and environmental conditions; they are expensive to produce and difficult to reuse. To overcome these and other limitations, efforts have been focused, for over 70 years now, on developing artificial enzymes – organic compounds that can perform enzymatic functions. The latest outcome from these attempts is a group of nanosized materials – both organic and inorganic – called nanozymes. The ability of nanomaterials to catalyze biochemical reactions was first recognized in 1996 when it was discovered that fullerene derivatives can scavenge free radicals. This was followed by a similar discovery in 2006 that cerium oxide nanoparticles can scavenge reactive oxygen. Definitive confirmation of nanoparticles possessing an intrinsic enzyme-mimetic activity was revealed in 2007. Since then, there has been a slew of research reporting a variety of nanomaterials (metals, metal oxides, metal-carbon compound nanomaterials, etc.) with catalytic properties mimicking natural enzymes peroxidase, haloperoxidase, peroxidase, catalase, oxidase, glucose oxidase, sulfite oxidase, superoxide dismutase, etc.

The field of nanozymes is very young, and in fact, a formal definition of nanozymes was not available until 2013. Nonetheless, there has been explosive growth in nanozymes-related research with a couple of hundred groups around the world pursuing some aspect of nanozyme, especially since nanozymes help overcome the stability and cost constraints of natural enzymes. Further advantages of nanozymes include small size, tunable properties, easy surface modification, high catalytic turnover number, targeted transfer, sequential catalysis, etc. In addition to these exciting properties, nanozymes also lend themselves to various applications in the broad fields of health, environment, and food. The further growth in nanozymes will have to take a more deliberate and rational approach to overcome limitations such as lack of specificity, potential toxicity, etc.

This book starts with a historical and practical account of enzymes (Chapter 1) followed by a broad overview of nanozymes (Chapter 2). Chapters 3 to 5 describe different nanozymes. In subsequent chapters, a detailed up-to-date summary of many applications of nanozymes in biomedicine (Chapters 7 to 10), environment (Chapters 11 and 12), and food (Chapters 13 to 15) fields are presented. Chapter 16 describes the rational design of nanozymes, with peroxidase as an example, to overcome their own set of limitations. The potential toxicological effects of nanozymes, presented in Chapter 17, are important to consider but have not received the attention they deserve, especially in certain biomedicine applications.

This book is a collective effort of several authors, who have made important contributions to the field of nanozymes. I sincerely thank them for supporting this project.

**Sundaram Gunasekaran**
*University of Wisconsin-Madison*

# Editor Biography

**Dr. Sundaram Gunasekaran** is a Professor in the Department of Biological Systems Engineering at the University of Wisconsin-Madison. He earned hid PhD in agricultural and biological engineering from the University of Illinois at Urbana-Champaign. His research focuses on the synthesis of metallic and non-metallic nanomaterials and their applications in biosensing, encapsulation, and delivery. He has developed various biosensors for the detection of targets such as pathogens, chemicals, heavy metals, disease biomarkers, and cancer cells. He has published nearly 250 peer-reviewed papers and has 12 patents.

# List of Contributors

**Syed Rahin Ahmed**
W Booth School of Engineering
   Practice and Technology
McMaster University
Ontario, Canada

**Loghman Alaei**
Department of Biology and
   Biotechnology
Faculty of Sciences
University of Kurdistan
Sanandaj, Iran

**Ebrahim Barzegari**
Medical Biology Research Center
Health Technology Institute
Kermanshah University of Medical
   Sciences
Kermanshah, Iran

**Ana Gomez Cardoso**
W Booth School of Engineering
   Practice and Technology
McMaster University
Ontario, Canada

**Ling Chen**
State Key Laboratory of Quality
   Research in Chinese Medicine
Institute of Chinese Medical Sciences
University of Macau
Macau, China

**Weilin Chen**
Institute of Molecular Sciences and
   Engineering
Institute of Frontier and
   Interdisciplinary Science
Shandong University
Shandong, China

**Zehua Cheng**
State Key Laboratory of Quality
   Research in Chinese Medicine
Institute of Chinese Medical Sciences
University of Macau
Macau, China

**Hossein Derakhshankhah**
Pharmaceutical Sciences Research
   Center
School of Pharmacy
Kermanshah University of Medical
   Sciences
Kermanshah, Iran

**Cem Erkmen**
Faculty of Pharmacy
Department of Analytical Chemistry
Ankara University
Ankara, Turkey

**Sundaram Gunasekaran**
Department of Biological Systems
   Engineering
University of Wisconsin-Madison
Madison, WI, USA

**Kadriye Özlem Hamaloğlu**
Chemical Engineering Department
Hacettepe University
Ankara, Turkey

**Kaiyu He**
State Key Laboratory for Managing
   Biotic and Chemical Threats to the
   Quality and Safety of Agro-Products
Institute of Agro-Product Safety and
   Nutrition
Zhejiang Academy of Agricultural
   Sciences
Hangzhou, China

**Lunjie Huang**
School of Food Science and Engineering
South China University of Technology
Guangzhou, China
and
Academy of Contemporary Food
    Engineering
Guangzhou Higher Education Mega
    Center
South China University of Technology
Guangzhou, China
and
Engineering and Technological
    Research Centre of Guangdong
    Province on Intelligent Sensing
    and Process Control of Cold Chain
    Foods, & Guangdong Province
    Engineering Laboratory for
    Intelligent Cold Chain Logistics
    Equipment for Agricultural Products
Guangzhou Higher Education Mega Centre
Guangzhou, China

**Zhila Izadi**
Pharmaceutical Sciences Research Center
School of Pharmacy
Kermanshah University of Medical
    Sciences
Kermanshah, Iran

**Samira Jafari**
Pharmaceutical Sciences Research Center
School of Pharmacy
Kermanshah University of Medical
    Sciences
Kermanshah, Iran

**Mehdi Jaymand**
Nano Drug Delivery Research Center
Health Technology Institute
Kermanshah University of Medical
    Sciences
Kermanshah, Iran

**Çiğdem Kip**
Chemical Engineering Department
Hacettepe University
Ankara, Turkey

**Satish Kumar**
W Booth School of Engineering
    Practice and Technology
McMaster University
Ontario, Canada

**Sevinc Kurbanoglu**
Faculty of Pharmacy
Department of Analytical Chemistry
Ankara University
Ankara, Turkey

**Chunxia Li**
Institute of Molecular Sciences and
    Engineering
Institute of Frontier and
    Interdisciplinary Science
Shandong University
Shandong, China

**Peng Li**
State Key Laboratory of Quality
    Research in Chinese Medicine
Institute of Chinese Medical Sciences
University of Macau
Macau, China

**Xin Li**
School of Chemistry and Chemical
    Engineering
Jiangsu University
Zhenjiang, China

**Biwu Liu**
Institute of Analytical Chemistry and
    Instrument for Life Science
The Key Laboratory of Biomedical
    Information Engineering of Ministry
    of Education
School of Life Science and Technology
Xi'an Jiaotong University
Xi'an, Shaanxi, China

**Juewen Liu**
Department of Chemistry
Waterloo Institute for Nanotechnology
University of Waterloo
Waterloo, Ontario, Canada

**Peng Liu**
School of Chemistry and Chemical
    Engineering
Jiangsu University
Zhenjiang, China

**Alireza Lotfabadi**
Pharmaceutical Sciences Research
    Center
School of Pharmacy
Kermanshah University of Medical
    Sciences
Kermanshah, Iran

**Mai Luo**
State Key Laboratory of Quality
    Research in Chinese Medicine
Institute of Chinese Medical
    Sciences
University of Macau
Macau, China

**Jean Louis Marty**
Université de Perpignan Via
    Domitia
Perpignan, France

**Seema Nara**
Department of Biotechnology
Motilal Nehru National Institute of
    Technology
Allahabad, India

**Xiangheng Niu**
School of Chemistry and Chemical
    Engineering
Jiangsu University
Zhenjiang, China

**Greter A. Ortega**
W Booth School of Engineering
    Practice and Technology
McMaster University
Ontario, Canada

**Haisheng Qian**
School of Biomedical Engineering
Research and Engineering Center of
    Biomedical Materials
Anhui Medical University
Hefei, China

**Amin Reza Rajabzadeh**
W Booth School of Engineering
    Practice and Technology
McMaster University
Ontario, Canada

**José I. Reyes De Corcuera**
Department of Food Science and
    Technology
University of Georgia
Athens, GA, USA

**Atul Sharma**
School of Chemistry
Monash University
Clayton, Melbourne, Australia
and
Department of Pharmaceutical
    Chemistry
SGT College of Pharmacy
SGT University
Budhera, Gurugram, Haryana,
    India

**Smriti Singh**
Department of Biotechnology
Motilal Nehru National Institute of
    Technology
Allahabad, India

**Seshasai Srinivasan**
W Booth School of Engineering
    Practice and Technology
McMaster University
Ontario, Canada

**Da-Wen Sun**
School of Food Science and
   Engineering
South China University of Technology
Guangzhou, China
and
Academy of Contemporary Food
   Engineering
Guangzhou Higher Education Mega
   Center
South China University of Technology
Guangzhou, China
and
Engineering and Technological
   Research Centre of Guangdong
   Province on Intelligent Sensing
   and Process Control of Cold Chain
   Foods, & Guangdong Province
   Engineering Laboratory for
   Intelligent Cold Chain Logistics
   Equipment for Agricultural Products
Guangzhou Higher Education Mega
   Centre
Guangzhou, China
and
Food Refrigeration and Computerized
   Food Technology (FRCFT)
Agriculture and Food Science Centre
University College Dublin
National University of Ireland
Belfield, Dublin, Ireland


**Swapnil Tiwari**
School of Studies in Chemistry
Pt Ravishankar Shukla University
Raipur, C.G., India


**Ali Tuncel**
Chemical Engineering Department
Hacettepe University
Ankara, Turkey


**Bengi Uslu**
Faculty of Pharmacy
Department of Analytical Chemistry
Ankara University
Ankara, Turkey


**Liu Wang**
State Key Laboratory for Managing
   Biotic and Chemical Threats to the
   Quality and Safety of Agro-Products
Institute of Agro-Product Safety and
   Nutrition
Zhejiang Academy of Agricultural
   Sciences
Hangzhou, China


**Man Wang**
Institute of Molecular Sciences and
   Engineering
Institute of Frontier and
   Interdisciplinary Science
Shandong University
Shandong, China


**Mengzhu Wang**
School of Chemistry and Chemical
   Engineering
Jiangsu University
Zhenjiang, China


**Ting Wang**
State Key Laboratory of Quality
   Research in Chinese Medicine
Institute of Chinese Medical Sciences
   University of Macau
Macau, China


**Weizheng Wang**
Department of Biological Systems
   Engineering
University of Wisconsin-Madison
Madison, WI, USA


**Xianwen Wang**
School of Food and Biological
   Engineering
Hefei University of Technology
Hefei, China
and
School of Biomedical Engineering
Research and Engineering Center of
   Biomedical Materials
Anhui Medical University
Hefei, China

**Xiaoyu Wang**
Department of Biomedical Engineering
College of Engineering and Applied
    Sciences
Nanjing National Laboratory of
    Microstructures
Jiangsu Key Laboratory of Artificial
    Functional Materials
Nanjing University
Nanjing, Jiangsu, China

**Hui Wei**
Department of Biomedical Engineering
College of Engineering and Applied
    Sciences
Nanjing National Laboratory of
    Microstructures
Jiangsu Key Laboratory of Artificial
    Functional Materials
Nanjing University
Nanjing, Jiangsu, China
and
State Key Laboratory of Analytical
    Chemistry for Life Science
School of Chemistry and Chemical
    Engineering
Chemistry and Biomedicine Innovation
    Center (ChemBIC)
Nanjing University
Nanjing, Jiangsu, China

**Jinchao Wei**
State Key Laboratory of Quality
    Research in Chinese Medicine
Institute of Chinese Medical Sciences
    University of Macau
Macau, China

**Long Wu**
Key Laboratory of Food Nutrition
    and Functional Food of Hainan
    Province
College of Food Science and
    Engineering
Hainan University
Haikou, Hainan, China

**Yulin Xie**
Institute of Molecular Sciences and
    Engineering
Institute of Frontier and
    Interdisciplinary Science
Shandong University
Shandong, China

**Xiahong Xu**
State Key Laboratory for Managing
    Biotic and Chemical Threats to the
    Quality and Safety of Agro-Products
Institute of Agro-Product Safety and
    Nutrition
Zhejiang Academy of Agricultural
    Sciences
Hangzhou, China

**Zhengbao Zha**
School of Food and Biological
    Engineering
Hefei University of Technology
Hefei, China

**Xiaoyan Zhong**
Department of Toxicology
School of Public Health
Jiangsu Key Laboratory of Preventive
    and Translational Medicine for
    Geriatric Diseases
Medical College of Soochow University
Suzhou, China

# 1 Enzymes—Inspiring Evolutionary Wisdom

*José I. Reyes De Corcuera*
Department of Food Science and Technology,
University of Georgia, Athens, GA, USA

## CONTENTS

## 1.1 INTRODUCTION

Since antiquity, humans have been intrigued by the mechanisms of natural processes. Early civilizations were particularly intrigued by the fermentation of wine, dough leavening, and digestion. It was not until the 19th century that Friedrich Wilhelm Kühne coined the term "enzyme" to name the entities that produced ferments in the absence of yeast. In the second half of the 20th century, enzyme structures began to be resolved and the mechanisms of regulation of enzyme catalysis began to be elucidated. Like with other marvels of the natural world, humans have tried to learn and harness the properties of enzymes. Enzymes are the muses that have inspired several biomimetic efforts. This metaphor is useful because enzymes have fascinated humans for thousands of years, and even today, they continue to mesmerize the minds of thousands of scientists. As catalysts present in all biological systems, enzymes are the engine of life, and to some extent, they are responsible for the

DOI: 10.1201/9781003109228-1

beauty of the living world. At the molecular level, the frequent symmetry and motion of these proteins is a structural ballet that adjusts its tempo with the environment and responds to the needs of living systems, regulating many of its processes.

Since the early 1970s, some scientists have tried to create synthetic enzymes that are stable by imitating some of the structural characteristics of natural enzymes (1). Indeed, many enzymes are not sufficiently stable to be of practical industrial use. Arguably, there are very few commercially available enzyme biosensors because of the poor stability of most bioanalytical enzymes (2). Some, including the author of this chapter, have researched the strategies to stabilize enzymes using conventional chemical modifications (3) and playing with one variable often ignored in enzyme stabilization: pressure (4). Nanozymes as defined by the consensus of the recent literature (5, 6) are not the product of biomimetics as the term might suggest. Rather, they are stable nanomaterials (NMs) that display high catalytic activity and may have other enzyme-like characteristics.

In this chapter, basic background on enzymes is presented to help the readers contextualize the current research efforts in nanozymes. Despite the over one million publications since 1900 that include the keyword "enzyme" (per Web of Science), science has not fully revealed all the mysteries of these proteins. It is impossible to do justice to enzymes in one chapter, especially in a book that is devoted to their human-made counterparts. Instead, after a brief history of enzymes and enzymology, we clarify some generalizations that have been done about enzymes, we overview chemical and enzyme catalysis, enzyme function, and biomimetics. We invite the reader to reflect and to explore in-depth the fundamentals of chemical and enzyme catalysis that are beyond the scope of this chapter as that will serve well in understanding nanozymes. We also hope that contemplating evolutionary wisdom revealed by thousands of enzyme reactions that have emerged through millions of years of evolution will help the scientific community leverage nanoscale research.

## 1.2   A BRIEF HISTORY/CHRONOLOGY ON ENZYMES AND ENZYMOLOGY

Fifteen years ago, Joseph Fruton published "Fermentation, Vital or Chemical Process?" (7), an excellent book that summarizes the history of enzymes. Most of this section is based on that book. For the benefit of the reader, we use the original references rather than the book but, credit should be given to Dr. Fruton for distilling through hundreds of most relevant publications. The dialectics of the title of that book could not be more pertinent to contextualize nanozymes. It is unclear when humans first observed and started using fermentation as a means to preserve and transform food. Archeological discoveries continue to push back that date. For many years, there was a consensus that beer had originated in Mesopotamia or Egypt shortly after agriculture began. However, recent findings suggest that the first man-made beer originated in China (8). Fermentation has fascinated humans not only because of the ability to leaven bread but because of the intoxicating effects of beverages resulting from this "effervescence."

The word enzyme has its origin in ancient Greece, ζύμη (zyme) meaning leaven or yeast. Of course, at that time, the nature of yeasts or ferments had not been discovered. Plato briefly refers to the bubbles produced during putrefaction and produce effervescence. Alchemists in Europe, northern Africa, and the Middle East developed multiple theories starting with knowledge exchanges in Alexandria. However, in the absence of a chemical understanding of the elements and the principle of conservation of mass, not much verifiable progress was made until the 17th century. Newton (9) hypothesized that strong attraction forces produced by acid particles were responsible for fermentation. Lavoisier (10) tested his principle of conservation of mass by fermenting sugar with "moût" (wort) and water. In 1810, Appert (11) published the book that revolutionized food preservation; he reported that food did not spoil when heated in sealed containers. Gay-Lussac (12) observed that putrefaction and fermentation occur when the heated containers were opened but he was unable to explain the reason. The development of the achromatic compound microscope allowed Caignard Latour, Schwann, and Kützing to discover almost at the same time that yeast consisted of "globular bodies able to reproduce themselves" that were not just chemical substances and were responsible for the fermentation of wine (13). Schwann wondered whether yeast fermentation could be compared to the effect of a chemical that he named pepsin, which is responsible for the gastric digestion of albumin. Friedrich Wilhelm Kühne coined the word enzyme in 1878 to refer in general to these unorganized ferments (different from organized ferments like yeasts) which led to the hypothesis that even within (the "en" of "enzymes) microorganisms, such compounds were responsible for the catalytic reaction in the cell. Twenty years later, Fisher observed that some enzymes (invertin and emulsin) hydrolyzed different stereoisomers and created the analogy of a "lock-and-key" to describe the specificity of enzymes toward the substrate (14). In 1907, Eduard Buchner received the Nobel Prize in Chemistry "for his biochemical researches and his discovery of cell-free fermentation." The extraction of the enzymes from the yeast cell was possible thanks to the use of a high hydraulic press, through mechanical maceration with sand and diatomaceous earth at 50 MPa. At that point, Buchner believed that only one enzyme "zymase" was responsible for alcoholic fermentation of sugar but Richard Neumeister hypothesized that multiple substances were involved. After the first World War, the 12-enzyme metabolic pathway that yeast uses to convert glucose into alcohol and carbon dioxide was fully elucidated. Like with other fields in science, the second half of the 20th century saw an accelerated rate of scientific discovery, and such acceleration continues along with the compartmentalization of subdisciplines. Enzymologists today can spend their entire careers in just one aspect of this immensely vast field discovering new enzymes, new metabolic pathways, new methods of purification, creating transgenic organisms that overexpress a given enzyme, studying the kinetics, thermodynamics, or the structure of a particular enzyme, etc.

## 1.3 CLARIFYING SOME GENERALIZATIONS OF THE PROPERTIES OF ENZYMES

### 1.3.1 STABILITY

In our efforts to highlight the relevance of our research on enzyme stabilization, we have stated that many enzymes are thermally unstable. It is true that enzymes like other proteins, unfold and lose their activity when exposed to elevated temperatures, pressures, or denaturants. However, the temperature, pressure, or concentration of denaturant that induces unfolding and the rate at which that occurs vary from protein to protein and depends on the amino acid sequence, the folding of the protein, and other environmental factors. Enzymes from hyperthermophiles, such as archaea and some bacteria that thrive at 80°C–110°C are thermostable. While hyperthermophiles are difficult to culture, sequencing and metagenomics have allowed the production of thermophilic enzymes in mesophiles (15). Piezophiles found in the deep sea, are also often thermophiles. Because of the very high pressure, in the deep sea, higher temperatures can be reached without phase change, which may result in increased thermophilicity (16). With the development of high hydrostatic pressure technology, the potential use of piezophilic/thermophilic enzymes may become economically viable. At the other end of the spectrum, enzymes from psychrophiles that are metabolically active in the range of –20°C to 10°C are of particular interest not only because of their catalytic activity at low temperatures, which represents energy savings compared to reaction that requires heating. Also, they appear to be more stable than their mesophilic homologs (17). Despite the advances in genomics, it is difficult to precisely ascertain the evolutionary route that has resulted in such a variety of enzymes with different properties (18) as microorganisms have adapted to different environments. Perhaps an important misconception is that "industrial conditions" are synonymous with high temperature and chemically harsh. About fifteen years ago talking to a friend whose company produces enzymes, he told me that actually, the industry would rather have enzymes that are highly catalytic at cold temperatures to save the equipment and energy costs of heating. Indeed, the "industrial conditions" are not dogmatic but set with the economic goal of reducing the cost of production. It is also true that many enzymes that have an economic potential have not reached that potential because of their poor stability. One such enzyme is alcohol oxidase, which our team is currently researching for its potential in biosensor development and the production of flavors (19, 20).

## 1.3.2 Cost

It is true that relative to the number of enzymes that have been discovered, very few have become commercially available. Cost of production, lack of a sufficiently large market, and sometimes poor stability have prevented the commercialization of many enzymes. However, many enzymes are inexpensive, including pectinases used in fruit juice clarification, amylases, enzymes used in the production of high fructose corn syrup, and proteases used in detergents. In some cases (e.g., pectinases), they are cheap enough that it is not worth immobilizing them for recovery. These enzymes end up being inactivated during fruit juice pasteurization. Enzymes used for analytical purposes vary widely in price. For example, per the Sigma-Aldrich website (accessed on March 18, 2021), 10 KU of glucose oxidase costs $51.30 while 5 U of xanthine oxidase costs the same $51.30 or 2000 times more! In further contrast ~2000–5000 KU of catalase costs $48.00. Of course, these prices are for small quantities for research laboratories, and the bulk pricing would be lower. The prices have changed over time as the cost of production of some enzymes has decreased. However, in some instances, prices have increased because enzyme companies probably have shifted production to enzymes with more lucrative markets. The quality and purity of enzymes, like any other chemical, also affect the price.

### 1.3.3 SELECTIVITY

Not all enzymes are very selective. However, all enzymes have some level of selectivity toward the substrate. For example, some enzymes are enantioselective. From an evolutionary perspective, these enzymes evolved to produce specific enantiomers that allow the production of building blocks of life and gave birth to the concept of "lock-and-key" mentioned earlier. Other enzymes, such as alcohol oxidase, can catalyze the oxidation of several different alcohols. That enzyme probably evolved to allow yeast like *Pichia pastoris* to grow in the presence of methanol or ethanol. However, it is unlikely that the presence of larger alcohols drove the evolution of this enzyme even though structurally, the enzyme can accommodate larger alcohols.

### 1.3.4 INHIBITION

Much has been written on enzyme kinetics to discuss enzyme inhibition and describe different mechanisms and methods to characterize it, in particular competitive, partially competitive, noncompetitive inhibition, and partially noncompetitive inhibition (21). Substrate and product inhibition are of particular interest because they are critical in the design and mode of operation of enzyme reactors. From an industrial, utilitarian point of view, enzyme inhibition is a problem as it limits yield and productivity. However, when considering that enzymes did not evolve in response to our industrial ingenuity but in response to environmental factors and the need to keep the delicate balance of the metabolism of all living organisms, one must recognize inhibition as a molecular mode of control. One should view this as a very efficient method of control that reduces the need for an additional mechanism to deal with the excess production of a particular metabolite. Likewise, the models for the mechanisms that explain the effect of pH and ionic strength on enzyme kinetics have been proposed and shed light on how enzymes have adapted to environments that sustain life as we know it. As observed in the early era of enzymology, cell-free fermentations were not always as productive as microbial fermentation. Arguably, this was in part due to different environments in different compartments that mixed as a result of homogenization and exposure of inhibitors that were not "intended" to be in the mix. In contrast, understanding and mimicking the mechanisms of inhibition may offer alternative process control strategies.

### 1.3.5 INCREASED REACTION RATE

Many enzymes are excellent catalysts and for many reactions, they are better than inorganic catalysts under similar temperature and pressure conditions. However, the turnover number ($k_{cat}$), that is, the number of moles of substrate that can be converted by one mole of enzyme per unit time range ranges approximately from 10 to $10^7$ s$^{-1}$. The rate of reactions typically increases exponentially with temperature. However, as discussed earlier, enzymes lose their activity at temperatures typically well below the boiling point. In contrast, inorganic catalysts can be often heated beyond that temperature and can catalyze reactions in the gas phase very efficiently.

## 1.4  ENZYME CATALYSIS

### 1.4.1  Basic Catalytic Mechanism

It seems pertinent to briefly overview some principles of chemical catalysis, enzyme catalysis, and reflect on homogeneous and heterogeneous catalysis. This is particularly important in the context of NMs because their catalytic properties at least in part, the result of their nanoscale dimensions and differ from their catalytic properties at the macroscale or if they were in true solution. This is also important because of the similarity that is found in the mechanisms of enzyme and heterogeneous catalysis. Entire textbooks on chemical kinetics and catalysis and enzyme kinetics have been published and we encourage the reader to consult them for an in-depth discussion and understanding of catalysis.

A catalyst is a substance that changes the rate of a chemical reaction but that itself is not produced or consumed during the reaction. However, to accelerate the reaction, the catalyst interacts with the reactants and products. The following basic mechanism exists behind any catalytic reaction:

$$\text{Reactants} + \text{Catalyst} \underset{k_2}{\overset{k_1}{\Longleftrightarrow}} \text{Complex}, \tag{1.1}$$

$$\text{Complex} \underset{k_4}{\overset{k_3}{\Longleftrightarrow}} \text{Products} + \text{Catalyst}, \tag{1.2}$$

where $k_1$, $k_2$, $k_3$, and $k_4$ are rate constants. The "complex" represents the association of the reactants with the catalyst. During the time of this association, the reactants are converted into products and then released as products. Enzyme kinetics is no exception. The mechanism in equations 1 and 2 probably was the starting point for Michaelis and Menten's proposed equation with the assumption the release of the product of the reaction was irreversible and the slow step of reaction:

$$E + S \underset{k_2}{\overset{k_1}{\Longleftrightarrow}} ES \tag{1.3}$$

$$ES \overset{k_3}{\rightarrow} E + P, \tag{1.4}$$

where $E$ is the enzyme, $S$ is the substrate, $ES$ is the enzyme–substrate complex, and $P$ is the product.

## 1.4.2 LOWERING THE ACTIVATION ENERGY

Catalysts accelerate reaction rates by decreasing the energy barrier required for the reactants to become products. The concept of an energy barrier was postulated by Faraday in 1834 who believed that there was an electrical resistance that needed to be overcome for reactants to react. That resulted in the chemical reaction not being instantaneous. However, at the end of the 19th century, Arrhenius correlated the rate of reactions with temperature assuming that molecules needed to be sufficiently hot to react. The well-known Arrhenius equation is:

$$r = Ae^{\frac{-E_a}{RT}},$$

where $r$ is the rate of reaction, $A$ is the pre-exponential factor, $E_a$ is the activation energy barrier, $R$ is the ideal gas constant, and $T$ is the absolute temperature. There are many deviations from this equation and often it is used to describe the effect of temperature in complex, multistep reactions, forgetting that it was intended to explain elementary chemical reactions. A group of researchers who studied the rate of killing of larvae in fruit using a particular thermal treatment noticed that the rate of larvae kill increased exponentially with temperature. Following which the researchers calculated the activation energy of the larvae kill using the Arrhenius equation. It is questionable if Arrhenius would be pleased by such use of his equation. The data fitted nicely the equation and served well the purpose of determining time–temperature combinations that were effective in killing the larvae but it cannot serve to interpret the mechanistic meaning of the activation energy (in kJ/mol) of larvae kill.

The precise origin of the activation energy is not perfectly defined but it includes bond stretching and distortion, orbital distortion, overcoming electron–electron repulsion, overcoming steric effects, and quantum effects. Sometimes the collision theory where reactants require minimum energy for a collision to be energetic enough to break or create a chemical bond helps us to imagine analogous collisions of everyday objects that might or might not break when dropped depending on the height from where they drop, the nature of the surface they hit, and the angle with which they hit that surface. The higher the energy barrier, the slower the reaction. Catalysts, therefore, help to lower the energy barrier. Notably, they stabilize the reversible transition state, that is, the state in which the reactant is sufficiently energetic to react. **Figure 1.1** contrasts the reaction of reactant A becoming B in the absence or the presence of a catalyst. The blue line and numbers represent the reaction in the absence of a catalyst and the red line and numbers represent a simple, one-substrate enzyme-catalyzed reaction. While the difference in energy ① between the reactants and the products is small and remains the same whether the reaction is catalyzed or not. That difference in energy can be calculated in terms of the equilibrium constant or from the difference in enthalpy and entropy between the reactants

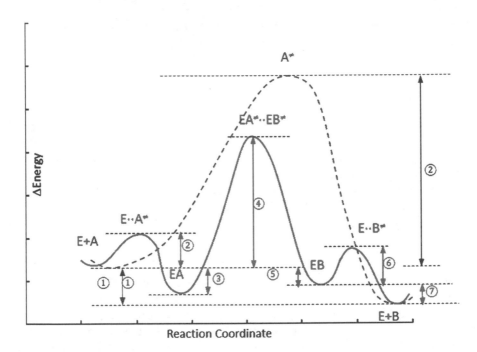

**FIGURE 1.1** Energy diagram for the noncatalytic (blue-dotted) and the enzymatic (red-continuous) conversion of A to B.

and the product. The energy barrier ② (blue) is larger than the energy barrier ④ (red) of the catalyzed reaction. That energy is associated with the changes in enthalpy, entropy, and free energy between the reactant and the activated reactant or activated complex. The catalyzed reaction lowers the barrier by adding steps that include the formation of the enzyme–reactant complex, the conversion of the reactant to the product within the complex, and the release of the product from the enzyme–product complex. Each of these has its energy barrier, but because these barriers are all smaller than the barrier for the noncatalytic reaction, then the rate of reaction is greater. In each of these steps, the catalyst contributes to reducing the amount of energy needed to stretch or distort bonds, distort orbitals, overcome electron–electron repulsion, overcome steric effects, and quantum effects. Whether the catalyst is an enzyme or other molecule, the efficiency of the catalyst depends on the catalyst's atomic and molecular structure. One must keep in mind that **Figure 1.1** is the simplest case. Enzyme reactions that involve two substrates, or in the presence of an inhibitor or denaturing conditions are less straightforward.

Cofactors are co-enzymes, prosthetic groups, or inorganic ions that contribute to enzyme catalysis. By themselves, most cofactors do not catalyze reactions and those that catalyze reactions by themselves, do that orders of magnitude less than with the enzyme. Cofactors often react during an enzyme reaction. For example, nicotinamide adenine dinucleotide (NAD+) is reduced to NADH in several enzyme reactions. In fact, it acts as a second substrate and if it is not replenished, the catalytic activity is lost. A second enzyme is often needed to regenerate the cofactor.

Coenzymes are typically not as tightly bound to the enzyme as prosthetic groups. Coenzymes can act as carriers of electrons, hydrogen, amino groups, phosphate, acyl, and other groups. Prosthetic groups often are responsible for oxidation/reduction reactions. Among other functions, inorganic metal cofactors may contribute to the enzyme conformation, as part of the active site, or as a part of a coenzyme. In different reactions, the order in which and the location where the substrates bind to the enzyme is different. Therefore, considering the contribution of cofactors in addition to inhibitors, one can see that the mechanisms by which enzymes lower energy barriers can be extremely complex. In contrast to nonbiological catalysts, the complex stereochemistry of enzymes and their cofactors is responsible for the selectivity and proper orientation of reactants, which also contributes to lowering the energy barrier. A detailed discussion of this is beyond the scope of this chapter but the reader should be aware of all these factors when studying enzymes and when reflecting on the potential of NMs to catalyze complex and stereospecific reactions.

### 1.4.3 HOMOGENEOUS AND HETEROGENEOUS CATALYSIS

In the paper by Gao et al. (22), frequently referred to as the first report of a nanozyme, the authors did not use that term. Instead, they compared the $k_{cat}$ of ferromagnetic ($Fe_3O_4$) nanoparticles (NPs) to that of horseradish peroxidase (HRP) for the reaction of hydrogen peroxide ($H_2O_2$) and 3,3,5,5-tetramethylbenzidine (TMB). The reported turnover number for the NPs was about one order of magnitude greater than that of the enzyme under similar reaction conditions. This was unexpectedly high. However, the comparison may not be justifiable when considering the stoichiometry of the reactions. More often than not, enzymes have one active site so the formation of the ES complex is 1:1. However, in the case of heterogeneous catalysis, the solid catalyst may have multiple sites for the reactants to react with it. For example, the particles that were used to calculate the turnover numbers were 300 nm. Thus, their surface area is approximately 280,000 $nm^2$. Assuming a kinetic diameter for $H_2O_2$ of 0.3 nm, a coarse approximation of the surface area that it would occupy on an NP would be 0.07 $nm^2$. Therefore, if only 1/10 of the surface area of the NP is used to catalyze the reaction, the NP to $H_2O_2$ stoichiometry would be approximately 1:400,000. A similar oversimplified calculation for TMB assuming its diameter is less than 3 nm, the projected area would be 7.06 $nm^2$, and therefore, the stoichiometry would be in the order of 1:4,000. These calculations are oversimplifications. Neither $H_2O_2$ nor TMB is spherical, the rate of collisions is affected by many factors. Finally, the concentration of TMB used for the experiments with HRP (~4 nm) was 60 times smaller than for the NPs. Therefore, mass action should also be considered. **Figure 1.2** shows a 2-D schematic representation of a 300-nm particle surrounded by a 3-nm particle.

Heterogeneous catalysis is quite complex. It requires the adsorption of the reactant on the solid catalyst. The rate of chemisorption depends on the concentration of vacant sites on the catalyst, the concentration of a reactant in solution, the concentration of reactants adsorbed onto the catalyst, and the adsorption equilibrium constant that is determined from adsorption experiments as reported in 1947 by Houghen and

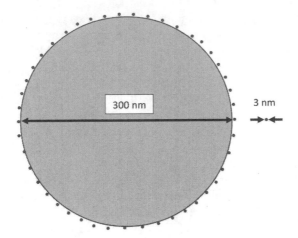

**FIGURE 1.2** Schematic representation of a $Fe_3O_4$ NP and a 3-nm molecule to illustrate that one $Fe_3O_4$ NP can catalyze the reaction of manifold more $H_2O_2$ or TNB molecules simultaneously.

Watson (23). The rate of desorption is similar. The overall mechanism for a simple heterogeneous reaction of reactant A being absorbed on a vacant site $l$, reacting to become B, and then desorbing can be expressed as:

$$A + l \underset{k_2}{\overset{k_1}{\Longleftrightarrow}} Al$$

$$Al \underset{k_4}{\overset{k_3}{\Longleftrightarrow}} Bl$$

$$Bl \underset{k_6}{\overset{k_5}{\Longleftrightarrow}} B + l.$$

The rate equation for this mechanism is given by:

$$r_A = \frac{C_t \left[ C_A - (C_B / K) \right]}{\left[ \left( \dfrac{1}{K_A k_{sr}} + \dfrac{1}{k_A} + \dfrac{1}{Kk_{RB}} \right) + \left( \dfrac{1}{K_A k_{sr}} + \dfrac{1 + K_{sr}}{Kk_B} \right) K_A C_A + \left( \dfrac{1}{K_A k_{sr}} + \dfrac{1 + K_{sr}}{K_{sr} k_B} \right) K_r C_B \right]},$$

where $k_A$ is the chemisorption rate coefficient, $k_B$ is the rate constant for the desorption of B, $k_{sr}$ is the surface reaction rate coefficient, $K_A$ is the adsorption equilibrium constant, $K_B$ is the adsorption equilibrium constant for the desorption step, $K_{sr}$ is the surface reaction equilibrium constant, $C_t$ is the concentration of absorption sites, $C_A$ is the concentration of A, $C_B$ is the concentration of B, $K = (K_A K_{sr}/K_B)$ (24). This equation is simplified if there is a limiting step. We present this to illustrate the differences between enzyme homogeneous and heterogeneous catalysis. Even though both show an elliptic behavior, the mechanisms are different.

## 1.5 ALLOSTERIC ENZYMES

The structure of enzymes not only contributes to the proper orientation of the substrate for stereoselectivity and enhanced catalysis as the rigid lock-and-key model suggested, but it also contributes to allosteric effects in which compounds other than the substrate can bind to the enzyme and regulate its activity. Initially, enzyme inhibition was believed to be the result of compounds that were similar to the substrate binding to or blocking the active site. However, it turned out that compounds that were very different from the substrate and that bound at locations away from the active state could inhibit enzymes. Allosteric inhibition was first reported in the early 1960s and defined as a "conformational alteration" (25). An excellent review on the history and explanation of allosteric interactions in enzymes was published by Cornish–Bowden (26). The existence of allosteric behavior shows one of the methods that nature has engineered, perhaps through evolution, control mechanisms of biological processes. The allosteric model assumes that the protein can exist in two or more conformations and the ligand binds to one and not to other conformations. This cooperative interaction can be positive or negative (allosteric activation of allosteric inhibition). In the case of polymeric enzymes, it also assumes symmetry, that is, that all the monomers change between conformations in a coordinated manner. **Figure 1.3** is a schematic representation of allosteric enzyme regulation. The question of how this additional ligand interaction takes place is being elucidated using modern methods, such as X-ray crystallography (27), nuclear magnetic resonance (NMR) (28), or transient infrared spectroscopy complemented with molecular dynamics simulations (29). Allosteric effects cannot occur in NPs because of their simple rigid structure.

## 1.6 THE UNIVERSE OF ENZYME FUNCTION

The immensely large number of compounds found in nature, the enzymes, and the metabolic pathways that produce them constitute a vast universe, most of which has not been explored in detail. That universe, although much younger than our galaxy, has spent millions of years of evolution building the fabric of life of all living organisms on Earth. The Enzyme Commission (EC) classifies enzymes using a 4-number system. The first number corresponds to seven main functions: oxidoreductases (26 subgroups), transferases (10 subgroups), hydrolases (13 subgroups), lyases (5 subgroups), isomerases (7 subgroups), ligases (6 subgroups), and translocases (6 subgroups). The second number corresponds to the subgroup, which in general, refers to the type of molecule or bond that the enzyme acts on. For example, EC 1.1 groups oxidoreductases that act on the CH–OH group of donors. Within

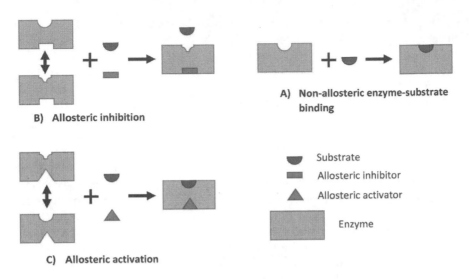

**FIGURE 1.3**  Schematic representation of different allosteric enzyme regulations.

each subgroup, enzymes with additional specificity are listed. For example, EC 1.1.1. uses $NAD^+$ or $NADPH^+$ as an acceptor. The last number corresponds to the specific enzyme and the specific reaction that it catalyzes. EC 1.1.1.1 represents alcohol dehydrogenase. For that enzyme, over 1600 substrates/products have been reported. Within EC 1.1.1, there are 424 enzymes. Each of these enzymes might have been detected in one or more organisms and there may exist multiple isozymes that catalyze the same reaction but under different conditions, due to different evolutionary conditions. A detailed list of enzymes, their properties, and the organisms of origin regarding the scientific literature can be found https://www.brenda-enzymes.org/. Browsing this database is as humbling as watching the stars in the sky on a clear night. From a functional perspective, because of their metallic nature, as of today, most nanozymes appear to fit a rather narrow range of redox functions. As nanotechnology and nanofabrication and artificial intelligence continue to develop, one would hope to see novel and fascinating nanostructures that in addition to having high catalytic activities, also display selective behavior and can reproduce metabolic pathways. This would have tremendous implications not only in biosensors but also in medicine, foods, environmental applications, etc.

## 1.7 BIOMIMETICS

"Biomimetic chemistry is the branch of organic chemistry, which attempts to imitate natural reactions and enzymatic processes as a way to improve the power of organic chemistry. In attempts to imitate some of the factors involved in enzymatic catalysis, i.e., the formation of an ES complex with subsequent polyfunctional catalysis by well-placed catalytic groups (and even the incorporation of special medium effects and strain effects), the emphasis has generally been on achieving the velocity of enzyme-catalyzed processes. However, for many practical purposes, a high speed of reaction is not as important as high selectivity, the other outstanding feature of an enzyme-catalyzed process" (1). In 2007, the term "nanozyme" appears in the title of a report of a self-assembled supramolecular structure with a hydrophobic core and a soluble charged surface (30). Even though the supramolecular structure might not have been inspired by a particular enzyme, structurally, the hydrophobic core and hydrophilic surface, just like that of cyclodextrins, justified the nickname. In the same year, when $Fe_3O_4$ NPs and the analogous kinetic behavior relative to substrate concentrations identified (22) were not called "nanozymes." Nevertheless, most of the recent literature and this book refer to these highly catalytic NPs as nanozymes. However, different approaches to produce highly catalytic and selective structures have been inspired by existing enzymes. For example, the extensive study of hydrogenases has led to the biomimetic design of transition metals guests incorporated into supramolecular scaffold hosts that modulate their catalytic activity (31).

## 1.8   SUMMARY AND FUTURE PERSPECTIVES

Understanding fermentation was of such interest that a 1-kg medal made of gold was offered to anyone that could establish the characteristics of the animal or vegetable substances that can act as ferments vs. those that cannot. The prize was offered in 1800 and 1804 but nobody was able to claim it (7). We cannot offer a 1-kg gold medal but it would be interesting to see whether nanozymes can be engineered to reproduce such fermentation with the desired specificity, selectivity, catalytic activity, and equivalent process regulation. This challenge may appear unattainable today within the current state of this emerging field, just like the challenge to characterize fermentations in 1800 was not achieved then. However, we are convinced that contemplating the evolutionary wisdom of enzymes will eventually allow humans to tailor synthetic enzymes to desired functionalities and stability by design. It appears that nanozymes have the potential of serving as one of the building blocks of either supramolecular structures or nano-assemblies that could achieve that (31). However, much more understanding from enzymes has to be gained. Great scientists, such as Lavoisier, made invaluable contributions thanks to their superior intelligence and their ability to question their understanding. "One can imagine how much it cost me to abandon my first ideas; it is only after several years of reflection, after long series of experiments and observations..." (10) p 150–51. In a world where an increasing number of scientists produce an overabundance of information, guided sometimes by the thirst for a greater number of publications rather than for knowledge and understanding, one can easily feel overwhelmed. However, human creativity has been preparing for this by developing artificial intelligence algorithms that will help sorting the most useful portions of current knowledge and device strategies to develop the next generation of catalysts.

## REFERENCES

1. Breslow R. 1972. *Chemical Society Reviews* 1: 553–80
2. Reyes-De-Corcuera JI, Olstad HE, Garcia-Torres R. 2018. In *Annual Review of Food Science and Technology, Vol 9*, ed. MP Doyle, TR Klaenhammer, pp. 293–322

3. Halalipour A, Duff MR, Howell EE, Reyes-De-Corcuera JI. 2017. *Enzyme and Microbial Technology* 103: 18–24
4. Eisenmenger MJ, Reyes-De-Corcuera JI. 2009. *Enzyme and Microbial Technology* 45: 331–47
5. Liang MM, Yan XY. 2019. *Accounts of Chemical Research* 52: 2190–200
6. Wang WZ, Gunasekaran S. 2020. *Trac-Trends in Analytical Chemistry* 126
7. Fruton JS. 2006. Fermentation: vital or chemical process? Leiden: Brill
8. Liu L, Wang JJ, Levin MJ, Sinnott-Armstrong N, Zhao H, et al. 2019. *Proceedings of the National Academy of Sciences of the United States of America* 116: 12767–74
9. Newton I, Turnbull HW. 1959. *The correspondence of Isaac Newton.* Cambridge [England]: Published for the Royal Society at the University Press
10. Lavoisier AL. 1789. *Traité élémentaire de chimie: présenté dans un ordre nouveau et d'après les découvertes modernes.* Paris: Cuchet
11. Appert N. 1810. *L'art de conserver, pendant plusieurs années, toutes les substances animales et végétales: ouvrage soumis au Bureau consultatif des Arts et Manufactures, revêtu de son approbation, et publié sur l'invitation de S. Ex. le Ministre de l'Interieur.* Paris: Patris
12. Gay-Lussac JL. 1810. *Annales de Chimie* 76: 243–59
13. Caignard de la Tour C. 1838. *Annales de Chimie* 68: 206–22
14. Fischer E. 1898. *Zeitschrift für physiologische Chemie* 26: 60–87
15. Elleuche S, Schafers C, Blank S, Schroder C, Antranikian G. 2015. *Current Opinion in Microbiology* 25: 113–9
16. Ohmae E, Miyashita Y, Kato C. 2013. *Extremophiles* 17: 701–9
17. Sarmiento F, Peralta R, Blamey JM. 2015. *Frontiers in Bioengineering and Biotechnology* 3
18. Poliakov E, Uppal S, Rogozin IB, Gentleman S, Redmond TM. 2020. *Biochim Biophys Acta Mol Cell Biol Lipids* 1865
19. Buchholz-Afari MI, Halalipour A, Yang DY, Reyes-De-Corcuera JI. 2019. *Journal of Food Engineering* 246: 95–101
20. Yang D, Reyes-De-Corcuera JI. 2021. *Enzyme and Microbial Technology* 145: 109751
21. Cavalieri RP, Reye-De-Corcuera JI. 2005. *In Food Engineering*, ed. GV Barbosa-Canovas, pp. 215–39: UNESCO
22. Gao LZ, Zhuang J, Nie L, Zhang JB, Zhang Y, et al. 2007. *Nature Nanotechnology* 2: 577–83
23. Houghen OA, Watson KM. 1947. *Kinetics and Catalysis.* New York
24. Froment GF, Bischoff KB. 1990. *Chemical Reactor Analysis and Design.* New York: John Wiley & Sons
25. Monod J, Changeux JP, Jacob F. 1963. *Journal of Molecular Biology* 6: 306-&
26. Cornish-Bowden A. 2014. *Febs Journal* 281: 621–32
27. Stieglitz K, Stec B, Baker DP, Kantrowitz ER. 2004. *Journal of Molecular Biology* 341: 853–68
28. East KW, Newton JC, Morzan UN, Narkhede YB, Acharya A, et al. 2020. *Journal of the American Chemical Society* 142: 1348–58
29. Bozovic O, Zanobini C, Gulzar A, Jankovic B, Buhrke D, et al. 2020. *Proceedings of the National Academy of Sciences of the United States America* 117: 26031–9
30. Pluth MD, Bergman RG, Raymond KN. 2007. *Angewandte Chemie-International Edition* 46: 8587–9
31. Simmons TR, Berggren G, Bacchi M, Fontecave M, Artero V. 2014. *Coordination Chemistry Reviews* 270–271: 127–50

# 2 Nanozymes— An Overview

*Loghman Alaei[1†], Zhila Izadi[2†], Samira Jafari[2],*
*Alireza Lotfabadi[2], Ebrahim Barzegari[3], Mehdi*
*Jaymand[4]\*, and Hossein Derakhshankhah[2]\**

[1]Department of Biology and Biotechnology, Faculty of
Sciences, University of Kurdistan, Sanandaj, Iran.
[2]Pharmaceutical Sciences Research Center,
School of Pharmacy, Kermanshah University
of Medical Sciences, Kermanshah, Iran.
[3]Medical Biology Research Center, Health
Technology Institute, Kermanshah University
of Medical Sciences, Kermanshah, Iran.
[4]Nano Drug Delivery Research Center, Health
Technology Institute, Kermanshah University
of Medical Sciences, Kermanshah, Iran

## CONTENTS

## 2.1 INTRODUCTION

Living beings are dynamic entities, both physically and chemically. From a chemist's standpoint, the dynamics of the living systems are characterized by chemical reactions. Like in many chemical conversions, the high activation energy of substrates is often an obstacle for biochemical reactions to occur spontaneously. Thus, cells require catalysts for promoting a majority of processes in their chemical life. In bioorganisms, enzymes are the molecular systems undertaking this task. These

---

† Contributed equally
* Corresponding authors: Hossein Derakhshankhah and Mehdi Jaymand

DOI: 10.1201/9781003109228-2

ubiquitous biocatalysts play a pivotal role by facilitating the majority of reactions that occur in living systems. Owing to the high substrate specificity, activity, and yield, enzymes are extremely efficient at catalyzing the biochemical reactions (1). Given their excellent properties, natural enzymes can catalyze biochemical reactions with extraordinary specificity and remarkable efficiency under mild reaction conditions (*e.g.,* aqueous solutions, room temperature, and ambient pressure). Hence, natural enzymes find applications in numerous fields, such as biosensing, biomedicine, and pharmaceutics, food, and environmental industries, agrochemical production, etc. (2).

In terms of chemical structure, natural enzymes are categorized as proteins or ribonucleic acids (RNAs), which confers them several intrinsic drawbacks. Enzymes require strict physiological conditions to perform their catalytic functions; they easily denature and prone to destabilization in harsh environmental conditions. Their preparation is highly costly and involves labor-intensive steps for synthesis, isolation, and purification (3). Besides, there are many difficulties in their reuse. These significant limitations have in turn limited their applications in practice (2).

To overcome the above-mentioned drawbacks of natural enzymes, developing efficient alternative enzymes has been an imperative need. Accordingly, research has been focused on utilizing the catalytic capabilities of chemical molecules as substances to mimic the catalytic functions of natural enzymes (3). In the 1950s, artificial enzymes were developed as stable, low-cost alternatives to natural enzymes (4). Porphyrins, cyclodextrins, metal-complexes, polymeric, and supramolecular structures were explored for their applicability as enzyme mimetics (5, 6). However, the utility of these artificial enzymes was hampered by concerns, such as biocompatibility and catalytic efficiency (3).

Recent progress in nanotechnology has led to an exponential growth in developing numerous nanomaterials. This has led to the development of nanomaterial-based catalysts, i.e., the systems involving immobilization of natural enzymes or catalytic ligands on nanomaterial surfaces, or nanosystems loaded with natural enzymes (7, 8). Nanozymes are nanomaterials demonstrating intrinsic enzyme-like characteristics. These nanosystems are distinct from the nanomaterial-based catalysts and exhibit outstanding features in comparison with conventional artificial biocatalysts and natural enzymes (8). Nanozymes demonstrate superior biocatalytic activity even under extreme temperature and pH conditions; they also offer resistance against digestion by proteases (3). **Table 2.1** is a comprehensive summary of various advantages and challenges of nanozymes, nanomaterial-based catalysts, artificial enzymes, and natural enzymes.

## 2.2 NANOZYMES

The term "nanozyme" first appeared in 2004 in a paper by Manea et al. (9). They reported the trans-phosphorylation activity of gold nanoparticles (Au NPs) functionalized by triazacyclononane. The definition of nanozyme, however, first appeared in 2007 in the landmark paper by Gao et al. (10). They discovered the intrinsic peroxidase (POD)-like property of iron oxide ($Fe_3O_4$) NPs toward typical POD substrates. They demonstrated that $Fe_3O_4$ NPs can catalyze the POD substrates oxidation in the

## TABLE 2.1

## Advantages and Challenges of Nanozymes, Nanomaterial-Based Catalysts, Conventional Artificial Enzymes, and Natural Biocatalysts[a,b]

| Advantages | Challenges |
|---|---|
| **Nanozymes** | |

| Advantages | Challenges |
|---|---|
| 1. High catalytic activity | 1. Still low efficiency |
| 2. Low cost | 2. Limited specificity |
| 3. Facile preparation and mass production | 3. Low substrate selectivity |
| 4. High operational stability and robustness under stringent conditions in harsh environments | 4. Limited catalytic types and reactions |
| 5. Long-term storage | 5. Ambiguous atomic 3D structure and mechanism |
| 6. Controllable catalytic activity and types | 6. *Difficulty rational designing of (efficient) nanozymes* |
| 7. *Size-, shape-, structure-, and composition-dependent properties* | 7. *Size-, shape-, structure-, and composition-dependent catalytic properties* |
| 8. Multi-enzyme mimetic activity | 8. *Biologically-directed (encoded) synthesis* |
| 9. **Multifunction – Other functions besides catalysis, particularly the unique features from the nanoscaled materials (such as magnetic properties for recycling, plasmonic properties for sensing, and physicochemical properties such as fluorescence, electricity, and paramagnetism)** | 9. Delivery and administration for nanomedicine |
| 10. **Larger surface area in comparison with molecular and bulk materials, allowing multifunctionalization and modifications such as bioconjugation** | 10. Potential nanotoxicity |
| 11. Smart response to external stimuli (heat, light, ultrasound, magnetic field, etc.) and tunable catalytic activity and type | 11. Limited types |
| 12. Self-assembly | 12. Lack of standards and reference materials |
| 13. Recyclable | |

| Advantages | Challenges |
|---|---|
| **Nanomaterial-based catalysts** | |

| Advantages | Challenges |
|---|---|
| 1. Low cost | 1. Limited efficiency |
| 2. Facile preparation and mass production | 2. Limited specificity |
| 3. High operational stability and robustness under stringent conditions in harsh environments | 3. Low substrate selectivity |
| 4. Long-term storage | 4. Limited catalytic types and reactions |
| 5. Controllable catalytic activity and types | 5. Ambiguous atomic 3D structure |
| 6. Size-, shape-, structure-, and composition-dependent properties | 6. Size-, shape-, structure-, and composition-dependent catalytic properties |
| 7. Multifunction – Other functions besides catalysis, particularly the unique features from the nanoscaled materials (such as magnetic properties for recycling, plasmonic properties for sensing, and physicochemical properties such as fluorescence, electricity, and paramagnetism) | 7. Poor biocompatibility |
| 8. Larger surface area in comparison with molecular and bulk materials, allowing multifunctionalization and modifications such as bioconjugation | |
| 9. Self-assembly | |
| 10. Exact catalytic mechanism | |

*(Continued)*

**TABLE 2.1  (Continued)**
**Advantages and Challenges of Nanozymes, Nanomaterial-Based Catalysts,**
**Conventional Artificial Enzymes, and Natural Biocatalysts[a,b]**

| Advantages | Challenges |
|---|---|
| **Conventional artificial enzymes** | |
| 1. Low cost | 1. Limited efficiency |
| 2. Facile preparation and mass production | 2. Limited specificity |
| 3. High operational stability and robustness to stringent conditions in harsh environments | 3. Low substrate selectivity |
| 4. Long-term storage | 4. Limited catalytic types and reactions |
| 5. Controllable catalytic activity and types | 5. Ambiguous atomic 3D structure and mechanism |
| 6. *Smaller size (compared with nanozymes)* | 6. *Difficulty rational designing of (efficient) artificial enzymes* |
| 7. *Uniform size and defined structures of molecular mimics* | 7. Separation and recycling |
| 8. *Established methods for preparation and characterization* | |
| **Natural enzymes** | |
| 1. High catalytic efficiency | 1. High cost |
| 2. High substrate specificity | 2. Hard to mass-produce |
| 3. High substrate (enantio)selectivity | 3. Time-consuming separation and purification |
| 4. Sophisticated 3D structures | 4. Limited operational stability |
| 5. Various catalytic types and a wide range of biocatalytic reactions | 5. Hard for long-term storage |
| 6. Tunable activity | 6. Sensitivity of catalytic activity to the environment, which makes it difficult to use for industrial catalysis in harsh environments (such as heat, extreme pH, salinity, and UV irradiation) |
| 7. Utmost biocompatibility | |
| 8. Rational design via gene manipulation and protein engineering, using computations | |
| 9. Wide range of applications | 7. Difficulties in recovery and recycling |

[a]  Items in italic are unique for nanozymes compared with conventional artificial enzymes. Items in bold are unique for nanozymes compared with natural enzymes.
[b]  Sources: (3, 9, 19, 35).

presence of hydrogen peroxide ($H_2O_2$) and bring about colorimetric reaction products. The discovery of this artificial POD enzyme based on ferromagnetic NPs upended the traditional notion that inorganic materials were biologically inert. This finding was the first report to show that the inorganic NPs could also catalyze an oxidation reaction similar to the natural horseradish peroxide (HRP) enzyme. These NPs have the potential use for antibody (Ab)-based identification, separation, and detection of analytes. It incentivized the researchers to extensively pursue investigations to identify other new enzyme-like nanomaterials (3, 11). The progression timeline of natural enzymes, artificial enzymes, and nanozymes is presented in **Figure 2.1**.

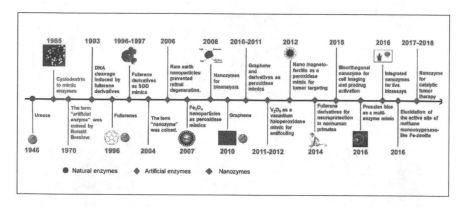

**FIGURE 2.1**   The timeline for the development of natural enzymes, artificial enzymes, and nanozymes. Reprinted from (1) with permission from The Royal Society of Chemistry.

Since 2007, numerous nanomaterials have been identified to possess intrinsic natural enzyme-like biocatalytic activities. Redox reaction catalysis, such as POD, oxidase (OXD), catalase (CAT), and superoxide dismutase (SOD) enzyme-like activities, has been the main catalytic function sought by researchers in the nanomaterials (3, 12–17). To date, over 300 nanomaterials have been discovered to have intrinsic enzyme-mimicking properties (18, 19). This rapid growth in nanozyme research was possible because of the various advantages of inorganic NPs in contrast to natural enzymes. Compared to naturally existing enzymes that are easily inactivated in extreme environments, nanozymes possess stable structure, robust catalytic performance, adjustable activity, and diverse functions. Nanozymes are also amenable to simple and low-cost methods of synthesis and allow smooth surface modification (4, 12).

Based on the material type, we can divide the nanozymes into three categories: 1) metal–oxide- or metal-sulfide-based; 2) metal-based; and 3) carbon-based. These nanozymes are mimetics of oxidoreductases, hydrolases, and lyases such as carbonic anhydrase (1, 12). As mentioned earlier, most nanozymes mimic oxidoreductase enzymes, which is attributable to their rough surface structure, thus they can catalyze only relatively simple chemical reactions. In general, the factors closely relevant to the surface properties, such as composition, size, morphology, and surface lattice and modification, determine the enzymatic properties of nanozymes (20, 21). Besides, factors, such as temperature, pH, and ionic strength, also have impacts on their catalytic features (12). As for the $Fe_3O_4$ nanozyme-based reaction, kinetic studies have indicated a ping-pong catalytic mechanism. Michaelis–Menten kinetic parameters show that nanozymes possess higher catalytic activity but lower substrate affinity than HRP (9). Studies to explain the catalytic mechanism have revealed rapid valence transition and electron transfer on the surface as the mechanisms for most nanozymes (12).

The exceptional advantages of nanozymes have made them valuable substitutes and prospective competitors for natural enzymes in many fields, such as industrial production, biochemical detection, disease treatment, and environmental

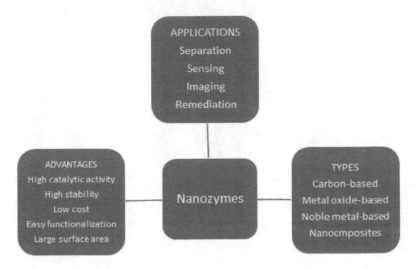

**FIGURE 2.2**  Nanozymes: types, advantages, and applications.

management (9, 12, 22–25). A general overview of nanozyme types, their advantages, and applications are depicted in **Figure 2.2**. Currently, nanozymes are being widely scrutinized to establish a broad range of applications in cell/tissue growth and proliferation, protection from oxidative stress, immunoassays, disease imaging, theranostics, biosensing, and removal of pollutants (3, 4, 26–28). Their applications in therapeutics, biosensor development, and environmental remediation have been demonstrated. There have been various applications of nanozyme in biomedicine (29). These biomedical applications of nanozymes can be divided into three types based on their mode of application such as self-acting, synergistic, and remotely controlled. Nonetheless, this field is actually in its infancy and faces many challenges, such as making the enzyme mimetic stimuli-responsive (8, 30).

The field of nanozymes still has much room for improvement in catalytic activity, substrate selectivity, and application diversity. The gaps between nanozymes and protein-based natural enzymes are still large. Thus, there are some challenges such as improving turnover and activity, augmenting specificity, and bioconjugation. In this regard, nanozyme research offers prospects and opportunities to explore new activities beyond redox, understanding enzyme-like reaction mechanisms, rational design of bio-inspired nanozymes, and exploring new biological and biomimetic applications (19, 27). Learning from nature provides us with effective strategies for enhancing the enzymatic properties of nanozymes. Identification of cofactor-like materials and constructing nanostructures similar to the active center of natural enzymes are some bio-inspired strategies to improve the performance of nanozymes (12).

With the advent of nanozymes, "nanozymology" has emerged as a new concept connecting nanotechnology and life sciences. Over the past decade, dozens of nanozymes have been identified based on hundreds of nanomaterials. There are more than 200 research groups actively pursuing nanozyme research, which has resulted in an exponential growth in the number of nanozyme-related publications from around the world (9). To attract and guide extensive and in-depth research on nanozymes, there is a need for standardization of nanozyme performance. Until now, the kinetics and catalytic mechanisms of nanozymes have been broadly investigated based on the theoretical system used in classic enzymology (31–33). For a deeper understanding and more precise regulation of their catalytic properties, it is critical to establish universal standards for quantitatively determining the catalytic mechanisms and kinetics of nanozymes. To date, some catalytic activity units have been defined specifically for nanozymes, and some standards have been established to facilitate the comparison of catalytic activity among various nanozymes (9, 34).

## 2.3   ENZYMATIC ACTIVITY

Enzymes are macromolecules that catalyze almost all biochemical reactions that occur in biological systems (36). These are generally protein-made, but also include some DNA and RNA, which have catalytic features. Such biological catalysts, work via lowering the activation energy barrier of the reaction and hence increase the reaction rate (37). These biocatalysts are proteins responsible for the catalysis of life. Proteins have a typical predecessor characterized by sequence and structure likelihood, which are grouped into families and superfamilies. The molecular actions of enzymes are characterized as their capacity to catalyze biochemical pathways.

The idea of enzymatic reactors was first introduced in 1833 during the revelation of the conversion of starch into sugars mediated by diastase (38). Although, it was not until the 20th century that researchers understood their maximum capacity about mediation and technology. Significant milestones in this development were the strategies for enzyme purification and isolation, the understanding that enzymes are proteins, including biochemical functionality, and their representation utilizing X-ray diffraction methods (39, 40). Research in the field of the dynamics of ribonuclease structure and related endeavors to unravel the catalytic mechanism of lysozyme introduced enzymology as a developing scientific area.

Proteins have numerous useful traits. At a molecular level, biocatalysts catalyze biochemical processes by quickening the change of substrates into products in a sepulture inside the active site of the protein. In the absence of catalysts, a lot of reactions would be too delayed, even though not all reactions in nature need catalysts (41). From the first studies by Krebs on the citric acid cycle (42) to the detailed exhaustive biochemical divider outlines and databases, scientists have understood that enzymes do not act autonomously; however, they balance metabolic pathways and systems. Biocatalysts play out their activity in specific cell segments. For example, hexokinase transforms D-glucose into α-D-glucose-6-phosphate in the glycolysis cycle, which happens in the cytosol of the cell.

## 2.4   BIOMEDICAL IMPORTANCE

Advancements in clinical applications of enzymes are at least as broad as those are for industrial applications, which mirrors the importance of the potential advantages. For instance, pancreatic enzymes are used since the 19th century for the treatment of stomach-related diseases. The assortment of enzymes and their potential therapeutic

## TABLE 2.2
## Some Important Therapeutic Enzymes (57–59)

| Enzyme | EC code | Reaction | Importance |
|---|---|---|---|
| Asparaginase | 3.5.1.1 | L-Asparagine $H_2O \rightarrow$ L-aspartate + $NH_3$ | Leukemia |
| Collagenase | 3.4.24.3 | Collagen hydrolysis | Skin ulcers |
| Glutaminase | 3.5.1.2 | L-Glutamine $H_2O \rightarrow$ L-glutamate + $NH_3$ | Leukemia |
| Hyaluronidase | 3.2.1.35 | Hyaluronate hydrolysis | Heart attack |
| Lysozyme | 3.2.1.17 | Bacterial cell wall hydrolysis | Antibiotic |
| Rhodanase | 2.8.1.1 | $S_2O_3^{2-} + CN^- \rightarrow SO_3^{2-} + SCN^-$ | Cyanide poisoning |
| Ribonuclease | 3.1.26.4 | RNA hydrolysis | Antiviral |
| β-Lactamase | 3.5.2.6 | Penicillin $\rightarrow$ penicilloate | Penicillin allergy |
| Streptokinase | 3.4.22.10 | Plasminogen $\rightarrow$ plasmin | Blood clots |
| Trypsin | 3.4.21.4 | Protein hydrolysis | Inflammation |
| Uricase | 1.7.3.3 | Urate + $O_2 \rightarrow$ allantoin | Gout |
| Urokinase | 3.4.21.31 | Plasminogen $\rightarrow$ plasmin | Blood clots |

applications are extensive (60). Several enzymes that afford significant therapeutic values are listed in **Table 2.2** (61). The best applications are extracellular: topical utilization, the expulsion of poisonous materials, and the treatment of hazardous issues in the blood circulatory tract.

Since the enzymes are explicit natural catalysts, they are the key to treat many metabolic disorders. Although, numerous factors seriously decrease this potential as described below:

i. They are very large molecules to be spread inside the cells of the body. This is a significant reason why these biocatalysts have not yet been effectively applied to a large number of human hereditary ailments (62). Various strategies are being pursued to overcome this by targeting enzymes. For example, ones with covalent-joined β-galactose adducts are focused at hepatocytes, and others covalently attached to target-explicit monoclonal Abs to dodge nonspecific side responses (63).

ii. They are foreign proteins to the body, called antigens, and can inspire immune reactions, which may cause unfavorable responses, especially upon prolonged use. It has been demonstrated that it is possible to dodge this issue, sometimes, by camouflaging a given enzyme as a nonprotein molecule using covalent change. For example, asparaginase (64), altered by the covalent connection of poly(ethylene glycol) (PEG), appeared to hold its anti-tumor impact while having no immunogenicity. Adding pyrogens, toxins, and other unsafe materials inside a therapeutic enzyme is prohibited. This supports the utilization of animal enzymes, despite their significant cost compared with microbial enzymes (65, 66).

iii. Their lifetime inside the circulation might be just in the order of minutes. But fortunately, this issue is simpler than the immunological issue to overcome, by camouflaging with covalent adjustment (67). Different techniques have been effective, especially those including entanglement of the enzyme inside fabricated liposomes, designed microspheres, and red blood cells. However, these techniques are effective at increasing the circulatory lifetime of the enzymes, they regularly cause an expanded immunological reaction and may cause blood clots (68).

Rather than the industrial-scale enzymes, remedially helpful enzymes are needed in moderately little quantities, though at an extremely high level of purity and (for the most part) explicitness (69). The suitable Michaelis–Menten kinetic properties of these enzymes are low $k_m$ and high $V_{max}$ to be maximally effective even at exceptionally low enzyme and substrate amounts. Therapeutically prepared aliquots of commercial enzymes are commonly prepared as a lyophilized pure powder with just biocompatible buffering salts and mannitol as the diluent additive agent. Although such enzymes are very expensive, and yet tantamount to those of contending restorative agents or medicines. For instance, urokinase (a serine protease) is extracted from human urine (70) (some hereditarily designed ones are being prepared) and used to disintegrate clots of blood.

Significant potential use of enzymes is to treat cancer. Asparaginase has been especially encouraging for the treatment of intense lymphocytic leukemia. Its activity relies on the way that tumor cells are inadequate in aspartate–ammonia ligase reaction, which confines their capacity to produce the typically insignificant amino acid L-asparagine. In this way, they are compelled to gain it from body liquids. The activity of the asparaginase does not influence the working of normal cells, which can orchestrate enough for their necessities, however, lessen the free exogenous amount thus instigates a condition of deadly starvation in the susceptible tumor cells (71). A 60% occurrence of complete abatement has been found in an investigation of around 6000 instances of intense lymphocytic leukemia. The enzyme is controlled intravenously. It is just powerful in decreasing asparagine levels inside the circulatory system, demonstrating a half-life of about a day. This half-life might be expanded by the use of PEG-altered asparaginase to about 20 times (72).

## 2.5 BIOMIMETIC AND ARTIFICIAL ENZYMES

At the interface between biochemistry and chemistry, data can stream in the two headings. Data from chemistry into biochemistry cause us to see how biochemical systems work and outfit a significant number of devices expected to investigate and comprehend biochemistry. Although, there is another perspective in which data from biochemistry streams into chemistry. This motivates a new chemistry area dependent on the criteria utilized by nature, a field that is called biomimetic chemistry (73–76). It reflects a movement that researchers have sought for a while, and that is developing new findings motivated by what nature uses. Overall, biomimicry is a field that covers any methodology planned for imitating fundamental properties of a biological framework. At the molecular level, molecularly imprinted polymers (MIPs) are a case of emulating molecular identification (69, 76).

Artificial enzymes might be characterized as organic, synthetic molecules designed to reproduce/imitate the active center of an enzyme. The interaction of a substrate near functional groups and important conformational centers in the enzyme does catalysis by a principle named closeness effect. Hence, it is conceivable to make comparative impetuses from a set of atoms that will mirror the enzyme active center (77).

Since the artificial enzymes work by binding the molecules, they are made dependent on the molecular structure of the host, for example, cyclodextrins, crown ethers or calixarene, etc. (78). Living cells frequently integrate complex molecules through multistep successive reactions, each catalyzed by its enzyme. To permit the entirety of the reactions to function admirably, nature utilizes separation or site segregation through which the individual reactions are spatially isolated to improve their activity. The way to accomplish site disengagement in liquid media is to use star polymers, macromolecules that can be functionalized so they can tie and encircle little catalytic molecules in their center, contiguous the active center of the reactant (79–81). There are several reports that various artificial enzymes catalyzing different reactions with rate increments up to $10^3$; this is, however, considerably lower than that of natural enzymes that regularly cause rate increments over $10^6$ (78).

The field of artificial biocatalysts is a quickly advancing domain. As the hindrances among biochemistry and chemistry become less particular, the scope of new techniques, which consolidate skills from the two areas, is growing (82). In recognition of both, the matter that the *de novo* configuration approach can be tedious and that a little erroneous conclusion will be calamitous, a pattern in all these ongoing strategies is the utilization of selection approaches. The natural procedure of determination and intensification is how enzymes have evolved their advanced function. The essential point in artificial enzyme synthesis is picking the choice occasion. From an experimental view, selection dependent on the affinity of binding is the least demanding technique to utilize. However, numerous techniques that utilize binding criteria have used trichostatin A (TSA) as a ligand (83) and have avoided delivering the rate-increasing speeds needed to be comparable to that of natural enzymes. This is maybe justifiable since the electrostatic and geometric devotion of TSA to the real transitional state cannot be altogether finished. Partly, the impact of this issue can be mitigated by bringing an element of the plan into the system (84).

Utilizing data accessible on the native enzyme mechanism and groups with catalytic activity, few scientists have elevated the increment of rates accessible with TSA strategies by joining catalytic groups into TSA binding, as it has seen with catalytic Abs and MIPs (85). Within the contrasting zones of enantioselective changes prompted by enzyme mimicry structures or by transition metal catalysts, a significant number of the most basic standards of design yet, apply to both. The jargon and accentuation utilized by every group are such that impressive interaction and transmission of helpful thoughts and ideas are nearly disheartening, although techniques, such as combinatorics are presently utilized by both. Now, when the transition state or intermediate in a catalyzed reaction may include halfway formation and rupture of a few bonds, and such factors as shape, polarity coordinate, electrostatic potential, basicity, and acidity versus molecular environment all must be accounted for, it would appear to be convenient to devise some new figurative method for speaking to and computing the relative steady estimation of these factors for different alternatives. Thus, albeit a tremendous informational collection is accessible, and breathtaking advances have been done, catalysis despite everything stays a magnificent region of disclosure (86).

## 2.6 SUMMARY AND FUTURE PERSPECTIVES

Enzymes possess chemical and biological properties. Their function and conformation together with sequences specify their role in levels of proteomics and genomics of living species and their sufficiency to catalyze chemical reactions. These properties expand their biochemical and biophysical functions to metabolic pathways and networks. Most of the enzymes perform numerous reactions and as the sequences evolve, enzymes can modify their reaction, too.

In this context, nanozymes have emerged as efficient biomimetic catalysts for various industrial as well as biomedical processes owing to their superior physicochemical as well as biological features that are summarized in **Table 2.1**. During the past decade, more than 200 research groups worldwide, working in the field of nanozymes, have developed numerous compounds, including hundreds of nanomaterials. Parallel to the significant successes in the nanozyme field, some other aspects, such as theoretical and kinetics mechanisms, fundamental concepts, and criteria of assaying their catalytic function, have also been studied. Especially, via the relation of distinguished physicochemical aspects and enzyme-mimicking catalytic functions of nanozymes, their applications have been many, from *in vitro* to *in vivo*.

Alongside the quick advancement and ever-extending comprehension of nanoscience and nanotechnology, nanozymes are sure to become immediate surrogates of conventional enzymes by emulating and further building the active sites of native enzymes. Interestingly, a wide assortment of nanomaterials displays double or multienzyme mimetic action. For instance, $Fe_3O_4$ NPs show POD- and CAT-like activities in a pH-dependent manner (87); Prussian blue NPs exhibit POD-, CAT-, and SOD-like activities at the same time; and $Mn_3O_4$ NPs emulate each of the three cellular antioxidant enzymes including SOD, CAT, and glutathione peroxidase (88). Exploiting the physicochemical features of nanomaterials, nanozymes have indicated an expansive scope of uses from *in vitro* detection to displace explicit enzymes in living cells. With the development of the new notion of nanozymology, nanozymes are now a rising area interfacing nanotechnology and biological sciences (89). Because of the high durability, low expense, huge surface area for modification, and tunable activity, nanozymes have the potential for a wide range of utilizations. Specifically, by joining physicochemical features and catalytic activity of nanozymes, a sequence of widespread technologies with applications in bioanalysis, disorder detection, and treatment (**Figure 2.2**) (90).

To drive more in the rapidly developing field of nanozyme research, it is necessary to establish a new definition of nanozymology and thereby promote nanozymes in nanozymological techniques. Even though the nanozyme field has been booming over the past few years, this area is a young discipline yet, which is faced with some challenges to overcome. Some of the challenges may be surmounted via more detailed and systematic nanozyme research and will accelerate the promotion of nanozyme area in basic research and medical usages, such as 1) elevating nanozymological concepts and standards; 2) organizing fundamental principles and mechanisms of nanozymology; 3) evaluating bioeffects of nanozymes; 4) translating clinical potential of nanozymes; and 5) multifunctionality of nanozymes. Also, molecular modeling could be considered as an efficient strategy to address these issues and development of more efficient nanozymes before experimental approaches. Finally, due to the high market potential of nanozymes, it is expected that more and more researches will be focused on this area. Overall, we think that the nanozyme field will have a high possibility of potential applications ranging from *in vitro* detection to *in vivo* monitoring and catalytic therapy in the near future.

## ACKNOWLEDGMENT

The authors gratefully acknowledge the partial financial support from Kermanshah University of Medical Sciences, Kermanshah, Iran.

## REFERENCES

1. Garcia-Viloca M, Gao J, Karplus M, Truhlar DG. 2004. *Science* 303: 186–95
2. Lin Y, Ren J, Qu X. 2014. *Acc Chem Res* 47: 1097–105
3. Singh S. 2019. *Front Chem* 7: 46
4. Breslow R. 2005. *Artificial Enzymes*. Weinheim: Wiley-VCH
5. Jeon WB, Bae KH, Byun SM. 1998. *J Inorg Biochem* 71: 163–9
6. Raynal M, Ballester P, Vidal-Ferran A, van Leeuwen PW. 2014. *Chem Soc Rev* 43: 1734–87
7. Jiang D, Ni D, Rosenkrans ZT, Huang P, Yan X, Cai W. 2019. *Chem Soc Rev* 48: 3683–704
8. Liang M, Yan X. 2019. *Acc Chem Res* 52: 2190–200
9. Manea F, Houillon FB, Pasquato L, Scrimin P. 2004. *Angew Chem Int Ed Engl* 43: 6165–9
10. Gao L, Zhuang J, Nie L, Zhang J, Zhang Y, et al. 2007. *Nat Nanotechnol* 2: 577–83
11. Zhang R, Fan K, Yan X. 2020. Sci China Life Sci
12. Karakoti A, Singh S, Dowding JM, Seal S, Self WT. 2010. *Chem Soc Rev* 39: 4422–32
13. Karim MN, Anderson SR, Singh S, Ramanathan R, Bansal V. 2018. *Biosens Bioelectron* 110: 8–15
14. Pirmohamed T, Dowding JM, Singh S, Wasserman B, Heckert E, et al. 2010. *Chem Commun (Camb)* 46: 2736–8
15. Singh S. 2016. *Biointerphases* 11: 04B202
16. Wang Q, Wei H, Zhang Z, Wang E, Dong S. 2018. *TrAC Trends in Analytical Chemistry* 105: 218–24
17. Zhao M, Tao Y, Huang W, He Y. 2018. *Phys Chem Chem Phys* 20: 28644–8
18. Wu J, Wang X, Wang Q, Lou Z, Li S, et al. 2019. *Chem Soc Rev* 48: 1004–76
19. Wei H, Wang E. 2013. *Chem Soc Rev* 42: 6060–93
20. Liu B, Liu J. 2017. *Nano Research* 10: 1125–48
21. Shi J, Yin T, Shen W. 2019. *Colloids Surf B Biointerfaces* 178: 163–9
22. Gao L, Yan X. 2016. *Sci China Life Sci* 59: 400–2
23. Liu Z, Qu X. 2019. *Sci China Life Sci* 62: 150–2
24. Zhang H, Liu XL, Zhang YF, Gao F, Li GL, et al. 2018. *Sci China Life Sci* 61: 400–14
25. Zhuang J, Zhang J, Gao L, Zhang Y, Gu N, et al. 2008. *Materials Letters* 62: 3972–4
26. Xie X, Xu W, Liu X. 2012. *Acc Chem Res* 45: 1511–20
27. Zhou Y, Liu B, Yang R, Liu J. 2017. *Bioconjug Chem* 28: 2903–9
28. Wang P, Wang T, Hong J, Yan X, Liang M. 2020. *Front Bioeng Biotechnol* 8: 15

29. Ghorbani M, Derakhshankhah H, Jafari S, Salatin S, Dehghanian M, et al. 2019. *Nano Today* 29: 100775

30. Golchin J, Golchin K, Alidadian N, Ghaderi S, Eslamkhah S, et al. 2017. *Artif Cells Nanomed Biotechnol* 45: 1–8

31. Li J, Liu W, Wu X, Gao X. 2015. *Biomaterials* 48: 37–44

32. Ma X, Zhang L, Xia M, Li S, Zhang X, Zhang Y. 2017. *ACS Appl Mater Interfaces* 9: 21089–93

33. Shen X, Liu W, Gao X, Lu Z, Wu X. 2015. *J Am Chem Soc* 137: 15882–91

34. Jiang B, Duan D, Gao L, Zhou M, Fan K, et al. 2018. *Nat Protoc* 13: 1506–20

35. Wang X, Guo W, Hu Y, Wu J, Wei H. 2016. In *Nanozymes: Next Wave of Artificial Enzymes*, pp. 4. Berlin Heidelberg: Springer Nature

36. Copeland RA. 2004. *Enzymes: a practical introduction to structure, mechanism, and data analysis*: John Wiley & Sons

37. Cui Q, Karplus M. 2003. In *Advances in Protein Chemistry*, pp. 315–72: Elsevier

38. Payen A, Persoz J-F. 1833. *Ann. Chim Phys* 53: 73–92

39. Sumner JB. 1926. *J Biol Chem* 69: 435–41

40. Blake C, Koenig D, Mair G, North A, Phillips D, Sarma V. 1965. *Nature* 206: 757–61

41. Keller MA, Piedrafita G, Ralser M. 2015. *Curr Opin Biotechnol* 34: 153–61

42. Krebs HA. 1940. *Biochem J* 34: 775

43. Thompson R. 1962. *Science* 137: 405–8

44. Tipton K, Boyce S. 2000. *Bioinformatics* 16: 34–40

45. Thompson R. 1962. *Nature* 193: 1227–31

46. Hoffmann-Ostenhof O, Thompson R. 1958. *Nature* 181: 452–

47. Duarte F, Amrein BA, Kamerlin SCL. 2013. *Phys Chem Chem Phy* 15: 11160–77

48. Gatti-Lafranconi P, Hollfelder F. 2013. *ChemBioChem* 14: 285–92

49. Pandya C, Farelli JD, Dunaway-Mariano D, Allen KN. 2014. *J Biol Chem* 289: 30229–36

50. Khanal A, Yu McLoughlin S, Kershner JP, Copley SD. 2015. *Mol Biol Evol* 32: 100–8

51. Aharoni A, Gaidukov L, Khersonsky O, Gould SM, Roodveldt C, Tawfik DS. 2005. *Nat Genet* 37: 73–6

52. Dellus-Gur E, Toth-Petroczy A, Elias M, Tawfik DS. 2013. *J Mol Biol* 425: 2609–21

53. Kaltenbach M, Tokuriki N. 2014. *J Exp Zool Part B: Mol Develop Evol* 322: 468–87

54. Consortium U. 2012. *Nucleic Acids Res* 41: D43–D7

55. Kersey PJ, Allen JE, Christensen M, Davis P, Falin LJ, et al. 2014. *Nucleic Acids Res* 42: D546–D52

56. Botstein D, Cherry JM, Ashburner M, Ball C, Blake J, et al. 2000. *Nat Genet* 25: 25–9

57. Cooney DA, Rosenbluth RJ. 1975. In *Advances in Pharmacology*, pp. 185–289: Elsevier

58. Kang TS, Stevens RC. 2009. *Hum Mutat* 30: 1591–610

59. Yari M, B Ghoshoon M, Vakili B, Ghasemi Y. 2017. *Curr Pharm Biotechnol* 18: 531–40

60. Chang TMS. 2013. *Biomedical applications of immobilized enzymes and proteins*: Springer Science & Business Media

61. Liang JF, Li YT, Yang VC. 2000. *J Pharm Sci* 89: 979–90

62. Liu X, Gao Y, Chandrawati R, Hosta-Rigau L. 2019. *Nanoscale* 11: 21046–60

63. Brynskikh AM, Zhao Y, Mosley RL, Li S, Boska MD, et al. 2010. *Nanomedicine* 5: 379–96

64. Fu CH, Sakamoto KM. 2007. *Expert Opin Pharmaco* 8: 1977–84

65. Keating MJ, Holmes R, Lerner S, Ho DH. 1993. *Leuk Lymphoma* 10: 153–7

66. Armstrong JK, Hempel G, Koling S, Chan LS, Fisher T, et al. 2007. *Cancer* 110: 103–11

67. Tian L, Qi J, Qian K, Oderinde O, Cai Y, et al. 2018. *Sensor Actuat B: Chem* 260: 676–84

68. Zhang P, Sun D, Cho A, Weon S, Lee S, et al. 2019. *Nat. Commun* 10: 1–14

69. Zhang Z, Zhang X, Liu B, Liu J. 2017. *J Am Chem Soc* 139: 5412–9

70. Novak L. 1973. Method for recovering urokinase from urine containing the same. Google Patents
71. Roberts J, Prager MD, Bachynsky N. 1966. *Cancer Res* 26: 2213–7
72. Abuchowski A, Kazo G, Verhoest JC, Van TE, Kafkewitz D, et al. 1984. *Cancer Biochem Biophys* 7: 175–86
73. Breslow R. 1972. *Chem Soc Rev* 1: 553–80
74. Breslow R. 1994. *Pure Appl Chem* 66: 1573–82
75. Breslow R. 1995. *Acc Chem Res* 28: 146–53
76. Breslow R. 1998. *Chem Biol* 5: R27–R8
77. Murakami Y, Kikuchi J-i, Hisaeda Y, Hayashida O. 1996. *Chem Rev* 96: 721–58
78. Sharma V, Bachwani M. 2011. *Curr Enzyme Inhib* 7: 178–89
79. Singla RK. 2012.
80. Chi Y, Scroggins ST, Fréchet JM. 2008. *J Am Chem Soc* 130: 6322–3
81. Helms B, Guillaudeu SJ, Xie Y, McMurdo M, Hawker CJ, Fréchet JM. 2005. *Angew Chem Int Ed* 44: 6384–7
82. Bjerre J, Rousseau C, Marinescu L, Bols M. 2008. *Appl Microbiol Biotechnol* 81: 1–11
83. Nomiya K, Yokoyama H, Nagano H, Oda M, Sakuma S. 1995. *J Inorg Biochem* 60: 289–97
84. Kulik V, Hartmann E, Weyand M, Frey M, Gierl A, et al. 2005. *J Mol Biol* 352: 608–20
85. Vanommeslaeghe K, Van Alsenoy C, De Proft F, Martins JC, Tourwé D, Geerlings P. 2003. *Org Biomol Chem* 1: 2951–7
86. Motherwell W, Bingham M, Six Y. 2001. *Tetrahedron* 22: 4663–86
87. Kıranşan KD, Aksoy M, Topçu E. 2018. *Mater Res Bull* 106: 57–65
88. Wickramaratne NP, Perera VS, Park B-W, Gao M, McGimpsey GW, et al. 2013. *Chem Mater* 25: 2803–11
89. Yan X, Gao L. 2020. In *Nanozymology*, pp. 3–16: Springer
90. Gao L, Wei H, Yan X, Qu X. 2020. In *Nanozymology*, pp. 557–62: Springer

# 3 Metal Oxide Nanozymes

*Biwu Liu[1] and Juewen Liu[2*]*
[1]Institute of Analytical Chemistry and Instrument for Life Science, The Key Laboratory of Biomedical Information Engineering of Ministry of Education, School of Life Science and Technology, Xi'an Jiaotong University, Xi'an, Shaanxi, P. R. China
[2]Department of Chemistry, Waterloo Institute for Nanotechnology, University of Waterloo, Waterloo, Ontario, Canada

## CONTENTS

* Corresponding author: Juewen Liu

DOI: 10.1201/9781003109228-3

## 3.1  INTRODUCTION

Sensors and biosensors are highly useful in many aspects of our daily life, such as biomedical diagnosis, environmental monitoring, and food safety (1–4). In the past few decades, nanomaterials have been widely used in designing sensors due to advancements in their synthesis and characterization (5). Among them, noble metals, such as gold (Au) and silver (Ag) (6–9), and carbon-based materials (10–13), have been the most frequently used. For example, Au nanoparticles (NPs) have attractive optical (14) and catalytic properties (15) that are useful for designing biosensors. Since 2007 (16), the intrinsic enzyme-like activities of many nanomaterials have been noticed, and many of them are metal oxides (MOs) (17, 18).

MO NPs are important materials with a diverse range of catalytic, magnetic, UV absorption, fluorescence quenching, and dielectric properties (19). For example, titanium dioxide ($TiO_2$) is a photocatalyst used for degrading organic contaminants; iron oxide ($Fe_3O_4$) NPs are superparamagnetic, useful for separation and drug delivery (20); and cerium oxide ($CeO_2$) is a powerful oxidative catalyst (21). These MOs are highly active, cost-effective, and stable, attractive for numerous interesting applications. MOs can serve as signal transduction and target recognition elements in sensors. For signal transduction, magnetic-, electric-, and optical-based sensing have been demonstrated. High-quality monodispersed MO NPs can be prepared in organic solvents with strong ligands (e.g., $Fe_3O_4$ NPs), but their surface chemistry is dominated by the capping ligands. Herein, we focus on sensing based on the enzyme-like activity of MO surfaces without strong ligands.

## 3.2  SURFACE PROPERTIES OF MO NPs

The surface property of nanozymes is critical for their catalytic and sensing performance. Dispersing MO NPs in water results in immediately the hydration of surface metal species via chemisorption of water, which then dissociates into surface hydroxide (22) (**Figure 3.1A**). Depending on the pH, the surface hydroxide can be further protonated/deprotonated, resulting in positively/negatively charged surfaces. The pH of transition from positive to negative potential is termed the point of zero charge (PZC), at which the overall charge is zero. Zhang et al. (23) reported the PZC values of some common MOs. Different materials have different PZCs, and depending on the method of preparation, surface treatment, particle size, the concentration of surface hydroxide, characterization method, and buffer conditions, the PZC of the same material may vary a few pH units (22). At physiological pH, most MOs are negatively charged with only a few exceptions [e.g., zinc oxide (ZnO), nickel oxide (NiO)] (24). The surface charge of MOs can affect their colloidal stability, adsorption of biomolecules (25), and nanozyme activities (26).

In addition to water molecules, the surface metal species on MO NPs can also interact with specific anions via coordination bonds. In this regard, the hard–soft–acid–base theory is a useful starting point (27). In general, metals that can form stable oxides tend to be hard or borderline metals, and they tend to adsorb harder ligands, such as oxygen and fluoride. For instance, arsenate strongly adsorbs on iron oxide surfaces with a few coordination modes (28, 29) (**Figure 3.1B**). Chemisorption

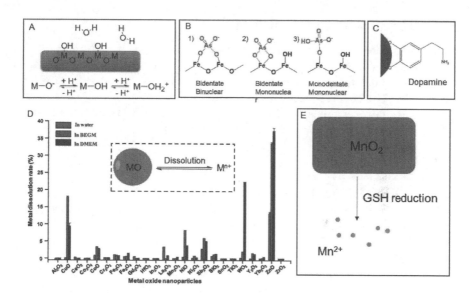

**FIGURE 3.1** Surface properties of MO NPs. (A) Chemisorption of water on an oxide surface and its protonation/deprotonation upon pH variation. (B) Different modes of arsenate complexing with iron oxide: 1) bidentate binuclear; 2) bidentate mononuclear; and 3) monodentate mononuclear. (C) Binding of dopamine on an oxide surface. (D) Dissolution of MO NPs in water, bronchial epithelial cell growth medium (BEGM), and Dulbecco's modified eagle medium (DMEM). (E) A scheme showing that $MnO_2$ nanosheets react with GSH to release $Mn^{2+}$ ions. Panel (D) reprinted from (23) with permission, copyright 2012 American Chemical Society.

of sulfate, phosphate, halides, nitrate, carbonate, selenate, and oxalate are also well-documented (22). Such anion adsorption could significantly alter the nanozyme activity of MO NPs (30, 31).

Besides anions, some biologically important small molecules can also strongly bind on the surface metal sites. For example, dopamine (32), catechol (33), amino acids (34), and nucleoside triphosphate (35) can adsorb on MO NPs and affect the nanozyme activity (**Figure 3.1C**). Finally, the adsorption of biomacromolecules on MO NPs may take place via various interaction forces (e.g., electrostatic, coordination, and hydrogen bonding) (25). For instance, DNA mainly relies on its phosphate backbone to adsorb on most MOs.

Most MO NPs are stable in water and even in complex biological fluids, while some may dissociate into free metal ions. **Figure 3.1D** shows the rate of dissolution of various oxides in water and cell culture media (23). Copper oxide (CuO) and ZnO dissolved significantly in a cell culture medium, followed by tungsten oxide ($WO_3$), NiO, antimony oxide ($Sb_2O_3$), and cobalt oxide (CoO), while other oxides are quite stable. Dissolution may be accelerated by lowering pH, and/or reacting with reducing agents (36). For example, dopamine as a ligand can cause Fe leaching from iron oxide (37). Biological thiols (e.g., glutathione and GSH) can reduce manganese oxide ($MnO_2$) and release free $Mn^{2+}$ ions (**Figure 3.1E**). Such dissolution of MO NPs and leaching of metal ions could cause a change in their activity over time and cellular toxicity.

## 3.3   ENZYME MIMICS OF MO NPs

Compared to a large number of chemical reactions catalyzed by natural (proteins) enzymes, currently, only limited reactions can be catalyzed by nanozymes. Though hundreds of nanomaterials have been identified as nanozymes, most mimic oxidoreductases (17). The effects to identify nanozymes with new activities are continuing. Some representative examples are highlighted herein (**Table 3.1**), and the Wei group (17) has published a more comprehensive survey on this broad topic.

### 3.3.1   PEROXIDASE

Yan group first reported that magnetic $Fe_3O_4$ NPs possess intrinsic peroxidase (POD)-like activity, facilitating the oxidation of many chromogenic substrates, such as 3,3′,5,5′-tetramethylbenzidine (TMB), di-azo-aminobenzene (DAB), and $o$-phenylenediamine (OPD) by hydrogen peroxide ($H_2O_2$) (16). The authors confirmed that the catalysis did come from the particles rather than any dissolved metal ions. Inspired by this pioneering work, many other MOs, such as ferric oxide ($Fe_2O_3$) (38), cobalt tetraoxide ($Co_3O_4$) (39), CuO (40), and vanadium oxide ($V_2O_5$) (41, 42), were also reported to mimic POD.

### 3.3.2   OXIDASE

Oxidase (OXD) can use dissolved oxygen to catalyze the oxidation of substrates, thus omitting the need for toxic and unstable $H_2O_2$. In 2009, Asati et al. (43) reported that $CeO_2$ NPs (nanoceria) were able to catalyze the oxidation of TMB, 2,2′-azino-bis(3-ethylbenzothiazoline-6-sulfonic acid (ABTS), and dopamine without $H_2O_2$. However, Peng et al. (44) challenged that the reaction mechanism was via oxidation

---

## TABLE 3.1
## Typical MO NPs-Based Nanozymes

| Enzyme activity | MO NPs | Substrate | Reference |
|---|---|---|---|
| Peroxidase | $Fe_3O_4$ | TMB, DAB, OPD | (16) |
| | $Fe_2O_3$ | TMB | (38) |
| | $V_2O_5$ | Bromide | (42) |
| | $Co_3O_4$ | TMB | (39) |
| | CuO | TMB | (40) |
| Oxidase | $CeO_2$ | TMB, ABTS, dopamine | (43) |
| | NiO | AR | (45) |
| | $MoO_3$ | Sulfite | (46) |
| Catalase | $CeO_2$ | $H_2O_2$ | (47) |
| | $Co_3O_4$ | $H_2O_2$ | (39) |
| SOD | $CeO_2$ | Superoxide free radical | (48) |
| Phosphatase | $CeO_2$ | pNPP, ATP, o-phospho-L-tyrosine | (51, 52) |
| DNase I | $CeO_2$ | 15-mer ssDNA | (54) |
| Photolyase | $CeO_2$ | cyclobutane pyrimidine dimers | (55) |

rather than catalysis. Wu et al. showed that the material alone cannot oxidize the substrate and $O_2$ is essential in their reaction (17). NiO is another OXD mimic, although so far it only reacts with Amplex Red (AR) to produce fluorescent resorufin (45). Interestingly, $CeO_2$ is not very efficient in catalyzing this reaction. Some more specific OXD-mimics have also been reported. For example, ultrasmall (2 nm) molybdenum oxide ($MoO_3$) NPs can catalyze the oxidation of sulfite to sulfate, mimicking sulfite oxidase (SuOx) activity (46).

### 3.3.3 CATALASE AND SUPEROXIDE DISMUTASE

Catalase (CAT) can decompose $H_2O_2$ into water and oxygen, while superoxide dismutase (SOD) catalyzes the decomposition of superoxide free radicals into water and $H_2O_2$. Both enzymes are important in cellular defense systems against reactive oxygen species (ROS). $CeO_2$ (47) and $Co_3O_4$ (39) have been reported to have CAT-like activity, and $CeO_2$ (48), NiO (49), and MnO (50) have been demonstrated to exhibit SOD activity, although they are less used for sensing applications.

### 3.3.4 HYDROLASE

MO NPs can also mimic hydrolases. Kuchma et al. (51) reported that $CeO_2$ showed phosphatase (PP)-like activity by breaking the phosphate ester bonds in p-nitrophenylphosphate (pNPP), ATP, o-phospho-L-tyrosine but not in plasmid DNA. The dephosphorylation of ATP and other nucleotides by self-made and commercial $CeO_2$ was further confirmed by Janos et al. (52). Yao et al. (53) revealed that porous $CeO_2$ nanorods were able to cleave the terminal phosphate ester of DNA. We recently found that $CeO_2$ can mimic deoxyribonuclease (DNase) I to cleave single-stranded (ss) oligonucleotides into shorter fragments (mostly 5-mer) (54). Incubation of DNA strands with $CeO_2$ at higher temperature is important for the cleavage likely due to the activation energy of the reaction. Analysis of the reaction product showed that the cleavage reaction was through the hydrolysis pathway instead of oxidation.

### 3.3.5 PHOTOLYASE

DNA photolyase can repair UV light-induced damage of DNA by splitting the pyrimidine dimers. Tian et al. (55) found that $CeO_2$ can cleave the cyclobutane bond in the thymidine dimer with the help of visible light. The porous $CeO_2$ with a higher $Ce^{3+}$ fraction showed higher activity.

## 3.4 MO NPs IN SENSING

A typical sensing process involves specific recognition of analytes followed by transduction into physically detectable signals. MO nanozymes can serve for target recognition and/or signal generation.

### 3.4.1  MO NPs for Signaling

#### 3.4.1.1  Immunoassays

Protein enzymes have been widely used in immunosorbent assays to achieve signal amplification taking advantage of their excellent catalytic activities. For instance, horseradish peroxidase (HRP)-coupled antibodies (Abs) are major reagents for immunoassays. However, such enzyme-Ab conjugates are costly to prepare and unstable, thus it is desirable to replace HRP with more stable nanozymes (**Figure 3.2A**). After discovering the POD-like activity of $Fe_3O_4$ NPs (16), Yan and

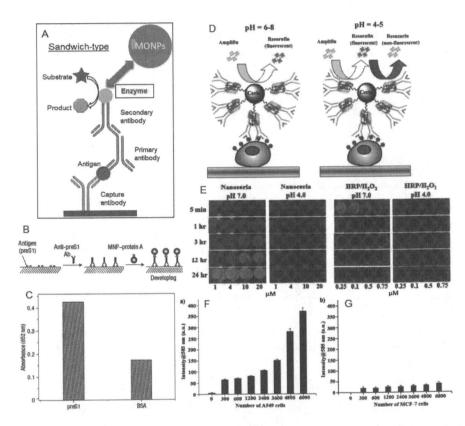

**FIGURE 3.2**  MO NPs replacing enzymes in immunoassays. (A) The design of a typical sandwich-type ELISA in which MO NPs replace the enzyme component. (B) The design of an indirect (no capture Ab) ELISA for the detection of antigen preS1. (C) The oxidation of TMB indicated by the absorbance at 652 nm correlated with the concentration of antigen preSA, and BSA was used as a control. (D) Schematic showing a nanoceria-involved ELISA can oxidize ampliflu into stable fluorescent products at neutral pH but not at acidic pH. (E) Images showing the oxidation of ampliflu catalyzed by either nanoceria or HRP with $H_2O_2$. Detection of folate receptor expressed in (F) lung carcinoma cells (A-549) and (G) MCF-7 breast carcinoma cells. Panel (B, C) reprinted from (16) with permission, copyright 2007 Springer Nature Publishing. (D–G) from (56) with permission, copyright 2011 American Chemical Society.

coworkers demonstrated such an immunoassay (**Figure 3.2B**). An anti-HBV preS1 Ab was attached to the immobilized antigen (hepatitis B virus surface antigen, preS1). The $Fe_3O_4$ NPs were functionalized with protein A, which can recognize the Ab. The substrates (TMB and $H_2O_2$) were then introduced to general a colorimetric signal. This assay was successfully used to detect preS1, and had a high selectivity against bovine serum albumin (BSA) (**Figure 3.2C**).

OXD-mimicking nanozymes have also been used in immunoassays to produce signals without $H_2O_2$. Asati et al. (56) prepared poly(acrylic acid) (PAA) modified $CeO_2$ nanoparticles (PAA-$CeO_2$), which could oxidize AR to a stable fluorescent product resorufin at pH 7.0 but not pH 4.0 (**Figure 3.2D and E**). It should be noted that most POD/OXD mimics show their optimal activity at pH 4 (17), which limits their applications. On the other hand, HRP also rapidly catalyzes AR into the nonfluorescent product by $H_2O_2$ even at pH 7. Thus, the OXD-like activity of PAA-$CeO_2$ is pH-tunable, allowing robust immunoassays for biomarkers at neutral pH. The PAA-$CeO_2$ was then modified with protein-G for attaching antifolate-receptor Ab, which can recognize the overexpressed folate receptors in tumors. A lung cancer cell line A-549 was then used as a model target, and the fluorescence intensity of resorufin was found to correlate well with the number of cancer cells (**Figure 3.2F**). Breast carcinoma cells (MCF-7) that do not overexpress the folate receptor were used as a control (**Figure 3.2G**).

### 3.4.1.2 Cascade Reactions

Another popular method to use nanozymes for signal generation is to couple them with natural enzymes. While Abs are excellent for recognizing macromolecular targets such as proteins, enzymes are powerful for targeting small molecules. In a typical design, the product of a natural enzyme can serve as the substrate of the nanozyme for signal generation. In this regard, $H_2O_2$ is the most common intermediate or by-product from many natural OXDs, such as glucose oxidase (GOx), lactate oxidase, cholesterol oxidase, xanthine oxidase, and urate oxidase (**Figure 3.3A**).

Early works simply carried out the reactions in two steps: 1) use natural enzymes to generate the intermediates and 2) add nanozymes and substrate to initiate the colorimetric assay. For example, Wei and Wang (57) reported this strategy using GOx and $Fe_3O_4$ NPs (ABTS as the chromogenic substrate) to detect glucose with a limit of detection (LOD) of 30 μM and a linear range from 50 μM to 1 mM (**Figure 3.3B**). This assay was highly selective to glucose due to the intrinsic selectivity of natural protein enzyme (**Figure 3.3C**).

The catalytic activity of many MO NPs nanozymes is pH-dependent, with higher activity at lower pH. Thus, enzymes generating/consuming protons can also be combined with nanozymes to develop bioassays. Using this strategy, Cheng et al. examined the hydrolysis of acetylcholine (ACh) into choline and acetic acid by acetylcholinesterase (AChE) (58). The intermediate acetic acid can lower the solution pH and activate the OXD-like activity of nanoceria using TMB as a substrate. This assay was used to detect the AChE with a linear response from 35 mU to 175 mU and a LOD of ~25 mU. Contrarily, the authors also determined the urease activity based on its proton-consuming ability.

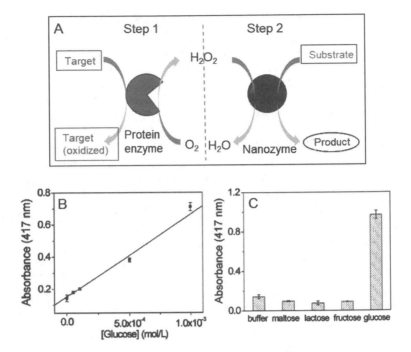

**FIGURE 3.3** Cascade reactions using protein enzymes and nanozymes. (A) A schematic showing the two steps in cascade reactions. (B) The linear calibration curve. (C) Specificity analysis for glucose using a two-step reaction strategy. (B, C) from (57) with permission, copyright 2008 American Chemical Society.

More elegant cascade reactions require positioning two or more enzymes/nanozymes in close proximity with precise control over distances and conformations (59). In this regard, cascade reactions between natural enzymes under the surface- or volume-confined environment have been reported (60, 61). It is however difficult to control the enzyme–nanozyme or nanozyme–nanozyme hybrids to achieve synergetic cascade reactions. Few reports have emphasized the precise controlling of the MO NPs nanozymes with either protein enzymes or other nanozymes (e.g., Au) (62, 63). Metal-organic frameworks (MOFs) seem promising in encapsulating multiple enzymes/nanozymes to form integrated systems (64–66).

## 3.4.2 MO NPs FOR BOTH RECOGNIZING AND SIGNALING

### 3.4.2.1 Intrinsic Optical Properties

Some MO NPs nanozymes possess intrinsic optical properties that are sensitive to their surface chemistry. For example, dilute $CeO_2$ is almost colorless, but it immediately turns yellow and then dark orange in the presence of $H_2O_2$ (**Figure 3.4A and B**) (67). Nanoceria was reported to have CAT activity to degrade $H_2O_2$, although this activity is quite low and the color change occurs much faster. This color change was ascribed to the increased percentage of surface Ce(IV), and capping by surface

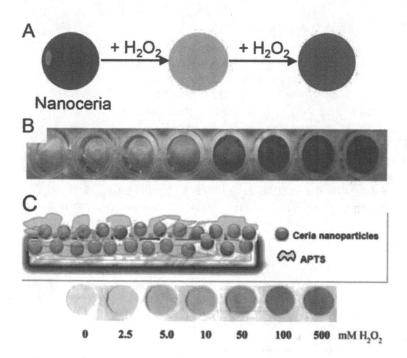

FIGURE 3.4  MO NPs with intrinsic optical properties as both recognition and signaling elements. (A) Scheme and photos of nanoceria (B) in a buffer and (C) deposited on filter paper showing the color change by $H_2O_2$. Panel (B and C) reprinted from (67) with permission, copyright 2011 American Chemical Society.

peroxide species. This colorimetric assay showed a linear range from 0.01 to 0.15 mM for detecting $H_2O_2$. Furthermore, a paper-based assay was designed by depositing $CeO_2$ NPs on filter paper silanized with aminopropyltriethoxysilane (APTES) (**Figure 3.4C**). This paper-based assay showed a linear range from 2.5 to 100 mM $H_2O_2$. When combined with GOx for producing $H_2O_2$ *in situ*, glucose can also be detected based on the color change.

The color change of nanoceria however is not unique to $H_2O_2$. Many antioxidants, including ascorbic acid, gallic acid, vanillic acid, epigallocatechin gallate, quercetin, and caffeic acid can also interact with nanoceria and result in a strong color change (68). For example, dopamine adsorbed on nanoceria and gave a dark color (68). Therefore, the application of this colorimetric method can only be in specialized cases where the sample matrix contains only one of these molecules. Nanozymes can be integrated with luminescent properties to light up the analyte binding. Pratsinis et al. (69) prepared europium ($Eu^{3+}$)-doped $CeO_2$ NPs ($CeO_2$:$Eu^{3+}$) possessing both CAT-like activity and luminescence properties with an emission peak at ca. 590 nm. The rapid adsorption of $H_2O_2$ by nanoceria resulted in a decrease of $CeO_2$:$Eu^{3+}$ luminescence. With this sensor, highly sensitive detection of $H_2O_2$ was demonstrated both in a buffer (LOD=150 nM) and bacterial cell culture (70).

### 3.4.2.2  Tuning Nanozyme Activities

Tuning the surface chemistry of MOs can dramatically change their nanozyme activity, which can also be used to detect the corresponding promotors or inhibitors (**Figure 3.5A**). We reported that fluoride can accelerate the OXD-mimicking activity of $CeO_2$ NPs up to 100 folds (**Figure 3.5B**) (31). The catalytic activity was evaluated using the steady-state kinetics of oxidation of TMB and ABTS. We found that the catalytic efficiency of $CeO_2$ NPs increased by 15 folds and 100 folds for ABTS and TMB, respectively. Mechanistic studies showed that fluoride capping altered the surface charge and oxygen vacancy levels of nanoceria (30). Using ABTS as the substrate and with this enhancement effect, we were able to detect fluoride down to 10 μM by the naked eyes (**Figure 3.5C**) and 0.64 μM by a spectrometer. This assay was highly selective for fluoride and common anions such as chloride did not produce any signal (**Figure 3.5D**). Finally, we showed fluoride in toothpaste can be accurately quantified.

The OXD-like activity of $CeO_2$ was also modulated by nucleoside triphosphates (NTPs). Xu et al. (35) reported that NTPs functioned as a cofactor, and its hydrolysis may further promote the oxidative reactions catalyzed by $CeO_2$ NPs. Among the four NTPs, GTP was the most efficient followed by ATP, UTP, and CTP. Based on

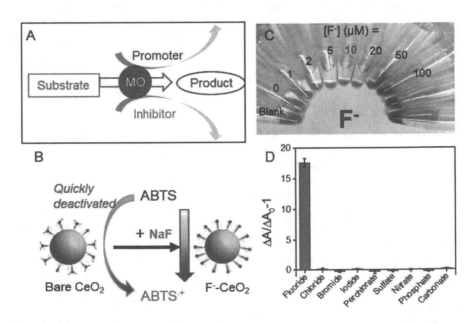

**FIGURE 3.5**  Sensing based on analytes tuning the nanozyme activity. (A) A scheme showing that analytes interfacing with nanozymes may alter their enzymatic properties by promoting or inhibiting. (B) A scheme of fluoride-boosted the OXD-like activity of nanoceria. (C) Photos showing the oxidation of ABTS with nanoceria and various concentrations of fluoride. (D) Selectivity test of different anions on oxidase activity of nanoceria using ABTS as a substrate. (B–D) reproduced from (31) with permission, copyright 2016 Royal Society of Chemistry.

the differential enhancing effect, the authors designed a colorimetric assay to type single-nucleotide polymorphism.

We recently reported another strategy to design sensors based on the analyte-induced recovery of poisoned nanozymes (**Figure 3.6A**) (71). We found that commonly used Good's buffer, including PIPES, HEPES, MOPS, Tris, and

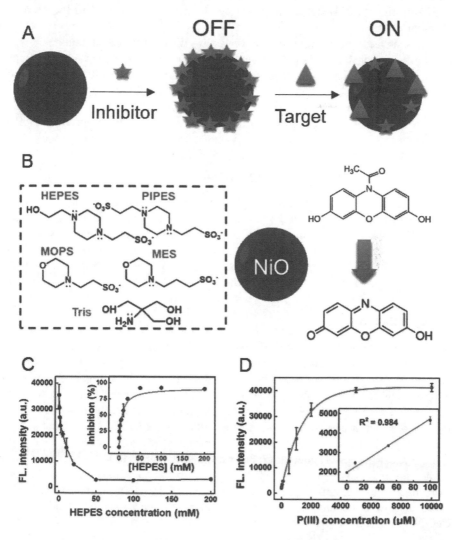

**FIGURE 3.6** Sensing based on analyte recovering the nanozyme activity. (A) A schematic showing that reversible inhibitors temperately block the active site of nanozymes (OFF state). Analytes can replace the inhibitors and recover the nanozymes (ON state). (B) A schematic showing the structures of Good's buffer and NiO-catalyzed oxidation of AR to resorufin. (C) Inhibition of AR oxidation by NiO as a function of HEPES concentration. (D) Recovery of the oxidase activity of NiO by phosphite (P(III)). (B-D) reproduced from (71) with permission, copyright 2020 American Chemical Society.

MES, could inhibit the OXD-like activity of NiO to different extents using AR as the substrate (**Figure 3.6B**). Mechanistic studies revealed that N-containing groups in Good's buffers coordinate with the surface Ni species, and block AR approaching the active sites (**Figure 3.6C**). Interestingly, the activity of NiO can be recovered only by P(III) ($HPO_3^{2-}$) among seven phosphorous (P)-containing anions and other interference ions. The developed sensor could detect P(III) with high sensitivity (LOD=1.46 μM) and a wide dynamic range (2 μM to 1 mM) (**Figure 3.6D**).

Many of the abovementioned discoveries are difficult to predict and some were randomly observed in the lab. Different results may come up in the same nanozyme system, which could be attributable to different experimental conditions such as buffer, pH, and concentration of MOs (72). Therefore, careful studies and systematic tests are needed to fully understand these systems. At the same time, such studies can offer interesting insights into the surface and catalytic properties of these nanozymes.

## 3.5 DNA-MODIFIED MO NANOZYMES

Compared to protein-based enzymes, MO NPs and other nanozymes lack the structural features to highly selectively recognize specific analytes. To improve the specificity in sensing, affinity ligands, including Abs, DNA aptamers (Apts), and molecularly imprinted polymers (MIPs) can be introduced. Some examples of Abs and protein enzymes were discussed above, and in this section, examples of DNA-modified nanozymes for sensor design are introduced.

### 3.5.1 DNA ADSORPTION

Since adsorption of DNA on MO NPs is needed in designing these sensors, it is important to understand the adsorption behavior of DNA. For sensing purposes, ssDNA oligonucleotide probes are typically used. Adsorption of DNA oligonucleotides by a large number of MO NPs was performed, and it was concluded that adsorption takes place mostly via the phosphate backbone to coordinate with nonsaturated surface metals and/or electrostatic interactions (18). Using ligand displacement assays, we confirmed that phosphate-binding predominates in the MOs tested (73). With Raman spectroscopy, Tian et al. (74) proved that all four types of DNA bases bind to the aluminum oxide ($Al_2O_3$) via the phosphate backbone. However, contributions from nucleobase adsorption can also be detected in some systems. For example, using photoelectron and X-ray absorption spectroscopies, adenine bonding with $CeO_2$ was observed (75).

### 3.5.2 EFFECT OF DNA ON NANOZYME ACTIVITY

The active sites of MO NPs nanozymes are mainly on their surfaces, which might be blocked by the adsorbed DNA (**Figure 3.7**). DNA strands may also crosslink different particles, resulting in aggregation, which may in turn decrease nanozyme activity. In some cases, adsorbed DNA may increase the binding affinity of

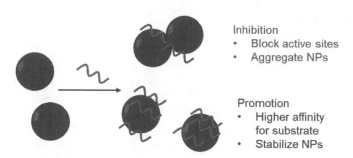

**FIGURE 3.7**    Complicated roles of DNA adsorption on nanozymes activity of MO NPs.

the substrate, which could accelerate reactions. Finally, if performed appropriately, DNA adsorption could enhance the colloidal stability of nanozymes.

Such complicated effects have yielded different results. Using nanoceria as an example, we found that its OXD-like activity for the oxidation of TMB was inhibited after attaching DNA (76). Control experiments showed the decrease of activity correlated with the DNA adsorption process. Anionic PAA and neutral polyethylene glycol (PEG) did not show an inhibition effect. Furthermore, up to 2% of polystyrene sulfonate (PSS) was needed to achieve close inhibition, while only 0.004% of DNA achieved the same effect. The strong binding between the DNA backbone and nanoceria may block the active site for the substrate, slowing down the catalytic process.

A subsequent study found that the inhibition was dependent on the buffer composition and DNA/$CeO_2$ ratio. In phosphate buffer, a low DNA concentration may even increase the kinetics of TMB oxidation (**Figure 3.7B**), but such acceleration was not observed in acetate buffer (**Figure 3.7C**). Such enhanced activity in phosphate buffer was previously observed by Bülbül et al. (77). In their assays, a nonlabeled DNA Apt for ochratoxin A (OTA) adsorbed by nanoceria can stabilize the dispersion and increase the OXD-like activity for the oxidation of TMB.

The different effects of DNA have also been observed on $Fe_3O_4$, a POD mimic. Park et al. (78) reported that the activity of $Fe_3O_4$ NPs was inhibited by DNA obtained from polymerase chain reaction (PCR) amplification. Using OPD as a substrate, the authors revealed that the negatively charged DNA may bind nonspecifically to the positively charged substrate, and then block its surface to inhibit peroxidation. However, we observed that the $Fe_3O_4$-catalyzed TMB peroxidation could be enhanced in the presence of DNA oligonucleotides, and the enhancement effect was positively correlated with DNA concentration (79). For peroxidation, $H_2O_2$ is activated for the reaction, and the TMB substrate does not need to reach the nanozyme surface. Therefore, DNA may block TMB for OXD nanozymes but not $H_2O_2$ for POD nanozymes. For POD nanozymes, DNA-mediated adsorption of TMB could then facilitate the reaction. Indeed, oxidation of negatively charged ABTS was inhibited due to electrostatic repulsion. Recently, Zeng et al. (80) performed a systematic study on various DNA secondary structures, including short double-stranded (ds)DNA, ssDNA, hairpin DNA, and hybridization chain reaction (HCR) products (similar to long dsDNA). They found that the largest rate enhancement was with the HCR products.

### 3.5.3    SENSOR DESIGN

#### 3.5.3.1    Displacement Assays

In the first method, DNA is reversibly adsorbed on nanozymes, and adding targets can desorb the DNA due to nanozyme–target interactions (**Figure 3.8A**). For example, nanoceria as a CAT mimic can bind $H_2O_2$ rapidly and change color to yellow-orange. However, this colorimetric reaction is not very sensitive (LOD: low mM range). We used fluorescently labeled DNA oligonucleotides to probe this fast and high-affinity binding (81). Upon adding $H_2O_2$, the quenched fluorescence of DNA was immediately recovered. Compared with the colorimetric assay, the fluorescence assay was more sensitive (LOD = 130 nM $H_2O_2$). More importantly, the signaling mechanism was revealed to be based on simple displacement. This assay was also very selective toward common metabolites, including some amino acids, sugars, and neurotransmitters, and can be further combined with GOx to detect glucose levels in serum samples (LOD=8.9 µM).

The Tang group also used this method to detect $H_2O_2$ in living cells, and wound-induced oxidative damages (82). This assay is not limited to fluorescent probes. Qi et al. (83) reported a liquid crystal (LC)-based platform for detecting $H_2O_2$ and glucose. A nonlabeled DNA was displaced by $H_2O_2$ from nanoceria, and it would interact with the positive layer (a cationic surfactant) on an LC surface. This DNA–surfactant

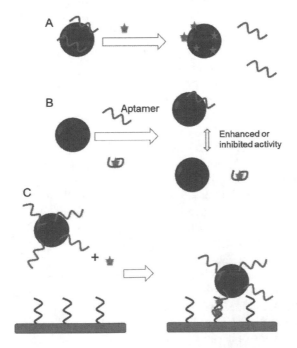

**FIGURE 3.8**  Sensors based on DNA-modified MO NPs nanozymes. Schematics showing that (A) the displacement of DNA by $H_2O_2$ from nanozymes resulted in free DNA strands, (B) free Apts and Apt-analyte complexes show differential binding affinity toward nanozymes, resulting in either enhanced or inhibited activity, and (C) nanozymes labeled with Apts bind to surfaces in the presence of analytes.

interaction disrupted the orientation of the LCs, resulting in an optical signal from dark to bright. The assay showed high sensitivity (LOD=28.9 nM) and selectivity.

### 3.5.3.2 Modulating Nanozyme Activity

In the second type of assay, DNA Apt or Apt-analyte complexes can adsorb on nanozymes with different affinities (**Figure 3.8B**). Depending on reaction conditions, the nanozyme activity could be either enhanced or inhibited. Bülbül et al. (77) designed an OTA sensor using OTA Apt to enhance the OXD-like activity of nanoceria. If the Apt formed a complex with its target, the adsorption of the Apt to $CeO_2$ was impeded and the Apt-free nanoceria showed lower activity. Using the OTA Apt, the authors were able to detect OTA with an LOD of 0.15 nM, and a dynamic range from 0.2 to 3.75 nM. This assay was quite selective to OTA since OTB and other analytes did not show any difference in TMB oxidation. Also, OTA did not show any effect using a random DNA sequence adsorbed on nanoceria.

### 3.5.3.3 High-Affinity Labeling

Similar to Ab-modified nanozymes, DNA can be potentially adsorbed on MO NPs nanozymes to fabricate sandwich type assays. For example, in **Figure 3.8C**, a split Apt-based sensor design is proposed. In this case, the nanozyme acts as a signaling label. However, for this idea to work effectively, reliable conjugation methods are required to label DNA Apts on MO NPs while still retaining the nanozyme activity.

## 3.6   SUMMARY AND FUTURE PERSPECTIVES

MOs represent a unique class of nanozymes for sensor development and its value was just beginning to be appreciated. Some oxides alone can be sensors since they have catalytic activities that can be modulated by target analytes. The strategies for MO NPs can in principle be used for other types of materials, such as Au and carbon. However, MOs also have their properties complementary to Au and carbon. For example, DNA adsorbs on Au- and carbon-based surfaces mainly via its nucleobases, while DNA uses its phosphate backbone on MO NPs. Another advantage is that there are many choices of the metal species, allowing distinct magnetic, catalytic, and optical properties for different applications. However, several problems need to be addressed before MO NPs-based system can be of practical use. For example, MOs can have different crystalline forms and sizes. These properties are likely to affect the activity of the oxides in terms of both catalysis and adsorption, and they need to be systematically investigated. Another challenge is bioconjugation. For using MOs as signaling labels, it is important to have active biomolecules linked to MO surfaces. In most cases, conjugation was achieved by first coating the oxide with a layer of polymer, and the intended biomolecules are then linked to the polymer layer. Developing robust yet easy-to-operate methods for this purpose is another challenge. Furthermore, most studies described here used only the redox catalytic activities of the nanozymes. It would be interesting to have PP- and nuclease-like nanozymes for sensing applications, as often demonstrated for their protein enzyme counterparts. Finally, developing nanozymes into practical sensor kits to solve real-world analytical problems is needed to fully demonstrate the usefulness of this technology.

## ACKNOWLEDGMENT

Funding for the related work in the Liu lab was mainly from the Natural Sciences and Engineering Research Council of Canada (NSERC).

## REFERENCES

1. Jayanthi VSPKSankara A, Das AB, Saxena U. 2017. *Biosensors and Bioelectronics.* 91: 15–23
2. Parolo C, Merkoci A. 2013. *Chemical Society Reviews* 42: 450–7
3. Rogers KR. 2006. *Analytica Chimica Acta* 568: 222–31
4. Howes PD, Chandrawati R, Stevens MM. 2014. *Science* 346
5. Rosi NL, Mirkin CA. 2005. *Chemical Reviews* 105: 1547–62
6. Giljohann DA, Seferos DS, Daniel WL, Massich MD, Patel PC, Mirkin CA. 2010. *Angewandte Chemie International Edition* 49: 3280–94
7. Zhao W, Brook MA, Li Y. 2008. *ChemBioChem* 9: 2363–71
8. Liu B, Liu J. 2017. *Analytical Methods* 9: 2633–43
9. Liu B, Liu J. 2019. *Matter* 1: 825–47
10. Zhang H, Zhang H, Aldalbahi A, Zuo X, Fan C, Mi X. 2017. *Biosensors and Bioelectronics* 89: 96–106
11. Xu H, Wang D, He S, Li J, Feng B, et al. 2013. *Biosensors and Bioelectronics* 50: 251–5
12. Lu C-H, Yang H-H, Zhu C-L, Chen X, Chen G-N. 2009. *Angewandte Chemie International Edition* 48: 4785–7
13. He S, Song B, Li D, Zhu C, Qi W, et al. 2010. *Advanced Functional Materials* 20: 453–9
14. Tan LH, Xing H, Lu Y. 2014. *Accounts of Chemical Research* 47: 1881–90
15. Xiao Y, Patolsky F, Katz E, Hainfeld JF, Willner I. 2003. *Science* 299: 1877–81
16. Gao L, Zhuang J, Nie L, Zhang J, Zhang Y, et al. 2007. *Nature Nanotechnology* 2: 577–83
17. Wu J, Wang X, Wang Q, Lou Z, Li S, et al. 2019. *Chemical Society Reviews* 48: 1004–76
18. Liu B, Liu J. 2019. *TRAC Trends in Analytical Chemistry* 121: 115690
19. Koziej D, Lauria A, Niederberger M. 2014. *Advanced Materials* 26: 235–57
20. Hao R, Xing R, Xu Z, Hou Y, Gao S, Sun S. 2010. *Advanced Materials* 22: 2729–42
21. Montini T, Melchionna M, Monai M, Fornasiero P. 2016. *Chemical Reviews* 116: 5987–6041
22. Blesa MA, Weisz AD, Morando PJ, Salfity JA, Magaz GE, Regazzoni AE. 2000. *Coordination Chemistry Reviews* 196: 31–63
23. Zhang H, Ji Z, Xia T, Meng H, Low-Kam C, et al. 2012. *ACS Nano* 6: 4349–68
24. Liu B, Liu J. 2015. *ACS Applied Materials & Interfaces* 7: 24833–8
25. Limo MJ, Sola-Rabada A, Boix E, Thota V, Westcott ZC, et al. 2018. *Chemical Reviews* 118: 11118–93
26. Liu B, Liu J. 2017. *Nano Research* 10: 1–24
27. Pearson RG. 1968. *Journal of Chemical Education* 45: 581–7
28. Manning BA, Fendorf SE, Goldberg S. 1998. *Environmental Science & Technology* 32: 2383–8
29. Liu C-H, Chuang Y-H, Chen T-Y, Tian Y, Li H, et al. 2015. *Environmental Science & Technology* 49: 7726–34
30. Zhao Y, Wang Y, Mathur A, Wang Y, Maheshwari V, et al. 2019. *Nanoscale* 11: 17841–50
31. Liu B, Huang Z, Liu J. 2016. *Nanoscale* 8: 13562–7
32. Liu Y, Ai K, Lu L. 2014. *Chemical Reviews* 114: 5057–115

33. Ye Q, Zhou F, Liu W. 2011. *Chemical Society Reviews* 40: 4244–58
34. Fan K, Wang H, Xi J, Liu Q, Meng X, et al. 2017. *Chemical Communications* 53: 424–7
35. Xu C, Liu Z, Wu L, Ren J, Qu X. 2014. *Advanced Functional Materials* 24: 1624–30
36. Blesa MA, Morando PJ, Regazzoni AE. 1994. *Chemical Dissolution of Metal Oxides*: CRC-Press
37. Shultz MD, Reveles JU, Khanna SN, Carpenter EE. 2007. *Journal of the American Chemical Society* 129: 2482–7
38. Chaudhari KN, Chaudhari NK, Yu J-S. 2012. *Catalysis Science & Technology* 2: 119–24
39. Mu J, Wang Y, Zhao M, Zhang L. 2012. *Chemical Communications* 48: 2540–2
40. Chen W, Chen J, Liu A-L, Wang L-M, Li G-W, Lin X-H. 2011. *ChemCatChem* 3: 1151–4
41. André R, Natálio F, Humanes M, Leppin J, Heinze K, et al. 2011. *Advanced Functional Materials* 21: 501–9
42. Natalio F, Andre R, Hartog AF, Stoll B, Jochum KP, et al. 2012. *Nature Nanotechnology* 7: 530–5
43. Asati A, Santra S, Kaittanis C, Nath S, Perez JM. 2009. *Angewandte Chemie International Edition* 121: 2344–8
44. Peng Y, Chen X, Yi G, Gao Z. 2011. *Chemical Communications* 47: 2916–8
45. Li D, Liu B, Huang P-JJ, Zhang Z, Liu J. 2018. *Chemical Communications* 54: 12519–22
46. Ragg R, Natalio F, Tahir MN, Janssen H, Kashyap A, et al. 2014. *ACS Nano* 8: 5182–9
47. Pirmohamed T, Dowding JM, Singh S, Wasserman B, Heckert E, et al. 2010. *Chemical Communications* 46: 2736–8
48. Korsvik C, Patil S, Seal S, Self WT. 2007. *Chemical Communications*: 1056–8
49. Mu J, Zhao X, Li J, Yang E-C, Zhao X-J. 2016. *Journal of Materials Chemistry B* 4: 5217–21
50. Ragg R, Schilmann AM, Korschelt K, Wieseotte C, Kluenker M, et al. 2016. *Journal of Materials Chemistry B* 4: 7423–8
51. Kuchma MH, Komanski CB, Colon J, Teblum A, Masunov AE, et al. 2010. *Nanomedicine: Nanotechnology Biology and Medicine* 6: 738–44
52. Janos P, Lovaszova I, Pfeifer J, Ederer J, Dosek M, et al. 2016. *Environmental Science Nano* 3: 847–56
53. Yao T, Tian Z, Zhang Y, Qu Y. 2019. *ACS Applied Materials & Interfaces* 11: 195–201
54. Xu F, Lu Q, Huang P-JJ, Liu J. 2019. *Chemical Communications* 55: 13215–8
55. Tian Z, Yao T, Qu C, Zhang S, Li X, Qu Y. 2019. *Nano Letters* 19: 8270–7
56. Asati A, Kaittanis C, Santra S, Perez JM. 2011. *Analytical Chemistry* 83: 2547–53
57. Wei H, Wang E. 2008. *Analytical Chemistry* 80: 2250–4
58. Cheng H, Lin S, Muhammad F, Lin Y-W, Wei H. 2016. *ACS Sensors* 1: 1336–43
59. Kuchler A, Yoshimoto M, Luginbuhl S, Mavelli F, Walde P. 2016. *Nature Nanotechnology* 11: 409–20
60. Tsitkov S, Hess H. 2019. *ACS Catalysis* 9: 2432–9
61. Wilner OI, Weizmann Y, Gill R, Lioubashevski O, Freeman R, Willner I. 2009. *Nature Nanotechnology* 4: 249–54
62. He X, Tan L, Chen D, Wu X, Ren X, et al. 2013. *Chemical Communications* 49: 4643–5
63. Qu K, Shi P, Ren J, Qu X. 2014. *Chemistry A European Journal* 20: 7501–6
64. Hu Y, Cheng H, Zhao X, Wu J, Muhammad F, et al. 2017. *ACS Nano* 11: 5558–66
65. Cheng H, Zhang L, He J, Guo W, Zhou Z, et al. 2016. *Analytical Chemistry* 88: 5489–97
66. Wang Q, Zhang X, Huang L, Zhang Z, Dong S. 2017. *Angewandte Chemie International Edition* 56: 16082–5
67. Ornatska M, Sharpe E, Andreescu D, Andreescu S. 2011. *Analytical Chemistry* 83: 4273–80
68. Sharpe E, Frasco T, Andreescu D, Andreescu S. 2013. *Analyst* 138: 249–62

69. Pratsinis A, Kelesidis GA, Zuercher S, Krumeich F, Bolisetty S, et al. 2017. *ACS Nano* 11: 12210–8
70. Henning DF, Merkl P, Yun C, Iovino F, Xie L, et al. 2019. *Biosensors and Bioelectronics* 132: 286–93
71. Chang Y, Liu M, Liu J. 2020. *Analytical Chemistry* 92: 3118–24
72. Zhao Y, Li H, Lopez A, Su H, Liu J. 2020. *ChemBioChem* 21: 2178–86
73. Liu B, Ma L, Huang Z, Hu H, Wu P, Liu J. 2018. *Materials Horizons* 5: 65–9
74. Tian S, Neumann O, McClain MJ, Yang X, Zhou L, et al. 2017. *Nano Letters* 17: 5071–7
75. Bercha S, Beranová K, Acres RG, Vorokhta M, Dubau M, et al. 2017. *The Journal of Physical Chemistry C* 121: 25118–31
76. Pautler R, Kelly EY, Huang P-JJ, Cao J, Liu B, Liu J. 2013. *ACS Applied Materials & Interfaces* 5: 6820–5
77. Bülbül G, Hayat A, Andreescu S. 2016. *Advanced Healthcare Materials* 5: 822–8
78. Park KS, Kim MI, Cho D-Y, Park HG. 2011. *Small* 7: 1521–5
79. Liu B, Liu J. 2015. *Nanoscale* 7: 13831–5
80. Zeng C, Lu N, Wen Y, Liu G, Zhang R, et al. 2019. *ACS Applied Materials & Interfaces* 11: 1790–9
81. Liu B, Sun Z, Huang P-JJ, Liu J. 2015. *Journal of the American Chemical Society* 137: 1290–5
82. Gao W, Wei X, Wang X, Cui G, Liu Z, Tang B. 2016. *Chemical Communications* 52: 3643–6
83. Qi L, Hu Q, Kang Q, Yu L. 2018. *Analytical Chemistry* 90: 11607–13

# 4 Noble Metal Nanozymes

*Chunxia Li*, Weilin Chen, Yulin Xie, and Man Wang*
Institute of Molecular Sciences and Engineering,
Institute of Frontier and Interdisciplinary Science,
Shandong University, Qingdao, China

## CONTENTS

## 4.1 INTRODUCTION

The insurmountable limitations, such as low stability, environmental sensitivity, and high cost have limited the applications of natural enzymes, which has also encouraged the emergence of artificial enzymes. Since, the peroxidase (POD)-like activity of iron oxide nanoparticles (NPs) was discovered in 2007 (1), several nanomaterials

---

* Corresponding author: Chunxia Li

DOI: 10.1201/9781003109228-4

(NMs) have been found to exhibit catalyst function. "Nanozyme" was first defined as "NMs with enzyme-like characteristics" in a review paper on nanozymes in 2013 (2). Among the many, noble metal-based nanozymes have become one of the most important groups of nanozymes, especially, in the field of biomedicine due to their unique optical characteristics, chemical stability, flexible enzyme-like activity, and good biocompatibility.

### 4.1.1  ENZYME ACTIVITY OF NOBLE METAL NANOZYMES

Noble metal NMs, such as those of gold (Au), platinum (Pt), palladium (Pd), and silver (Ag) and their multimetallic alloys and composites that possess enzyme-like activities are used for therapy and biosensing. In most cases, there are four kinds of enzyme mimics, namely, POD, oxidase (OXD), superoxide dismutase (SOD), catalase (CAT), which in some cases are dependent on environmental factors, such as pH and temperature (3, 4). Besides, Au NPs may also have glucose oxidase (GOx) functionality (5, 6). To obtain multienzyme mimics, multimetallic nanozymes are fabricated using noble metals and other kinds of nanozymes (7).

### 4.1.2  MECHANISM OF NOBLE METAL NANOZYMES

The catalytic mechanisms of noble-metal nanozymes that have been well analyzed. Different from the catalytic mechanism of metal oxide nanozymes, the valence of metal elements in noble metal nanozymes does not change during the catalytic reaction (8, 9). As for OXD-mimic, the mechanism could be explained as the decomposition of oxygen ($O_2$) molecule on the surface of noble metal NPs and the formation of strong oxidizing monoatomic oxygen as shown below (10):

$$O_2 = 2O^*.$$

The SOD catalyst is generated from thermodynamics and kinetics, which can be explained as $O_2^{\cdot-}$ could be protonated at the surface and then react with water to produce $HO_2^{\cdot}$, and then reorganized to hydrogen peroxide ($H_2O_2$) and $O_2$ (11, 12). The procedure could be explained by the following reaction:

$$O_2^{\cdot-} + H_2O = HO_2^{\cdot} + OH^-$$

$$2H_2* = O_2* + H_2O_2*.$$

Different from these two kinds of enzyme-like activities, POD and CAT could be affected by the pH of the environment (13). In an acid environment, it would be POD catalyst and $H_2O_2$ would be bound with hydrogen bond cluster with water molecules on the surface of noble metal NPs and then decomposed to $H_2O$ and monoatomic oxygen:

$$H_2O_2* = H_2O* + O*.$$

When it comes to basic conditions, noble metals would be CAT catalysts, which have no difference with the decomposition of $H_2O_2$ in the air (14, 15). However, in this circumstance, the addition of water molecules on the surface of noble metal NPs would promote decomposition

$$2H_2O_2* = 2H_2O*+O_2*.$$

### 4.1.3 Regulating Noble Metal Nanozyme Activity

The catalytic activity of noble metal nanozymes could be adjusted by environmental factors, such as temperature and pH. Besides, size, construction, and surface modification are also important effect factors.

The catalytic activity of noble metal nanozymes is almost in line with those of natural enzymes (16). The pH dependence of CAT and POD catalysts is different (17). For example, at pH 4.5 Ag NPs exhibited POD-like activity but at pH 7.4, it was CAT-like (18). The temperature can also help alter the catalytic activity of noble metals. For example, Pt NPs fabricated using apoferritin (Ft) as nucleation substrate (Pt-Ft NPs), exhibited CAT activity with $H_2O_2$ as substrate; but in organic dyes with $H_2O_2$ as substrate, the same NPs exhibited POD activity (19). The two kinds of catalytic activities presented different responsiveness to pH and temperature. The CAT activity of Pt-Ft NPs increased with pH up to 12 and temperature up to 85°C, with a synergistic effect at 60°C and pH 12. The POD activity was optimal at acidic conditions (pH=4) and physiological temperature (37°C). Besides pH and temperature, particle size is an another important factor. In general, the smaller the size is, the larger the specific surface area and the more substrate binding is. For example, smaller NPs of Au and Pt showed better catalytic activities (20–22).

Because the catalytic reaction mainly takes place on the surface of a nanozyme, the metal composition could affect exposed facets. For instance, Au (111) and Ag (111) facets only have little OXD-like activity, but Pt (111) and Pd (111) have OXD-like activity because $O_2$ could easily dissociate at Pt (111) and Pd (111) thermodynamically and kinetically (10). As for bimetallic alloy NPs, the catalytic activities of different substrates are different with the composition ratio of alloy. For example, the catalyst activity of Au@Pt nanorods (NRs) would be better with the addition of the Pt component. Pt-Pd alloy could catalyze the oxidation of ascorbic acid (AA), 3,3′, 5,5′-tetramethyl benzenediamine (TMB), and o-nitrophenol with $O_2$. The component ratio could affect these catalytic activities, in which the more the Pt content, the stronger the catalytic activity of o-nitrophenol has; however, the catalytic activities of AA and TMB are just the opposite (23).

The surface modification of nanozymes is also of great importance to improve the activity and selectivity of nanozyme. The deposition of some other metal on Au NPs could also present catalyst-like activity. Au NPs co-deposited with $Pd^{2+}$ and mercury ($Hg^{2+}$) has POD-like activity. In another case, $Hg^{2+}$ and bismuth ($Bi^{3+}$) deposited on Au NPs could rise the CAT activity of Au NPs 100 times (24). Meanwhile, using micro-molecules to modify the surface could also adjust the catalytic activity of noble metal nanozymes. As Liu et al. reported, Au nanoclusters (NCs) lost the original POD activity when being covered with polyamide amine dendrimer (PAMAM);

but they still kept the CAT activity. The covered PAMAM suppressed the intermediate product •OH in the POD process (25). Eventually, the Au NCs could be used in the tumor microenvironment (TME) to generate $O_2$ and enhance photodynamic therapy (PDT) (26).

Furthermore, integrated nanozymes (INAzymes) could be a meaningful way to adjust the catalyst activity of noble metal nanozymes (27). INAzymes have been developed by encapsulating two or more different biocatalysts together within confined frameworks, which could gain higher cascade reaction efficiency. For example, Wu et al. fabricated a POD-mimicking nanozyme AuNPs@MIL-101 and assembled it with natural enzymes to obtain INAzymes, which could continue to oxidize leucomalachite green into Raman-active malachite green via the catalysis of Au NPs (28). The modification of INAzymes could improve stability and promote cascade efficacy. Therefore, INAzymes indisputably could become a new way of designing multifunctional nanozymes.

## 4.2  NOBLE METAL NANOZYMES

### 4.2.1  Gold-Based Nanozymes

Au NPs are usually used as the core of noble metal NMs for enzyme-catalytic reactions. The catalytic activities of Au NMs have been observed to mimic POD, CAT, SOD, and to some extent GOx. It should be noted, however, that Au (111) only had little OXD-like activity, which meant that Au NPs were seldom applied as OXD mimics.

#### 4.2.1.1  Gold as GOx Mimic

Rossi et al. were the first ones to report GOx-like activity of Au NPs, while other noble metals, such as Pt and Ag did not show a similar activity (5, 6). GOx could catalyze the oxidation of β-D-glucose into D-glucono-1, 5-lactone and then hydrolyze to gluconic acid (29–31). The Au NPs with GOx activity could catalyze glucose in the presence of $O_2$ to produce gluconic acid and $H_2O_2$. The hydrated glucose anion interacted with the surface of Au atoms, which activate molecular oxygen by a nucleophilic attack. $Au^+$-$O^{2-}$ or $Au^{2+}$-$O_2^{2-}$ couples are considered as a bridge for the two electron-transfer from glucose to dioxygen. The mechanism of molecular activation is presented in **Figure 4.1**.

The GOx activity of Au NPs could be easily adjusted by size and shape, which are controlled during synthesis. Luo et al. induced the growth of Au NPs with $HAuCl_4$, which used the size-dependent activity decrease of Au NPs and product (gluconic acid)-induced surface passivation to adjust the GOx activity of Au NPs (32). Meanwhile, Au NPs showed resistance to $O_2$, and the reaction products showed a lower affinity to adsorption onto the Au surface (33). Cooperating with a ligand or adjuvant could also improve the efficiency of GOx-mimic rather than naked Au NPs. To obtain a higher affinity towards glucose as a substrate, Ortega-Liebana et al. developed a feasible and straightforward strategy of supporting Au NPs onto mesoporous silica via electrostatic attraction (34). The GOx activity of Au NPs improved due to the homogeneous distribution of active sites of Au in the mesoporous carrier.

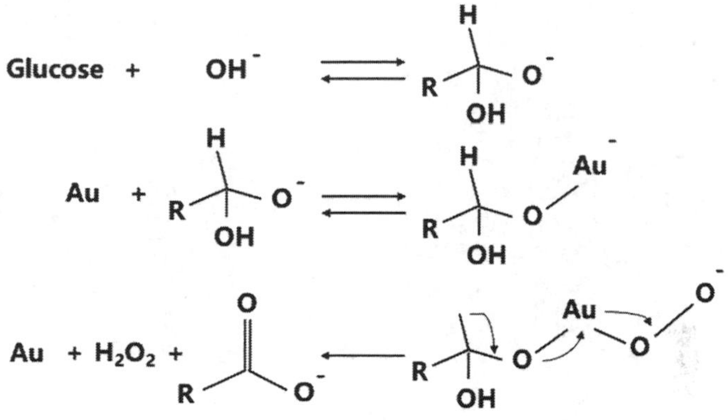

**FIGURE 4.1** The mechanism of GOx activity of Au NPs.

The surface ligand was also a key factor to increase the affinity to glucose, as Fan et al. reported, aminophenyl boronic acid (APBA) could be used to improve GOx activity as surface ligand, which could also be used to build molecularly imprinted polymer (MIP) shells to realize the selectivity for template molecules of glucose (35). Constructed by molecular imprinting technology, the highly selective and efficient Au NPs enzyme obtained specific-binding pockets to recognize, capture, and enrich glucose, which was polymerized by adjacent hydroxyls-binding APBA. In addition, using the matrix as a structural component could also improve the enzyme mimic activity. Lin et al. used expanded mesoporous silica-encapsulated Au NPs to realize GOx and POD artificial enzymes (36). The expanded mesoporous silica could induce well-dispersed Au NPs and exhibited extraordinary stability.

The GOx activity of Au NPs has been extensively used in artificial cascade reactions. This kind of hybrid NM could be applied to molecule detection by colorimetry. He et al. reported $Fe_3O_4$–Au microspheres could present GOx and POD activities to realize the function of an enzymatic cascade system (37). As soon as $H_2O_2$ was entered into the microsphere, the $Fe_3O_4$ drove it to catalyze TMB and lead to color change (**Figure 4.2A**). The microsphere was applied to target and visualize tissues as cell probes or detect biomolecules. With a similar function, Huang et al. developed a kind of 2-D metalloporphyrinic metal-organic framework (MOF) nanosheets (NSs) with ultrasmall Au NPs (38). The 2-D MOF could serve as POD mimics, while the Au NPs could act as GOx. The MOF could fully use the $H_2O_2$ produced from the reaction with Au NPs to catalyze TMB to oxidized TMB (oxTMB), which led to changing the solution color blue. The NS was designed to mimic the natural enzymes and catalyze the cascade reactions. Meanwhile, the NM could also be applied as a glucose indicator.

Besides colorimetry, a sensor could also be designed for the high stability of Au NPs, which has low cost, quick response, high sensitivity, and good selectivity. Cao et al. fabricated ternary layers of indium tin oxide (ITO)/PbS/SiO$_2$/Au NPs nanostructure to develop a photoelectrochemical (PEC) glucose sensor (**Figure 4.2B**) (39). The thioglycolic acid-capped lead sulfide (PbS) quantum dots were employed as an active probe, which was sensitive to $O_2$ (**Figure 4.2C**). Silicon dioxide ($SiO_2$)

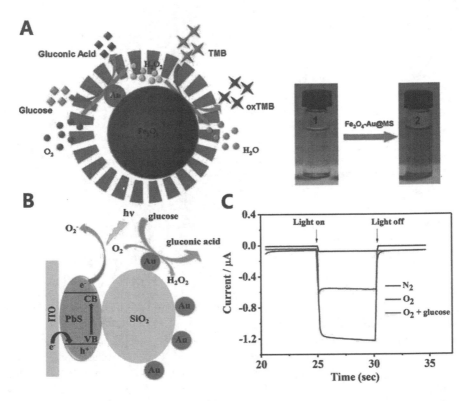

**FIGURE 4.2** (A) The principle of the artificial enzymatic cascade system based on $Fe_3O_4$–Au@MS microspheres. Copyright 2013, Royal Society of Chemistry (37) (B) Illustration of the photoelectrochemical strategy for detection of glucose at ITO/PbS/SiO$_2$/Au NPs electrode. (C) Photocurrent responses of the ITO/PbS/SiO$_2$/Au NPs electrode in an N$_2$ (black), oxygen (red), and after addition of 1 mM glucose at an applied potential of −0.2 V (versus time) under visible light irradiation. Copyright 2019, Royal Society of Chemistry (39).

was designed as the insertion layer between Au NPs and PbS to lower the base current and improve the limit of detection (LOD) according to its low electroconductivity. The response was highly sensitive and linear in the range of 1.0 μM to 1.0 mM with an LOD of 0.46-mM glucose. Au could also be used as a surface coating to enhance electrochemical properties in sensor design. Baek et al. used Au NPs and copper (Cu) nanoflower (NF) to coat the surface of graphene oxide (GO) nanofiber as an electrochemical biosensor for glucose detection (40). Due to the Au-Cu layer, the conductivity of GO NFs and sensitivity for glucose detection were improved, which exhibited a wide linear range (0.001 to 0.1 mM) with an LOD of 0.018 μM for glucose detection. The Au GOx activity was also applied in the indicator system, which provided a promising way to monitor glucose levels.

A new abiotic glucose indicator system (sensitivity, 0.616 μA.mM$^{-1}$; linear dynamic range up to 50 mM) was designed by Baingane and Slaughter (41). The core of this system is an abiotic glucose biofuel cell comprising colloidal Pt-decorated Au microwire anode and a 2 mg.cm$^{-2}$ Pt catalyst GOx cathode. The power output of the cell was affected by the glucose concentration. Meanwhile, the output was interfaced to a light-emitting diode (LED) circuit consisting of a charge pump circuit to amplify the nominal voltage generated by the biofuel cell to power the LED. The blinking of the LED could be easily measured by a smartphone application.

Because of the identical GOx activity of Au, studies about using Au GOx mimic in tumor sensors or treatment have attracted much attention. Similarly, it could be used as a biosensor for point-of-care (POC) testing of other tumor markers. Li et al. fabricated a paper-based electrochemical device by sequentially growing Au NPs and manganese oxide ($MnO_2$) nanowire network on a freestanding three-dimensional (3-D) origami device (42). The 3-D structure was obtained by growing the Au NPs layer upon the surfaces of cellulose fibers in the screen-printed paper working electrode and then electrodeposited $MnO_2$ nanowire on the surface. The NMs could be utilized in the detection of prostate-specific antigen (PSA) protein, a biomarker of prostatic cancer, which used GOx as an enzyme label, TMB as a redox terminator, and glucose as a substrate. In short, $MnO_2$ could oxidize TMB to oxTMB in the presence of $H_2O_2$, which is generated from the GOx activity of Au NPs. The enzymatic redox cycling could be exploited to measure PSA (linear range: 0.005 to 100 ng.mL$^{-1}$; LOD: 0.0012 ng mL$^{-1}$). Meanwhile, the material showed a reliable performance in human serum assay.

Besides being used in biosensors, Au GOx material is also be used in cancer treatment as a vital material for starvation therapy, since glucose is the major energy source in a tumor cell. Starvation therapy is a new alternative therapy for cancer, which can inhibit the growth of a tumor by cutting off its energy supply (43–46). Because the metabolism and proliferation of tumor cells are faster than the normal cells, nutrients are essential to tumor cells. In addition, the existence of the Warburg effect increases the glucose demand of cancer cells (47). Therefore, inspired by the enzyme catalytic reaction of GOx, it is feasible to devise a cascade catalytic reaction to treat tumors. The starvation therapy can also produce $H_2O_2$ to increase $O_2$ production, which could be incorporated with Fenton reaction or phototherapy. Cai et al. developed a kind of covalent organic framework (COF) –Au–$MnO_2$ therapeutic platform to catalyze endogenous $H_2O_2$ to produce $O_2$ and consume glutathione (GSH) to enhance the $O_2$-dependent PDT, and the generated $O_2$ could also facilitate the decomposition of glucose by Au NPs (48).

The relieving intratumoral hypoxia strategy with the GOx catalytic cascade reactions could combine with a variety of reactions. For example, Ding et al. combined MOFs and Au NPs to build a hybrid nanomedicine for cancer chemo/chemodynamic therapy (CDT) (**Figure 4.3**) (49). Camptothecin (CPT) encapsulated in MOF was the main chemotherapeutic drug, and it got released after the collapse of the Fe-MOF (Fe-tris (chlorisopropyl) phosphate) triggered by the intracellular phosphate. On the other hand, the Fe-MOF would start the Fenton reaction and generate •OH, which could be incorporated with the GOx starvation strategy of Au NPs. The intracellular glucose oxidization by Au NPs would elevate the endogenous $H_2O_2$ level, which is the fuel for the Fenton reaction. The excellent synergy of chemotherapy and CDT could suppress the tumor growth and produce a satisfactory antitumor effect. Au GOx materials could also cooperate with phototherapy. Liu et al. developed a novel

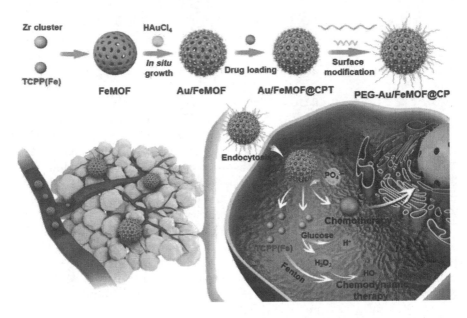

**FIGURE 4.3** Hybrid nanomedicine PEG-Au/FeMOF@CPT and its application in cancer chemo/chemodynamic therapy. Copyright 2020, John Wiley & Sons (49).

*in situ* polymerized hollow mesoporous organosilica (HMONs) biocatalysis nano-reactor for synergistic CDT/PDT (50). Au NPs were immobilized inside the hollow cavity of HMONs, while Cu complexes were then coated onto the surface of the HMONs. The Au NPs catalyzed glucose into $H_2O_2$, which could be further con-verted into •OH by a Fenton-like reaction via the catalysis of Cu complexes. Still, the material integrated the synergistic effect of PDT/CDT and enhanced ROS-mediated antitumor efficacy.

### 4.2.1.2   Gold as POD Mimic

POD mimicking is a vital property for Au nanozymes; however, the POD activity is restricted by pH, which limits their application (pH = 3). Tao et al. developed a kind of synergistic GO–Au NCs hybrid, which overcame the pH limitation to some extent (51). In the presence of GO, the lysozyme-stabilized Au NCs tended to be readily adsorbed onto the surface of GO via electrostatic interactions. As the result, the GO–Au NCs exhibited a high POD mimic activity in a broad pH range, which widened its application, especially for biocatalysts.

Jv et al. provided a simple approach to colorimetric detection of $H_2O_2$ and glucose using Au NPs (20). The positively charged Au NPs could be used to catalyze the oxi-dation of TMB by $H_2O_2$ and result in a blue solution. Similarly, Liu et al. fabricated $Au/Co_3O_4$–$CeO_x$ nanocomposite for colorimetric detection of $H_2O_2$ (**Figure 4.4A, B**) (52). TMB was chosen to create a blue-colored indication solution. Because of the striking POD activity, the colorimetric sensor presented a sensitive and efficient performance ($H_2O_2$ detection range: 10–1000 μM; LOD: 5.3 μM).

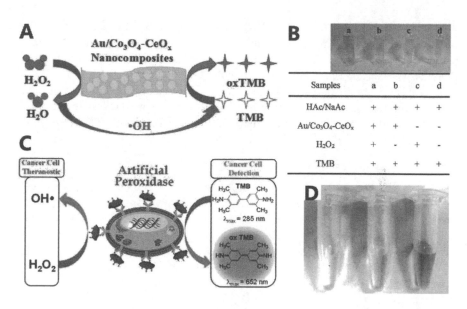

**FIGURE 4.4** (A) Illustration of colorimetric detection of $H_2O_2$ catalyzed by using Au/$Co_3O_4$–CeOx nanocomposites. (B) Visual photograph of different reaction system: a. Au/$Co_3O_4$–CeOx NCs + $H_2O_2$+ TMB; b. Au/$Co_3O_4$–CeOx NCs + TMB; c. $H_2O_2$ + TMB; d. TMB. Copyright 2018, Elsevier (52). (C) Illustration of peroxidase activity of GSF@AuNPs for cancer cell detection and therapeutic cancer treatment. (D) Typical photographs for cancer cell detection using the colorimetric method developed from GSF@AuNPs. From left to right: buffer, HEK 293 cells, and HeLa cells. Copyright 2015, American Chemistry Society (53).

On basis of the POD activity, other bioentities have also been detected. For example, Zhao et al. used folic acid (FA) to modify Au NPs upon mesoporous silica-coated nanosized reduced graphene oxide (rGO) (53). This nanohybrid could detect cancer cells *in vitro*, which was monitored by catalytic oxidation of TMB, while FA could fulfill tumor cell targeting duty to exhibit tumor-selective activity (**Figure 4.4C**). A significant visual color change could occur with the oxidation of TMB for HeLa cancer cell detection with an LOD of 50 cells (**Figure 4.4D**). Owing to its chemical stability, Au NPs could be used in environmental applications for long-term catalytic activity. Kuo et al. reported the synthesis of Au@$Cu_2O$ core@shell NCs for effective inactivation of *Escherichia coli* (*E. coli*) (54). The Au NPs played the role of POD mimic while the $Cu_2O$ performed as a Fenton reagent, and the charge separation of Au@$Cu_2O$ NCs provided photocatalytic capability, so the NM could inactivate *E. coli* with and without visible light illumination simultaneously. The sustainable function and stable performance provide a practical strategy for real-world environmental purification.

The application of Au NMs with POD mimic in cancer treatment is also of growing interest. The POD process could decompose $H_2O_2$ and generate •OH to cause oxidation therapy. Generally, it would combine with other therapeutic methods to gain a better antitumor effect. For example, Liu et al. reported multifunctional Au NPs with Cu–tannic acid core-shell nanostructures for tumor treatment (55). The Au

NPs with near-infrared radiation (NIR) absorption exhibited a universally known photothermal effect, therefore, the nanostructure could convert light into heat for photothermal therapy (PTT) (56). The photothermal effect could also improve the POD activity and produce high levels of •OH. On the other hand, due to the high-level GSH and acidic microenvironment in a tumor, the Cu-tannic acid shell would degrade and release $Cu^{2+}$ to consume GSH and amplify oxidative stress of tumor cells. Eventually, the nanostructure could kill cancer cells with PTT and CDT *in vitro* and *in vivo*.

### 4.2.1.3   Gold as CAT and SOD Mimic

CAT and SOD are important for antioxidant defense. These enzymes present complementary functions. Specifically, SOD catalyzes the dismutation of superoxide into $O_2$ and $H_2O_2$, and later on the toxic intermediates. $H_2O_2$ generated by SOD can be promptly eliminated by CAT. He et al. reported that with the catalysis of Au, the decomposition of $H_2O_2$ was accompanied by the formation of •OH at lower pH and $O_2$ at higher pH (4). The SOD mimetic activity of Au NPs is related to their adsorption and electron transfer of superoxide. This work has provided a considerable way to adjust cell viability and ROS-mediated treatment.

Hypoxia is a hallmark of solid tumors, owing to the aberrant vasculature for burgeoning tumor growth (57–59). The hypoxic circumstance causes inevitable challenges for oxygen-dependent therapy like PDT and CDT. On the other hand, high $H_2O_2$ level in the TME has attracted attention from researchers, which may provide $O_2$ for treatment under the assistance of CAT catalyst. Au nanozyme, with stable chemical stability and significant CAT activity, has become a key element in antitumor material design. However, the pH inside cellular organelles, such as endosomes (pH $\approx$ 5.5) and lysosomes (pH $\approx$ 4.8) is not the best pH for CAT or POD activity. Chang et al. prepared the 2D copper molybdenum sulfide ($Cu_2MoS_4$, labeled as CMS) NSs with ultrasmall Au NPs deposited on the surface (60). Under NIR irradiation, the CMS/Au heterostructures showed enhanced NIR absorption compared with CMS, resulting in an excellent photothermal conversion and ROS generation. The photoacoustic/computed tomography (PA/CT) dual-mode imaging was obtained due to the strong NIR absorption ability of CMS/Au and the prominent X-ray attenuation ability of Au NPs. In addition, CMS/Au with CAT-like activity relieved tumor hypoxia by catalyzing superfluous $H_2O_2$ to produce $O_2$ in TME, thereby heightening the therapeutic effect of $O_2$-dependent PDT. Above all, the released tumor-associated antigens (TAAs) mediated by CMS/Au-based phototherapy of the primary tumor exhibited vaccine-like functions, which could stimulate intense immune responses via accelerating dendritic cells (DCs) maturation, cytokine secretion, and increasing the amount of cytotoxic CD8+ T cells as well as helper CD4+ T cells. Thus, the CMS/Au heterostructures could be well-suited for photoimmunotherapy for the treatment of primary and distant cancer. Similarly, Liu et al. fabricated amine-terminated, PAMAM dendrimer-encapsulated Au NCs, which could generate $O_2$ for PDT and overcome the pH limitation (26). The enriched tertiary amines of dendrimers in the material could be protonated in acidic solutions to facilitate the preadsorption of •OH on the metal surface, subsequently triggering the CAT-like reaction. Due to the presence of amine-terminated PAMAM, the CAT activity of Au NPs would be extended to acidic conditions and, therefore, could overcome hypoxia to enhance tumor treatment. Wang et al. developed a new bimetallic and biphasic rhodium (Rh)-based core–shell nanosystem (Au@Rh-ICG) to overcome hypoxia challenge and enhance PDT (61). The Au@Rh structure could decompose $H_2O_2$ and generate $O_2$, which could enhance the PDT efficacy of the loaded photosensitizer indocyanine green (ICG). Meanwhile, the Au@Rh-ICG could generate a mild photothermal effect thus improving the intracellular uptake of ICG and nanozyme efficacy. As a result, partly similar to Wang's project, Dan et al. chose ICG as photosensitizer and Au NPs as CAT mimic to gain enhanced PDT (**Figure 4.5A**) (62). The major difference is that Dan et al. focused on the X-ray absorption capacity of Au NPs to enhance radiotherapy. The Au NCs-ICG also exhibited an outstanding antitumor effect *in vitro* and *in vivo* (**Figure 4.5B**).

The photothermal effect of Au NPs could also be used in PTT. Luo et al. developed a CAT-like nanovesicle with NIR response, that is, Pt/Au nanoshell-encapsulated chlorin e6 (Ce6) (Pt@Au-Ce6) resveratrol liposome, which contained multiple functions, chemotherapy, PTT, and PDT (64). Under 808 nm irradiation, the photothermal effect of Au NPs could cause hyperthermia to a tumor and induce the release of photosensitizer Ce6 and chemotherapeutic agent resveratrol. Meanwhile, the CAT mimic NPs could catalyze $H_2O_2$ in the tumor site and generate vast amounts of $O_2$ for further enhancement of the PDT. The NM showed acceptable potency for destroying tumor cells due to the trimodal therapeutic modality.

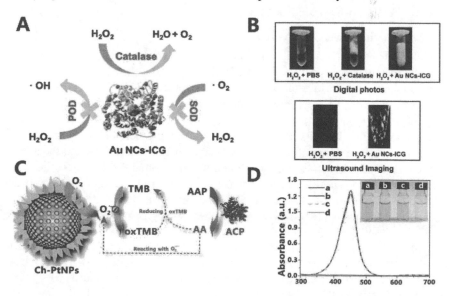

**FIGURE 4.5** (A) Illustration for three types of activities of Au NCs-ICG. (B) Digital photos and ultrasound images of $H_2O_2$ under different conditions. Copyright 2020, Royal Society of Chemistry (62). (C) Proposed detection process for ACP based on the Ch-PtNP-catalyzed TMB reporting system. (D) The UV–vis spectra of (a) Ch-PtNPs + TMB, (b) Ch-PtNPs + TMB + AAP, (c) Ch-PtNPs + TMB + ACP, and (d) Ch-PtNPs + TMB + AAP + ACP. Inset: corresponding photographs of each solution. Copyright 2017, Royal Society of Chemistry (63).

CAT activity of Au NPs could also be used in other biocatalytic functions, which are also closely related to ROS. Wang et al. developed activity-controllable nanozymes, which could be used to change cell viability (65). Encapsulated in azobenzene-modified mesoporous silica and combined with cyclodextrin, the catalytic of Au NPs inside was blocked by cyclodextrin, and could be activated by ultraviolet (UV) or visible light. Inside the mesoporous silica, the modified nanozyme combined with cyclodextrin resulted in blocking the catalytic sites. Simultaneously, because of the light-responsive ability of azobenzene, the azobenzene-modified mesoporous silica could respond to illumination and control the release of cyclodextrin to adjust the CAT activity of AuNPs. The CAT mimic activity could be easily adjusted by radiation, and eventually, it could adjust the ROS level in cells to control cell viability. Different from this work, the Au nanozyme could also be used in cell protection because it could scavenge ROS to avoid oxidative stress. Dashtestani et al. designed apoferritin containing Au-AG NPs and used them as a protective agent for human sperm against oxidative stress (66). During cryopreservation of sperm, high levels of $O_2^{\cdot-}$ and $H_2O_2$ are generated, which cause OXD stress and the loss of sperm motility and viability. The Au-AG NPs could attract $O_2^{\cdot-}$ into its cavity and assist the electron transferring process; further, it could catalyze the dismutation of $O_2^{\cdot-}$ to $H_2O_2$ and the reduction of $H_2O_2$ to $H_2O$. Thus, sperm cryopreservation can proceed more safely with the apoferritin-containing Au–Ag NPs.

## 4.2.2 PLATINUM-BASED NANOZYMES

### 4.2.2.1 Platinum as OXD Mimic

Pt nanozyme has inherent OXD-like activity, which could catalyze the rapid oxidation of TMB in the presence of dissolved $O_2$. Acid phosphatase (ACP) has been used as a biomarker for certain diseases. The development of ACP detection methods could be a breakthrough, especially in disease diagnosis and drug screening (67–69). Inspired by this property, Deng et al. designed a colorimetric assay for ACP detection (**Figure 4.5C, D**) (63). They prepared chitosan-protected Pt NPs in a one-pot process for ACP detection. Based on the OXD activity of these NPs and the antioxidant capacity of AA, a colorimetric method was developed for the determination of ACP. This method is highly selective, sensitive, simple, rapid, and of low cost; hence, it has a broad application prospect in clinical diagnosis and drug discovery.

### 4.2.2.2 Platinum as CAT Mimic

Pt NMs have CAT-like activity and can decompose $H_2O_2$ into $O_2$ and $H_2O$. Studies have shown that hypoxia is one of the main characteristics of TME (57). Hypoxia affects many molecular changes and ultimately leads to the activation of hypoxia-inducible factors (HIFs). HIFs can induce the transcription of many key genes involved in glucose metabolism, angiogenesis, tumor invasion, and metastasis, leading to the poor clinical efficacy of tumor therapy (70, 71). In addition, the excess $H_2O_2$ in TME provides a potential opportunity to solve this issue (72). To relieve tumor hypoxia, researchers achieved satisfactory results via applying Pt NMs in tumor therapy. Zhang et al. modified Pt nanozyme on photosensitizer-integrated MOF to alleviate tumor hypoxia and enhance the effect of PDT (**Figure 4.6A, B**) (31).

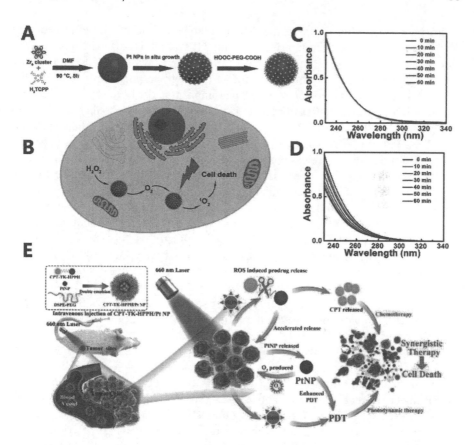

**FIGURE 4.6** (A) Illustration of the preparation of PCN-224-Pt and (B) the use of PCN-224-Pt for enhanced PDT. UV–vis spectra of remainder $H_2O_2$ were recorded after reaction with (C) PCN-224-Pt and (D) PCN-224 for different times in pH 7.4. Copyright 2018, American Chemistry Society (74) (E) Illustration of colon cancer treatment using CPT-TK-HPPH/Pt NP under 660-nm laser irradiation for 5 min. Copyright 2020, John Wiley & Sons (75).

Pt nanozyme oxidized and decomposed excess $H_2O_2$ in TME into $O_2$ and $H_2O$ (**Figure 4.6C, D**). MOFs could prevent the aggregation of neighboring Pt nanozymes and hold them steady, which afforded the Pt nanozyme higher stability and CAT-like activity. Similarly, Wang et al. used a combination of Pt nanozyme and MOFs for tumor therapy, which could not only alleviate tumor hypoxia but also target tumor cells to improve the therapeutic effect (73). Using polydopamine (PDA) as the nucleus, Pt NPs were grown *in situ* and coated with zirconium (Zr)-porphyrin MOFs to modify the tumor-targeting FA and finally obtained the PDA-Pt@PCN-FA nanoplatform. PDA-Pt@PCN-FA seems like an efficient nanometer factory, and each link plays its role. Because of the core-shell structure, the interference between the reactions is reduced and the ROS diffusion distance is shortened. Under irradiation, the $O_2$ produced by Pt nanozyme was converted into singlet oxygen ($^1O_2$) by photosensitizer and significantly inhibited the tumor growth.

To realize CDT/PDT synergistic tumor treatment, Hao et al. developed a Pt nanozyme to load ROS responsive prodrug NPs (CPT-TK-HPPH/Pt NPs) (75). The ROS-responsive prodrug consisted of a thioketal bond bound to camptothecin and photosensitizer-2-(1-hexyloxyethyl)-2-devinyl pyropheophorbide-a (HPPH) (**Figure 4.6E**). Pt NPs could catalyze the decomposition of $H_2O_2$ into $O_2$ and relieve hypoxia. Under the irradiation of 660 nm laser, the $O_2$ generated could meet the consumption of HPPH release CPT on-demand, which is conducive to enhancing PDT. CPT-TK-HPPH/Pt NPs could be used as an anticancer drug, thanks to its outstanding ROS-responsive drug-release behavior and PDT efficiency.

With CAT-like activity, Pt nanozyme could combine with PDT and PTT to realize the synergistic effect of various therapeutic methods. Hypoxic tumor cells are susceptible to heat, and mild photothermal action (e.g.,~43°C) can enhance the endocytosis of photosensitizers or drugs, so combining PDT and PTT could achieve a better tumor therapeutic effect with "1 + 1 > 2" effect (76–78). Our group synthesized a novel Pt-Ce6 nanocomposite with photothermal effect and CAT activity (79). Due to its inherent CAT-like activity, Pt-Ce6 could catalyze the decomposition of excess $H_2O_2$ in TME into $O_2$, relieve tumor hypoxia and enhance PDT. Moreover, Pt-Ce6 showed an excellent photothermal conversion ability under 1064 nm light. This simple nanoplatform achieved the synergistic effect of PDT and PTT guided by CT imaging. We also studied the mechanism of Pt-Ce6-mediated PDT apoptosis. Similarly, Yang et al. designed a self-supplied oxygen nanoplatform (BP/Pt-Ce6@ PEG NSs) based on black phosphorus (BP) to enhance PDT and PTT. Pt nanozyme provided sufficient $O_2$ for Ce6 (80). The activity of the Pt nanozyme was enhanced by BP under irradiation. The components of the nanoplatform could interact and influence each other. The experimental results showed that BP/Pt-Ce6@PEG NSs could relieve tumor hypoxia and eliminate tumor cells, showing the considerable effect of oxygen self-supplied PDT combined with PTT.

Pt NPs could also augment the effect of radiotherapy apart from CAT-like activity. The success of radiotherapy depends on the total radiation dose. However, radiation energy absorption by normal tissues can cause harmful radiotoxicity to the skin and organs, thereby limiting the total radiation dose. Therefore, it is important to develop metal and metal oxide NPs with a high molecular number as radiosensitizers to heighten the radiotherapy effect of tumor sites (81–84). Taking advantage of the high atomic number property, Li et al. designed and synthesized porous Pt NPs which could enhance radiotherapy (**Figure 4.7A**) (85). Porous Pt NPs could not only significantly lead to radiation-induced DNA damage, cell cycle arrest, and ROS stress by emitting electron radiation after interacting with X-rays in cancer cells, but also could increase conversion from endogenous $H_2O_2$ to $O_2$ (**Figure 4.7B**), thus greatly strengthening the efficacy of conventional RT. This NM with high molecular number element and enzyme activity provided a new nanomedicine strategy for enhancing the radiotherapy effect.

### 4.2.2.3   Platinum as POD Mimic

Pt NPs can catalyze the reaction of POD substrate TMB with $H_2O_2$, showing excellent POD simulation activity. Jin et al. prepared ultrafine Pt NCs using yeast extract as reductant and stabilizer (**Figure 4.7C**) (87). Based on the POD-like activity,

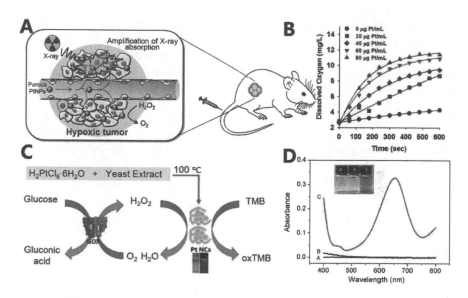

**FIGURE 4.7** (A) Illustration of enhanced radiotherapy using porous PtNPs. (B) Oxygen generation at various PtNPs contents in the presence of $H_2O_2$. Copyright 2018, Elsevier (86). (C) Illustration of Pt NCs as a highly sensitive colorimetric sensor for $H_2O_2$ and glucose. (D) Typical absorption spectra of the different solutions: A. TMB + Pt NCs, B. TMB + $H_2O_2$, C. TMB + $H_2O_2$ + Pt NCs. (inset) The color of corresponding solutions. Copyright 2017, American Chemistry Society (87).

Pt NCs combined with TMB and GOx to establish a highly sensitive colorimetric sensor for $H_2O_2$ and glucose (**Figure 4.7D**). To detect $H_2O_2$ and glucose, Li et al. prepared a novel Pt/EMT nanocomposite using ultrafine EMT zeolite as a carrier for Pt NPs (88). Compared with EMT zeolite and Pt/Y zeolite catalyst, Pt/EMT nano-catalysts had better POD-like performance and catalytic stability in the presence of $H_2O_2$. The Pt/EMT nanocatalysts could accurately monitor the content of $H_2O_2$ and glucose in buffer solution and real samples (human blood serum and fruit juices) with a wide linear range and a low LOD. Similarly, Wang et al. synthesized Pt/UiO-66 nanocomposite in which the UiO-66 MOF structure served as the carrier for Pt NPs (89). The OXD- and POD-like activities were dependent on the percentage of Pt. Compared with the commercially available Pt/carbon catalysts, Pt/UiO-66 had stronger enzyme-like activity.

Pt NPs were also used to catalyze the reaction of TMB and $H_2O_2$ to detect $Hg^{2+}$, which are virulent and can cause serious damage to the human body through food and water pollution. Xiang et al. loaded Pt NPs on the surface of Si NPs through a mixing step to obtain silica-based nanozyme, which could specifically reduce $Hg^{2+}$ to inhibit the catalytic ability of nanozymes (90). By monitoring the color change of TMB, the concentration of $Hg^{2+}$ was detected within 20 min.

Platinum dioxide ($PtO_2$) also has OXD- and POD-like activities. Liu et al. synthesized $PtO_2$ NPs with a clean surface and high dispersion in water (91). Catalytic oxidation of several enzymatic substrates, such as $o$-ophenylenediamine (OPD), TMB, and 2,20 -azino-bis (3-ethylbenzothiazoline-6-sulfonic acid) diammonium salt (ABTS) displayed distinguishable color change, demonstrated the intrinsic enzyme activity of $PtO_2$ NPs.

The free radicals in tumor cells are important for their proliferation, metastasis, and other tumor events (92, 93). However, high levels of ROS make tumor cells more sensitive to the external oxidative environment than normal cells (94–96). In the presence of $H_2O_2$, chemokinetic therapy produces large amounts of •OH through Fenton or Fenton-like reactions. On this basis, Shi et al. prepared a nanoplatform (FePt@FeOx@TAM-PEG) with a regulated catalytic activity using polymeric matrix poly(styrene-co-maleic anhydride) (PSMA)-encapsulated core-shell FePt@FeOx NPs and pH-responsive tamoxifen (TAM) drugs (94). In slightly acidic TME, FePt@ FeOx@TAM-PEG could be dissociated to release FePt@FeOx and TAM. TAM could enhance glycolysis and lactic acid content as an inhibitor of mitochondrial complex I, leading to intracellular $H^+$ accumulation in cancer cells and thereby could overcome acid-limited CDT efficiency. As a kind of POD-mimic, FePt@FeOx could react with $H_2O_2$ to generate extensive •OH, and further inhibit the growth of tumors.

### 4.2.2.4 Platinum as SOD Mimic

Pt nanozyme can also be used to remove ROS to treat acute kidney injury (AKI). Significant clinical features of AKI include a rapid decline in renal excretion, decreased urine volume, and increased nitrogen metabolism (97). Several reactive oxygen/nitrogen species (RONS) would react with biomolecules during AKI, triggering oxidative stress and inflammation, leading to renal tubular necrosis and renal insufficiency, respectively (98–100). Zhang et al. developed ultrasmall (~3 nm) Pt NPs-polyvinylpyrrolidone (PVP) complex as multienzyme simulators (CAT, POD, and SOD) and RONS scavengers to alleviate AKI (87). Besides, Pt NPs-PVP exhibited rapid excretion in healthy mice with relatively low toxicity and side effects due to its small size. Thus, ultrasmall Pt NPs-PVP was a novel antioxidant that is promising for dual-mode imaging to guide the AKI treatment.

### 4.2.3 SILVER-BASED NANOZYMES

Ag NPs are effective electron trapping agents for inhibiting electron-hole pair recombination due to their relatively low cost and low Fermi level (101). Lian et al. developed a simple one-pot solvothermal method to obtain Ag–cobalt oxide (CoO) NPs with highly dispersed core-shell structures (102). Compared with the bare CoO NPs and other composite catalysts, the Ag–CoO NPs showed stronger POD-like activity. Based on this, a novel colorimetric sensor with high sensitivity and selectivity for $H_2O_2$ and OPD detection was established.

Similarly, silver tungstate ($Ag_2WO_4$) could be exploited as an OXD mimic, which could catalyze the color reaction between TMB and dissolved oxygen to produce blue oxTMB. Ju et al. introduced Ag NPs on the surface of $Ag_2WO_4$ NRs to facilitate rapid electron transfer and enhance the OXD-like activity of $Ag_2WO_4$ NRs (103). $Hg^{2+}$ could selectively stimulate and improve the OXD-like properties of Ag@ $Ag_2WO_4$ NRs. Then, TMB was oxidized with obvious color change. The released $Ag^+$ interacted with $Hg^{2+}$ to form Ag-Hg amalgam, which enhanced OXD-like activity, providing the feasibility for the naked-eye observation and signal amplification detection of $Hg^{2+}$. The Ag@$Ag_2WO_4$ NRs also had POD- and CAT-like activities.

Koyappayil et al. prepared Ag@Ag$_2$WO$_4$ NRs by modified solvothermal method (104). The dual-enzyme activity of Ag@Ag$_2$WO$_4$ NRs changed with pH. The •OH produced by Ag@Ag$_2$WO$_4$ NRs under acidic conditions, which could be used to cause tumor damage. In addition, the dual-enzyme activity of Ag@Ag$_2$WO$_4$ NRs could be exploited to detect and measure H$_2$O$_2$.

Polyaniline (PANI) is a suitable supporter for inorganic NPs due to its rich chemical and imine groups. In particular, hybrid products composed of PANI and functional molecular modified inorganic NPs often exhibit better properties than independent components due to their synergistic effects. Tang et al. prepared Ag@ PANI nanocomposites with cascaded enzyme activities (saccharide-oxidase- and POD-like activities) by one-step self-assembly redox polymerization method (105). The nanocomposite could act as a tandem enzyme to produce H$_2$O$_2$ from saccharides and catalyze the oxidation of TMB. At the same time, it could be used as a surface-enhanced Raman scattering (SERS) substrate to obtain the characteristic peak of oxTMB. Based on these activities, ultra-sensitive detection of various sugars under unlabeled conditions was realized.

### 4.2.4 IRIDIUM-BASED NANOZYMES

Under acidic conditions, as a noble metal electrocatalyst, Ir is highly active in oxygen reduction and oxygen evolution reactions (106). As shown in **Figure 4.8A, B**, Su et al.

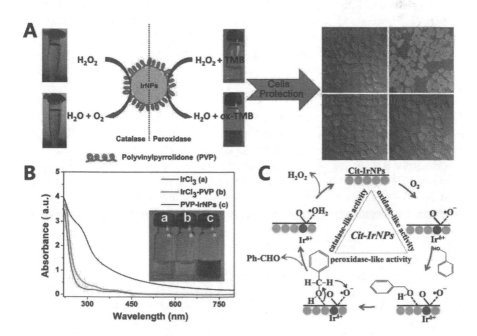

**FIGURE 4.8** (A) The CAT and POD activity of PVP-Ir NPs. (B) UV–vis absorbance of PVP-Ir NPs. Insets were optical images of aqueous solutions of iridium chloride (IrCl$_3$), a mixture of IrCl$_3$ and PVP without heating (IrCl$_3$-PVP), and PVP-Ir NPs. Copyright 2015, American Chemistry Society (107). (C) Proposed mechanism of the oxidation of benzyl alcohol to benzaldehyde. Copyright 2020, Elsevier (110).

synthesized PVP-stabilized Ir NPs using PVP as a protective agent by alcoholic reduction method (107). The PVP-Ir NPs with CAT and POD activities were the first Ir NPs with two simulated enzyme activities. However, the enzyme activity is pH-dependent. The CAT activity was higher under neutral and alkaline pHs, while the POD activity was higher under slightly acidic pHs. Zhen et al. prepared bovine serum albumin (BSA)-based iridium oxide ($IrO_2$) NPs by one-step biomineralization (108). BSA-$IrO_2$ NPs had extremely high photothermal conversion efficiency (67.8%), CAT activity, and X-ray absorption capacity, which could completely destroy tumors under NIR irradiation with PA/CT/thermal imaging.

The enzyme activity based on Ir NMs could also be used in the removal of RONS rather than the degradation of $H_2O_2$ and other substances. (109). PVP-Ir NPs have SOD, POD, CAT activities, and other enzyme-like mimics to remove various RONS *in vitro*. Also, PVP-Ir NPs could be rapidly excreted in urine and showed good bio-safety due to the small size.

Ir NMs are also be used for selective catalysis of organic matter. Jin et al. designed and synthesized citric acid-coated Ir NPs and studied their CAT-, POD-, and OXD-like activities, kinetics, and catalytic mechanism (**Figure 4.8C**) (110). They found that the synthesized NPs were highly selective and efficient in converting aromatic alcohols to corresponding aldehydes in an aqueous solution. Density-functional theory (DFT) calculation was employed to elucidate the reaction mechanism and it was found that the alcohol is initially bound to Ir(0) and subsequently forms Ir $\delta^+$-alkoxide species and a carbonyl product. Meanwhile, the Ir $\delta^+$-hydride species reductively eliminate $O_2^-$ and returns to Ir(0). This is the first report that explained how metallic NMs can convert aromatic alcohols into corresponding aldehydes under environmental conditions without the need for external energy input.

## 4.2.5 OTHER NOBLE METAL NANOZYMES

The unique structure and coordination environment of monoatomic nanocatalysts enhance their catalytic activity in many reactions with superior stability (111–113). In addition, monoatomic catalysts have become very useful for organismic biochemical reactions due to their high atomic availability and abundant active sites. Wang et al. used $Mn_3[Co(CN)_6]_2$ MOF as the carrier material and added single-atom ruthenium (Ru) into the skeleton, in which Ru could partially replace Co as the single-atom catalytic site of endogenous $O_2$ (114). Then, Ru-substituted MOF self-assembled with chlorin e6 (Ce6) and PVP to form a well-defined and uniform single-atom nano-zyme (SAzyme), OxgeMCC-r SAE. OxgeMCC-r SAE offered excellent advantages including high Ce6 loading capacity, outstanding catalytic capacity, and catalytic durability, which enabled rapid generation of $O_2$ from endogenous $H_2O_2$ without being self-consumed or requiring external activation. OxgeMCC-r SAE also had T1-weighted magnetic resonance imaging, which allowed the tracking of therapeutic agents *in vivo*.

It was reported that heat eliminated tumor cells and caused damage to nearby normal cells (115, 116). The use of mild-temperature PTT (38 °C to 43 °C) can avoid damage to normal tissue. Based on the highly efficient catalytic activity of SAzyme, Chang et al. reported an innovative strategy for ferroptosis-boosted mild

PTT based on SAzyme (117). The Pd SAzyme in the catalytic centers exhibited the activity of POD and glutathione oxidase simulants and the photothermal conversion performance, which could lead to ferroptosis characterizing the upregulation of lipid peroxides and ROS. The production of a large amount of lipid peroxides and ROS could neutralize the expression of heat shock proteins, thereby enhancing the therapeutic effect of mild-temperature PTT. This was the first report about ferroptosis enhancing mild PTT.

## 4.2.6 NOBLE METAL ALLOY-BASED NANOZYMES

Bimetallic nanocatalysts have attracted much attention because of their excellent catalytic activity and selectivity. Alloying or the formation of bimetallic NPs will affect their catalytic activity from the perspective of the chemical composition and structural properties of NPs (118–122).

### 4.2.6.1 Au@Pt-Based

He et al. prepared Au@Pt nanostructure and studied its OXD-, POD-, and CAT-like activities (123). They used the Au@Pt nanostructures instead of HRP to detect mouse interleukin 2 (IL-2) in a conventional enzyme-linked immunosorbent assay (ELISA). Zan et al. designed and prepared Au@Pt NRs (124). They found that Au@Pt NRs could reduce the ability of AA to scavenge 1,1-diphenyl-2-picryl-hydrazyl radicals, superoxide radicals, and hydroxyl radicals. Therefore, they hypothesized that Au@Pt NRs have properties similar to ascorbic acid oxidase, finally confirming the OXD-like activity of Au@Pt NRs. Gan et al. designed a kind of Au@Pt NRs with a similar function, which could be applied in the detection of AA with a selective colorimetric method (125). They used a spectrophotometer and chromogenic substrate TMB to study optical and catalytic properties of Au-tipped Pt NRs. With the presence of AA, the POD-like activity of Au-tipped Pt NRs was significantly reduced. The generated $O_2$ reacted with AA to produce ascorbyl radicals (AA center dot) instead of oxidizing TMB. On this basis, the selective colorimetry based on Au-Pt NRs to detect AA was established.

Zhu et al. designed a simple and universal quantitative POC testing method by combining target-responsive hydrogel and Au@Pt NPs with CAT activity (126). In this, each component of the nanoplatform plays a different role, such as target-response hydrogels for target recognition, Au@Pt NPs for robust yet efficient signal transduction and amplification, and a volumetric bar-chart chip for visual quantitative readout. This was a rapid, convenient, and inexpensive quantitative visual method to detect a wide range of targets without any external electronic instrumentation.

The synergistic effects of multiple therapeutic modalities can help to overcome the limitations of single therapy and enhance tumor suppression with minimal side effects (60, 127–129). Based on the unique enzyme activity of $Au_2Pt$ NMs, our group designed and synthesized a multifunctional therapeutic nanoplatform ($Au_2Pt$-PEG-Ce6) (130). This nanoformulation not only had CAT-like activity to relieve tumor hypoxia and improve PDT efficiency but also had POD mimic activity to generate •OH for CDT (**Figure 4.9A**). In addition, $Au_2Pt$-PEG-Ce6 is an excellent photothermal agent for PTT due to the strong NIR absorption. The system realized

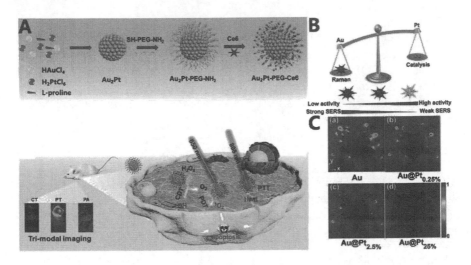

**FIGURE 4.9** (A) Illustration of the fabrication of Au$_2$Pt-PEG-Ce6 nanoformulation and multimodal imaging-guided synergistic PTT/PDT/CDT by employing tumor microenvironment. Copyright 2020, Elsevier (130). (B) Rational design of high-performance Au@Pt NP bifunctional nanozymes by controlling the Pt amount. (C) Simulated electric-field distributions of AuNPs (a) and Au@Pt NPs with increased Pt amount (b–d) under X-polarized illumination at a wavelength of 633 nm. Copyright 2018, American Chemistry Society (134).

the integration of diagnosis and treatment with PA/PT/CT imaging and multi synergistic effects of multiple therapeutic modalities.

Based on the CAT-like activity of Au@Pt NPs, Liang et al. first combined Au@Pt NPs with cytokine-induced killer (CIK) cell immunotherapy for tumor treatment. (131) This work achieved the synergistic effect of regulating tumor hypoxic microenvironment and immunotherapy. Au@Pt NPs catalyzed endogenous H$_2$O$_2$ to produce O$_2$, downregulated HIF-1α, a key factor related to hypoxia, and enhanced the cytotoxicity mediated by CIK cells. Liu et al. designed and synthesized a nanoplatform (Pt@UiO-66-NH$_2$@Au shell-Ce6) with CAT-like activity (132). Under light irradiation, the photosensitizer Ce6 converted generated O$_2$ into $^1$O$_2$ for PDT. Porous Au nanoshells were used as photothermal agents for PTT. Thus, this nanoplatform realized the synergistic effect of PDT and PTT, restrained tumor cells, and prolonged the survival time of mice. Furthermore, Au@Pt NPs can also be used as a radiosensitizer to enhance the therapeutic effect of radiotherapy. Yang et al. synthesized Au@Pt NPs nanozymes with uniform nanosphere at room temperature (133). Au-Pt nanozymes have the radiosensitivity to enhance the X-ray deposition and catalyze the conversion of H$_2$O$_2$ to O$_2$. Compared with the control group, Au@Pt NPs significantly reduced hypoxia and inhibited tumor growth under 8 Gy of X-ray irradiation.

Au NPs have SERS activity and Pt NPs have various enzyme activities (28). Their combination can prepare high-performance nanozymes with sensitive SERS performance. Wu et al. obtained monodisperse bimetallic NPs (Au@Pt NPs) by a seed-mediated method. They studied the effect of Pt content with POD-like activity and SERS function of multi-branched AuNPs (134). Au@Pt NPs with an optimal Pt provided high catalytic activity and SERS activity, and was applied in $H_2O_2$ sensing (**Figure 4.9B, C**). Besides, it has been reported that Au@Pt bimetallic NCs as a biosensor to detect target organisms. Pebdeni et al. designed a novel biosensor (DNA-Au@Pt NCS) using Au@Pt NCs as an enzyme mimic. Au@Pt NCs showed outstanding POD-like activity, and the catalytic activity of the colorimetric probe would change with *Staphylococcus aureus (S. aureus)* (135). *S. aureus* in food could be detected quickly and sensitively by evaluating this reaction. Long et al. used the intrinsic POD-like activity of Au@Pt NRs to replace HRP and linked antigen conjugate to monitor the specific interaction between measles antigen and measles-specific antibody (IgM isotype), which could simulate the capture-ELISA method (136). Even in harsh environments, the Au@Pt NRs-antigen conjugate showed strong robustness, indicating that this nanozyme-antigen conjugate is promising for clinical diagnosis.

### 4.2.6.2   Pd@Pt-Based

Pathogenic bacterial infection is a major problem for humans (137, 138). Although the use of antibiotics had excellent results against bacterial infections, antibiotic resistance in mutant bacteria limits the effect of antibiotics and leads to high mortality rates (139). Sonodynamic therapy (SDT) is a promising alternative for treating multidrug-resistant bacterial infections. Sun et al. designed an ultrasound-switchable nanosystem (Pd@Pt-T790) by using T790 (mesotetra(4-carboxyphenyl)porphine) as a sound sensitizer for SDT (**Figure 4.10A**) (140). The modification of T790 on Pd@Pt could significantly block the CAT activity, possibly due to the coating of T790 affecting the diffusion of $H_2O_2$ and decrease its contact with Pd@Pt. The nanozyme activity could be restored under ultrasound, catalyzing the decomposition of endogenous $H_2O_2$ to $O_2$. This ultrasound-controlled change in enzyme activity helped to decrease the toxicity and side effects of nanosystems on normal tissues. Also, due to ultrasound-controlled $O_2$ generation, the SDT efficacy of Pd@Pt-T790 was greatly improved and could eradicate deep-seated myositis induced by methicillin-resistant *S. aureus.*

### 4.2.6.3   Ag@Pt-Based

Wu et al. established a sensitive colorimetric method for detecting copper ions ($Cu^{2+}$) by modifying the surface of Ag@Pt NCs and regulating the activity of POD (141). It was found that 3-mercaptopropionic acid (MPA) had an inhibitory effect on the catalytic capacity of the Ag@Pt NCs. However, with the catalytic action of $Cu^{2+}$, MPA oxidized by oxygen would lose its inhibition of the catalytic capacity of Ag@Pt NCs. On this basis, a colorimetric method for detecting $Cu^{2+}$ was established by measuring the colorimetric signal of the TMB-$H_2O_2$ reaction.

### 4.2.6.4   Ag@Pd-Based

Aghahosseini et al. prepared a novel Ag@Pd alloy-based semi-heterogeneous magnetic nanostructure and used it as a nanocatalyst for the conversion of 4-nitrophenol into 4-aminophenol by $NaBH_4$ (118). The synergistic effects of Ag@Pd NPs as catalytic active sites, the semi-heterogeneous properties of the catalyst as an important organic substrate microenvironment, and the structure of magnetite make it

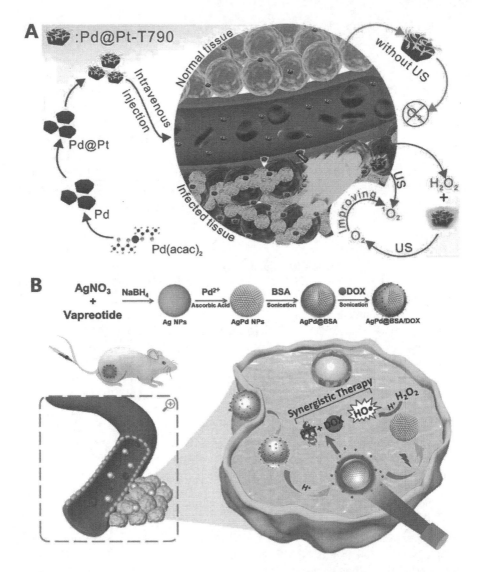

**FIGURE 4.10** (A) Illustration of the main synthesis procedure of the Pd@Pt-T790 nanoplatform and its ultrasound-switchable nanozyme catalytic oxygen-generation-enhanced SDT of bacterial infection. Copyright 2020, American Chemistry Society (140) (B) Illustration of synthesizing AgPd@BSA/DOX and antitumor mechanism. Copyright 2020, Elsevier (142).

highly selective, easy to recycle and reuse, and high turnover frequency. Li et al. used the POD-like activity of Ag@Pd NPs in combination with doxorubicin (DOX) for the synergistic treatment of tumors (**Figure 4.10B**) (142). They designed and synthesized the Ag@Pd@BSA/DOX nano-therapeutic platform. Ag@Pd NPs could catalyze the generation of •OH from excessive $H_2O_2$ in the TME and generate a fairly high heating effect under NIR irradiation to promote the release of DOX and realize the combination of ROS killing tumor therapy, PTT, and chemotherapy. This kind of nanomedicine based on bimetallic nanozyme has great potential for clinical applications.

### 4.2.6.5 Au@Ag-Based

Au@Ag bimetallic alloys have POD-like activity, which could catalyze the oxidation of $H_2O_2$ to •OH under acidic conditions. Also, Au@Ag alloys can generate hot electrons through local surface plasmon resonance (SPR) to boost the energy of chemical processes due to strong red-shift spectral absorption (143). Au-Ag hollow nanotriangles (Au@Ag HNTs) exhibited strong absorption in the NIR-II region due to their special morphology, which could induce the SPR effect and generate hot electrons in deep tissue. The weak absorption and scattering of biological tissues in the NIR-II biological window (1000–1700 nm) can greatly reduce the signal background and improve the image quality and penetration depth (144–146). Xu et al. prepared Au@Ag HNTs using Ag nanoprisms as templates with GOx-loaded nanocarriers (147). Au@Ag-GOx HNTs could not only consume glucose in tumor cells but also catalyze $H_2O_2$ to produce •OH to kill the tumor cells. In addition, the pH reduction caused by the production of gluconic acid accelerated the degradation of Ag NPs, thereby destroying the intact structure and avoiding long-term toxicity. The reaction is as follows:

$$Glucose + O_2 + H_2O \xrightarrow{GOx} Gluconic\ acid\ (H^+) + H_2O_2$$

$$H_2O_2 + e^- + H^+ \xrightarrow{Au@Ag} •OH + H_2O$$

$$Ag + H_2O_2 + H^+ \rightarrow Ag^+ + H_2O.$$

### 4.2.6.6 Ir@Ru-Based

Ir@Ru materials have been demonstrated with CAT and POD activities. Wei et al. designed ultrasmall Ir@Ru NPs with CAT and POD activities (148). The combination of Ir@Ru NPs and GOx could carry out a series of cascade catalytic reactions (**Figure 4.11A, B**). Ir@Ru-GOx@PEG NPs decomposed glucose in the tumor cells into gluconic acid and $H_2O_2$ and then catalyzed the oxidation of $H_2O_2$ to form $O_2$ and $^1O_2$. The synergistic effect of starvation therapy and oxidation therapy could inhibit tumor cells, relieve the hypoxia state of the tumor, and facilitate the degradation of glucose. This strategy of a cyclic catalytic system guided by multiple enzymes could add new perspectives for tumor therapy.

## 4.3 SUMMARY AND FUTURE PERSPECTIVES

Noble metal-based nanozymes exhibit GOx, CAT, POD, SOD, and OXD activities. During the past few years, interest in these nanozymes has grown, and their performance has been significantly improved. However, these materials are still not the same as their natural counterparts. The following aspects need to be investigated for advancing the future of nanozyme research.

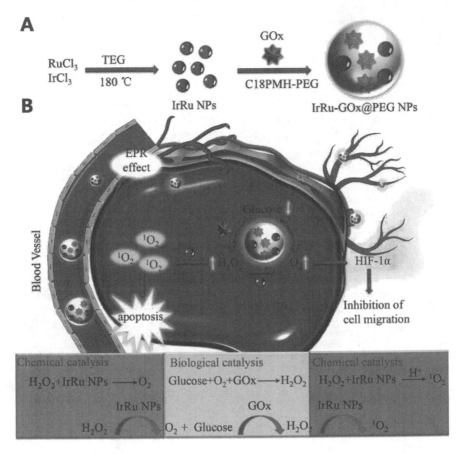

**FIGURE 4.11** (A) Scheme of IrRu-GOx@PEG NPs nanosystem and (B) Illustration of the cycle-like nanosystem IrRu-GOx@PEG NPs including catalyzing efficient glucose depletion, $O_2$ cycle-like support, and starvation therapy for enhanced oxidation therapy in a hypoxic tumor microenvironment. Copyright 2020, Elsevier (148).

1. Natural enzyme can only catalyze a single reaction, while noble metal-based nanozymes are generally multiple enzyme mimics. The diversified catalyst from one kind of NM could interact with each other and result in an unsatisfactory effect. On the other hand, the natural enzyme systems could contain an enzyme to coordinate and organize systematic functions (2, 149). In the aspect of noble metal nanozyme, although there has been an attempt to build an industrial enzyme cascade, the diversified catalysts have incommoded the process. It could be a key issue by adjusting the enzyme mimic of noble metal-based nanozyme with environment or composition to realize a balance of functions.

2. Other characteristics besides catalyst activity of noble metal nanozyme should not be ignored. For example, Au NPs could be used as photothermal and imaging agents (150, 151). Although there are materials that use the

physical, chemical, and catalytic properties of noble metals, the internal connection between these properties still needs to be examined. Making full use of the special nature of noble metals may widen their applications and lead to better performance.

3. Over the past few years, the researchers mostly have been focused on redox reaction with noble metal-based nanozymes. The studies about other kinds of enzyme-like activities of noble metal-based nanozymes may find more potential applications.

4. The toxicity and bio-capacity of noble metal nanozymes used *in vivo* or as biocatalysts could be a problem, no matter where it was used, in cell protection or cancer treatment. The safety of noble metal nanozymes is still a gap between them and natural enzymes. Developing low-toxic material and well-understanding the toxicity is meaningful for the clinical applications of noble metal nanozymes.

5. Inside the natural enzyme systems, there exist active agents and inhibitors that focus on active sites to adjust catalytic activity (152–154). Besides adjusting the metal part, using adjuvant like surfactants or mesoporous substrates could also change catalytic function. We should pay more attention to exploring their catalytic kinetics and mechanisms to benefit the regulation of catalytic activities. Some of these unsolved issues will be the frontier for future research.

# REFERENCES

1. Gao L, Zhuang J, Nie L, Zhang J, Zhang Y, et al. 2007. *Nat Nanotechnol* 2: 577–83
2. Wei H, Wang E. 2013. *Chem Soc Rev* 42: 6060–93
3. Gao LZ, Yan XY. 2013. *Progress Biochem Biophys* 40: 892–902
4. He W, Zhou YT, Wamer WG, Hu X, Wu X, et al. 2013. *Biomaterials* 34: 765–73
5. Comotti M, Della Pina C, Matarrese R, Rossi M. 2004. *Angew Chem Int Ed Engl* 43: 5812–5
6. Comotti M, Della Pina C, Falletta E, Rossi M. 2006. *Adv Synth Catalysis* 348: 313–6
7. Huang Y, Ren J, Qu X. 2019. *Chem Rev* 119: 4357–412
8. Yi X, Chen L, Zhong XY, Gao RL, Qian YT, et al. 2016. *Nano Res* 9: 3267–78
9. Xi J, Da L, Yang C, Chen R, Gao L, et al. 2017. *Int J Nanomed* 12: 3331–45
10. Shen X, Liu W, Gao X, Lu Z, Wu X, et al. 2015. *J Am Chem Soc* 137: 15882–91
11. Goel S, Wu Z, Zones SI, Iglesia E. 2012. *J Am Chem Soc* 134: 17688–95
12. Tian B, Gao W, Ning XF, Wu YQ, Lu GX. 2019. *Appl Catalysis B Environ* 249: 138–46
13. Li J, Liu W, Wu X, Gao X. 2015. *Biomaterials* 48: 37–44
14. Tan LL, Ong WJ, Chai SP, Mohamed AR. 2015. *Appl Catalysis B Environ* 166: 251–9
15. Lv C, Yan C, Chen G, Ding Y, Sun J, et al. 2018. *Angew Chem Int Ed Engl* 57: 6073–6
16. Gao L, Fan K, Yan X. 2017. *Theranostics* 7: 3207–27
17. He W, Wu X, Liu J, Hu X, Zhang K, et al. 2010. *Chem Mater* 22: 2988–94
18. He W, Zhou YT, Wamer WG, Boudreau MD, Yin JJ. 2012. *Biomaterials* 33: 7547–55
19. Fan J, Yin JJ, Ning B, Wu X, Hu Y, et al. 2011. *Biomaterials* 32: 1611–8
20. Jv Y, Li B, Cao R. 2010. *Chem Commun (Camb)* 46: 8017–9
21. Chen C, Fan S, Li C, Chong Y, Tian X, et al. 2016. *J Mater Chem B* 4: 7895–901
22. Moglianetti M, De Luca E, Pedone D, Marotta R, Catelani T, et al. 2016. *Nanoscale* 8: 3739–52
23. Zhang K, Hu X, Liu J, Yin JJ, Hou S, et al. 2011. *Langmuir* 27: 2796–803

24. Lien CW, Chen YC, Chang HT, Huang CC. 2013. *Nanoscale* 5: 8227–34
25. Liu CP, Wu TH, Lin YL, Liu CY, Wang S, et al. 2016. *Small* 12: 4127–35
26. Liu CP, Wu TH, Liu CY, Chen KC, Chen YX, et al. 2017. *Small* 13: 1700278
27. Wu J, Li S, Wei H. 2018. *Chem Commun (Camb)* 54: 6520–30
28. Hu Y, Cheng H, Zhao X, Wu J, Muhammad F, et al. 2017. *ACS Nano* 11: 5558–66
29. Xian Y, Hu Y, Liu F, Xian Y, Wang H, Jin L. 2006. *Biosens Bioelectron* 21: 1996–2000
30. Mani V, Devadas B, Chen SM. 2013. *Biosens Bioelectron* 41: 309–15
31. Zhang L, Wan SS, Li CX, Xu L, Cheng H, et al. 2018. *Nano Lett* 18: 7609–18
32. Luo W, Zhu C, Su S, Li D, He Y, et al. 2010. *ACS Nano* 4: 7451–8
33. Stasyuk N, Smutok O, Demkiv O, Prokopiv T, Gayda G, et al. 2020. *Sensors (Basel)* 20
34. Ortega-Liebana MC, Bonet-Aleta J, Hueso JL, Santamaria J. 2020. *Catalysts* 10: 333
35. Fan L, Lou D, Wu H, Zhang X, Zhu Y, et al. 2018. *Adv Mater Interfaces* 5: 1870107
36. Lin Y, Li Z, Chen Z, Ren J, Qu X. 2013. *Biomaterials* 34: 2600–10
37. He X, Tan L, Chen D, Wu X, Ren X, et al. 2013. *Chem Commun (Camb)* 49: 4643–5
38. Huang Y, Zhao M, Han S, Lai Z, Yang J, et al. 2017. *Adv Mater* 29: 1700102
39. Cao L, Wang PP, Chen L, Wu Y, Di JW. 2019. *Rsc Adv* 9: 15307–13
40. Baek SH, Roh J, Park CY, Kim MW, Shi R, et al. 2020. *Mater Sci Eng C Mater Biol Appl* 107: 110273
41. Baingane A, Slaughter G. 2021. *IEEE Sensors J* 21: 5751–7
42. Lang NJ, Liu B, Liu J. 2014. *J Colloid Interface Sci* 428: 78–83
43. Li SY, Cheng H, Xie BR, Qiu WX, Zeng JY, et al. 2017. *ACS Nano* 11: 7006–18
44. Yu Z, Zhou P, Pan W, Li N, Tang B. 2018. *Nat Commun* 9: 5044
45. Zhang MK, Li CX, Wang SB, Liu T, Song XL, et al. 2018. *Small* 14: e1803602
46. Zhang R, Feng L, Dong Z, Wang L, Liang C, et al. 2018. *Biomaterials* 162: 123–31
47. Warburg O. 1956. *Science* 123: 309–14
48. Liu C, Cai Y, Wang J, Liu X, Ren H, et al. 2020. *ACS Appl Mater Interfaces* 12: 42521–30
49. Ding Y, Xu H, Xu C, Tong Z, Zhang S, et al. 2020. *Adv Sci (Weinh)* 7: 2001060
50. Liu T, Zhao Q, Xie Y, Jiang D, Chu Z, et al. 2020. *Biosens Bioelectron* 156: 112145
51. Tao Y, Lin Y, Huang Z, Ren J, Qu X. 2013. *Adv Mater* 25: 2594–9
52. Liu H, Ding YN, Yang BC, Liu ZX, Liu QY, Zhang X. 2018. *Sensors Actuators B Chem* 271: 336–45
53. Maji SK, Mandal AK, Nguyen KT, Borah P, Zhao Y. 2015. *ACS Appl Mater Interfaces* 7: 9807–16
54. Kuo MY, Hsiao CF, Chiu YH, Lai TH, Fang MJ, et al. 2019. *Appl Catalysis B Environ* 242: 499–506
55. Liu YH, Shi QY, Zhang Y, Jing JL, Pei J. 2020. *New J Chem* 44: 19262–9
56. Grabowska-Jadach I, Kalinowska D, Drozd M, Pietrzak M. 2019. *Biomed Pharmacother* 111: 1147–55
57. Noman MZ, Hasmim M, Messai Y, Terry S, Kieda C, et al. 2015. *Am J Physiol Cell Physiol* 309: C569–79
58. Vuillefroy de Silly R, Dietrich PY, Walker PR. 2016. *Oncoimmunology* 5: e1232236
59. Zhu S, Gu ZJ, Zhao YL. 2018. *Adv Therapeutics* 1: 1800050
60. Chang M, Hou Z, Wang M, Wang M, Dang P, et al. 2020. *Small* 16: e1907146
61. Wang J, Sun J, Hu W, Wang Y, Chou T, et al. 2020. *Adv Mater* 32: e2001862
62. Dan Q, Hu D, Ge Y, Zhang S, Li S, et al. 2020. *Biomater Sci* 8: 973–87
63. Deng HH, Lin XL, Liu YH, Li KL, Zhuang QQ, et al. 2017. *Nanoscale* 9: 10292–300
64. Luo L, Li L, Cong C, He Y, Hao Z, Gao D. 2020. *Sci China Mater* 64: 1021–34
65. Lian X, Fang Y, Joseph E, Wang Q, Li J, et al. 2017. *Chem Soc Rev* 46: 3386–401
66. Dashtestani F, Ghourchian H, Najafi A. 2019. *Mater Sci Eng C Mater Biol Appl* 94: 831–40
67. Schiffer E. 2007. *World J Urol* 25: 557–62

68. Leman ES, Getzenberg RH. 2009. *J Cell Biochem* 108: 3–9
69. Makarov DV, Loeb S, Getzenberg RH, Partin AW. 2009. *Annu Rev Med* 60: 139–51
70. Semenza GL. 2003. *Nat Rev Cancer* 3: 721–32
71. Manalo DJ, Rowan A, Lavoie T, Natarajan L, Kelly BD, et al. 2005. *Blood* 105: 659–69
72. Gao S, Wang G, Qin Z, Wang X, Zhao G, et al. 2017. *Biomaterials* 112: 324–35
73. Wang XS, Zeng JY, Zhang MK, Zeng X, Zhang XZ. 2018. *Adv Funct Mater* 28
74. Zhang Y, Wang F, Liu C, Wang Z, Kang L, et al. 2018. *ACS Nano* 12: 651–61
75. Hao Y, Chen Y, He X, Yu Y, Han R, et al. 2020. *Adv Sci (Weinh)* 7: 2001853
76. Wang Y, Huang X, Tang Y, Zou J, Wang P, et al. 2018. *Chem Sci* 9: 8103–9
77. Zhang Y, Dai C, Liu W, Wang Y, Ding F, et al. 2019. *Microchimica Acta* 186: 1–9
78. Chen D, Zhong Z, Ma Q, Shao J, Huang W, et al. 2020. *ACS Appl Mater Interfaces* 12: 26914–25
79. Chen Q, He S, Zhang F, Cui F, Liu J, et al. 2020. *Sci China Mater* 64: 510–30
80. Yang XY, Liu RG, Zhong ZH, Huang H, Shao JJ, et al. 2021. *Chem Eng J* 409: 127381
81. Porcel E, Liehn S, Remita H, Usami N, Kobayashi K, et al. 2010. *Nanotechnology* 21: 85103
82. Su XY, Liu PD, Wu H, Gu N. 2014. *Cancer Biol Med* 11: 86–91
83. Retif P, Pinel S, Toussaint M, Frochot C, Chouikrat R, et al. 2015. *Theranostics* 5: 1030–44
84. Song G, Chen Y, Liang C, Yi X, Liu J, et al. 2016. *Adv Mater* 28: 7143–8
85. Su C, Bai L, Zhang H, Chang K, Li G, et al. 2019. *Chem Res Chinese Univ* 35: 163–70
86. Li Y, Yun KH, Lee H, Goh SH, Suh YG, et al. 2019. *Biomaterials* 197: 12–9
87. Jin L, Meng Z, Zhang Y, Cai S, Zhang Z, et al. 2017. *ACS Appl Mater Interfaces* 9: 10027–33
88. Li X, Yang X, Cheng X, Zhao Y, Luo W, et al. 2020. *J Colloid Interface Sci* 570: 300–11
89. Wang H, Zhao J, Liu C, Tong Y, He W. 2021. *ACS Omega* 6: 4807–15
90. Xiang KK, Chen G, Nie AX, Wang WJ, Han HY. 2021. *Sensors Actuators B Chem* 330: 129304
91. Liu X, Zhou Y, Liu J, Xia H. 2021. *Spectrochim Acta A Mol Biomol Spectrosc* 248: 119280
92. Xu X, Saw PE, Tao W, Li Y, Ji X, et al. 2017. *Adv Mater* 29: 1700141
93. Xuan W, Xia Y, Li T, Wang L, Liu Y, et al. 2020. *J Am Chem Soc* 142: 937–44
94. Shi L, Wang Y, Zhang C, Zhao Y, Lu C, et al. 2021. *Angew Chem Int Ed Engl*
95. Zhao C, Chen J, Zhong R, Chen DS, Shi J, et al. 2020. *Angew Chem Int Ed Engl*
96. Wang S, Yu G, Wang Z, Jacobson O, Lin LS, et al. 2019. *Angew Chem Int Ed Engl* 58: 14758–63
97. Chawla LS, Eggers PW, Star RA, Kimmel PL. 2014. *N Engl J Med* 371: 58–66
98. Nath KA, Norby SM. 2000. *Am J Med* 109: 665–78
99. Ozturk E, Demirbilek S, Koroglu A, But A, Begec ZO, et al. 2008. *Prog Neuropsychopharmacol Biol Psychiatry* 32: 81–6
100. Heemskerk S, Masereeuw R, Russel FG, Pickkers P. 2009. *Nat Rev Nephrol* 5: 629–40
101. Kumar A, Paul B, Boukherroub R, Jain SL. 2020. *J Hazard Mater* 387: 121700
102. Lian JJ, Yin DX, Zhao S, Zhu XX, Liu QY, et al. 2020. *Colloids Surfaces A Physicochem Eng Aspects* 603: 125283
103. Ju P, Wang Z, Zhang Y, Zhai XF, Jiang FH, et al. 2020. *Colloids Surfaces A Physicochem Eng Aspects* 603
104. Koyappayil A, Berchmans S, Lee MH. 2020. *Colloids Surf B Biointerfaces* 189: 110840
105. Tang RY, Lei Z, Weng YJ, Xia XM, Zhang X. 2020. *New J Chem* 44: 16384–9
106. Antolini E. 2014. *Acs Catalysis* 4: 1426–40
107. Su H, Liu DD, Zhao M, Hu WL, Xue SS, et al. 2015. *ACS Appl Mater Interfaces* 7: 8233–42

108. Zhen W, Liu Y, Lin L, Bai J, Jia X, et al. 2018. *Angew Chem Int Ed Engl* 57: 10309–13
109. Zhang DY, Younis MR, Liu H, Lei S, Wan Y, et al. 2021. *Biomaterials* 271: 120706
110. Jin GX, Liu J, Wang C, Gu WX, Ran GX, et al. 2020. *Appl Catalysis B Environ* 267: 118725
111. Lin L, Zhou W, Gao R, Yao S, Zhang X, et al. 2017. *Nature* 544: 80–3
112. Liu G, Robertson AW, Li MM, Kuo WCH, Darby MT, et al. 2017. *Nat Chem* 9: 810–6
113. Geng Z, Liu Y, Kong X, Li P, Li K, et al. 2018. *Adv Mater* 30: e1803498
114. Wang D, Wu H, Phua SZF, Yang G, Qi Lim W, et al. 2020. *Nat Commun* 11: 357
115. Hu K, Xie L, Zhang Y, Hanyu M, Yang Z, et al. 2020. *Nat Commun* 11: 2778
116. Li S, Gu K, Wang H, Xu B, Li H, et al. 2020. *J Am Chem Soc* 142: 5649–56
117. Chang M, Hou Z, Wang M, Yang C, Wang R, et al. 2021. *Angew Chem Int Ed Engl*
118. McLaren A, Valdes-Solis T, Li G, Tsang SC. 2009. *J Am Chem Soc* 131: 12540–1
119. Cao S, Tao FF, Tang Y, Li Y, Yu J. 2016. *Chem Soc Rev* 45: 4747–65
120. Verma AD, Mandal RK, Sinha I. 2016. *Rsc Adv* 6: 103471–7
121. Khan I, Saeed K, Khan I. 2019. *Arabian J Chem* 12: 908–31
122. Bawaked S, Narasimharao K. 2020. *Sci Rep* 10: 518
123. He W, Liu Y, Yuan J, Yin JJ, Wu X, et al. 2011. *Biomaterials* 32: 1139–47
124. Zan X, Fang Z, Wu J, Xiao F, Huo F, et al. 2013. *Biosens Bioelectron* 49: 71–8
125. Gan H, Han WZ, Liu JD, Qi JT, Li H, et al. 2020. *Catalysts* 10: 1282
126. Zhu Z, Guan Z, Jia S, Lei Z, Lin S, et al. 2014. *Angew Chem Int Ed Engl* 53: 12503–7
127. Li J, Li Y, Wang Y, Ke W, Chen W, et al. 2017. *Nano Lett* 17: 6983–90
128. Nishimura T, Sasaki Y, Akiyoshi K. 2017. *Adv Mater* 29: 1702406
129. Wang WL, Guo Z, Lu Y, Shen XC, Chen T, et al. 2019. *ACS Appl Mater Interfaces* 11: 17294–305
130. Wang M, Chang M, Chen Q, Wang D, Li C, et al. 2020. *Biomaterials* 252: 120093
131. Liang H, Wu Y, Ou XY, Li JY, Li J. 2017. *Nanotechnology* 28: 465702
132. Liu C, Luo L, Zeng L, Xing J, Xia Y, et al. 2018. *Small* 14: e1801851
133. Yang S, Han G, Chen Q, Yu L, Wang P, et al. 2021. *Int J Nanomed* 16: 239–48
134. Wu J, Qin K, Yuan D, Tan J, Qin L, et al. 2018. *ACS Appl Mater Interfaces* 10: 12954–9
135. Pebdeni AB, Hosseini M. 2020. *Microchem J* 159: 105475
136. Long L, Liu J, Lu K, Zhang T, Xie Y, et al. 2018. *J Nanobiotechnol* 16: 46
137. Rizzello L, Pompa PP. 2014. *Chem Soc Rev* 43: 1501–18
138. Ji H, Dong K, Yan Z, Ding C, Chen Z, et al. 2016. *Small* 12: 6200–6
139. Alekshun MN, Levy SB. 2007. *Cell* 128: 1037–50
140. Sun D, Pang X, Cheng Y, Ming J, Xiang S, et al. 2020. *ACS Nano* 14: 2063–76
141. Wu LL, Qian ZJ, Xie ZJ, Zhang YY, Peng CF. 2017. *Chinese J Anal Chem* 45: 471–5
142. Li L, Liu H, Bian J, Zhang X, Fu Y, et al. 2020. *Chem Eng J* 397: 125438
143. Yin Z, Wang Y, Song C, Zheng L, Ma N, et al. 2018. *J Am Chem Soc* 140: 864–7
144. Li C, Li F, Zhang Y, Zhang W, Zhang XE, et al. 2015. *ACS Nano* 9: 12255–63
145. Lin H, Gao S, Dai C, Chen Y, Shi J. 2017. *J Am Chem Soc* 139: 16235–47
146. Cao Y, Wu T, Zhang K, Meng X, Dai W, et al. 2019. *ACS Nano* 13: 1499–510
147. Xu M, Lu QL, Song YL, Yang LF, Ren CC, et al. 2020. *Nano Res* 13: 2118–29
148. Wei C, Liu Y, Zhu X, Chen X, Zhou Y, et al. 2020. *Biomaterials* 238: 119848
149. Wu J, Wang X, Wang Q, Lou Z, Li S, et al. 2019. *Chem Soc Rev* 48: 1004–76
150. Jain PK, Lee KS, El-Sayed IH, El-Sayed MA. 2006. *J Phys Chem B* 110: 7238–48
151. Boisselier E, Astruc D. 2009. *Chem Soc Rev* 38: 1759–82
152. Toullec D, Pianetti P, Coste H, Bellevergue P, Grandperret T, et al. 1991. *J Biol Chem* 266: 15771–81
153. Jang M, Cai L, Udeani GO, Slowing KV, Thomas CF, et al. 1997. *Science* 275: 218–20
154. Anand P, Kunnumakkara AB, Newman RA, Aggarwal BB. 2007. *Mol Pharm* 4: 807–18

# 5 Glucose Oxidase-Mimicking Nanozymes

*Atul Sharma[1,2], Swapnil Tiwari[3], and Jean Louis Marty[4]*
[1]School of Chemistry, Monash University (Clayton Campus), Melbourne, VIC, Australia
[2]Department of Pharmaceutical Chemistry, SGT College of Pharmacy, SGT University, Budhera, Gurugram, Haryana, India (Current Address)
[3]School of Studies in Chemistry, Pt Ravishankar Shukla University, Raipur, C.G., India
[4]Université de Perpignan Via Domitia, Perpignan, France

## CONTENTS

DOI: 10.1201/9781003109228-5

## 5.1 INTRODUCTION

In the past decade, certain metal nanoparticles (NPs), such as that of gold (Au) (1) and iron (Fe) (2) obeyed enzyme kinetics, i.e., Michaelis–Menten equation and ping-pong mechanism (3). At present, there is a large number of inorganic nanomaterials that possess enzyme-like activity, especially, oxidoreductase-like activity, such as oxidases (OXDs) and catalases (CATs) (4). The Fe oxide ($Fe_2O_3$) NPs were first discovered to mimic the natural enzyme, horseradish peroxidase (HRP) (5). They fit the role of an enzyme perfectly because these NPs contain an active structure or electron transfer properties, and electronic processes like surface plasmon resonance (6). Owing to their high catalytic activity, nanozymes mimicking oxidoreductase- and CAT-like activities are commonly used in the biosensors field (7).

Nanozymes with intrinsic enzyme-like activity are easier to synthesize and functionalize than conventional artificial enzymes, and they have greater stability and catalytic activity (8). Their high catalytic activity allows them to be used in biological detection instead of natural enzymes (9). Several novel nanozyme-based techniques for detecting bioactive molecules, such as hydrogen peroxide ($H_2O_2$) and glucose, and macromolecules, such as nucleic acids and proteins, have been developed (10, 11). As a result, nanozymes play an important role in disease detection and environmental protection (12).

## 5.2 REGULATION OF NANOZYME ACTIVITIES

Nanozymes have the advantage of being quick to refine and modulate. Since their catalytic activity occurs at the surface of NPs, various factors affecting the particle surface properties can be used to control the enzymatic activity.

The surface area of NPs increases drastically as their size decreases, and the electrons on their surfaces become highly active at the same time (13). By affecting the active site on the surface of NPs, the size-dependent effect can indirectly affect the catalytic activity of nanozymes (11).

In addition to its size, the morphology of nanozymes influences their enzymatic behavior (14). By comparing the behavior of three different nanoclusters with different structures, the effect of structure on $Fe_3O_4$ nanozymes has been studied by Liu et al. (15). The most active form was the spherical structure, while the least active was the octahedral shape. Jiang et al. investigated the CAT-like behavior of various forms of cobalt oxide nanozymes and discovered that nanoplates of cobalt oxide have the highest catalytic activity (16). Similarly, the morphologies of NPs affect vanadium pentoxide ($V_2O_5$) nanozymes (17). $V_2O_5$ nanospheres have substantially higher catalytic activity than $V_2O_5$ nanowires due to the various crystal facets revealed. Given the importance of morphology in nanozyme behavior, it is worthwhile to investigate the behaviors of nanozymes with sufficient morphology to maintain high catalytic activity and stability (17).

The surface microenvironment, such as intermolecular bonds, viscosity, hydrophobicity, etc., affects the enzymatic effects of morphology in addition to size and morphology (18). Nanozymes are essential nanomaterials and they have a profound impact on the ambient microenvironmental conditions. pH is an important factor in determining nanozyme catalytic activity (19). As with natural enzymes, the enzymatic reactions of nanozymes occur under acidic conditions (19).

## 5.3   GLUCOSE OXIDASE

### 5.3.1   MODE OF ACTION OF GLUCOSE OXIDASE

The glucose oxidase enzyme (GOx), also known as notatin, belongs to the class of oxidoreductases (20). It catalyzes the conversion of glucose to $H_2O_2$ and D-glucono-$\delta$-lactone (21). It is a dimeric protein, formed by two complex protein monomers. The single polypeptide chain of one subunit has 583 amino acid residues (22). In GOx-catalyzed reactions, molecular oxygen is the normal electron acceptor. However, several other natural and synthetic electron acceptors can also be used in GOx reactions. GOx is a hollow enzyme with an active site of flavin adenine dinucleotide (FAD) as a cofactor. Flavin is a group of enzyme cofactors that participate in electron- and proton-coupled electron transfer reactions (23). GOx catalyzes the oxidation of D-glucose to D-glucono-$\delta$-lactone, which is nonenzymatically hydrolyzed to gluconic acid in the reductive half-reaction. GOx FAD ring is reduced to $FADH_2$ as a result (24). The reduced GOx is reoxidized by oxygen in the oxidative half-reaction, yielding $H_2O_2$. CAT breaks down $H_2O_2$ to create water and oxygen (20). GOx is favored over other glucose-oxidizing enzymes because of its high specificity.

### 5.3.2   GLUCOSE OXIDASE NANOZYMES

These enzymes are a subclass of oxidoreductases. More, precisely they catalyze the electron transfer reactions. OXD nanozymes use the mechanism of activating molecular oxygen to yield reactive oxygen species (ROSs) which subsequently oxidize the substrate (25). However, OXD nanozymes show relatively less specificity compared to the POD nanozymes. The most common example of this category is MNPs reported by Gao et al., exhibiting POD-like activity (5). Another example of OXD nanozymes is nanoceria showing the SOD activity.

Glucose is the fuel for our body. It is the main source of energy that gives the capacity and strength to work. However, excess glucose in the blood can cause endocrine and metabolic disorders including diabetes. It is estimated that diabetes affects 200 million people globally (26). As a result, it is important to develop new methods for determining blood glucose levels in an easy, fast, and accurate manner (27). Besides, glucose is extensively used commercially in various fields, such as the production of sucrose, the beverage industry, and fuel production. Hence, oxidation of glucose is a significant process both metabolically and commercially. The oxidation of glucose in the body takes place by an oxidoreductase enzyme GOx (28). Apart from cellular function, GOx is also used in food industries and as a biosensing tool (29). This shows the wider need for the availability of the enzyme as it is a potent biosensor for glucose. Despite their widespread use, free enzymes are often limited in their use due to low operating reliability and recovery difficulties.

Nanozymes have emerged as potent artificial enzymes mimicking the catalytic activity of GOx. Various nanomaterials excellently serve the purpose of GOx. Under controlled conditions, Au nanozymes show GOx activity (30). In 2004, Comotti et al. oxidized the D-glucose to D-gluconic acid using naked Au NPs possessing OXD-mimicking activity (31). Kinetic measurement suggests that the enzymatic Ely–Rideal mechanism for Au nanozyme-based mimetics is followed (30). Another analog of GOx mimic is the nanozymes of copper oxide (CuO) composites (32). It is reported that CuO-based nanomaterial imitates the OXD activity under basic conditions; however, there is still room for improvement from commercial aspects (32). Although these types of enhancements can be overcome by forming new complexes or hybrids. For instance, Cheng et al. developed integrated nanozymes by simultaneously embedding two cascade groups, namely, hemin and GOx, inside a metal-organic framework (MOF) (33). This cascade system boosted the overall catalytic activity and provided a facile platform for the colorimetric determination of glucose. In commercial samples, such as beverages, glucose is determined by a combination of peroxide detection. In the biomedical analysis and diabetes monitoring, glucose detection is critical. GOx colorimetry is currently used primarily in clinical glucose detection, and its concept is based on a dual enzyme system that combines HRP and GOx to create a color reaction. For instance, the $Fe_3O_4$ nanozyme has a POD catalytic function, it can not only replace HRP in colorimetry but also conjugate GOx directly onto the surface of $Fe_3O_4$ NPs, allowing the nanozyme to directly exert its POD catalytic activity while GOx catalyses glucose to produce $H_2O_2$. This establishes a notion in which one type of nanozyme can be used in conjunction with the natural enzymes.

MOF-based nanozymes are widely used as glucose sensors. MOFs are compounds consisting of metal ion clusters linked to organic ligand via coordinated bonds. Li et al. (25), synthesized an MOF-based nanomaterial (MOF 818), which shows efficient catechol oxidase mimicking activity with no POD-like activity. This novel catechol oxidase nanozyme has trinuclear copper centers. The enzyme kinetic constants Michaelis–Menton constant ($K_m$) and catalytic constant ($K_{cat}$) were $8.10 \times 10^{-4}$ M and $0.383$ s$^{-1}$, respectively, which show good catalytic activity.

In general, the nanozyme works with multiple substrates functioning and properties. Nanozymes are generally categorized into two types: a) enzyme-associated nanomaterials and b) nanomaterials having an intrinsic enzyme-like activity like $Fe_3O_4$ NPs possessing POD activity (34). After that, an in-depth description was given, which served as the foundation for nanozyme mechanisms. Nanozymes based on $Cu_2O$ NPs have also been found to mimic OXDs (35), and hydrothermal methods were used to reduce Cu ions into $Cu_2O$ NPs (36).

## 5.4 GLUCOSE DETECTION WITH DIFFERENT NANOZYMES

Structurally, nanozymes are chemically synthesized nanomaterials designed to mimic the biological enzymatic activity (8). An enzyme catalyzes or speeds up the reaction rates of specific molecules via its active site, which constitutes a very small portion of the total enzyme. Similarly, nanozymes function by mimicking the receptors involved in catalysis at the active site of an enzyme, but they are much smaller and can easily be synthesized. In the absence of an active substrate molecule site for enzyme binding, several attempts have been made to endow nanozymes with increased selectivity and specificity toward target molecules (10, 12).

The strategies are the OXD-coupled and the surface-modification methods. Nanozymes with POD-like activity achieve their specificity in the OXD-coupled system by being coupled with an OXD, which generates $H_2O_2$ as a result of a catalytic reaction that only occurs in the presence of the target molecule. Subsequently, POD-like nanozymes catalyze the oxidation of colorimetric substrates and produce $H_2O_2$. In a colorimetric immunoassay, an antibody is usually conjugated on the surface of the nanozyme to provide specificity for the target antigen molecules. The nanozyme can act as a target-specific probe by conjugating the target antigen-specific antibody to the surface of the nanozyme, generating a colorimetric signal in the presence of the colorimetric substrate and $H_2O_2$. In the same way, when the targeted molecules bind to the nano-molecules, ligand-conjugated nanozymes can specifically bind to target receptors and produce a colorimetric signal.

The intrinsic enzyme-like activities of nanozymes are generally believed to be produced by atoms present on the surface and in the inner core of the nanozyme. The atomic composition of nanozymes is, therefore, the most important factor in determining their catalytic activity, although other factors, such as size, morphology, surface coating and modification, pH, and temperature, can also affect (11). In the following, we summarize the literature available for nanozymes integrated with GOx-based biosensing platforms for the detection of glucose.

## 5.4.1 METAL-BASED

In general, noble metals are transition metals that are resistant to corrosion and oxidation in the humid air. Noble metal nanomaterials (NMs) containing one or more elements, such as Pt, Au, palladium (Pd), rhodium (Rh), and ruthenium (Ru), may be classified on various substrates as unsupported NMs (monometallic, bimetallic, and multimetallic) and immobilized NMs (37). Herein, various noble metal nanozymes with special reference to GOx for glucose determination are discussed.

In 2004, Rossi et al. reported the conversion of glucose to gluconic acid and $H_2O_2$ in the presence of oxygen using Au NPs (31). Au NPs were produced as a colloidal sol by reducing chloroauric acid ($HAuCl_4$), where a large amount of glucose acting as either a reagent or a protector with a molar activity of $1.804 \times 10^{-4}$ mol gluconate [mol Au]$^{-1}$ h$^{-1}$. However, the control experiments demonstrated that NMs of other metals (Pd, Ag, Pt, and Cu) did not exhibit any significant catalytic ability for glucose oxidation (38). Based on the promotive effect by alkali, and the generation of $H_2O_2$, the mechanism of molecular activation for Au catalysis is shown in **Figure 5.1**. The hydrated glucose anion interacting with the surface of Au atoms could form electron-rich Au species, which activates the molecular oxygen by a nucleophilic attack. The formation of $Au^+-O_2^-$ or $Au^{2+}-O_2^{2-}$ couples of dioxogold ($AuO_2$) intermediate could serve as the bridge to transform electrons from glucose to dioxygen ($O_2$).

Lee et al. reported the first example of colorimetric assay employing a nanozyme for the detection of glucose without sample pretreatment (26). In this study, a facile design of preparing new GOx nanozymes constructed on HRP-mimic GOx-conjugated with GO/manganese oxide ($MnO_2$) to detect glucose concentration in

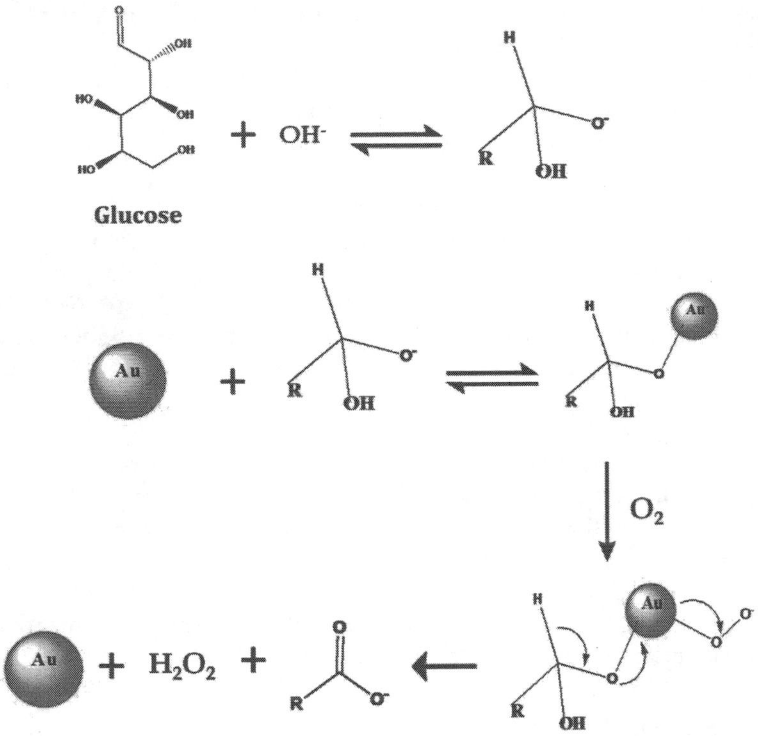

**FIGURE 5.1** Catalytic mechanism of Au NPs as GOx mimics [Adopted from Comotti et al. (38)].

whole blood was presented. The detection principle employed was the oxidation of 3,3′,5,5′-tetramethylbenzidine (TMB) catalysis by HRP-mimicking activity. The $MnO_2$ NPs embedded in bovine serum albumin (BSA)-coated GO by *in situ* growth were evaluated focusing on the principle of HRP-mimic activity catalyzing the oxidation of TMB in the presence of $H_2O_2$. Furthermore, we constructed dual-sensing platforms based on a combination of a plasma separation pad and GOx-GO/$MnO_2$ for direct detection of glucose concentration in whole blood by colorimetric assay without blood sample pretreatment. As a proof-of-concept, a limit of detection (LOD) of 3.1 mg $dL^{-1}$ for glucose was obtained with a wide linear quantification range from 25 to 300 mg $dL^{-1}$ through visual observation and quantitative analysis, suggesting potential clinical applications of blood glucose monitoring for diabetic patients.

NPs of Au and Pt have been reported to possess the catalytic activities of GOx. Additionally, nanocomposites comprising a combination of metals have gained significant attention. Furthermore, metal-based nanozymes often exhibit synergistic effects that primarily improve catalytic performance when coupled with other nanozymes (39). When loaded on conductive graphite carbon nitride (GCN) support, manganese selenide (MnSe) NPs as nanocatalysts can exhibit enhanced POD-like catalysis (40). By calcinating a mixture of pure MnSe, dicyandiamide, and cyanuric acid, MnSe NPs were successfully loaded on the surface of polymeric GCN as a co-catalyst using a thermal condensation process. The prepared MnSe-GCN NSs (NSs) had higher aqueous stability, and in particular, much greater POD-like catalysis than the initial MnSe and GCN NSs possibly due to the synergetic effects of conductive GCN and lamellate MnSe nanocatalysts effectively loaded. MnSe-GCN NSs were found to be novel POD mimics, capable of rapidly catalyzing the oxidation of the POD substrate TMB in the presence of $H_2O_2$ resulting in a blue-colored solution. According to kinetic analysis, the catalytic activity assumes a ping-pong mechanism and follows standard Michaelis–Menten kinetics. At 652 nm, the MnSe-GCN nanosheets (NSs) were superior in sensitivity with a glucose concentration from 0.16 to 1.6 mM and an LOD of 8 μM over to previously reported POD mimetics based on $Fe_3O_4$ NPs (0.022 mM) (41) and carbon NPs (20 μM) (42). Thus, MnSe-GCN NSs can be used as enzymatic mimics for potential medical diagnostics and biotechnology applications.

Nonetheless, several MOs have lower activity and specificity than natural enzymes, owing to inhomogeneous elemental composition and low density of catalytic activity sites (43, 44), which severely limits nanozyme use. Size reduction, surface adjustment, structure alteration, and composition optimization have all been proposed to overcome these problems, but they are still far from satisfactory (43, 45). Reducing the size of NPs increases their surface free energy, causing significant accumulation and rapid loss of activity. Some active sites on the surface of nanozymes may be shielded by surface alteration, resulting in low atomic utilization. As a consequence, developing a new form of nanozyme with a homogeneous atomic composition and high densities of activity sites is a top priority.

Because of their high atomic utilization efficiency and well-defined coordination structure, single-site nanozyme (SSN) catalysts can help bridge the gap between natural enzymes and nanozymes. In light of this, a new self-supporting atomically distributed single iron site nanozyme (Fe SSN) with high POD-like efficiency was proposed utilizing a support-sacrificed strategy (43). The Fe(phen)x complex was formed when ferrous acetate (Fe(OAc)$_2$) reacted with 1,10-phenanthroline monohydrate (O-phen) in ethanol. The as-prepared hybrid sample (Fe(phen)x/MgO) was dried and pyrolyzed at 600 °C in argon (Ar) atmosphere to obtain Fe-N-C/MgO, after which magnesium oxide powder (MgO) was added. Finally, MgO was extracted using acid pickling, resulting in Fe SSN. The Fe SSN performs prominent POD-like action by efficiently activating $H_2O_2$ into hydroxyl radical (•OH) species, thanks to its well-defined coordination structure and high density of active sites. The Fe SSN-GOx-TMB system could detect glucose in solution (linear range=10 to $60 \times 10^{-6}$ M and LOD = $2.1 \times 10^{-6}$ m) and an improved hydrogel film was able to quantify $8.20 \times 10^{-6}$ M glucose with a linear range of 10 to $100 \times 10^{-3}$ M in human serum. These results not only open up new possibilities for developing single-site catalysts-based biosensors but also open up the possibility of point-of-care (POC) glucose detection in biomedical diagnosis.

## 5.4.2 Nonmetal-Based

Photocatalytic generation of $H_2O_2$ through proton-coupled electron transfer to $O_2$ is preferable to conventional $H_2O_2$ development methods, such as anthraquinone

(46) and noble metal-based (47) catalysis because it needs no hydrogen gas reagent, and operates in an environmentally friendly manner (Eq. 1). However, enhancing the selectivity of two-electron transfer to $O_2$ and minimizing the decomposition of *in situ* derived $H_2O_2$ are two major challenges. Since it has lower adsorption for $H_2O_2$, GCN is an ideal material for preventing *in situ* decomposition of $H_2O_2$ (48). Furthermore, the chemical functional groups and electronic properties of GCN can be easily modified, making it a promising photocatalyst for the development of $H_2O_2$. While GCN has been used as a POD-mimicking nanozyme for glucose detection, its GOx-mimicking behavior in enzymatic tandem cascade (domino) reactions for colorimetric glucose detection has never been investigated

$$O_2 + 2H^+ + 2e^- \rightarrow H_2O_2;\; E^o = 0.659\; V_{NHE} \qquad (5.1).$$

A bifunctional metal-free modified GCN nanozyme that functions as an OXD mimic in glucose oxidation and a POD mimic in chromogenic substrate oxidation under irradiation and darkness was proposed (46). *In situ* photogeneration of $H_2O_2$ from glucose oxidation under visible light is supported by the selectivity for $O_2$ reduction and effective charge separation. Furthermore, *in situ* derived $H_2O_2$ is then used to complete the bifunctional OXD-POD mimicking glucose detection by peroxiding a chromogenic substrate on the same changed GCN. The bifunctional modified GCN had a near 100% quantum efficiency of $H_2O_2$ generation, allowing for colorimetric glucose detection through coupled cascade reactions. In microfluidics, the bifunctional cascade catalysis has been successfully demonstrated for real-time colorimetric detection of glucose with an LOD of 0.80 M in 30 s. Nanozymes that can support physiological functions provide viable strategies to mimic natural enzymes for biomedical applications. The advantages of the current nanozyme-microfluidic sensor make it an excellent candidate for POC diagnosis. Overall, the efficiency of the microfluidic reactor for biomimetic cascade catalysis reaction as a miniaturized method for rapid and simple real-time glucose monitoring has been successfully demonstrated.

Sengupta et al. (49) developed a bifunctional metal-free nanozyme as a hybrid of chemically modified GCN, chitin, and acetic acid (AcOH). The modified GCN mimicked GOx activity, while chitin–AcOH mimicked POD activity. When in contact with glucose, modified GCN chitin–AcOH oxidized glucose to gluconic acid and $H_2O_2$, whereas chitin–AcOH decomposed the produced $H_2O_2$, as demonstrated separately by the concurrent oxidation of TMB. This results in the establishment of the dual-role of modified GCN–chitin–AcOH hybrid as a POD-OXD nanozyme. The UV–vis absorption (A) measurements showed a linear relationship with an increase in the glucose concentration (C, μM) from 5.0 to 1000 μM as follows: A=0.00140C+0.1119 ($R^2$=0.995) at 375 nm and A=0.00084C+0.0458 ($R^2$=0.995) at 659 nm. Lineweaver-Burk plots were used to assess the applicability of catalytic activity for modified GCN–chitin–AcOH. In contrast to natural GOx and most other GOx mimicking nanozymes, the $K_m$ and $V_{max}$ were found to be 4.54 mM, and 4.67 × $10^{-6}$ M.s$^{-1}$, respectively.

### 5.4.3 CARBON-BASED

Since the discovery of fullerene and its derivatives in 1996, various carbon-based nanomaterials, such as carbon nanotubes (CNTs), GO, graphene quantum dots (GQDs), and carbon quantum dots (CQDs), have been considered as carbon-based nanozymes (50). Pristine fullerene, CNTs, and graphene are water-insoluble, making them unsuitable as nanozymes. However, the multiform binding modes of carbon atoms have made it easy to modify carbon-based nanozymes resulting in improved water solubility (51–53). Carbon-based nanozymes can be classified into two groups based on the enzymatic behavior they mimic: 1) SOD mimics and 2) POD mimics. The time-dependent advancements in the production of carbon-based nanozymes are depicted in **Figure 5.2**.

Carbon-based nanozymes have promising potential to catalyze the oxidation of TMB or ABTS by $H_2O_2$ and exhibit POD-like activity (42, 54, 55). For example, modified-GO (GO-COOH) could catalyze the colorimetric reaction of POD substrate TMB in the presence of $H_2O_2$ (54). Analogous to HRP, GO-COOH catalytic activity also depended upon pH, temperature, and $H_2O_2$ concentration (54). Various modified and doped carbon-based nanozymes have been proven as potential candidates displaying improved enzymatic activity (56–58). The parameter of $V_{max}$ and $K_m$ calculated from the Michaelis–Menten model for $H_2O_2$ catalysis of different carbon-based nanozymes are listed in **Table 5.1**. It was worth noting that, despite the relatively high POD-like activity of carbon-based nanozymes, there is still a significant difference when compared to normal PODs such as HRP as tabulated in **Table 5.1**.

As described above, $H_2O_2$ is an important signaling molecule, especially in glucose metabolism. In the absence of $O_2$, glucose can be catalyzed to produce gluconolactone and $H_2O_2$. As a result, glucose can be quantified indirectly by measuring the concentration of enzymatically liberated $H_2O_2$ (40, 59, 60). Zhang et al. created POD-like nanozymes out of 3-D Fe- and N-doped carbon structures (Fe-Phen-CFs) (61) for the detection of glucose and $H_2O_2$. The prepared Fe-Phen-CFs can catalyze the POD substrate terephthalic acid into a fluorescent hydroxyterephthalate in the presence of $H_2O_2$, allowing for quantitative detection of $H_2O_2$ with an LOD of

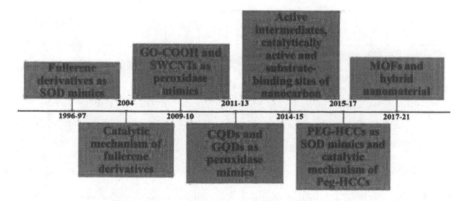

**FIGURE 5.2** A brief timeline for the development of carbon-based nanozymes [adapted from Sun et al. (50)].

**TABLE 5.1**

**Parameters of Michaelis–Menton Kinetics of Some Typical Carbon-Based Materials for the Catalysis of $H_2O_2$**

| Material | $V_{max}$ ($10^{-8}$ M s$^{-1}$) | $K_m$ (mM) | HRP ($V_{max}$ ($10^{-8}$ M s$^{-1}$) | HRP ($K_m$, mM) | Reference |
|---|---|---|---|---|---|
| GQDs | 2.62 | 0.49 | - | - | (57) |
| GO-COOH | 3.85 | 3.99 | $2.46 \pm 0.32$ | $0.214 \pm 0.014$ | (54) |
| $C_{60}[C(COOH)_2]_2$ | 4.01 | 24.58 | - | - | (55) |
| CQDs | 30.61 | 26.77 | $12.1 \pm 2.60$ | $0.276 \pm 0.057$ | (56) |
| Carbon nanohorn | 2.07 | 49.80 | - | - | (58) |

~68 nM and a linear range of 0.1 to 100 mM. Recently, Bao et al. (62) reported the preparation of Pt-doped carbon NPs with intrinsic POD-like activity for colorimetric detection of glucose and $H_2O_2$. This sensor displayed an excellent sensitivity for glucose detection with an LOD of 0.30 mM.

Ding et al. (63) proposed a hybrid of iron disulfide ($FeS_2$) NPs encapsulated by two-dimensional (2-D) carbon NSs with superior POD activity and excellent stability. The incorporation of 2-D NSs increases the specific surface area of the proposed $FeS_2$@carbon nanozymes, allowing for more active sites to come into contact with the substrate. Furthermore, the embedded $FeS_2$ NPs are prevented from aggregating due to the encapsulation and confinement of 2-D carbon sheets, avoiding the traditional failure of single-component nanozymes. A colorimetric method for glucose detection based on GOx and the intricately designed $FeS_2$@carbon nanozymes exhibited excellent simplicity and sensitivity with an LOD of 0.19 μM (**Figure 5.3**).

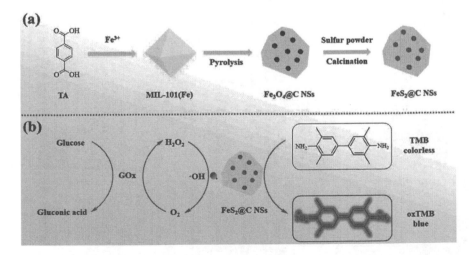

**FIGURE 5.3** (a) Synthesis of $FeS_2$@carbon NSs, and (b) colorimetric detection of glucose based on $FeS_2$@carbon nanozymes as the sensing platform. (Reprinted with permission from Ding et al., (63) Copyright 2020 American Chemical Society.)

More importantly, this method was successful in performing glucose assays in some real samples, indicating its potential in biotechnology and clinical diagnostics.

A multifunctional hemin@CQDs hybrid nanozymes with simultaneous POD-like activity and fluorescence signaling property was reported by Su et al. (64). Inspired by their dual nature, hemin@CQDs were utilized for the development of dual-channel fluorescent probes for $H_2O_2$ and $H_2O_2$-based biocatalytic systems. The oxidative coupling of 4-aminoantipyrine with phenol in the presence of $H_2O_2$ can be catalyzed by the hemin@CQDs, resulting in a pink-red quinoneimine dye with a maximum absorbance of 505 nm. The green fluorescence of hemin@CQDs peaks at 540 nm under a 480 nm excitation wavelength and is quenched by the produced quinoneimine dye due to an inner filter effect, as well as by $H_2O_2$ due to dynamic quenching. As a result, a dual-channel colorimetric and fluorimetric optical probe for $H_2O_2$ was developed. The probe could detect glucose due to the transformation of glucose under the formation of $H_2O_2$ by the related OXD catalysis. An LOD of 0.15 μM of glucose was obtained for colorimetric and fluorimetric detections. Thus, the hemin@CQDs is a low-cost and simple-to-use technique for detecting a variety of species involved in the $H_2O_2$-generating reaction, which is a major drawback of the proposed strategy. The merits and demerits of carbon-based nanozymes are summarized in **Table 5.2**.

### 5.4.3.1 Mechanism of GOx-Like Carbon Nanozymes

Natural GOx is capable of catalyzing the oxidation of glucose to $H_2O_2$ and D-glucono-δ-lactone (59). Zhang et al. created a GOx-mimicking nanozyme using functionalized porous carbon (FPC) as a growth substrate for ultrasmall Au NPs and -FeOOH microcrystals (61). Carbon atoms aided glucose oxidation by promoting $O_2$ adsorption via unpaired electrons on the porous carbon edges and glucose oxidation occurred on the surface of Au NPs. The adsorbed $O_2$ increased the likelihood of a reaction between glucose and $O_2$, speeding up the formation of $H_2O_2$. Furthermore, as an electron acceptor, α-FeOOH was able to extract electrons from excited Au NPs, which helped to prevent electron–hole pair recombination. The photoexcited α-FeOOH electrons were then transferred from $Fe^{3+}$ to $Fe^{2+}$ (65).

---

**TABLE 5.2**
**Merits and Demerits of Carbon-Based Nanozymes**

| Merits | • Facile production on large-scale production |
|---|---|
| | • Low-cost of production |
| | • Long-term storage |
| | • High stability in harsh environments |
| | • Large surface area |
| | • Improved surface chemistry |
| **Demerits** | • Unclear catalytic mechanism |
| | • Difficulties in rational design and construction of carbon-based nanozymes |
| | • Unclear catalytic mechanism |
| | • Lower catalytic activity |

## 5.4.4 MOFs and Other Materials

Enzymes typically work collectively in biological systems to enhance the catalytic efficiency of their reactions through synergy. Nanozymes with POD-like activity and natural enzymes have recently been reported to function synergistically, broadening the application of cascade catalysis (66, 67). The natural enzymes precisely identify substrate molecules in these types of interactions and the products serve as substrates for the nanozyme catalytic reaction, thereby causing a color change of a particular probe. This technique effectively blends nanozyme stability with the specificity of natural enzymes (8, 11). Despite widespread availability, due to poor operational stability and difficult recovery, the use of natural enzymes is often limited (68, 69). To resolve these restrictions, concerted efforts have been made to enhance natural enzyme reusability and stability through porous support immobilization (70).

For enzyme immobilization, MOFs with uniform porosity and a large surface area provide excellent support (71). Two methods that are commonly used to immobilize enzymes based on MOF are co-precipitation and post-synthesis modification (72). In the co-precipitation process, a natural enzyme is immobilized onto the surface of MOF under mild reaction conditions (73). This process is limited to a few MOFs, such as ZIF-8 (NiPd) (74) and MIL-100 (Fe) (75). Whereas in the post-synthesis modification process, the MOF is immersed into an enzyme solution to convert into enzyme@MOF. Mostly, the MOFs are microporous, and the tiny pore size restricts the penetration and embedding of enzymes in the interior space (76). Therefore, due to their cage-like mesoporous structure, mesoporous MOFs are usually favored for enzyme immobilization (77).

However, due to the small pore size of the initial MOF, the long response time of 30 min restricts substrate diffusion (78). Therefore, hierarchically porous MOF assemblies are recommended as ideal supports for enzyme immobilization (79). Leaching of an immobilized enzyme from a hierarchically porous MOF during the reaction is a common problem, which is due to a lack of specific interactions between the enzyme and support. The above problem can be altered by functional modification of MOF that can specifically adhere to enzymes. GOx-integrated MOFs-based nanozymes with biomimetic activity to oxidize glucose to gluconic acid and the ability of MOFs to mimic the POD activity is of current interest (80, 81). POD-like activity in the reaction of glucose to gluconic acid and $H_2O_2$ by GOx triggers a chromogenic reaction with the addition of chromogenic agents (27). Here, the efficiency and selectivity depend upon the biological activity of GOx and nanozymes integrated into MOFs.

Inspired by the above hypothesis, Xu et al. (27) designed an iron-based MOF (Fe-MIL-88B-NH$_2$) via amidation of GOx with intrinsic POD-like activity and improved stability. The presence of numerous amino groups in Fe-MOF (82) eases the immobilization of GOx via cross-coupling reaction, which further initiates cascade reaction to detect glucose (**Figure 5.4a**). The nanoscale size of MOF results in immediate oxidation of $H_2O_2$ generated from the GOx-catalysed oxidation of glucose in the presence of $O_2$, which minimizes the decomposition of $H_2O_2$ and decreases the effect of diffusion resistance (**Figure 5.4b**) (83). The GOx@Fe-MOF showed promising results over a free enzyme system (Fe-MOF/GOx) with higher temperature

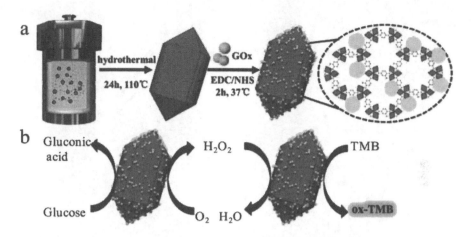

**FIGURE 5.4** (a) Schematic on of the synthetic approach of Fe-MOF-GOx and (b) corresponding cascade catalytic detection of glucose by Fe-MOF-GOx. (Reprinted with permission from Xu et al. (27), Copyright 2019 American Chemical Society.)

and acid-base tolerance for the detection of glucose. The designed GOx@ Fe-MIL-88B-NH$_2$ MOF exhibited a linear range of 1–500 µM with a detection limit of 0.48 µM for glucose in the human serum sample.

A universal enzyme-immobilized MOF was prepared for simple and rapid immobilization of enzyme using a post-modification method by refluxing a mixture of HP-MIL-88B and 4-formylphenylboronic acid in ethanol (80 °C for 12 h) as shown in **Figure 5.5** (84). This results in the formation of a boronic acid (BA)-functionalized hierarchically porous HP-MIL-88B-BA matrix, which was dispersed in a GOx solution to prepare GOx@ HP-MIL-88B-BA. This HPR-mimicking nanozyme architecture was used for the detection of glucose in human blood with a short analysis time (LOD = 0.98 µM; linear range = 2–100 µM). Therefore, the GOx@ HP-MIL-88B-BA integrated nanozyme architecture was used for rapid analysis of glucose.

Platinum-based nanostructures mimicking the enzymatic activity as an effective catalyst for OXD, POD, and SOD have been reported (85). Unfortunately, the accumulation and aggregation of Pt NPs in the reaction solution decreases their catalytic activity. A successful approach to solve this problem is to grow Pt NPs on 2-D support substrates, such as GO (86), Pd NSs (87), and Mo(88), to form hybrid nanomaterials, which provide enhanced catalytic activity due to the synergistic effect between their single components. Inspired by these, Chen et al. (89) used a porphyrin-like ligand, i.e., Fe(III)tetra(4-carboxyphenyl)porphine chloride (TCPP(Fe)) to synthesize MOF NSs (as Cu-TCPP(Fe) by surfactant-assisted method for high-yield and decorated with Pt NPs via photochemical reduction method and obtained Pt NPs/Cu-TCPP(Fe) as a biomimetic nanozyme for glucose detection (**Figure 5.6**). Based on the colorimetric absorbance at 652 nm, a linear relation was established from 2 to 200 µM with an LOD of 0.994 µM. The response of this glucose sensor was insensitive to other sugars, such as fructose, lactose, and maltose. Liu et al. (90) described an artificial enzyme cascade bio-platform constructed on MOF-derived

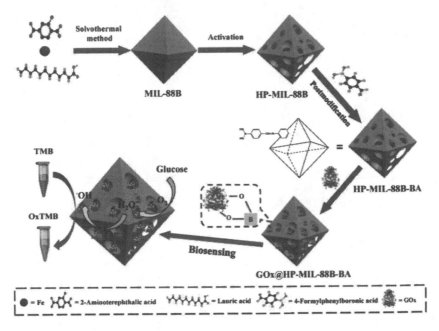

**FIGURE 5.5** Construction of GOx@HP-MIL-88B-BA synthesis and catalytic oxidation of glucose. (Reprinted with permission from Zhao et al. (84), Copyright 2020 American Chemical Society.)

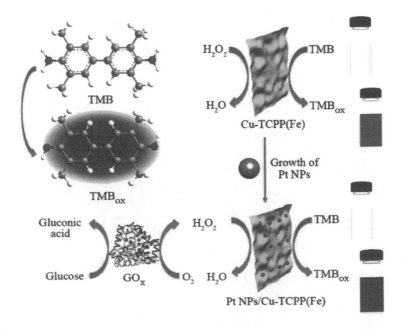

**FIGURE 5.6** Schematic illustration of the synthesis method of PtNPs/Cu-TCPP(Fe) hybrid NSs, and its application in colorimetric detection of glucose and $H_2O_2$. (Reprinted with permission from Chen et al. (89), Copyright 2018 American Chemical Society.)

bimetal nanocomposite with improved efficiency. The BSA-Pt NPs@MnCo$_2$O$_4$ MOF was both a nanozyme and a scaffold for GOx immobilization. Combining the advantages of a nanozyme and natural enzyme, this sensor provided an LOD of 8.1-μM glucose. In addition to extending the application of nanozyme in natural enzyme catalysis, the tandem catalytic system provided a simple, effective, and organized bio-platform enzyme cascade for biosensing and other applications.

Molybdenum trioxide (MoO$_3$) NSs, which are solution-processable, were used as models for direct liquid-phase growth of Pt NPs in ambient conditions. Compared to MoO$_3$, the Pt-MoO$_3$ hybrid was a better POD-like nanozyme and afforded an ultrasensitive colorimetric detection of glucose (LOD = 187.4 nM; linear range = 5 to 500 μM) (88). Furthermore, H$_2$O$_2$ produced, during the conversion of O$_2$ to peroxide, was detected as low as 44.6 nM. This research suggests a promising strategy for designing and developing biomimetic catalysts based on a clever assembly of various dimensional nanomaterials.

Zhang et al. (91) developed a protocol for encapsulating two closely related sequential biocatalysts into MOFs and demonstrating their improvement in cascade reactions. This protocol consists of two steps: 1) coupling two sequential biocatalysts, OXD and Hemin, with proximity using a bifunctional polymer called poly(1-vinyl imidazole) (PVI) and 2) encapsulating the coupled biocatalysts (GOx) in ZIF-8 (**Figure 5.7a**). As illustrated in **Figure 5.7b**, GOx oxidizes the glucose molecule into gluconic acid with the production of H$_2$O$_2$. Then, the reaction of H$_2$O$_2$ and ABTS can be catalyzed by hemin with POD-mimic activity to give H$_2$O and ABTS+, which is detectable at 420 nm. They examined the POD-like catalytic behavior of the GOx/PVI-Hemin@ZIF-8 composite. H$_2$O$_2$ oxidizes ABTS to ABTS+ with colorless to

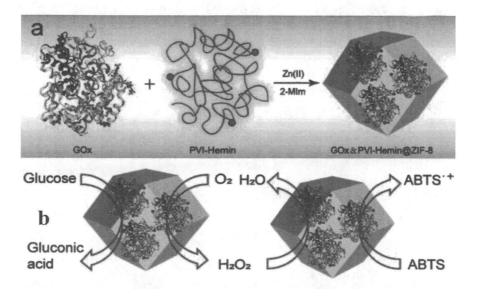

**FIGURE 5.7** (a) Schematic illustration of the preparation of GOx&PVI-Hemin@ZIF-8 composite and (b) schematic illustration of the proximity effects on the enhanced cascade catalysis for GOx, and Hemin in GOx&PVI-Hemin@ZIF-8. (Reprinted with permission from Zhang et al. (91), Copyright 2020 American Chemical Society.)

green in the presence of GOx/PVI-Hemin@ZIF-8. The GOx&PVIHemin@ZIF-8 material showed not only enhanced the catalytic activity in this design but also long-term, reusable cascade catalytic activity attributable to the ZIF-8 protective host.

Incorporating 2-D MOF NSs with other functional materials is a well-known approach for producing 2-D MOF-based hybrid nanomaterials (92). Because Au NPs have GOx-like activity that can catalyze glucose oxidation to produce gluconic acid and $H_2O_2$ in the presence of $O_2$ (93), integration of metalloporphyrin-based MOF NSs with Au NPs can mimic enzymatic cascade. The 2-D Cu-TCPP(M) NS is used as a metal nanostructure growth template such as Au NPs. Using Au NPs/Cu-TCPP(Fe) hybrid NS as an example, the first 2-D Cu-TCPP(Fe) NSs with a thickness of sub-10 nm were synthesized based on a surfactant-assisted synthetic process (94). Later, the Au NPs/Cu-TCPP(Fe) NSs were synthesized by reduction of $HAuCl_4$ with sodium borohydride ($NaBH_4$) in the presence of Cu-TCPP(Fe) NSs. In the presence of dissolved $O_2$ (in equilibrium with air), Au NPs/Cu-TCPP(M) hybrid NSs catalyze glucose oxidation, releasing gluconic acid, and $H_2O_2$ in the reaction solution. The obtained supernatant contained gluconic acid and $H_2O_2$ after centrifuging the reaction solution to eliminate Au NPs/Cu-TCPP(M) hybrid NSs. A particular colorimetric assay was used to analyze gluconic acid at 652 nm. The absorption results established a good linear relationship from 10 μM to 300 μM with an LOD of 8.50-μM glucose.

The lack of external influence can eventually cause NPs to develop uncontrollably and lose their nanoscale properties. Luo et al. reported a self-catalyzed and self-limiting system based on Au NPs that takes advantage of Au NPs GOx-like catalytic action (93). The Au NPs-catalyzed glucose oxidation creates $H_2O_2$ *in situ*, which induces the seeded growth of the Au NPs in the presence of $HAuCl_4$ (**Figure 5.8**). The two negative feedback factors—size-dependent activity decreases of Au NPs and product (gluconic acid)-induced surface passivation internally control this crystal growth of Au NPs—lead to a rapidly self-limiting system. In this method, the scale, shape, and catalytic activity of Au NPs are all regulated at the same time.

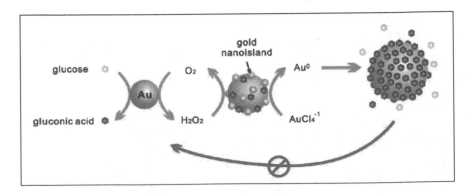

**FIGURE 5.8** Schematic of the Au NPs-based self-limiting growth system. The size, shape, and catalytic activity of Au NPs are self-limited by the integrated influence from the catalytic reaction, seeded enlargement, and surface passivation of Au NPs. (Reprinted with permission from Luo et al. (93), Copyright 2010 American Chemical Society.)

This research contributes to the development of a new method for the controlled synthesis of novel nanomaterials, the design of "smart" self-limiting nanomedicine, and a deeper understanding of self-limiting systems in nature. A standard Michaelis–Menten behavior was accompanied by the catalysis of Au NPs and $K_m = 6.97$ mM, which was slightly greater than that for GOx ($K_m = 4.87$ mM), signifying slightly lower affinity; however, Au NPs had a twofold higher catalytic constant ($K_{cat}$) than GOx, indicating a faster reaction rate.

## 5.5 CHALLENGES IN NANOZYME APPLICATIONS AND POTENTIAL SOLUTIONS

While nanozyme-based detection is a promising platform for quickly and reliably detecting a variety of analytes, such as glucose, heparin, biomarkers, etc., it suffers from the combined technological and clinical challenges that both nanozymes and electrochemical biosensors face.

### 5.5.1 LOW SPECIFICITY

Nanozymes, unlike natural enzymes, lack specific binding sites that allow them to interact with a substrate properly. High specificity is crucial in biomolecular sensing for a wide range of biomedical applications, especially, disease diagnosis and monitoring. Therefore, finding ways to improve nanozyme substrate specificity may be just as critical as improving catalytic activity. Also, there are some lacunae in understandings of deep mechanisms of nanozyme involved in an enzymatic reaction. Lots of emphases is still needed for a comprehensive understanding of the change in the orientation of molecules during enzymatic catalysis. By studying the natural enzymatic mechanism, there is an opportunity for scientists to look deeper into the mechanism of artificial enzymes.

### 5.5.2 LOW CATALYTIC ACTIVITY

While nanozymes have unrivaled stability and large-scale preparation capabilities, they are not without flaws. The catalytic activity of nanozymes is still inferior to that of most natural enzymes, making it more difficult to fully substitute nanozymes in most applications. Bioconjugation of nanozymes is greatly hindered by their low catalytic activities (95). This restriction can be solved by using molecularly imprinted polymers (MIPs) (96) on nanozymes and synthesizing "integrated nanozymes" (97). MIPs increase the specificity and catalytic activity of enzymes by polymerizing binding sites on the substrate. Natural enzymes are combined with nanozymes in a 3-D network structure to increase selectivity and catalytic activity in integrated nanozymes. MOFs hold great promise among the various 3-D network structures needed to fabricate such a hybrid enzyme mimicking nanomaterial (71). Utilizing MOFs- or MIPs-based hybrid nanozymes will significantly improve the selectivity.

### 5.5.3   Limited Enzyme-Mimicking Activity

The aspect of nanozymes that needs to be most improved is their enzyme-mimicking abilities. Synthesizing more robust nanozymes that better exhibit the properties of natural enzymes is needed to achieve this goal. The morphology of some typical nanozymes should also be improved compared to their natural counterparts. In addition to enzyme-like activities, nanozymes have special physical and chemical properties, such as magnetic and thermal properties. Combining these characteristics with nanozyme catalytic activity may be a breakthrough in nanozyme application. Nanotechnology, artificial intelligence, and computational chemistry can dramatically increase nanozyme activity.

### 5.5.4   Poor Reproducibility

Poor reproducibility of nanozymes is a significant issue that could stymie the widespread use of nanozyme-based sensing protocols or strategies. This problem occurs primarily for two reasons. First, small-scale synthesis in a single lab cannot guarantee the size, shape, or porosity of NPs from different batches, which results in significant variations in activity. Second, bioconjugation of the recognition factor and nanozyme is highly subjective and is dependent on the knowledge and considerations of the person. As a result, substantial efforts must be made to industrialize and streamline successful bioconjugation protocols.

### 5.5.5   Potential Toxicity

Nanozymes are exogenous compounds, so their toxicity must be carefully considered. Nanozymes have so far been studied primarily for their catalytic function in comparison to enzymatic systems, but they can also be used to improve the body's immune system. It appears that this is only the beginning and that much further research is needed in the field of nanozyme technology.

## 5.6   SUMMARY AND FUTURE PERSPECTIVES

We have summarized representative enzyme mimics and possible catalytic mechanisms in this paper, with a special emphasis on recent advances in the nanozyme-based schemes of GOx for glucose determination. A plethora of literature has been reported based on the integration of metal, metal-free, MOFs-based, and hybrid nanozymes mimicking the enzymatic activity of OXD cascade reaction in glucose metabolism. However, the inherent characteristics and constraints of limited selectivity, low catalytic activity, and deprived reproducibility of nanozymes limit their further applications over the standalone stability of the GOx enzyme.

Nanozymes are being endowed with enormous functionalities, such as nanocarriers, robust catalytic behavior, probe immobilizers, conductive surface modifiers, and signal generators or tracer tags as a result of dynamic progress in this area. Until now, only a few nanozymes have demonstrated catalytic activity in the same way their natural counterparts do, but the vast majority have moderate to low activity. While heteroatom doping, composites, and bimetal formation can significantly increase activity, the improvement in substrate selectivity is still modest. Molecular imprinting or surface modifications, on the other hand, increase molecular recognition and substrate selectivity at the expense of action. To elucidate the catalytic mechanism and impart maximum activity and selectivity at the same time or balancing them for a specific application, a deeper understanding of structure–activity relationships, the logical design of nanomaterials, experimental and computational studies are critical. One of the most relevant factors is the multienzymatic property, which is effective in therapeutic applications.

Also, it is unclear how this could help with the design and fabrication of solid-state immunoassays and different sensing strategies. Furthermore, most sensors have used HRP-mimicking nanomaterials over the years. As a result, the vast majority of nanozymes have remained unstudied. The creation of multifunctional nanozymes may be a difficult and fascinating topic to pursue. Aside from catalysis, unique physicochemical properties such as magnetic, optical, or thermal properties may allow enzyme mimics to be realized for ultra-sensitive and user-friendly biomolecule detection in complex body fluids. Furthermore, integration with microfluidics will speed up many time-consuming, subjective synthesis, and bioconjugation processes. The automation and standardization of this area can be aided by replacing laboratory shakers, centrifuge machines with reliable micromixers, and microfluidic-based particle separation systems. Furthermore, combining the isolation, separation, and detection of pathogenic targets on a single chip could revolutionize the use of nanozyme-based electrochemical biosensors for disease diagnosis and therapy effectiveness monitoring.

Herein, we propose the necessary suggestions for nanozymes to be positioned as an innovative source technology effectively overcoming the limitations of natural enzymes. For this, it is necessary to synthesize or design nanozymes structured with improved activity and structural integrity. Rather than a random screening of enzyme-like activities of existing unspecified nanomaterials, future research on developing nanozymes will use a strategy of logical screening of enzyme-like activity based on certain atomic compositions that are required to catalyze enzymatic reactions. In this regard, combining the synergistic effect of nanozymes with low catalytic activity to promote electron transfer between composite materials during redox reactions, a strategy for preparing nanocomposites or hybrid materials can potentially help to overcome the current major limitations of nanozymes with low catalytic activity. Synthesis of bioinspired nanozymes will offer a way to make nontoxic nanozymes by avoiding toxic chemicals from traditional chemical synthesis. Design and development of surface immobilization or new surface chemistry will enable nanozymes to be used for highly selective target determination.

## CONFLICT OF INTEREST

The authors declare no financial or commercial conflict of interests

## ACKNOWLEDGMENTS

A.S. would like to acknowledge the library search engine of SGT University, Gurugram, India, to provide continuous support. The authors would also to thank the editor for his valuable suggestions to improve the quality of the chapter.

# REFERENCES

1. Lang NJ, Liu B, Liu J. 2014. *Journal of Colloid and Interface Science* 428: 78–83
2. Li X, Lu X, Xing M, Yang X-H, Zhao T-T, et al. 2012. *Bioorganic & Medicinal Chemistry Letters* 22: 3589–93
3. Meng Y, Li W, Pan X, Gadd GM. 2020. *Environmental Science: Nano* 7: 1305–18
4. Wang F, Chen L, Liu D, Ma W, Dramou P, He H. 2020. *TrAC Trends in Analytical Chemistry* 133: 116080
5. Gao L, Zhuang J, Nie L, Zhang J, Zhang Y, et al. 2007. *Nature Nanotechnology* 2: 577–83
6. Zhang Z, Zhang C, Zheng H, Xu H. 2019. *Accounts of Chemical Research* 52: 2506–15
7. Stasyuk N, Smutok O, Demkiv O, Prokopiv T, Gayda G, et al. 2020. *Sensors (Basel, Switzerland)* 20: 4509
8. Wu J, Wang X, Wang Q, Lou Z, Li S, et al. 2019. *Chemical Society Reviews* 48: 1004–76
9. Sun H, Zhou Y, Ren J, Qu X. 2018. *Angewandte Chemie International Edition Engl* 57: 9224–37
10. Shin HY, Park TJ, Kim MI. 2015. *Journal of Nanomaterials* 2015: 756278
11. Wei H, Wang E. 2013. *Chemical Society Reviews* 42: 6060–93
12. Wang H, Wan K, Shi X. 2019. *Advanced Materials* 31: 1805368
13. Liu P, Wang Y, Han L, Cai Y, Ren H, et al. 2020. *ACS Applied Materials & Interfaces* 12: 9090–7
14. Chen W-F, Malacco CMDS, Mehmood R, Johnson KK, Yang J-L, et al. 2021. *Materials Science and Engineering: C* 120: 111663
15. Liu S, Lu F, Xing R, Zhu J-J. 2011. *Chemistry – A European Journal* 17: 620–5
16. Jiang B, Yan L, Zhang J, Zhou M, Shi G, et al. 2019. *ACS Applied Materials & Interfaces* 11: 9747–55
17. Ghosh S, Roy P, Karmodak N, Jemmis ED, Mugesh G. 2018. *Angewandte Chemie International Edition* 57: 4510–5
18. Wang L, Hu Z, Wu S, Pan J, Xu X, Niu X. 2020. *Analytica Chimica Acta* 1121: 26–34
19. Hu L, Liao H, Feng L, Wang M, Fu W. 2018. *Analytical Chemistry* 90: 6247–52
20. Bankar SB, Bule MV, Singhal RS, Ananthanarayan L. 2009. *Biotechnology Advances* 27: 489–501
21. Pluschkell S, Hellmuth K, Rinas U. 1996. *Biotechnology and Bioengineering* 51: 215–20
22. Gökçal B, Kip Ç, Tuncel A. 2020. *Journal of Alloys and Compounds* 843: 156012
23. Roth JP, Klinman JP. 2003. *Proceedings of the National Academy of Sciences* 100: 62–7
24. Witt S, Wohlfahrt G, Schomburg D, Hecht HJ, Kalisz HM. 2000. *Biochemical Journal* 347: 553–9
25. Wang L, Li S, Zhang X, Huang Y. 2020. *Talanta* 216: 121009
26. Lee P-C, Li N-S, Hsu Y-P, Peng C, Yang H-W. 2019. *Analyst* 144: 3038–44
27. Xu W, Jiao L, Yan H, Wu Y, Chen L, et al. 2019. *ACS Applied Materials & Interfaces* 11: 22096–101
28. Lee LG, Whitesides GM. 1985. *Journal of the American Chemical Society* 107: 6999–7008
29. Ghoshdastider U, Wu R, Trzaskowski B, Mlynarczyk K, Miszta P, et al. 2015. *RSC Advances* 5: 13570–8
30. Wong ELS, Vuong KQ, Chow E. 2021. *Sensors* 21: 408
31. Comotti M, Della Pina C, Matarrese R, Rossi M. 2004. *Angewandte Chemie International Edition* 43: 5812–5
32. Periasamy AP, Roy P, Wu W-P, Huang Y-H, Chang H-T. 2016. *Electrochimica Acta* 215: 253–60

33. Cheng H, Zhang L, He J, Guo W, Zhou Z, et al. 2016. *Analytical Chemistry* 88: 5489–97
34. Huang Y, Ren J, Qu X. 2019. *Chemical Reviews* 119: 4357–412
35. Liang M, Yan X. 2019. *Accounts of Chemical Research* 52
36. Jiao A, Xu L, Tian Y, Cui Q, Liu X, Chen M. 2021. *Talanta* 225: 121990
37. Cai S, Yang R. 2020. In *Nanozymology: Connecting Biology and Nanotechnology*, ed. X Yan, pp. 331–65. Singapore: Springer Singapore
38. Comotti M, Della Pina C, Falletta E, Rossi M. 2006. *Advanced Synthesis & Catalysis* 348: 313–6
39. Kim MI, Ye Y, Woo M-A, Lee J, Park HG. 2014. *Advanced Healthcare Materials* 3: 36–41
40. Qiao F, Qi Q, Wang Z, Xu K, Ai S. 2016. *Sensors and Actuators B: Chemical* 229: 379–86
41. Wang H, Li S, Si Y, Sun Z, Li S, Lin Y. 2014. *Journal of Materials Chemistry B* 2: 4442–8
42. Wang X, Qu K, Xu B, Ren J, Qu X. 2011. *Nano Research* 4: 908–20
43. Chen M, Zhou H, Liu X, Yuan T, Wang W, et al. 2020. *Small* 16: e2002343
44. Fan K, Wang H, Xi J, Liu Q, Meng X, et al. 2017. *Chemical Communications* 53: 424–7
45. Qian M, Zhang L, Pu Z, Xia J, Chen L, et al. 2018. *Journal of Materials Chemistry B* 6: 7916–25
46. Zhang P, Sun D, Cho A, Weon S, Lee S, et al. 2019. *Nature Communications* 10: 940
47. Edwards JK, Solsona B, N EN, Carley AF, Herzing AA, et al. 2009. *Science* 323: 1037–41
48. Moon G-h, Kim W, Bokare AD, Sung N-e, Choi W. 2014. *Energy & Environmental Science* 7: 4023–8
49. Sengupta P, Pramanik K, Datta P, Sarkar P. 2020. *Biosensors and Bioelectronics* 154: 112072
50. Sun H, Ren J, Qu X. 2020. In *Nanozymology: Connecting Biology and Nanotechnology*, ed. X Yan, pp. 171–93. Singapore: Springer Singapore
51. Sun H, Zhao A, Gao N, Li K, Ren J, Qu X. 2015. *Angewandte Chemie International Edition Engl* 54: 7176–80
52. Liu Q, Zhang L, Li H, Jia Q, Jiang Y, et al. 2015. *Materials Science and Engineering: C* 55: 193–200
53. Qian J, Yang X, Yang Z, Zhu G, Mao H, Wang K. 2015. *Journal of Materials Chemistry B* 3: 1624–32
54. Song Y, Qu K, Zhao C, Ren J, Qu X. 2010. *Advanced Materials* 22: 2206–10
55. Li R, Zhen M, Guan M, Chen D, Zhang G, et al. 2013. *Biosensors and Bioelectronics* 47: 502–7
56. Shi W, Wang Q, Long Y, Cheng Z, Chen S, et al. 2011. *Chemical Communications* 47: 6695–7
57. Zhang Y, Wu C, Zhou X, Wu X, Yang Y, et al. 2013. *Nanoscale* 5: 1816–9
58. Samuel ELG, Marcano DC, Berka V, Bitner BR, Wu G, et al. 2015. *Proceedings of the National Academy of Sciences* 112: 2343
59. Ding H, Hu B, Zhang B, Zhang H, Yan X, et al. 2021. *Nano Research* 14: 570–83
60. Wang Q, Zhang X, Huang L, Zhang Z, Dong S. 2017. *ACS Applied Materials & Interfaces* 9: 7465–71
61. Zhang R, He S, Zhang C, Chen W. 2015. *Journal of Materials Chemistry B* 3: 4146–54
62. Bao Y-W, Hua X-W, Ran H-H, Zeng J, Wu F-G. 2019. *Journal of Materials Chemistry B* 7: 296–304
63. Ding W, Liu H, Zhao W, Wang J, Zhang L, et al. 2020. *ACS Applied Bio Materials* 3: 5905–12
64. Su L, Cai Y, Wang L, Dong W, Mao G, et al. 2020. *Microchimica Acta* 187: 132
65. Zhang Q, Chen S, Wang H. 2018. *Green Chemistry* 20: 4067–74

66. Wang Z, Zhang R, Yan X, Fan K. 2020. *Materials Today* 41: 81–119
67. Liu Q, Yang Y, Li H, Zhu R, Shao Q, et al. 2015. *Biosensors and Bioelectronics* 64: 147–53
68. Lin Y, Ren J, Qu X. 2014. *Accounts of Chemical Research* 47: 1097–105
69. Zhu J, Peng X, Nie W, Wang Y, Gao J, et al. 2019. *Biosensors and Bioelectronics* 141: 111450
70. Vriezema DM, Comellas Aragonès M, Elemans JAAW, Cornelissen JJLM, Rowan AE, Nolte RJM. 2005. *Chemical Reviews* 105: 1445–90
71. Lian X, Fang Y, Joseph E, Wang Q, Li J, et al. 2017. *Chemical Society Reviews* 46: 3386–401
72. Mehta J, Bhardwaj N, Bhardwaj SK, Kim K-H, Deep A. 2016. *Coordination Chemistry Reviews* 322: 30–40
73. Wu J, Li S, Wei H. 2018. *Chemical Communications* 54: 6520–30
74. Wang Q, Zhang X, Huang L, Zhang Z, Dong S. 2017. *Angewandte Chemie International Edition* 56: 16082–5
75. Gascón V, Jiménez MB, Blanco RM, Sanchez-Sanchez M. 2018. *Catalysis Today* 304: 119–26
76. Ariga K, Vinu A, Yamauchi Y, Ji Q, Hill JP. 2012. *Bulletin of the Chemical Society of Japan* 85: 1–32
77. Koh K, Wong-Foy AG, Matzger AJ. 2009. *Journal of the American Chemical Society* 131: 4184–5
78. Zhao Z, Lin T, Liu W, Hou L, Ye F, Zhao S. 2019. *Spectrochimica Acta Part A: Molecular and Biomolecular Spectroscopy* 219: 240–7
79. Sun Y, Shi J, Zhang S, Wu Y, Mei S, et al. 2019. *Industrial & Engineering Chemistry Research* 58: 12835–44
80. Xia Y, Ye J, Tan K, Wang J, Yang G. 2013. *Analytical Chemistry* 85: 6241–7
81. Vázquez-González M, Torrente-Rodríguez RM, Kozell A, Liao W-C, Cecconello A, et al. 2017. *Nano Letters* 17: 4958–63
82. Ma M, Noei H, Mienert B, Niesel J, Bill E, et al. 2013. *Chemistry – A European Journal* 19: 6785–90
83. Zhao Z, Fu J, Dhakal S, Johnson-Buck A, Liu M, et al. 2016. *Nature Communications* 7: 10619
84. Zhao Z, Huang Y, Liu W, Ye F, Zhao S. 2020. *ACS Sustainable Chemistry & Engineering* 8: 4481–8
85. Li W, Chen B, Zhang H, Sun Y, Wang J, et al. 2015. *Biosensors and Bioelectronics* 66: 251–8
86. Li Y, Gao W, Ci L, Wang C, Ajayan PM. 2010. *Carbon* 48: 1124–30
87. Wei J, Chen X, Shi S, Mo S, Zheng N. 2015. *Nanoscale* 7: 19018–26
88. Wang Y, Zhang X, Luo Z, Huang X, Tan C, et al. 2014. *Nanoscale* 6: 12340–4
89. Chen H, Qiu Q, Sharif S, Ying S, Wang Y, Ying Y. 2018. *ACS Applied Materials & Interfaces* 10: 24108–15
90. Liu M, Mou J, Xu X, Zhang F, Xia J, Wang Z. 2020. *Talanta* 220: 121374
91. Zhang X, Zhang F, Lu Z, Xu Q, Hou C, Wang Z. 2020. *ACS Applied Materials & Interfaces* 12: 25565–71
92. Zhu Q-L, Xu Q. 2014. *Chemical Society Reviews* 43: 5468–512
93. Luo W, Zhu C, Su S, Li D, He Y, et al. 2010. *ACS Nano* 4: 7451–8
94. Wang Y, Zhao M, Ping J, Chen B, Cao X, et al. 2016. *Advanced Materials* 28: 4149–55
95. Mahmudunnabi RG, Farhana FZ, Kashaninejad N, Firoz SH, Shim Y-B, Shiddiky MJA. 2020. *Analyst* 145: 4398–420
96. Zhang Z, Li Y, Zhang X, Liu J. 2019. *Nanoscale* 11: 4854–63
97. Wu J, Li S, Wei H. 2018. *Chem Commun (Camb)* 54: 6520–30

# 6 Bioaffinity-Based Nanozymes

*Çiğdem Kip, Kadriye Özlem Hamaloğlu, and Ali Tuncel*
Chemical Engineering Department,
Hacettepe University, Ankara, Turkey

## CONTENTS

## 6.1  INTRODUCTION

Enzymes can catalyze a variety of reactions with high substrate specificity, activity, and yield under mild conditions (1, 2). Hence, there is special interest in utilizing enzymes in different applications, such as biosensing, pharmaceutical processes, and the food industry (3–5). However, problems related to low operational stability, difficulties in recovery and recycling, and the high cost of preparation and purification, etc., greatly limit applications of natural enzymes (6). To overcome these limitations, extensive research is underway to design functional nanomaterials that have intrinsic enzyme-mimicking properties (7, 8). Nanozymes are a type of nanomaterials with enzyme-like activities; they have shown great potential to replace natural enzymes in numerous fields, including biosensing, immunoassays, cancer diagnostics, and therapy (9). Zinc(II)-triazacyclonane-functionalized gold (Au) nanoparticles (NPs) with phosphoesterase-like activity (10) and iron oxide ($Fe_3O_4$) NPs with POD-like activity (11) are two pioneering examples of nanozymes. Following these, nanozymes have attracted considerable attention in recent years.

DOI: 10.1201/9781003109228-6

## 6.2 NANOZYME TYPES

Most nanozymes are transition MOs-, noble metals-, and lanthanides-based nanomaterials and possess excellent peroxidase (POD)- or oxidase (OXD)-like properties. The nanozymatic properties vary according to the structure and composition of nanomaterials. In this section, some representative nanomaterials for different types of nanozyme are described along with their properties and applications (**Table 6.1**).

**TABLE 6.1**
**Selected POD-Like Nanozymes and Their Applications**

| Nanozyme | Shape Structure | Application | Ref. |
|---|---|---|---|
| Nanomagnet-silica shell (Fe$_3$O$_4$@ SiO$_2$) decorated with Au@Pd NPs (Fe$_3$O$_4$@SiO$_2$-NH$_2$-Au@PdNPs) | Nanoparticles | Determination of glucose concentrations in serum samples | (12) |
| Au/Fe$_3$O$_4$/GO hybrid material | Nanosheet | Colorimetric detection of Hg$^{2+}$ | (13) |
| Gold nanoparticles (AuNPs) supported by cationic cellulose (C.CNF) (AuNPs@C.CNF) | Nanofibrils | Colorimetric detection methods for H$_2$O$_2$ and glucose | (14) |
| Ni-V mixed metal oxide (MMO) | Nanosheets | Determination of H$_2$O$_2$ | (15) |
| CoFe$_2$O$_4$ | Irregular nanoparticles | Colorimetric glucose detection in one pot | (16) |
| Cobalt-based metal oxides nanomaterials ZnCo$_2$O$_4$ | Nanosheets | Detection of pyrophosphate (PPi) and pyrophosphatase (PPase) | (17) |
| Monodisperse-porous cerium oxide (CeO$_2$) | Microspheres | Detection of large phosphorylated molecules | (18) |
| Human serum albumin@ polydopamine/Fe nanocomposites (HSA@PDA/Fe NCs) | Nanosheet | In vitro H$_2$O$_2$ detection/in situ detection of H$_2$O$_2$ generated from the cells | (19) |
| Pepsin-templated copper (Cu NCs) | Nanoclusters | For hydrogen peroxide and glucose detection | (20) |
| Hep-stabilized Pt nanozyme | Nanocluster | Directly monitoring glucose | (21) |
| Glucose oxidase immobilized-Au nanoparticle attached-magnetic SiO$_2$ (GOx@Au@MagSiO$_2$)) | Microspheres | Direct determination of glucose level in human whole blood | (22) |
| Gold nanoparticle decorated, monodisperse porous silica microspheres in the magnetic form (Au@SiO$_2$@Fe$_3$O$_4$@SiO$_2$) | Microspheres | Determination of glutathione concentration in human serum | (23) |
| A platinum (II)-doped graphitic carbon nitride (Pt$^{2+}$@g-C$_3$N$_4$) nanozyme | Nanosheet | Detection of glucose | (24) |
| Citric acid-modified bimetallic PtNi (CA@PtNi hNS) | Hollow nanospheres | Colorimetric detection of human serum albumin | (25) |
| Perovskite Lanthanum ferrite (LaFeO$_3$) nanozyme | Microspheres | Colorimetric detection of gallic acid | (26) |

*(Continued)*

**TABLE 6.1 (Continued)**
**Selected POD-Like Nanozymes and Their Applications**

| Nanozyme | Shape Structure | Application | Ref. |
|---|---|---|---|
| CuO tandem nanozyme | Nanoparticles | Ascorbic acid and alkaline phosphatase detection | (27) |
| FeS$_2$/SiO$_2$ Double Mesoporous nanozyme | Hollow spheres | Determination of H$_2$O$_2$ and Glutathione | (28) |
| Homogeneous Copper (Cu NCs) nanozyme | Nanoclusters | Colorimetric sensing of H$_2$O$_2$ and GSH | (29) |
| Bimetallic Au@Pt nanozymes | Nanoparticles | Detection of streptomycin (STR) | (30) |
| One-dimensional core–shell Fe$_3$O$_4$@C/Ni nanocomposites | Nanotubes | Colorimetric detection of H$_2$O$_2$ and cholesterol | (31) |
| Hyaluronic acid attached-silica microspheres containing accessible magnetite nanoparticles (HA@Fe$_3$O$_4$@SiO$_2$) | Microparticles | Colorimetric determination of tumor cells | (32) |
| Polythiocyanuric acid-functionalized MoS$_2$ NS (PTCA–MoS$_2$ NS). | Nanosheets | Detection of H$_2$O$_2$ (direct) and glucose (indirect *via* glucose oxidase) | (34) |
| The magnetic Fe$_3$O$_4$-TiO$_2$/reduced graphene oxide (Fe$_3$O$_4$-TiO$_2$/rGO) nanocomposite | Tetragonal crystalline TiO$_2$ NPs on rGO sheets. | Detection of any pesticides in an aqueous medium | (35) |
| AuPd nanozyme | Nanocluster | Quantitative determination of acid phosphatase (ACP) | (24) |
| Polyallylamine-stabilized IrO$_2$/ graphene oxide nanozyme | nanosheets | Ascorbic acid in real samples | (36) |
| Silica microspheres functionalized with the iminodiacetic acid/copper(II) | Microspheres | Colorimetric determination of histidine-tagged proteins | (37) |

## 6.2.1 Transition MOs-Based

Transition MOs [MeO$_x$, Me = manganese (Mn), zinc (Zn), iron (Fe), copper (Cu), cobalt (Co), and nickel (Ni)] have been widely used in the field of colorimetric determination of various biomolecules due to their POD-like or OXD-like activity (38–42). Generally, it may be necessary to provide functional groups to chemically and biologically inert MO NPs by combining them with reactive substances (41). Iron oxide (Fe$_x$O$_y$)-based (including Fe$_3$O$_4$ and Fe$_2$O$_3$) NPs are the most widely used nanozymes. However, in recent years, there have been many studies reporting enzyme-like activities, such as cobalt oxide (CoO), manganese dioxide (MnO$_2$), vanadium oxide (VO), and copper oxide (CuO) NPs (41, 43). Gao et al. (11) reported that oxidation of several POD substrates was catalyzed in the presence of H$_2$O$_2$ using Fe$_3$O$_4$ magnetic NPs (MNPs). The studies in which 3,3′,5,5′-tetramethylbenzidine (TMB), o-phenylenediamine dihydrochloride (OPD), (2,2′-Azinobis [3-ethylbenzothiazoline-6-sulfonic acid]-diammonium salt) (ABTS) are preferred as POD substrates and the biological molecules, such as proteins, nucleic acids, and different types of cells, are determined using colorimetric protocol using iron oxide NPs have attracted great interest (44, 45). $Fe_xO_y$ NPs, which have high chemical stability in a wide temperature and pH range and magnetic functions, can be synthesized at a low cost (43, 46, 47). On the other hand, it is necessary to modify the surface of $Fe_xO_y$ NPs since they can be easily agglomerated in biological samples due to their size and inappropriate surface charge (48). The detection sensitivity in the presence of $H_2O_2$ is strongly dependent on the oxidation ability of $Fe_xO_y$ NPs against the POD substrate selected. However, the POD-like activity of $Fe_xO_y$ NPs decreases with the formation of a surface coating around them. For this reason, some metals, such as Au and platinum (Pt), are deposited onto $Fe_xO_y$ NPs or integrated with other nano–micro materials. These $Fe_xO_y$ NPs-based hybrid materials are widely preferred to increase the activity of $Fe_xO_y$-based NPs (49, 50). Öğüt et al. reported that $Fe_3O_4$ NPs immobilized in the porous interior of monodisperse-porous silica microspheres (pSiO2) provided enhanced POD-like activity (51). The nanozyme prepared by immobilizing $Fe_3O_4$ NPs in the porous monodisperse silica microspheres exhibited POD-like activity while bare $Fe_3O_4$ NPs did not show any significant activity due to the aggregation in the aqueous medium containing human genomic DNA (hgDNA) (**Figure 6.1A–C**) (51). Kip et al. (32) also used the above $Fe_3O_4$ NPs immobilized in pSiO2 as POD-like nanozyme for a colorimetric determination of tumor cell concentration with T98G glioblastoma and HeLa cells.

$Fe_3O_4$ NPs-based hybrid materials with enhanced POD-like activity, such as $Fe_3O_4@Cu@Cu_2O$ nanocomposite, meso-tetrakis (4-carboxyphenyl)-porphyrin-functionalized $\gamma$-$Fe_2O_3$ NPs ($H_2$TCPP-$\gamma$-$Fe_2O_3$), yolk-shell nanostructured $Fe_3O_4@$

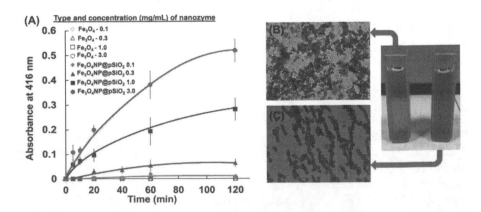

**FIGURE 6.1** (A) The variation of absorbance of the reaction medium at 416 nm over time in the presence of hgDNA using bare $Fe_3O_4$ NPs or $Fe_3O_4$ NPs@pSiO2 as the nanozyme. hgDNA concentration: 150 ng/μL (10.7 nM). The concentration of both nanozymes varied between 0.1 and 3.0 mg/mL in a reaction volume of 4.0 mL at pH 5.0. OPDA concentration: 100 μM, 100 rpm, Room temperature. (B) The optical micrograph of the aqueous dispersion containing bare $Fe_3O_4$ NPs (3 mg/mL) and hgDNA (150 ng/μL). (C) The optical micrograph of the aqueous dispersion containing $Fe_3O_4$NP@pSiO2 microspheres (3 mg/mL) and hgDNA (150 ng/μL). Magnification: X400. (Copyright©, Reproduced from (51) with permission from Elsevier Inc.)

carbon NPs, core-shell $Fe_3O_4$@carbon/Ni nanocomposites, and the magnetic $Fe_3O_4$-$TiO_2$/reduced graphene oxide (rGO) nanocomposite, have been successfully prepared and applied in the colorimetric detection of $H_2O_2$, glucose, and cholesterol (31, 35, 52–54).

The POD-like activity of $Fe_3O_4$ NPs can also be increased by combining with various metals to form MO complexes, such as $Fe_3O_4$@Pt NPs, Au/$Fe_3O_4$/GO hybrid material, and Au-loaded ferric oxide ($Fe_2O_3$) nanocubes, $Fe_3O_4$-Pt/core-shell NPs, $Fe_3O_4$@$SiO_2$-$NH_2$-Au@Pd NPs, Au@$SiO_2$ microspheres. These materials were evaluated in the colorimetric detection of biomarkers, $Hg^{2+}$, glucose, and various cells (12, 13, 22, 49, 55, 56). Gökçal et al. synthesized Au NPs-decorated magnetic, $pSiO_2$ with high POD-like activity. Based on the decrease of the activity with the increasing glutathione (GSH) adsorption onto the nanozyme, the nanozyme was applied for the determination of the GSH concentration in biological samples (23).

$MnO_x$ (MnO, $MnO_2$, $Mn_2O_3$, $Mn_3O_4$, $Mn_5O_8$)-based nanomaterials, which can be obtained in various shapes and morphologies, have high POD-, OXD-, and catalase (CAT)-like activities probably originated from their highly porous special crystal structures (57, 58). Compared to natural enzymes, such as horseradish peroxidase (HRP), $MnO_x$-based nanozymes showed high stability in addition to their low cost and simple preparation. $MnO_x$-based nanozymes are capable of oxidizing various substrates (TMB or OPD) in the absence of $H_2O_2$ (57, 58). This property eliminates the possible instability problems that may originate from $H_2O_2$. With all these features, these nanozymes are widely used as colorimetric or fluorometric biosensors for the determination of biomolecules, such as proteins, vitamins, GSH, etc., with high sensitivity and selectivity. $MnO_x$-based nanozymes have intrinsic POD-like activity and catalyze the oxidation of OPDA to 2,3-diaminophenazine in the absence of $H_2O_2$ (59). By using this property, $MnO_x$ microspheres were evaluated as an OXD mimic for colorimetric detection of ascorbic acid (AA) (59).

$MnO_2$-based nanozymes provide high and efficient analyte adsorption due to their highly porous structures and exhibit an effective catalytic activity (60–63). This property makes it easier to use these materials as the nanozymes for detecting various biological agents. $MnO_2$ NPs MnO nanosheets and $MnO_2$ nanoflakes also exhibit POD-like activity for the detection of metal ions, bacteria, protein, and glucose (60–63).

$Co_3O_4$ NPs have more efficient catalytic activity and have better stability at high temperatures and extreme pH values compared to natural catalysis (64–68). $Co_3O_4$-based nanozymes having different morphologies, such as NPs, nanoplates, nanotubes, and nanocrystals, were synthesized with excellent catalytic activity for the sensing of glucose, $H_2O_2$, and GSH (64, 65, 67, 68).

Other MO-based nanozymes, such as CuO, NiO, and ZnO, have also been reported (27, 69–71). CuO NPs provide intrinsic POD-like activity (27). He et al. developed CuO NPs, which displayed intrinsic glutathione oxidase- and POD-like activities as a dual-functional nanozyme with high sensitivity (69). Yan et al. prepared NiO assembled on ordered mesoporous carbon, which exhibited excellent POD-like activity for colorimetric detection of gallic acid with high selectivity and sensitivity (70). Tripathi et al. developed colorimetric sensors based on ZnO-Pd nanosheets, that oxidize TMB in the presence of $H_2O_2$ (71).

## 6.2.2 NOBLE METAL-BASED

Noble metals (Au, Pt, etc.)-based materials mimic natural enzymes, similar to transition MO-based materials. The nanocomposites which are synthesized by combining a noble metal-based nanozyme with other nanozymes exhibit synergistic effects that significantly increase their catalytic performance (72–75). Au NPs are widely used in biomedical applications with their physical and chemical, tunable optical properties, large surface-to-volume ratios, low toxicity, ease of surface functionalization, and excellent biocompatibility. The biosensing applications of Au-based nanozymes are remarkable for the detection of proteins, ions, nucleic acids, small molecules, and cells (76). Chen et al. developed Au nanoclusters (NCs) for the detection of $H_2O_2$ with colorimetric and fluorescence methods. In their study, Au NCs were used as a template to obtain Au NPs encapsulated by Au NCs. This composite nanozyme exhibited glucose oxidase (GOx)-like activity and was used for glucose sensing (77). Deng et al. investigated the synthesized cerium ($Ce^{3+}$) bound Au NPs as a POD-like nanozyme for the detection of $Ce^{3+}$. They demonstrated that the POD-like activity of the designed nanozyme increased with $Ce^{3+}$ concentration (78). Das et al. developed an Au nanozyme (an aptamer-mediated tunable Au nanozyme sensor) with POD- and ascorbate oxidase-like activities for potential detection of a bacterial pathogen (79). Ye et al. demonstrated the intrinsic POD-like activity of thin 2-D Au nano seaweeds for colorimetric detection of $H_2O_2$ with high sensitivity (80).

Also, alloying Au NPs with other metals or combining them with other nanozymes to form composites is the most effective way to improve the catalytic properties of metal-based nanozymes exhibiting synergistic effects. The high POD-like activity of Au@Pt nanozyme has been applied for the detection of streptomycin (30). Au-tipped Pt nanorods (NRs) have very strong POD-mimicking activity and have been used to construct colorimetric assays for the detection of AA (81). Biogenic Au Pd NCs exhibited synergistic effects, which significantly enhanced the catalytic performance for colorimetric determination of acid phosphatase (24). The intrinsic POD-like activity of Au NPs supported by cationic cellulose nanofibrils for glucose detection has also been reported (14). Qi et al. developed a colorimetric detection platform for ultrasensitive DNA detection by using POD mimetics of graphene oxide (GO)/Au NPs nanocomposite (82). A hybrid catalyst consisting of "naked" Au NPs *in situ* grown on graphitic carbon nitride (GCN) nanosheets (NSs) (Au NPs@GCN NSs) was developed (83). This nanozyme showed high POD activity compared to pure GCN NSs and naked Au NPs and was used as a colorimetric detection platform for $H_2O_2$ and glucose detection (83).

Pt NPs are widely used as a POD-mimicking sensing platform (21, 84–86). Gu et al. developed heparin-stabilized Pt NPs for the detection of glucose with high sensitivity (21). Su et al. synthesized a new nanozyme by decorating magnetic carbon nanospheres with PtNPs for the detection of $H_2O_2$ (85). Li et al. developed a novel and ultrasensitive system for heparin detection in both aqueous solution and biological fluid using N-acetyl-L-cysteine-stabilized Pt nanozyme (NAC–Pt NCs). The cluster size and the charge state of NAC–Pt NCs mainly contributed to their POD-like activity (84). A platinum (II)-doped GCN was synthesized by thermal polymerization showed an enhanced POD-like activity compared to GCN (86).

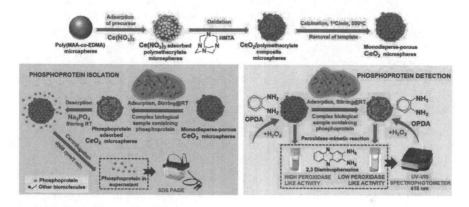

**FIGURE 6.2** The schematic representation of synthesis CeO$_2$microspheres with POD-like activity for colorimetric detection of phosphoproteins. (Copyright©, Reproduced from (18) with permission from Elsevier Inc.)

### 6.2.3 LANTHANIDE OXIDE-BASED

Cerium oxide (CeO$_2$) has recently emerged as a possible agent for biosensing applications, with its fluorite crystal structure and enzyme-like activities of CAT, OXD, and POD. CeO$_2$-based nanozymes have the advantage of having adjustable catalytic activity compared to the natural enzymes, and their POD-like activity is increasingly investigated especially for the detection of H$_2$O$_2$ and glucose (87).

Yıldırım et al. synthesized monodisperse-porous CeO$_2$ microspheres with a large surface area and a considerable pore volume (18). These microspheres showed dual functions including selective adsorption of phosphoproteins and intrinsic POD activity (**Figure 6.2**) (18, 88).

Li et al. reported that Pt nanocube-CeO$_2$ nanocomposite has intrinsic POD-like activity and use it to detect metabolites, including H$_2$O$_2$ and glucose (89). Liu et al. designed Pt/CeO$_2$ nanocomposites by using a polyol reduction process for the detection of AA with high sensitivity and selectivity (90). Bhagat et al. designed an Au core/ceria (CeO$_2$) shell-based colorimetric sensor for the detection of H$_2$O$_2$. Compared with natural HRP, Au/CeO$_2$ exhibited higher POD-like activity at extreme reaction conditions (91). The results also demonstrated that Au/CeO$_2$ can be used as a POD-like nanozyme for easy and rapid detection of the blood glucose level of both normal and diabetic persons (91).

## 6.3 BIOSENSING APPLICATIONS

### 6.3.1 SMALL BIOMOLECULES

Nanozymes have received much attention for the detection of small molecules, such as H$_2$O$_2$, glucose, GSH, and ascorbic acid. H$_2$O$_2$, which is produced by an incomplete reduction of metabolite oxygen, is a byproduct of numerous biological reactions. Therefore, the detection of H$_2$O$_2$ is important in different fields, such as medicine, biology, and food science (92). Different nanozymes have been used for the colorimetric detection of $H_2O_2$. Wang et al. synthesized Au–Hg amalgam-loaded rGO nanosheets as a nanozyme (93). Zhang et al. designed hollow $Co_3O_4/MO_3$ (M = Mo, W) hybrid by Mo or W doping of ZIF-67 for the detection of $H_2O_2$ both with OXD-like and POD-like activities by catalyzing the oxidation of TMB (94). Liu et al. synthesized human serum albumin@polydopamine/Fe nanocomposites (HSA@ PDA/Fe NCs) for the *in vitro* and *in situ* colorimetric detection of $H_2O_2$ generated from live cells (29). Yao et al. synthesized bimetallic Ag–Pt NPs-decorated rGO by UV-assisted one-pot method (95). Chen et al. fabricated vanadium tetrasulfide ($VS_4$) submicrospheres by hydrothermal method (96). Xi et al. synthesized Fe-doped GCN nanoflakes by one-step pyrolysis and showed that it exhibited POD-like activity (97).

Glucose plays different roles in some cerebral functions like learning and memory and for this reason, it is important to measure the glucose level in brain tissue. Also, easy and quick measurement of glucose in human blood is an important point for diabetes patients (2). However, the high dilution of biological samples makes it difficult for colorimetric sensors to detect glucose levels in a complex sample. Gökçal et al. designed a new magnetic nanozyme with POD- and OXD-like activities by immobilizing GOx on Au NPs attached-magnetic $SiO_2$ microspheres (GOx@Au@ mMagSiO$_2$) and used to measure glucose concentration directly in human blood without any sample pretreatment. (**Figure 6.3**) (22).

Yin et al. synthesized $SO_4^{2-}/CoFe_2O_4$ nanozyme for colorimetric glucose detection at physiological pH by combining POD mimic with GOx (16). $CeO_2@MnO_2$ core-shell hollow nanosphere was synthesized growing $MnO_2$ nanolayer on hollow $CeO_2$ nanospheres. The prepared nanospheres exhibited GOx-like photoenzyme property and were used for photoelectrochemical sensing of glucose in pH-7.0 PBS buffer (98). Au@Pd NPs decorated nanomagnet-silica shell NPs ($Fe_3O_4@SiO_2$-NH$_2$-Au@

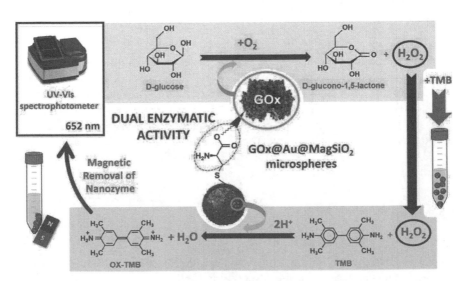

**FIGURE 6.3** The mechanism for one-pot colorimetric detection of glucose using the dual enzymatic activity of GOx@Au@MagSiO$_2$ microspheres. (Copyright©, Reproduced from (37) with permission from Elsevier Inc.)

PdNPs) were synthesized and used for the colorimetric detection of glucose (12). Cai et al. fabricated two-dimensional (2D) Pd nanosheet-supported zero-dimensional (0D) Au NPs for the detection of glucose (99). An MOF-based integrated nanozyme was synthesized by encapsulating GOx within Cu 1,4-benzenedicarboxylate MOF nanozyme via a one-step biomimetic mineralization process. This nanozyme was used for the detection of glucose (15). GOx-immobilized boronic acid-functionalized porous MIL-88B (GOx@HPMIL-88B-BA) was prepared for rapid one-step detection of glucose (100). Atomically dispersed single iron site nanozyme with high POD-like performance was synthesized for glucose detection (17).

GSH takes part in some important processes, such as redox balance, signal transmission, and gene regulation. Also, the wrong expression of GSH may result in different diseases, such as inflammation, cancer, or cardiovascular diseases (28). Gökçal et al. synthesized Au NPs- immobilized $pSiO_2$ ($Au@SiO_2@Fe_3O_4@SiO_2$) as a nanozyme that has POD-like activity and was used for the detection of GSH in human serum (**Figure 6.4**) (37). There are several other GSH detection schemes: $CoSe_2$ hollow microspheres via self-templated synthesis (101); carbon nanodots

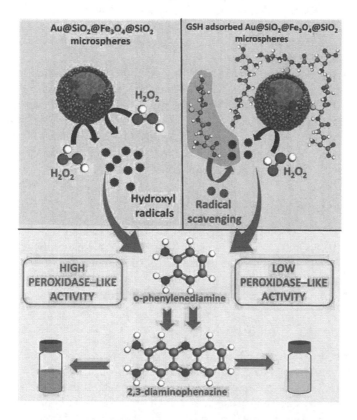

**FIGURE 6.4**    The scheme for colorimetric detection of GSH using $Au@SiO_2@Fe_3O_4@SiO_2$ microspheres. (Copyright©, Reproduced from (23) with permission from Royal Society of Chemistry).

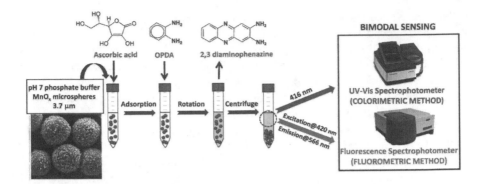

**FIGURE 6.5** The bimodal sensing protocol for colorimetric and fluorometric determination of the AA by MnOx microspheres. (Copyright©, Reproduced from (59) with permission from Royal Society of Chemistry).

(C-dots) with POD activity (102); sodium lignosulfonate-loaded Cu peroxide composites produced by a simple two-step method (29); monodisperse, homogeneous Cu NCs (19); $FeS_2/SiO_2$ double mesoporous hollow spheres (28); OXD-mimicking $Mn_3O_4$ microspheres (103); $Cu-CuFe_2O_4$ nanozyme synthesized by a facile hydrothermal method (104); and Mn–Co-containing nanosheets MOF synthesized by the ultrasonic hydrothermal method (105).

Vitamins are involved in different physiological functions and their lack or excess will cause risk on human health. Thus, the measurement of vitamin concentration is necessary. Tosun et al. synthesized monodisperse-porous MnOx microspheres and used them as a nanozyme for bimodal sensing of AA (vitamin C) via colorimetric and fluorometric methods (59). (**Figure 6.5**) Some other nanozymes, such as Pt NPs-decorated $CeO_2$ NRs (90), $CuO_2$ NPs (27), and N-doped carbon nanostructure (106) were also used for the colorimetric detection of AA.

### 6.3.2  NUCLEIC ACIDS (DNA)

Nucleic acids can be colorimetrically detected using different POD-like nanozymes (51, 82, 107, 108). Öğüt et al. used monodisperse porous magnetic silica microspheres ($Fe_3O_4NP@pSiO_2$) as a nanozyme for the colorimetric detection of hgDNA (51). Au NPs on GO (82), Pt NPs on GO (108), mesoporous Si, and Pt NPs (107) have also been used for the colorimetric detection of nucleic acids.

### 6.3.3  TUMOR CELLS AND BACTERIA

An antibody or ligand immobilized nanozymes can be used for the colorimetric detection of cancer cells by recognizing the overexpressed receptors which are the biomarkers (32, 109–112). Kip et al. designed a nanozyme-functionalized with hyaluronic acid (HA) as a ligand sensitive to CD44 receptors of tumor cells (32). In this study, monodisperse-porous magnetic silica microspheres were synthesized and HA was immobilized on microspheres by using carbodiimide activation ($HA@Fe_3O_4@SiO_2$) as a nanozyme. (**Figure 6.6**)

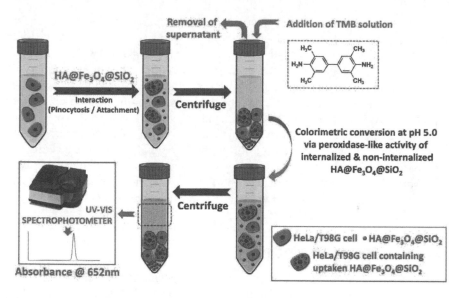

**FIGURE 6.6** The scheme for colorimetric determination of HeLa or T98 G cell concentration with HA@Fe$_3$O$_4$@SiO$_2$ microspheres. (Copyright©, Reproduced from (32) with permission from Elsevier Inc.)

Tian et al. synthesized CuO$_2$-immobilized rGO/Au NPs composite and used them as a nanozyme for the detection of circulating tumor cells by an ultrasensitive electrochemical detection method (112). Fluorescence hybrid nanozyme with flower-like nanostructures integrated with C-dots were conjugated with folic acid (FA) to obtain Fe$_3$(PO$_4$)$_2$·8H$_2$O–CDs–FA hybrid nanoflowers (hNFls). The hNFls exhibited POD-like activity and were used for the colorimetric detection of cancer cells (109). Li et al. described the colorimetric detection of circulating tumor cells by bifunctional MNPs (111). Cu$_2$–xSe NPs-immobilized on rGO hybrids (Cu$_2$–xSe/rGO) as an efficient nanozyme for visual detection of cancer cells (110). The nanozymes have been also used for the colorimetric detection of bacteria such as *Escherichia coli* O157:H7 (113–115) and *Staphylococcus aureus* (116, 117).

## 6.3.4 Proteins

Detection of proteins has great importance in clinical diagnosis, treatment, and biological research. Different nanozymes have been used for the colorimetric detection of proteins with POD reactions (23, 94, 118–121). Gökçal et al. synthesized iminodiacetic acid-Cu$^{2+}$ complex functionalized-porous silica microspheres (Cu(II)@IDA-GPTMS@SiO$_2$) and used as a POD nanozyme for the colorimetric detection of green fluorescent protein (GFP) as a histidine-tagged protein in *E. coli* lysate (37). Yıldırım et al. reported the usage of monodisperse-porous CeO$_2$ microspheres as a new POD nanozyme for the colorimetric detection of phosphoprotein from complex biological samples, such as milk and human serum (18) **(Figure 6.2)**.

Other examples include that of Wang et al., who reported a simple colorimetric sensor array for the detection of phosphorylated proteins using a Zr-based MOF as a POD-mimicking nanozyme in the presence of $H_2O_2$ and TMB (33). Son et al. synthesized 3-aminophenylboronic acid (APBA) modified PB NPs with POD-like activity and used for the detection of glycated albumin by catalyzing the oxidation of TMB in the presence of $H_2O_2$ (119). Citicoline bovine serum albumin-conjugated and aptamer-functionalized Au NPs were synthesized as a new nanozyme for the colorimetric detection of C-reactive protein in the blood (121). Nanoceria-linked GCN quantum dots (QDs) were used for colorimetric and fluorescent detection of cardiac troponin I (118). 1-D $Fe_3O_4$@carbon core-shell nanowires with POD activity were synthesized and used for ultrasensitive colorimetric detection of target protein (42). Various nanozymes used for the detection of different analytes and their performance metrics are given in **Table 6.2**.

## 6.4  SUMMARY AND FUTURE PERSPECTIVES

Nanozymes have attracted significant attention as potential candidates in place of natural enzymes in various biotechnological applications. Different types of MO NPs have been tried in various biotechnological and biomedical applications. The nanozymes with POD-like activity are the strong candidates that can be utilized instead of POD particularly in ELISA-based detection kits developed for different biological agents.

In general, the enzyme mimetic activities of most nanozymes are lower than those of natural enzymes. The surface modifications of nanozymes aiming to increase their specificities against target molecules mostly result in lower enzyme-mimetic activities. To develop surface modification techniques aiming to increase their specificity without decreasing the enzyme mimetic activity is an important topic extensively investigated for improving the performances of current nanozymes. The synthesis of target-specific ligand attached or molecularly imprinted (i.e., plastic antibody attached) nanomaterials with enzyme-mimetic activity is another challenge for improving the performance. The preparation of composite nanomaterials by integrating/attaching nanomaterials with different functions at the molecular level is a current approach to synthesize nanozymes with synergistic enzyme-mimetic activity. The development of biomimetic synthesis protocols will also allow obtaining more biocompatible, nontoxic nanozymes that can be more commonly utilized in biomedical applications.

The development of surface and bulk analysis techniques, such as X-ray photoelectron spectroscopy and X-ray fluorescence spectroscopy, enables a better understanding of the atomic structure, the reversible switching ability between valence states, and the presence of oxygen vacancies of nanomaterials. Hence, the molecular design of nanomaterials with higher enzyme mimetic activity and higher specificity can be achieved by utilizing the information from advanced structural analyses. Imaging, cancer diagnosis and therapy, and immunoassays are the most prospective areas for active future nanozymes research.

## TABLE 6.2
## Applications of Different Nanozymes in Biosensing

| Target Analyte | Nanozyme | Enzyme-like Activity | Linear Range (µM) | LOD (µM) | Ref. |
|---|---|---|---|---|---|
| $H_2O_2$ | Au–Hg/rGO | Peroxidase | 5–100 | 3.25 | (92) |
| | $Co_3O_4/MoO_3$ | Oxidase/Peroxidase | 0.1–200 | 0.08 | (93) |
| | HSA@PDA/Fe NCs | Peroxidase | 1–200 | 0.06 | (42) |
| | Ag-Pt/rGO | Peroxidase | 10–100 | 0.90 | (122) |
| | $VS_4$ | Peroxidase | 50–100 | 5.00 | (95) |
| | Fe@GCN NFs | Peroxidase | 2–100 | 1.18 | (96) |
| Glucose | GOx@Au@MagSiO$_2$ | Oxidase/Peroxidase | 2.8–38.9[a] | 1.78[a] | (22) |
| | $SO_4^{2-}/CoFe_2O_4$ | Peroxidase | 100–300 | 6.40 | (17) |
| | $CeO_2@MnO_2$ | Oxidase | 0.1–300 | 0.07 | (16) |
| | $Fe_3O_4@SiO_2$-NH$_2$-Au@PdNPs | Peroxidase | 0.01–60 | 0.60 | (98) |
| | Au$_x$Pd$_{100-x}$ NCs | Peroxidase | 5–400 | 0.85 | (12) |
| | GOx@CuBDC | Oxidase/Peroxidase | 10–500 | 4.10 | (99) |
| | GOx@HPMIL-88B-BA | Oxidase/Peroxidase | 2–100 | 0.98 | (15) |
| | Fe SSN | Peroxidase | 10–60 | 2.10 | (100) |
| Glutathione | Au@SiO$_2$@Fe$_3$O$_4$@SiO$_2$ | Peroxidase | 0–5 | 0.24 | (23) |
| | CoSe$_2$ hollow MS | Peroxidase | 0.005–10 | 4.62[b] | (17) |
| | CDs | Peroxidase | 0–7 | 0.30 | (123) |
| | Fe$_3$O$_4$@CP | Peroxidase | 0.2–40 | 0.05 | (102) |
| | CuNCs | Peroxidase | 1–150 | 0.89 | (29) |
| | FeS$_2$/SiO$_2$ DMHSs | Peroxidase | 1–40 | 0.16 | (19) |
| | Mn$_3$O$_4$ MSs | Oxidase | 5–60 | 0.90 | (28) |
| | Cu-CuFe$_2$O$_4$ | Peroxidase | 2.5–10 | 0.31 | (103) |
| | Mn-Co NS | Peroxidase | 0.1–25 | 0.07 | (104) |
| Ascorbic acid | MnO$_x$ MSs | Oxidase | 0.57–4.5[a] | 0.74[a] | (59) |
| | Pt/CeO$_2$ NCs | Peroxidase | 0.5–30 | 0.08 | (105) |
| | CuO$_2$ NPs | Oxidase | 0.75–7.5 | 0.03 | (90) |
| | N-doped carbon nanozyme | Peroxidase | 8–80 | 8.00 | (27) |
| Nucleic acid | Fe$_3$O$_4$NP@pSiO$_2$ | Peroxidase | 0–21.5[b] | 1.10[b] | (51) |
| | GO/AuNPs nanocomposite | Peroxidase | 0.4–120[b] | 8.00[c] | (106) |
| | GO–PtNPs | Peroxidase | 25–5000[c] | 14.60[c] | (82) |
| | MS-PtNPs | MS-PtNPs | 500–100000[c] | 2.60[c] | (108) |
| Tumor cells | HA@Fe$_3$O$_4$@SiO$_2$ MSs | Peroxidase | 0.25–4.0×10$^6$[d] | 2×10$^{-6}$[d] | (32) |
| | CuO/ rGO/AuNPs | Peroxidase | 50–10000[d] | 27.00[d] | (107) |
| | Fe$_3$(PO$_4$)$_2$·8H$_2$O–CDs–FA hNFs | Peroxidase | 0–130000[d] | 25.00[d] | (112) |
| | MNPs | Peroxidase | 50–5×10$^4$[d] | 13.00[d] | (109) |
| | Cu$_2$–xSe/rGO | Peroxidase | - | 45.00[d] | (111) |
| Bacteria | AuNP-ICA | Peroxidase | 5000–250000[e] | 12.50[e] | (110) |
| | AuNRs | Peroxidase | 10$^2$–10$^5$ [e] | 22.00[e] | (114) |
| | Ap@PtNp | Peroxidase | 10–10$^7$ [e] | 14.00[e] | (115) |

(Continued)

**TABLE 6.2 (Continued)**
**Applications of Different Nanozymes in Biosensing**

| Target Analyte | Nanozyme | Enzyme-like Activity | Linear Range (μM) | LOD (μM) | Ref. |
|---|---|---|---|---|---|
| | IgY-Fe$_3$O$_4$/Au NCs | Peroxidase | 10– 10$^{6}$ $^e$ | 10.00$^e$ | (113) |
| | Co$_3$O$_4$ MNE | Peroxidase | 10–10000$^e$ | 8.00$^e$ | (117) |
| Proteins | Cu(II)@IDA-GPTMS@SiO$_2$ | Peroxidase | 9.0–92$^f$ | 6.20$^f$ | (37) |
| | CeO$_2$ | Peroxidase | 0–800$^f$ | 21.20$^f$ | (18) |
| | Zr-MOF | Peroxidase | 0.17–5.0$^f$ | 0.16$^f$ | (120) |
| | APBA-modified PBNPs | Peroxidase | 10–2000$^f$ | 7.30$^f$ | (119) |
| | cBSA-aptamer@AuNPs | Peroxidase | 0.0001–0.2$^f$ | 8.00$^g$ | (121) |
| | nCeO2 linked-GCN QDs | Peroxidase | 1–10000$^g$ | 0.41$^g$ | (118) |
| | Fe$_3$O$_4$@CNWs | Peroxidase | 10–100000$^g$ | 10.00$^g$ | (124) |

$^a$Concentration in mM.
$^b$Concentration in nM.
$^c$Concentration in pM.
$^d$Concentration in cells/mL.
$^e$Concentration in CFU/mL.
$^f$Concentration in μg/mL.
$^g$Concentration in pg/mL.

# REFERENCES

1. Wang Q, Wei H, Zhang Z, Wang E, Dong S. 2018. *TrAC Trends in Analytical Chemistry* 105: 218–24
2. Huang Y, Ren J, Qu X. 2019. *Chemical Reviews* 119: 4357–412
3. Choct M. 2006. *World's Poultry Science Journal* 62: 5–16
4. Gurung N, Ray S, Bose S, Rai V. 2013. *BioMed Research International* 2013
5. Posorske L. 1984. *Journal of the American Oil Chemists' Society* 61: 1758–60
6. Zhou Y, Liu B, Yang R, Liu J. 2017. *Bioconjugate Chemistry* 28: 2903–9
7. Lin Y, Ren J, Qu X. 2014. *Accounts of Chemical Research* 47: 1097–105
8. Wei H, Wang E. 2013. *Chemical Society Reviews* 42: 6060–93
9. Wang X, Hu Y, Wei H. 2016. *Inorganic Chemistry Frontiers* 3: 41–60
10. Manea F, Houillon FB, Pasquato L, Scrimin P. 2004. *Angewandte Chemie* 116: 6291–5
11. Gao L, Zhuang J, Nie L, Zhang J, Zhang Y, et al. 2007. *Nature Nanotechnology* 2: 577–83
12. Adeniyi O, Sicwetsha S, Mashazi P. 2020. *ACS Applied Materials & Interfaces* 12: 1973–87
13. Zhang S, Li H, Wang Z, Liu J, Zhang H, et al. 2015. *Nanoscale* 7: 8495–502
14. Alle M, Park SC, Bandi R, Lee S-H, Kim J-C. 2021. *Carbohydrate Polymers* 253: 117239
15. Cheng X, Zheng Z, Zhou X, Kuang Q. 2020. *ACS Sustainable Chemistry & Engineering* 8: 17783–90
16. Yin X, Liu P, Xu X, Pan J, Li X, Niu X. 2021. *Sensors and Actuators B: Chemical* 328: 129033
17. Chen M, Zhou H, Liu X, Yuan T, Wang W, et al. 2020. *Small* 16: 2002343

18. Yıldırım D, Gökçal B, Büber E, Kip Ç, Demir MC, Tuncel A. 2021. *Chemical Engineering Journal* 403: 126357
19. Wang F, Chen L, Liu D, Ma W, Dramou P, He H. 2020. *TrAC Trends in Analytical Chemistry* 133: 116080
20. Maity S, Bain D, Chakraborty S, Kolay S, Patra A. 2020. *ACS Sustainable Chemistry & Engineering* 8: 18335–44
21. Gu H, Huang Q, Zhang J, Li W, Fu Y. 2020. *Colloids and Surfaces A: Physicochemical and Engineering Aspects* 606: 125455
22. Gökçal B, Kip Ç, Tuncel A. 2020. *Journal of Alloys and Compounds* 843: 156012
23. Gökçal B, Hamaloğlu KÖ, Kip Ç, Güngör SY, Büber E, Tuncel A. 2020. *Analytical Methods* 12: 5219–28
24. Zheng S, Gu H, Yin D, Zhang J, Li W, Fu Y. 2020. *Colloids and Surfaces A: Physicochemical and Engineering Aspects* 589: 124444
25. Gupta PK, Son SE, Seong GH. 2020. *Materials Science and Engineering: C* 116: 111231
26. Chen L, Yang J, Chen W, Sun S, Tang H, Li Y. 2020. *Sensors and Actuators B: Chemical* 321: 128642
27. He S-B, Balasubramanian P, Hu A-L, Zheng X-Q, Lin M-T, et al. 2020. *Sensors and Actuators B: Chemical* 321: 128511
28. Huang X, Xia F, Nan Z. 2020. *ACS Applied Materials & Interfaces* 12: 46539–48
29. Liu G, Liu H, Xu H, Zhu L, Su C, et al. 2020. *Spectrochimica Acta Part A: Molecular and Biomolecular Spectroscopy* 239: 118544
30. Wei D, Zhang X, Chen B, Zeng K. 2020. *Analytica Chimica Acta* 1126: 106–13
31. Peng H, Zhang J, Zeng C, Zhou C, Li Q, et al. 2020. *ACS Applied Bio Materials* 3: 5111–9
32. Kip Ç, Akbay E, Gökçal B, Savaş BO, Onur MA, Tuncel A. 2020. *Colloids and Surfaces A: Physicochemical and Engineering Aspects* 598: 124812
33. Wang Q, Hong G, Liu Y, Hao J, Liu S. 2020. *RSC Advances* 10: 25209–13
34. Sreeramareddygari M, Somasundrum M, Surareungchai W. 2020. *New Journal of Chemistry* 44: 5809–18
35. Boruah PK, Das MR. 2020. *Journal of Hazardous Materials* 385: 121516
36. Sun H, Liu X, Wang X, Han Q, Qi C, et al. 2020. *Microchimica Acta* 187: 1–9
37. Gökçal B, Kip Ç, Şahinbaş D, Çelik E, Tuncel A. 2020. *Microchimica Acta* 187: 1–9
38. Alizadeh N, Salimi A. 2021. *Journal of Nanobiotechnology* 19: 1–31
39. Attar F, Shahpar MG, Rasti B, Sharifi M, Saboury AA, et al. 2019. *Journal of Molecular Liquids* 278: 130–44
40. Liang M, Yan X. 2019. *Accounts of Chemical Research* 52: 2190–200
41. Shin HY, Park TJ, Kim MI. 2015. *Journal of Nanomaterials* 2015
42. Zhang X, Lin S, Liu S, Tan X, Dai Y, Xia F. 2020. *Coordination Chemistry Reviews*: 213652
43. Gao L, Fan K, Yan X. 2020. *Nanozymology*: 105–40
44. Gao Y, Zhou Y, Chandrawati R. 2020. *ACS Applied Nano Materials* 3: 1–21
45. Wei H, Wang E. 2008. *Analytical Chemistry* 80: 2250–4
46. Gao L, Yan X. 2019. *Biological and Bio-inspired Nanomaterials*: 291–312
47. Shi C, Li Y, Gu N. 2020. *ChemBioChem* 21: 2722–32
48. Ali A, Hira Zafar MZ, ul Haq I, Phull AR, Ali JS, Hussain A. 2016. *Nanotechnology, Science and Applications* 9: 49
49. Ma M, Xie J, Zhang Y, Chen Z, Gu N. 2013. *Materials Letters* 105: 36–9
50. Wang X, Ouyang F, Cui L, Xiong T, Guan X, et al. 2019. *Journal of Nanoparticle Research* 21: 1–13
51. Öğüt E, Kip Ç, Gökçal B, Tuncel A. 2019. *Journal of Colloid and Interface Science* 550: 90–8

52. Liu Q, Zhang L, Li H, Jia Q, Jiang Y, et al. 2015. *Materials Science and Engineering: C* 55: 193–200
53. Lu N, Zhang M, Ding L, Zheng J, Zeng C, et al. 2017. *Nanoscale* 9: 4508–15
54. Wang Z, Chen M, Shu J, Li Y. 2016. *Journal of Alloys and Compounds* 682: 432–40
55. Boriachek K, Masud MK, Palma C, Phan H-P, Yamauchi Y, et al. 2019. *Analytical Chemistry* 91: 3827–34
56. Kim MS, Kweon SH, Cho S, An SSA, Kim MI, et al. 2017. *ACS Applied Materials & Interfaces* 9: 35133–40
57. Wan Y, Qi P, Zhang D, Wu J, Wang Y. 2012. *Biosensors and Bioelectronics* 33: 69–74
58. Wu C-W, Unnikrishnan B, Tseng Y-T, Wei S-C, Chang H-T, Huang C-C. 2019. *Journal of Colloid and Interface Science* 541: 75–85
59. Tosun RB, Kip Ç, Tuncel A. 2019. *New Journal of Chemistry* 43: 18505–16
60. Han L, Zhang H, Chen D, Li F. 2018. *Advanced Functional Materials* 28: 1800018
61. Li Y, Wu J, Zhang C, Chen Y, Wang Y, Xie M. 2017. *Microchimica Acta* 184: 2767–74
62. Sun K, Liu Q, Zhu R, Liu Q, Li S, et al. 2019. *International Journal of Analytical Chemistry* 2019
63. Wu M, Hou P, Dong L, Cai L, Chen Z, et al. 2019. *International Journal of Nanomedicine* 14: 4781
64. Mu J, Wang Y, Zhao M, Zhang L. 2012. *Chemical Communications* 48: 2540–2
65. Wang Q, Chen J, Zhang H, Wu W, Zhang Z, Dong S. 2018. *Nanoscale* 10: 19140–6
66. Wei X, Chen J, Ali MC, Munyemana JC, Qiu H. 2020. *Microchimica Acta* 187: 1–9
67. Li W, Wang J, Zhu J, Zheng Y-Q. 2018. *Journal of Materials Chemistry B* 6: 6858–64
68. Wang T, Su P, Li H, Yang Y, Yang Y. 2016. *New Journal of Chemistry* 40: 10056–63
69. He L, Lu Y, Gao X, Song P, Huang Z, et al. 2018. *ACS Sustainable Chemistry & Engineering* 6: 12132–9
70. Yan L, Ren H, Guo Y, Wang G, Liu C, et al. 2019. *Talanta* 201: 406–12
71. Tripathi RM, Ahn D, Kim YM, Chung SJ. 2020. *Molecules* 25: 2585
72. Ahmed SR, Chen A. 2020. *ACS Applied Nano Materials* 3: 9462–9
73. Biswas S, Tripathi P, Kumar N, Nara S. 2016. *Sensors and Actuators B: Chemical* 231: 584–92
74. Stasyuk N, Smutok O, Demkiv O, Prokopiv T, Gayda G, et al. 2020. *Sensors* 20: 4509
75. Yu Z, Lou R, Pan W, Li N, Tang B. 2020. *Chemical Communications*
76. Sharifi M, Hosseinali SH, Yousefvand P, Salihi A, Shekha MS, et al. 2020. *Materials Science and Engineering: C* 108: 110422
77. Chen J, Wu W, Huang L, Ma Q, Dong S. 2019. *Chemistry–A European Journal* 25: 11940–4
78. Deng H-H, Luo B-Y, He S-B, Chen R-T, Lin Z, et al. 2019. *Analytical Chemistry* 91: 4039–46
79. Das R, Dhiman A, Kapil A, Bansal V, Sharma TK. 2019. *Analytical and Bioanalytical Chemistry* 411: 1229–38
80. Ye S, Brown AP, Stammers AC, Thomson NH, Wen J, et al. 2019. *Advanced Science* 6: 1900911
81. Gan H, Han W, Liu J, Qi J, Li H, Wang L. 2020. *Catalysts* 10: 1285
82. Qi Y, Chen Y, He J, Xiu F. 2020. *Microchemical Journal* 159: 105546
83. Li D, Garisto SL, Huang P-JJ, Yang J, Liu B, Liu J. 2019. *Inorganic Chemistry Communications* 106: 38–42
84. Xu X, Zou X, Wu S, Wang L, Pan J, et al. 2019. *Microchimica Acta* 186: 815
85. Su C, Bai L, Zhang H, Chang K, Li G, Li S. 2019. *Chemical Research in Chinese Universities* 35: 163–70
86. Zeng G, Duan M, Xu Y, Ge F, Wang W. 2020. *Spectrochimica Acta Part A: Molecular and Biomolecular Spectroscopy* 241: 118649
87. Singh S. 2016. *Biointerphases* 11: 04B202

88. Kang T, Kim YG, Kim D, Hyeon T. 2020. *Coordination Chemistry Reviews* 403: 213092
89. Li Z, Yang X, Yang Y, Tan Y, He Y, et al. 2018. *Chemistry – A European Journal* 24: 409–15
90. Liu X, Wang X, Qi C, Han Q, Xiao W, et al. 2019. *Applied Surface Science* 479: 532–9
91. Bhagat S, Vallabani NS, Shutthanandan V, Bowden M, Karakoti AS, Singh S. 2018. *Journal of Colloid and Interface Science* 513: 831–42
92. Wang T, Zhu H, Zhuo J, Zhu Z, Papakonstantinou P, et al. 2013. *Analytical Chemistry* 85: 10289–95
93. Kong F-Y, Yao L, Lu X-Y, Li H-Y, Wang Z-X, et al. 2020. *Analyst* 145: 2191–6
94. Zhang X, Lu Y, Chen Q, Huang Y. 2020. *Journal of Materials Chemistry B* 8: 6459–68
95. Yao L, Kong F-Y, Wang Z-X, Li H-Y, Zhang R, et al. 2020. *Microchimica Acta* 187: 1–8
96. Chen C, Wang Y, Zhang D. 2019. *Microchimica Acta* 186: 1–8
97. Kong W, Guo X, Jing M, Qu F, Lu L. 2020. *Biosensors and Bioelectronics* 150: 111875
98. Wang H, Yang W, Wang X, Huang L, Zhang Y, Yao S. 2020. *Sensors and Actuators B: Chemical* 304: 127389
99. Cai S, Fu Z, Xiao W, Xiong Y, Wang C, Yang R. 2020. *ACS Applied Materials & Interfaces* 12: 11616–24
100. Zhao Z, Huang Y, Liu W, Ye F, Zhao S. 2020. *ACS Sustainable Chemistry & Engineering* 8: 4481–8
101. Sun H, Cai S, Wang C, Chen Y, Yang R. 2020. *ChemBioChem* 21: 2572–84
102. Shamsipur M, Safavi A, Mohammadpour Z. 2014. *Sensors and Actuators B: Chemical* 199: 463–9
103. Xi J, Zhu C, Wang Y, Zhang Q, Fan L. 2019. *RSC Advances* 9: 16509–14
104. Xia F, Shi Q, Nan Z. 2020. *Dalton Transactions* 49: 12780–92
105. Zhang Y, Dai C, Liu W, Wang Y, Ding F, et al. 2019. *Microchimica Acta* 186: 1–9
106. Lou Z, Zhao S, Wang Q, Wei H. 2019. *Analytical chemistry* 91: 15267–74
107. Chen W, Fang X, Ye X, Wang X, Kong J. 2018. *Microchimica Acta* 185: 1–10
108. Chen W, Zhang X, Li J, Chen L, Wang N, et al. 2020. *Analytical Chemistry* 92: 2714–21
109. Guo J, Wang Y, Zhao M. 2019. *Sensors and Actuators B: Chemical* 297: 126739
110. Guo QJ, Pan ZY, Men C, Lv WY, Zou HY, Huang CZ. 2019. *Analyst* 144: 716–21
111. Li J, Wang J, Wang Y, Trau M. 2017. *Analyst* 142: 4788–93
112. Tian L, Qi J, Qian K, Oderinde O, Liu Q, et al. 2018. *Journal of Electroanalytical Chemistry* 812: 1–9
113. Bu S, Wang K, Wang C, Li Z, Hao Z, et al. 2020. *Microchimica Acta* 187: 679
114. Fu J, Zhou Y, Huang X, Zhang W, Wu Y, et al. 2020. *Journal of Agricultural and Food Chemistry* 68: 1118–25
115. Zhou J, Tian F, Fu R, Yang Y, Jiao B, He Y. 2020. *ACS Applied Nano Materials* 3: 9016–25
116. Liu P, Wang Y, Han L, Cai Y, Ren H, et al. 2020. *ACS Applied Materials & Interfaces* 12: 9090–7
117. Yao S, Li J, Pang B, Wang X, Shi Y, et al. 2020. *Microchimica Acta* 187: 1–8
118. Miao L, Jiao L, Tang Q, Li H, Zhang L, Wei Q. 2019. *Sensors and Actuators B: Chemical* 288: 60–4
119. Son SE, Gupta PK, Hur W, Choi H, Lee HB, et al. 2020. *Analytica Chimica Acta* 1134: 41–9
120. Wang L, Hu Z, Wu S, Pan J, Xu X, Niu X. 2020. *Analytica Chimica Acta* 1121: 26–34
121. Xie J, Tang M-Q, Chen J, Zhu Y-H, Lei C-B, et al. 2020. *Talanta* 217: 121070
122. Chen M, Zhou H, Liu X, Yuan T, Wang W, et al. 2020. *Small* 16: e2002343
123. Wang L, Li S, Zhang X, Huang Y. 2020. *Talanta* 216: 121009
124. Zhang R, Lu N, Zhang J, Yan R, Li J, et al. 2020. *Biosensors and Bioelectronics* 150: 111881

# 7 Nanozymes in Biosensing and Bioimaging

Syed Rahin Ahmed, Ana Gomez Cardoso, Satish Kumar, Greter A. Ortega, Seshasai Srinivasan*, and Amin Reza Rajabzadeh*
W Booth School of Engineering Practice and Technology, McMaster University, Ontario, Canada

## CONTENTS

---

* Corresponding authors: Seshasai Srinivasan and Amin Reza Rajabzadeh

DOI: 10.1201/9781003109228-7

## 7.1 INTRODUCTION

Nanozymes, the nanomaterials that possess enzymatic properties, have generated huge research interest over the last few years (1–9). Several types of nanomaterials with enzyme-like qualities have been discovered. Nanozymes are emerging in different sectors of the biomedical fields, such as biosensors, bioimaging, and disease treatments (10, 11). In 2004, Scrimin et al. introduced the word "nanozyme" and used triazacyclonane-functionalized gold (Au) nanoparticles (NPs) as a nanozyme to catalyze a transphosphorylation reaction (12). The horseradish peroxidase (HRP)-like activity of iron oxide ($Fe_3O_4$) NPs as an artificial enzyme was first reported in 2007 (13). Since then, extensive research has revealed excellent nanozymatic activities of various nanomaterials and nanocomposites, which are making a bridge between nanotechnology and biotechnology.

Nanozymes have gained prominence due to their advantages over natural enzymes (14). They possess unique features, such as a large surface-to-volume ratio, ease of bioconjugation, and stability over a wide range of temperatures and pHs. These characteristics of nanozymes ultimately assist in reducing some drawbacks of natural enzymes. The rapid advancement of nanotechnology has expanded the novel applications of nanozymes in biomedical and related fields to achieve improved sensitivity and specificity. This in turn enables the understanding of bio/nano interfaces and has become an interesting research topic in disciplines, such as biology, physics, chemistry, and engineering. In this chapter, the characteristics of nanozymes and their recent applications in different biosensing techniques (fluorescence, colorimetric, electrochemical, and Raman), bioimaging, and therapeutics development are discussed.

## 7.2 DIFFERENT NANOZYMES

The most commonly used nanozymes are oxidoreductase- and hydrolases-mimics, such as OXD, POD, CAT, SOD, PP, and nuclease. Moreover, the magnetic and electrical properties of nanomaterials integrated with their nanozymatic activity give them extensive potential applications in bioimaging, biosensing, and therapeutics compared to natural enzymes (79–82).

The morphology and chemical composition of nanozymes highly affect their activity and selectivity. The size-, shape-, facet-, and coordination-dependent enzyme-like activities of nanomaterials are inconsistent and sometimes challenging to regulate and control. Moreover, the inhomogeneous chemical composition and various facet structures on the surface of the nanomaterials lead to complex catalytic mechanisms and multiple catalytic pathways. Hence, the understanding of the enzyme-like specificity, the active surface sites, and the origin of nanozymatic activity is complicated (8, 11, 83–85).

### 7.2.1 METAL-BASED

Several metal nanomaterials were recognized as candidates for sensing applications owing to their unique nanozymatic characteristics. Based on structural characteristics, the metallic nanozymes can be categorized as single-metal and multi-metal nanozymes. Single-metal-based nanozymes have widespread importance because they are easier to synthesize and are cheaper. The nanozymatic activity depends mainly on the size of the nanomaterials. Au NPs are well-known for their strong nanozymatic activity and received a lot of research interest due to their stability and ease of bioconjugation for biosensing and bioimaging applications. Moreover, Au NPs are biologically inert and their characteristics could easily be altered by changing their structural properties (15–19). Besides Au NPs, NPs of silver (Ag), palladium (Pd), copper (Cu), platinum (Pt), iridium (Ir), and ruthenium (Ru) show nanozymatic activity (**Table 7.1**). These metal NPs primarily mimic peroxidase (POD), oxidase (OXD), catalase (CAT), and superoxide dismutase (SOD) enzymes.

Two or more metals in a single entity, as a metal hybrid, are also gaining research interest, allowing to overcome the drawbacks, such as aggregation of nanomaterials during bioconjugation and weak enzyme-like activity. The recent biosensing applications of hybrid nanozymes are listed in **Table 7.2**.

## 7.2.2 METAL OXIDE-BASED

A considerable amount of research has been focused on the synthesis of metal oxide-based nanozymes. The intrinsic POD-like activity of $Fe_3O_4$ showed promise for many bio-related applications due to its catalytic capability to oxidize not

**TABLE 7.1**
**The Enzyme-Like (Colorimetric) Activity of Single-Metal Nanoparticles**

| Metal NPs | Enzyme-mimic | Reference |
|-----------|--------------|-----------|
| Au | POD | (20) |
| Au | OXD | (21) |
| Au | CAT | (22) |
| Au | SOD | (23) |
| Ag | POD | (24) |
| Ag | OXD | (25) |
| Ag | CAT | (26) |
| Cu | POD | (27) |
| Pt | POD | (28) |
| Pt | OXD | (29) |
| Pt | CAT | (30) |
| Ru | POD | (31) |
| Ru | OXD | (31) |
| Ir | POD | (32) |
| Ir | OXD | (33) |
| Ir | CAT | (34) |
| Pd | POD | (35) |
| Pd | OXD | (36) |
| Pd | CAT | (37) |

## TABLE 7.2
## The Enzyme-Like (Colorimetric) Activity of Hybrid Nanomaterials

| Metal hybrid[#] | Enzyme-mimic activity | Detection* | Reference |
|---|---|---|---|
| Au-Ag | POD | Haptoglobin | (38) |
| Au-Pt | POD | PSA | (39) |
| Au-Pd | POD | Malathion | (40) |
| Pt-Pd | POD | Glucose | (41) |
| Pt-Ru | Multiple | $Fe^{2+}$ ions | (42) |
| Pt-Co | OXD | Cancer cells | (43) |
| Pd-Ir | POD | Carcinoembryonic | (44) |
| Pt-Cu | POD | Hydrogen peroxide | (45) |
| Graphene-Au | POD | Norovirus | (15) |
| CNT-Au | POD | Influenza virus | (17) |
| Graphene-Pt | OXD | Dihydroxybenzene | (46) |
| Ni-Pd | POD | Glucose | (47) |
| Ce-MOF | OXD | Biothiols | (48) |
| MOF (Ce/Fe) | POD | Hydrogen peroxide | (49) |
| Au-MOF | OXD | Glucose | (50) |

[#] Carbon nanotubes (CNT), Metal-organic framework (MOF)
* Prostate-specific antigen (PSA)

only 3,3′,5,5′-tetramethylbenzidine (TMB) but also diazoaminobenzene (DAB), and o-phenylenediamine (OPD). Studies on the kinetic nature of $Fe_3O_4$ nanozymes revealed that they possess a lower Michaelis–Menten constant ($K$m) value with TMB than HRP, which indicates the higher affinity of the $Fe_3O_4$ nanomaterials for TMB than HRP (13, 51, 52). Similarly, hydrothermally synthesized $Fe_3O_4$ QDs have been shown to possess high POD-like activity and exhibited a higher affinity towards TMB than HRP. The X-ray photoelectron spectroscopy revealed that the Fe (II) to Fe (III) ratio in $Fe_3O_4$ QDs is higher than $Fe_3O_4$ NPs, which might have a positive effect on the enhanced nanozymatic activity (53).

Cerium oxide ($CeO_2$) is another promising metal-oxide nanozyme. It has intrinsic POD-, OXD-, CAT-, SOD-, and phosphatase (PP)-like activities. These features have extended $CeO_2$ nanozyme applications in biosensing and medical therapy (54–56). For example, Li et al. reported the OXD-like activity of $CeO_2$ NPs for the fluorescent detection of fluoride is very crucial for environmental and biological applications. The oxidation activity of $CeO_2$ is enhanced in the presence of amplex red (AR) (substrate) and fluoride. As a result, the concentration of fluoride is correlated to the fluorescent production of resorufin. Most importantly, compared to other metal-oxide nanozymes, the oxidation of only $CeO_2$ nanozyme can be enhanced by fluoride, which could inversely be used for the detection of $CeO_2$ (57).

Recently, the POD-like activities of $CeO_2$ nanozymes have been studied by Liu et al. (58). This research might also be helpful to understand the more complex DNA or RNA cleavage reactions and colorimetric biosensor development. The authors compared the PP-like activities of $CeO_2$ (considering $CeO_2$ has both Ce (III) and Ce (IV) species) with that of alkaline phosphatase (ALP). Results revealed that $CeO_2$ nanozymes have good activity in presence of p-nitrophenyl phosphate (p-NPP) as a substrate, while other metal ions cannot demonstrate such activities. Furthermore, the ALP lost its enzymatic activity under heat treatment while $CeO_2$ remained active, showing superior characteristics of $CeO_2$ nanozyme for biosensing and chemical biology applications (58). The nanozymatic performance of dextran- and polyacrylic-acid-coated $CeO_2$ NPs depend on the pH of the reaction media and the size of synthesized $CeO_2$ NPs. Experimental results showed that $CeO_2$ NPs exhibited better OXD-like activity in acidic media (pH 4.0) with smaller $CeO_2$ NPs. The rod-structured $CeO_2$ nanomaterial also exhibited an enzyme-mimicking nature that has promising advantages in terms of cost-effectiveness, biocompatibility, and stability (59).

Vanadium oxide $(V_2O_5)$ nanowires and vanadium dioxide $(VO_2)$ nanobelts also showed similar intrinsic POD-like properties (60–63). Similarly, various shapes of manganese oxide $(MnO_2)$ nanomaterials, for example, nanosheets, nanorods, and porous microspheres, and hollow $MnCo_2O_4$ nanofibers have been reported for their OXD-mimicking properties (64–66).

### 7.2.3 METAL-ORGANIC FRAMEWORK-BASED

Metal-organic frameworks (MOF) and their derivatives open up a new avenue for constructing stable and active mesoporous nanozymes (67–70). Besides pristine MOF, MOF-based composites (e.g., $MOF/Fe_3O_4$, MOF/Au, and MOF/enzyme complex), and MOF-based derivatives including carbon-based nanomaterials (e.g., heteroatom-doped carbon or carbon with metal-nitrogen-carbon moiety), metal oxide/carbon NPs and metal/carbon nanomaterials, are among the most effective substitutes for conventional enzymes.

Various methods to synthesize catalytically active MOF-derived mesoporous carbon nanostructures have been reported in the literature. In general, pristine carbon that is bonded with sp2 carbon atoms has no catalytic activity; however, the introduction of intrinsic defects or edge oxidation on carbon materials could change the localized electronic structure of carbon with abundant active sites for catalytic reactions (71). A way to synthesize multifunctional enzyme mimicking nitrogen (N)-doped carbon nanospheres (N-PCNs) has been reported by Goa and co-workers in which the N-PCNs have four (OXD, POD, CAT, and SOD) enzyme-mimicking activities with intracellular reactive oxygen species (ROS) generation for cancer therapy (72). Moreover, MOF enables the construction of heterogeneous atom-doped carbon materials. Single-atom nanomaterials with a universal metal-nitrogen-carbon moiety seem to be a great catalyst for a variety of reactions. For example, Chen and co-workers reported the synthesis of graphene-based N-coordinated metal cofactors centered with main group metals (Mg, Ca, and Al) through direct carbonization of MOF, showing extremely high oxygen reduction activity in alkaline media (73). Single-atom catalysts have also become one of the main areas of research focus (74, 75). Liu and co-workers reported the synthesis of $Zn-N_4$ single-atom nanozymes using zeolitic imidazolate framework-8 (ZIF-8) MOF as a precursor. This precursor serves as a photosensitizer and it displays POD-mimicking activity (76). A way to synthesize single-atom Fe–$N_4$ nanozyme anchored within N-doped porous carbon has also been reported (77). This synthesis is performed through the one-step carbonation of ZIF-8 MOF and it has excellent CAT- and SOD-mimicking activities. Shi et al. reported a Fe-based single-atom nanocatalyst through high-temperature carbonization of MOF followed by PEGlyation, exhibiting an excellent Fenton reaction activity toward hydrogen peroxide ($H_2O_2$) for hydroxyl radical (•OH) generation (78).

### 7.2.4  SINGLE-ATOM NANOZYMES

Flytzani-Stephanopoulos, Gates, and Zhang were the first to encounter the instability of single-atom catalyst (SAC) nanozymes (86–88). The atomically dispersed active metal sites of the SACs, which are similar to the active centers of the metalloenzymes, provide excellent selectivity and activity (89–95). The new concept of single-atom nanozymes (SAzymes) was inspired by the specific spatial structures of SACs and metalloenzymes, which integrated the state-of-the-art single-atom technologies with inherent active sites of enzyme mimics. SAzymes and their applications are essential breakthroughs and promising next-generation nanozymes, where the performance of the nanozymes is strongly dependent on the morphology of the nanomaterials.

### 7.2.5  LIGHT-RESPONSIVE NANOZYMES

Nanomaterials with light-responsive capacity can be utilized for oxidizing enzymatic substrates and constructing photoactive nanozyme-based biosensors. The photocatalytic properties of some nanomaterials originate from the nanomaterials themselves. This can generate ROS by absorbing light and subsequently oxidizing enzymatic substrates. In this case, superoxide anion (•$O^{2-}$), •OH, singlet oxygen ($^1O_2$), and photogenerated holes ($h^+$) are involved during the photocatalytic reactions. Photocatalytic nanozymes can catalyze challenging reactions that hardly proceed without light. The disadvantage of photocatalytic reactions is the low efficiency under the sunlight, which is overcome by other light sources such as xenon (Xe) lamps (96). In another type, the nanomaterials provide photocatalytic activities due to the introduction of functional photoactive molecules on their structure. For example, photoisomerization, photo-induced pH-changing, and photothermal molecules are tagged on the nanomaterials. The enzyme-like activities of nonphotoactive nanozymes may be impacted by the introduction of such functional molecules. Researchers are still in the pursuit of more types of photoactive molecules (96).

Although carbon-based photosensitizers are very useful photoactive nanozymes, their low efficiency and lack of rational design prevent them from being efficient photo-oxidative nanozymes (97). Wu group has approached this by designing a way to synthesize a series of N-doped carbon dots (C-dots) and studying the correlation between photo-oxidation activity and phosphorescence quantum yield. Their research showed that the synthesized C-dots exhibited enzyme-like activity under light irradiation. Moreover, C-dots exhibited better performance for the activation of oxygen than other carbon-based nanomaterials as well as dyes of phloxine B and rose bengal (98).

Another critical factor to consider is the long excited-state lifetime of the nanozymes that are light-responsive. Liu group used Mn(II) to interact with C-dots to activate the catalysis of C-dots for TMB oxidation at a neutral pH in the presence of singlet oxygen produced via photosensitization. Mn(II) can be oxidized to Mn(III) by the photo-generated singlet oxygen, enhancing the electron transfer upon light irradiation. In comparison to other metal ions, only Mn(II) could enhance the oxidation of TMB in a physiological buffer. The Mn-regulated oxidation method resolved a major problem for the nanozymes that lacked efficient activity levels at a physiological pH (99). •OH is another type of ROS in photocatalytic reactions. Xia group reported that Au NPs exhibit POD-like activity under visible-light irradiation. This study suggests that the excitation of localized surface plasmon resonance in Au NPs leads to the activation of hot carriers (electrons and holes), and the injection of those hot electrons into the $H_2O_2$ molecule could produce more •OH, leading to an enhanced enzyme-like performance (100). Superoxide anion can also be generated by activating oxygen by injecting hot electrons. Besides Au NPs, other photocatalytic nanozymes, including graphitic carbon nitride ($g$-$C_3N_4$), gold-bismuth tungstate ($Au$–$PdBi_2WO_6$), and indium sulfide ($\beta$-$In_2S_3$) rely on the photo-generated superoxide anion for the oxidation of substrates (101–103).

Generally, nonphotocatalytic modulation strongly affects the activity of nanozymes in the absence of ROS. When photoactive molecule azobenzene (Azo)-modified mesoporous silica NPs were used as a host to encapsulate Au NPs and cyclodextrin (Au–Si–Azo), the catalytic activity was inhibited due to the trans conformations of Azo in Au–Si–Azo. While UV light was irradiated, Azo underwent the isomerization from trans to cis conformation and led to the enzyme-like activity of Au NPs. On the other hand, under visible light irradiation, the transformation of Azo from cis to trans conformation inhibited the CAT-like activity of Au NPs (22). By switching the light source, the hydrolysis of Au NPs can be controlled. Au NPs have a higher affinity toward the trans isomer of the photoactive molecule while functionalized with C9-thiol-based molecules. Therefore, the photoactive molecule with the trans conformation inhibits the absorption of the substrate 2-hydroxypropyl-4-nitrophenylphosphate and decreases the hydrolysis activity. The trans isomer of photoactive molecules transform into a cis isomer upon irradiation at 365 nm, which reduces their affinity to the surface of Au NPs, and therefore the transphosphorylation rate of 2-hydroxypropyl-4-nitrophenylphosphate was upregulated (104). It can be concluded that light-responsive nanozymes will open a new window in the field of biosensing with high sensitivity and low background signal.

## 7.2.6 CHIRAL NANOZYMES

The specific reaction of nanozyme-substrate is essential to minimize the gap between nanozymes and natural enzymes (6). For example, many natural enzymes are stereospecific and work only when the substrates possess stereoisomers. The chiral discrimination on substrates' enantiomers is another important characteristic of enzymes' stereospecificity. For example, $L$-amino acid OXD can only catalyze the oxidation of $L$-amino acid but does not affect D-amino acid (105). Hence, the synthesis of enantioselective nanozymes may broaden their applications in the biomedical fields, which might require more selectivity.

In general, most of the nanozymes are prepared from achiral molecules and have no enantioselectivity properties. However, the introduction of chiral ligands (amino acids, nucleic acids, and some chiral chemical compounds) on the surface of nanozymes may generate enantioselectivity. As an example, graphene oxide (GO) nanozyme showed enantioselective POD-like activity in the presence of $H_2O_2$ and TMB while chiral zinc (Zn) finger protein-like alpha-helical supramolecular complexes ($[Fe_2L_3]^{4+}$) has been conjugated on its surface (106).

Au NPs have been reported for suitable transphosphorylation catalytic activity when thiols and triazacyclononane $Zn^{2+}$-binding head groups are assembled on its surface. When cysteine (Cys) chiral ligand was attached to the surface of Au NPs and loaded into mesoporous silica carrier, the results revealed that D-Cys@AuNPs-mesoporous Si NPs catalyzes the oxidation of L-dopa whereas L-Cys@AuNPs-mesoporous Si NPs was more effective for the oxidation of D-dopa (12, 107–109). Moreover, DNA-modified Au NPs have exhibited different enantioselectivities in catalyzing the oxidation of glucose enantiomers (110). Phenylalanine modified-$CeO_2$ NPs have also shown excellent catalytic and enantioselective properties (111). Surprisingly, chiral Cys-modified molybdenum disulfide ($MoS_2$) QDs exhibited remarkable POD-like activity in the presence of copper (Cu) ions though neither unmodified $MoS_2$-QDs nor Cys-modified $MoS_2$-QDs showed any POD-like catalytic activity (112–114).

### 7.2.7 Oxydase Mimics

In general, OXD enzymes catalyze an oxidation–reduction reaction using $O_2$ as the electron acceptor. The reaction involves the donation of a hydrogen atom, and subsequently, the reduction of an oxygen molecule to $H_2O$ or $H_2O_2$. For example, Au NPs are well-known OXD mimic nanomaterials that could catalyze glucose to form gluconic acid and $H_2O_2$ in the presence of $O_2$ (115). The kinetic study has revealed that the glucose molecule is first absorbed on the surface of Au NPs, which then attacks the dissolved oxygen to generate gluconic acid and $H_2O_2$. Depending on the type of nanomaterials, different enzyme-like activities are expected.

Molybdenum trioxide ($MoO_3$) NPs possess an intrinsic sulfite OXD-like activity that might be useful for potential therapeutic in case of sulfite OXD deficiency. Steady-state kinetic studies suggest that the $MoO_3$ nanozyme first accepts two electrons from sulfite that reduces $Mo^{6+}$ to $Mo^{4+}$ in the presence of $[Fe(CN)_6]^{3-}$. Such an oxidation–reduction reaction was reported to have higher efficiency than native human sulfite OXD (116).

### 7.2.8 Peroxidase Mimics

Many nanomaterials have been reported to possess POD-like activity and catalyze the oxidation of substrates in the presence of $H_2O_2$. $Fe_3O_4$ was the first POD-like nanozyme that was reported to have higher activity, performance at different pH, temperature stability, and reaction rate than the natural HRP (13). This finding has inspired many researchers to develop different nanozymes with POD-like activity for biomedicine applications (**Table 7.3**).

## 7.2.9 SUPEROXIDE DISMUTASE MIMICS

ROS-scavenging enzymes, such as CAT, SOD, and glutathione peroxidase (GPx), exist in the human body and act as an antioxidant system. Of these, SOD is one of the most exclusive and acts as a first-line defense to treat diseases caused by ROS. Natural SOD is in charge of protecting the body from superoxide anions (7). However, the high production cost and low stability of this enzyme make it less than desirable for mass production.

SOD-containing nanozymes are useful in therapy for anti-inflammatory purposes. They have also proven to be effective in a variety of applications, such as drug development and biosensing. SOD, much like CAT is a good ROS scavenger in the body. Many highly efficient ROS-scavenging enzymes have been used but there are still some improvements that need to be made. These enzymes are very susceptible to environmental conditions and they are also difficult to mass-produce. This is where nanozymes, such as SOD can make a big difference because of their enhanced stability and multifunctionality (155). Shen et al. suggested that the functionality of these SOD-mimicking NPs depends on the type of metal used (157).

The most researched SOD-mimics are Ce NPs. They mimic SOD due to the valance states of $Ce^{3+}$ and $Ce^{4+}$. It has been proven that a high $Ce^{+3}/Ce^{+4}$ ratio portrays SOD-mimetic activities, whereas a low ratio would exhibit CAT-mimetic activities. Together, with ROS-scavenging activities and biocompatibility, Ce NPs are an excellent replacement for natural enzymes (156).

Kajita et al. were the first to report the scavenging properties of superoxide and $H_2O_2$. Although the mechanism is still unclear, it has been shown that Pt NPs increased the lifespan of the nematode *Caenorhabditis elegans* (157). Another use for SOD-mimicking nanozymes is to protect exposed cells from ROS caused by cigarette smoke (158). In a study by Onizawa et al., Pt NPs were administered intranasally to prevent antioxidant depletion. This study proved that the Pt NPs were able to control the antioxidant depletion and neutrophilic inflammation after three days of exposure to cigarette smoke (158). Although this experiment was somewhat successful, it showed that the Pt concentration in the subjects' lungs increased by 400% but not in any other organs. Thus, the toxic effects of NPs are still not well understood and further research is required.

Besides being used during photosynthesis, it is also known that at higher oxidation states, Mn is an important part of redox reactions in enzymes, such as CAT and SOD. Besides Ce, manganese phosphate ($MnPO_4$) was among the first reported SOD-mimic (158). The NPs composed of $Mn_3O_4$ can be shaped as flakes, cubes, polyhedrons, or hexagonal plates. Since, the morphology of nanozymes affects the way they interact, NPs with flake-like morphology has the lowest rate of activity, lower by 50% than the rest. Other NPs that exhibit SOD-mimic activity include Cu, Co, Fe, and carbon-based nanomaterials. **Table 7.4** is a list of SOD-mimic nanomaterials and their applications.

## TABLE 7.3
## Nanozymes with POD-Like Activity for Biomedicine Applications

| Nanozyme* | Detection | Technique | Reference |
|---|---|---|---|
| Hemin–graphene | Single nucleotide polymorphism | Colorimetric | (117) |
| GO and Au | Cancer cell detection | Colorimetric | (118) |
| GO | Cancer biomarker | Colorimetric | (119) |
| Hemin-graphene | $H_2O_2$ | Electrochemical | (120) |
| GQDs | $H_2O_2$ and glucose | Colorimetric | (121) |
| GQDs-Au | $H_2O_2$ | Electrochemical | (122) |
| Graphene-ferric porphyrin | DNA biosensing | Electrochemical | (123) |
| Carbon NP-porphyrin | Glucose | Colorimetric | (124) |
| GO-$Co_3O_4$ | Glucose | Colorimetric | (125) |
| $Fe_3O_4$-GO | Acetylcholine | Colorimetric | (126) |
| $Co_3O_4$-GO | $H_2O_2$ | Colorimetric | (127) |
| GQDs | Cholesterol | Colorimetric | (128) |
| Graphene–CuO | Bisphenol A | Colorimetric | (129) |
| Pt NP-GO | Cysteine | Colorimetric | (130) |
| GO-Prussian blue | $H_2O_2$ | Electrochemical | (131) |
| $Fe_2O_3$–graphene | Glucose | Colorimetric | (132) |
| Hemin-GO-CNTs | $H_2O_2$, ascorbic acid, dopamine, uric acid, and tryptophan | Colorimetric | (133) |
| GO-Au NPs-mercury | Syncytial virus | Colorimetric | (134) |
| GO /$MnO_2$ | $H_2O_2$ | Electrochemical | (135) |
| Pt NPs-GO | Cancer cells | Colorimetric | (136) |
| $Fe_3O_4$ NPs-GO-CNT | $H_2O_2$ and glucose | Electrochemical | (137) |
| PtPd-Graphene | $H_2O_2$ | Colorimetric | (138) |
| $CeO_2$ | $H_2O_2$ and glucose | Colorimetric | (139) |
| $TiO_2$-CeOx | $H_2O_2$ | Colorimetric | (140) |
| $Cu_2(OH)_3Cl$-$CeO_2$ | $H_2O_2$, glucose, and cholesterol | Colorimetric | (141) |
| Porphyrin-$CeO_2$ | Glucose | Colorimetric | (142) |
| Fe-doped $CeO_2$ | Glucose | Colorimetric | (143) |
| Montmorillonite$CeO_2$ | $H_2O_2$ | Colorimetric | (144) |
| $Co_3O_4$ | $H_2O_2$ and glucose | Colorimetric | (145) |
| $Co_3O_4$ | Sulfite | Colorimetric | (146) |
| PB@$Co_3O_4$ - $SiO_2$@$Co_3O_4$ | $H_2O_2$ and glucose | Colorimetric | (147) |
| Porphyrin-$Co_3O_4$ | $H_2O_2$ | Colorimetric | (148) |
| Co-magnetoferritin | Tumor tissue | Colorimetric | (149) |
| $Co_3O_4$-montmorillonite | $H_2O_2$ and glutathione | Colorimetric | (150) |
| Pt NPs-$MoO_3$ | Glucose | Colorimetric | (151) |
| Pt NPs | Choline and acetylcholine | Colorimetric | (152) |
| Pt NPs | rabbit IgG | Colorimetric | (153) |
| Au-Pt | Prostate-specific antigen | Colorimetric | (154) |

* Graphene Oxide (GO), Graphene Quantum Dots (GQDs)

## TABLE 7.4
## SOD-Mimic Nanozymes and Their Applications

| Nanozyme | Activity | Applications | Reference |
|---|---|---|---|
| CeO$_2$ | SOD, CAT | Cell protection in radiation therapy | (159) |
| | | Anti-inflammation | |
| | | Neuroprotection | |
| | | Anti-cancer treatment | |
| | | Wound healing | |
| Apoferritin-encapsulated Pt NPs | SOD, CAT | Protection against oxidative stress | (160) |
| Pt NPs | SOD, CAT | Scavenging UV-induced cellular ROS | (161) |
| Au-Pt NPs | SOD, CAT | Glucose | (162) |
| SiO$_2$-Mn$_2$O$_4$ & Mn/(PO$_4$)$_2$ | SOD | Electrochemical detection of superoxide ion | (163, 164) |
| Mn$_2$O$_4$ nanoflowers | SOD, CAT, GPx | Cytoprotection in Parkinson disease | (165) |
| MnO | SOD, CAT | Enhance MRI contrast | (166) |
| Gly-Cu (OH)$_2$ NPs | SOD | Reducing ROS in cigarette smoke | (167) |
| Co$_3$O$_4$ NPs | POD, SOD, CAT | Immunohistochemistry detection | (168) |

### 7.2.10 CATALASE MIMICS

The main function of CAT in organisms is to catalyze the conversion of H$_2$O$_2$ into oxygen and water and has the potential to be therapeutic as an antioxidizing agent (169, 170). Aside from decomposing H$_2$O$_2$, CAT has an important role in protecting the cells in the body from oxidative stress. It has been proven that CAT deficiency in the body is related to degenerative disorders, such as diabetes and Alzheimer's (171). The formation of H$_2$O$_2$ due to mitochondrial superoxide leakage causes and continues the oxidative stress in neuronal injury.

Although CAT therapy has made great advances, it is still in the need of improvements. The difficulty in this process is in delivering the desired amount of CAT to the desired area. Other negatives reported by researchers include a short half-life and inadequate cellular uptake (172). Various methods to improve the half-life have been attempted, such as delivery with polyethylene glycosylation and lecithinization. Unfortunately, the methods mentioned earlier were rejected due to low enzymatic uptake by neuronal cells. For the therapeutic effect to work to the best of its abilities, it is necessary to design a delivery system that protects CAT from degradation along the way and that also makes it across the blood-brain barrier (BBB). The main fault of the natural catalase is its inability to travel across the BBB. Using the NPs mode of transportation, CAT will be protected from degradation in the biological milieu and it will be able to cross the BBB (173).

To synthesize the CAT-covered NPs, it is important to research the CAT activity. This is usually measured with a CAT assay kit and the decomposition reaction rate of H$_2$O$_2$ is determined. The triglyceride and phosphatidylcholine formulated solid lipid NPs are prepared using a double emulsion method and using evaporation techniques. It was proven that free CAT was only 30% effective after an hour of being incubated and was unmeasurable after 5 h, whereas CAT activity in CAT-loaded solid lipid NPs was 48% of their initial activity at 5 h (174).

CeO$_2$ NPs, also known as nanoceria, are popular for CAT therapy. The level of CAT activity of nanoceria depends on the Ce$^{3+}$/Ce$^{4+}$ ratio (175, 176). ROS can often denature proteins. A high concentration of ROS will destroy the balance of redox reactions and are a big cause of oxidative stress. Nanoceria is known for neutralizing this kind of stress on cells. When this occurs, nanoceria is used to remove ROS inside and outside of the cell. These nanozymes act as antioxidants and anti-inflammatory agents by protecting the cells from ongoing oxidative stress.

CAT therapy for tumors is a popular and indirect way to kill malignant cells (177). CAT relieves the hypoxia of a tumor and prevents the bad cells from growing and obtaining nutrients. It has been hypothesized that the sensitivity and weakness of tumor cells compared to regular cells was their lower potential to metabolize H$_2$O$_2$. The regular cells (treated with CAT) removed the overload of H$_2$O$_2$ with double the efficiency of cancer cells. In this experiment, the CAT was transported to the target site using an adenovirus. Although the adenovirus CAT worked, it was not able to properly target the desired cells. Nanozyme-based tumor therapy could potentially kill tumors directly by being more specifically targeted to the desired area.

Some researchers also used CAT-covered poly (lactic-co-glycolic acid) NPs, often referred to as nano-CAT. Singhal et al. (172) determined that 200 µg/mL was the optimal dose of CAT that would protect the neurons from H$_2$O$_2$. Cells were treated with H$_2$O$_2$ and/or nano-CAT to analyze the ability of nano-CAT to protect the cells from toxicity. The cells that had both H$_2$O$_2$ and nano-CAT conserved and guarded cell viability. Not only do CAT NPs protect cells from cytotoxicity but they can also reduce the oxidative stress of cells that have already been exposed. CAT nanozymes have also been proven to have many advantages over free CAT therapy and they continue to be widely used in the diagnosis and treatment of tumors.

## 7.3   KINETIC BEHAVIOR OF NANOZYMES

The kinetic study of nanozymes indicated that the reaction follows the Michaelis–Menten behavior. The apparent Michaelis–Menten constants ($K$m) obtained using a Lineweaver–Burk plot of different nanozymes reactions are shown in **Table 7.5**. The $K$m value of different nanozymes is higher than that of HRP toward H$_2$O$_2$, indicating that the nanozymes have a lower affinity toward H$_2$O$_2$ than HRP. In contrast, the $K$m value is lower than that of HRP toward TMB, indicating that the nanozymes have a higher affinity toward TMB than HRP. These results indicate that nanozymes possess relatively high POD-like activity than natural enzymes

## 7.4   NANOZYMES IN BIOSENSING

### 7.4.1   COLORIMETRIC BIOSENSING

The colorimetric detection method could significantly reduce the cost of analysis and allows on-site screening possibilities. This method has gained huge research interest after the introduction of nanozymes, and until now, most of the nanozyme-based

TABLE 7.5

Michaelis–Menten Constant (Km) of HRP and Nanozymes
Against TMB and $H_2O_2$

| Nanozyme | Substrate | $K_m$ (mM) | Reference |
|---|---|---|---|
| HRP | TMB | 0.43 | (13) |
| | $H_2O_2$ | 3.7 | |
| $Fe_3O_4$ | TMB | 0.1 | (13) |
| | $H_2O_2$ | 154 | |
| $Co_3O_4$ | TMB | 0.04 | (145) |
| | $H_2O_2$ | 140 | |
| PB-$Fe_2O_3$ | TMB | 0.31 | (178) |
| | $H_2O_2$ | 323.6 | |
| Pt NPs | TMB | 0.12 | (153) |
| | $H_2O_2$ | 769 | |
| Pd NPs | TMB | 0.165 | (179) |
| | $H_2O_2$ | 1064 | |

articles reported are based on the colorimetric method. Visual observation of an analyte based on color has provided the first screening results for the target analysis (161, 180–184). After confirming the positive results, other instruments, such as UV–vis spectroscopy or electrochemical detection can be used to quantify the concentration of a target analyte. The typical reaction mechanism involves the oxidation of chromogenic substrates (e.g., TMB, ABTS, and OPD) using nanozymes. The development of color in the presence of $H_2O_2$ enables the quantification of $H_2O_2$ directly or indirectly. Ahmed et al. reported the direct detection of $H_2O_2$ using nanozymatic activity of $Fe_3O_4$ QDs with the LOD value of 3.87 nM. Indirect quantification of $H_2O_2$ needs enzyme-substrate (glucose, lactose, or alcohol) reaction. For example, Zhang and co-workers developed an indirect approach to detect $H_2O_2$ using $gC_3N_4$ nanozyme (185). A list of POD-mimicking nanomaterials for $H_2O_2$ detection is presented in **Table 7.6**.

## 7.4.2 FLUORESCENCE BIOSENSING

The fluorescence-based target analytes detection has gained popularity because of the fast response and sensitive detection (215–225). Recent studies have shown that several fluorescent nanomaterials possess nanozymatic activity. For example, Li et al. reported the fluorescent detection of fluoride using OXD-like activity of $CeO_2$ and AR as the substrate (57). This method allowed to detect fluoride up to 1.8 μM with high specificity under optimized conditions within 2 min, compared to the 10-min detection time via the conventional colorimetric method.

Wang et al. reported an approach to synthesize three fluorescent $C_3N_4$-based nanozymes (i.e., $C_3N_4$–Ru, $C_3N_4$–Cu, and $C_3N_4$–hemin) (226). These POD-mimicking nanozymes can catalyze the oxidation of OPD to form OPDox in the presence of $H_2O_2$, which results in fluorescence emission and quenching at 564 nm and 438 nm,

## TABLE 7.6
## $H_2O_2$ Detection with POD Mimics

| Nanozyme | LOD (μM) | Reference |
|---|---|---|
| $Fe_3O_4$ MNPs | 3 | (186) |
| $Fe_3O_4$ MNPs | 0.25 | (187) |
| $Fe_3O_4$ MNPs | 0.5 | (188) |
| $Fe_3O_4$ GO composite | 0.32 | (189) |
| Fe-substituted SBA-15 microparticles | 0.2 | (190) |
| Fe phosphate microflowers | 0.010 | (191) |
| [$Fe^{III}$(biuret-amide)] on mesoporous silica | 10 | (192) |
| FeTe nanorods | 0.055 | (193) |
| Fe(III)-based coordination polymer | 0.4 | (194) |
| $Fe_3O_4$ nanocomposite | 1.07 | (195) |
| $Fe_3O_4$ nanocomposite | 0.2 | (196) |
| Glucose oxidase (GOx)/$Fe_3O_4$/GO magnetic nanocomposite | 0.04 | (197) |
| $Fe_3H_9(PO_4)_6 \cdot 6H_2O$ crystals | 1 | (198) |
| MIL-53(Fe) | 0.13 | (199) |
| CuO NPs | N/A | (200) |
| AuNPs | 4 | (20) |
| AuNC@BSA | 0.020 | (201) |
| Au@Pt core/shell nanorods | 45 | (202) |
| NiTe thorny nanowires | 0.025 | (203) |
| Graphene oxide | 0.050 | 106) |
| Hemin-graphene hybrid nanosheets | 0.020 | (204) |
| Carbon nanodots | 0.2 | (205) |
| Carbon nitride dots | 0.4 | (206) |
| Tungsten carbide nanorods | 60 nM | (207) |
| CoFe nanoplates | 0.4 | (208) |
| $Co_3Fe_{3-x}O_4$ | 0.4 | (209) |
| $Co_3O_4$ nanostructures | 0.1 | (210) |
| Pt-DNA complexes | 392 | (211) |
| PB NPs | 0.031 | (212) |
| MWCNTs-Prussian blue NPs | 0.100 | (213) |
| Polyoxometalate | 0.134 μM | (214) |

respectively. The ratiometric fluorescence intensity (F564/F438) exhibited a broad dynamic range for the $H_2O_2$ concentration from 10 to 1000 μM with a LOD of 4.20 μM. Moreover, by coupling GOx with $C_3N_4$–Ru, glucose was detected by this ratiometric fluorescent sensor. The fluorescent peak at 438 nm was gradually quenched, while the peak at 564 nm increased with increasing glucose concentration. The calibration curve of glucose detection was linear over 10 and 250 μM glucose with an LOD of 4.73 μM.

Another study reported a fluorescent "turn-on" sensor for the quantitative and highly selective analysis of phosphite (P(III)) through the recovery of the OXD-like activity of nickel oxide (NiO) nanozyme inhibited by a Good's buffer (227). HEPES

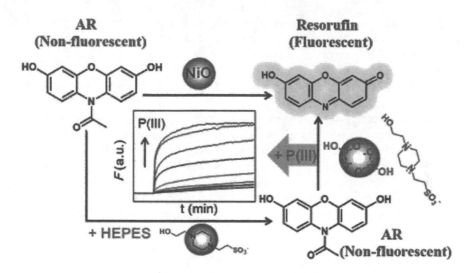

**FIGURE 7.1** OXD-like activity of NiO NPs results in the fluorescent resorufin for P(III) detection [reused with permission from (227)].

was the most effective inhibitor for the OXD-like activity of NiO NPs for the oxidation of AR that resulted in fluorescent resorufin. Under the optimal condition, the sensor detected P(III) up to 1 mM (LOD= 1.46 μM) (**Figure 7.1**). The P(III) analysis with recovery rates ranged from 74.2 ± 2.6% to 107.5 ± 0.5% in water and biological samples respectively, suggesting the potential applicability of this sensor.

### 7.4.3 ELECTROCHEMICAL BIOSENSING

The electrochemical biosensing technique provides a cost-effective and rapid way of target analyte detection (228). The application of nanozymes in electrochemical detection strategy either as an electrode material or as a signal amplifier is vital to develop sensitive and stable biosensors. In the conventional electrochemical immunoassay, the enzyme-labeled antigen and enzyme-labeled antibody form a sandwich structure on the electrode surface that can be measured by an electrochemical readout. However, the separation and purification of enzyme-labeled antigen or antibody is a laborious and challenging process. The application of nanozymes helps overcome some of the disadvantages; for example, nanozyme-labeled antigen or antibody could easily separate from unconjugated part through centrifugation. Moreover, the conjugation between nanozyme and antigen or antibody can be simply achieved via either electrostatic interactions or covalent linkers. As an example, an electrochemical immunosensor has been reported for the squamous cell carcinoma antigen detection where the amino groups of secondary antibodies electrostatically interacted with the nanozymes. The sensor revealed an excellent sensitivity with a LOD of 33 fg mL$^{-1}$ (229).

In general, the sensitivity of traditional enzyme-based biosensors is compromised when applied in the blood sample due to the presence of electroactive species, such as ascorbic acid, uric acid, and 4-acetaminophen. The use of nanozyme could be helpful to overcome this drawback. For example, the electrochemical detection of glucose is a well-known approach where the enzymatic oxidation of $H_2O_2$ directly occurs at the GOx-modified electrode. A glucose sensor was developed based on the co-immobilization of PB and GOx on titanium dioxide ($TiO_2$) nanotube. In this sensor, PB reduces $H_2O_2$ and enables the detection of glucose with LOD of 3.2 mM within 1 s (230).

Nanozymes can also be used as an electrochemical signal blocking material in sandwich-based electrochemical immunosensing strategies. This sensing strategy involves a nanozyme-catalyzed generation of a nonconducting substrate that blocks the working area and obstructs the electron transfer reaction. Recently, the detection of α-fetoprotein has been reported based on electrochemical signal off strategy, i.e., iron disulfide ($FeS_2$)-Au NPs nanozymes catalyze 4-chloro-1-naphthol in the presence of $H_2O_2$ to form an insoluble precipitate, which reduces the DPV response of the electroactive nickel hexacyanoferrate NPs (231).

Aptamer-based biosensors are popular because of their high specificity, smaller size, stability, and ease of modification. An electrochemical sensor for the detection of *Pseudomonas aeruginosa (P. aeruginosa)* using the nanozymatic activity of Au NPs and *P. aeruginosa*-specific aptamer has been reported (232). Here, the aptamer adsorption onto the surface of Au NPs inhibits the nanozymatic-activity of Au NPs, however, the POD-like activity of Au NPs resumes in the presence of the target molecule and enables the oxidation of TMB at the working electrode. The proposed method facilitated the detection of *P. aeruginosa* with an LOD of 60 CFU mL$^{-1}$. The nanozymatic activity of Au–Pt and Au–Cu bimetallic nanomaterials has also been reported for aptamer-based electrochemical detection of cardiac troponin I (cTnI) (233, 234). **Table 7.7** presents a list of nanozyme-based electrochemical detection applications.

### 7.4.4 SURFACE-ENHANCED RAMAN SCATTERING (SERS) BIOSENSING

SERS is an advanced Raman spectroscopy, which allows to detect analytes with high sensitivity and provides precise fundamental information. In particular, the introduction of surface plasmon properties of noble NPs, such as Au NPs and Ag NPs, plays a vital role in improving the LOD and providing a promising approach in developing SERS-based bioassays. For example, Hu and co-workers used the nanozymatic properties of Au NPs for SERS-based *in vitro* detection of glucose and lactate (262). In this study, they *in situ* synthesized Au NPs into MOF (AuNPs@MIL-101), which acted as POD-mimic and oxidized leucomalachite green (Raman-inactive reporter) into the active malachite green (MG) in the presence of $H_2O_2$. The *in vitro* sensing performance revealed that the SERS signal increased with the increase of glucose and lactate concentration, enabling glucose detection and lactate with an LOD of 4.2 µM and 5.0 µM, respectively (**Figure 7.2**).

A biomimetic nanozyme-linked immunosorbent assay (BNLISA) based on molecularly imprinted polymers and nanozymatic properties of Pt NPs have been reported for triazophos detection. Here, the POD-like activity of Pt NPs catalyzed the oxidation of colorless TMB into an ideal SERS marker in the presence of Au NPs@MIL-101 as the SERS-enhanced substrate. The proposed BNLISA strategy enabled the detection of triazophos with an LOD of 1 ng mL$^{-1}$ (263).

## TABLE 7.7
## Nanozymes-Based Electrochemical Detection of Various Target Analytes

| Nanozyme | Target analyte | LOD | Reference |
|---|---|---|---|
| CoFe$_2$O$_4$ MNPs | microRNA-21 | 0.3 fM | (235) |
| PdNPs@Fe-MOFs | microR-122 | 0.003 fM | (236) |
| Fe$_3$O$_4$/Cu(II) | microR-21 | 33 aM | (237) |
| FeTCPP@MOF | DNA | 0.48 fM | (238) |
| Au@PtNPs | DNA | 0.3 aM | (239) |
| ZrHCF MNPs | DNA | 0.43 fM | (240) |
| Hemin/G-quadruplex DNAzyme | HBV DNA | 0.5 pM | (241) |
| Mesoporous iron oxide | Global DNA methylation | 10% of methylation in genomic DNA | (242) |
| Au@NPFe$_2$O$_3$NC | p53 autoantibodies | 0.02 U mL$^{-1}$ | (243) |
| Au–NPFe$_2$O$_3$NC | p53 autoantibody | 0.08 U mL$^{-1}$ | (244) |
| Fe$_3$O$_4$/Au@Pt | cTnI | 7.5 pg mL$^{-1}$ | (245) |
| Fe$_3$O$_4$@UiO-66/Cu@Au | cTnI | 16 pg mL$^{-1}$ | (234) |
| Mn$_3$O$_4$/Pd@Pt | HER2 | 0.08 ng mL$^{-1}$ | (246) |
| Pt–Cu HTBNFs | PSA | 0.03 pg mL$^{-1}$ | (247) |
| Au@ZIF-8(NiPd) | Thrombin (TB) | 15 fM | (248) |
| Au@MGr | Tissue polypeptide antigen | 7.5 fg mL$^{-1}$ | (249) |
| Pt@P-MOF(Fe) | Telomerase activity | 20 HeLa cells mL$^{-1}$ | (250) |
| Au–NPFe$_2$O$_3$NC | Exosome | 10$^3$ mL$^{-1}$ | (251) |
| CuO/WO$_3$-GO | Cancer cells | 18 cells mL$^{-1}$ | (252) |
| NGQD@NC@Pd HNS | Cancer cells | - | (253) |
| CuO | Circulating tumor cells (CTCs) | 27 cells mL$^{-1}$ | (254) |
| rGO/MoS$_2$/ Fe$_3$O$_4$NP | CTCs | 6 cells mL$^{-1}$ | (255) |
| GQD | *Yersinia enterocolitica* | 5 CFU mL$^{-1}$ | (256) |
| Au NPs | *Pseudomonas aeruginosa* | 60 CFU mL$^{-1}$ | (232) |
| Co$_3$(PO$_4$)$_2$ NRs | Superoxide anion | 2.25 nM | (256) |
| Mn-MPSA-HCS & Mn-MPSA-HCC | Superoxide anion | 1.25 nM | (257) |
| GS@ZIF-67 | Glucose | 0.36 µM | (258) |
| CeO$_2$ | Norepinephrine | 66 nM | (259) |
| h-CuS NCs | Glucose | - | (260) |
| Au/Co@HNCF | UA | 0.023 µM | (261) |

### 7.4.5 NANOZYME-BASED MICROFLUIDIC DEVICE FOR BIOSENSING

The integration of nanozyme into microfluidics devices can lead to a promising real-time biosensing platform for the rapid detection of numerous analytes. To date, only a few articles have been reported using such an analytical method. Koo et al. integrated Fe$_3$O$_4$ nanozyme with a microfluidic device for electrochemical detection of circulating tumor nucleic cancer (264). The nanozymatic properties of immobilized Au NPs and Pt NPs with GO were integrated with a microfluidic point-of-care (POC) device for the real-time electrochemical detection of H$_2$O$_2$ (LOD = 1.62 µM) (265).

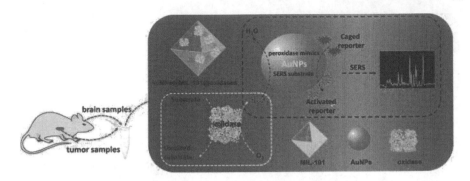

**FIGURE 7.2** SERS-based detection of glucose using the POD-like activity of Au NPs [reused with permission from (262)].

A microfluidic fluorescence sensor for in vivo $H_2O_2$ detection in cells has been reported using ZIF-8 nanozyme (266). Moreover, a droplet-based microfluidic platform for fluorescence $H_2O_2$ detection into cells has also been developed where Au NCs were trapped in a droplet and enhanced the detection sensitivity (267).

The incorporation of nanozymes into microfluidic paper-based analytical devices allows a simple and cost-effective analytical platform with an outstanding real-life application. Moreover, microfluidic paper-based analytical devices can be combined with smartphones for further digital data processing (185). The use of Au NPs in microfluidic paper-based analytical devices has been reported for the colorimetric detection of mercury ions ($Hg^{2+}$) (268). In another article, the POD-like MOF was integrated with a microfluidic paper-based analytical device for the colorimetric detection of glucose (269).

## 7.5   NANOZYMES IN THERAPEUTICS

Nanozymes have a lot of promise in therapeutics for treating a wide range of diseases. A low concentration of ROS in the body is useful as a critical secondary messenger in various signaling pathways, but at high concentrations, ROS can be detrimental (270). Common ROS are superoxide and $H_2O_2$. Research has proven that nanozymes could be used to eliminate any threat of ROS in large quantities. Nanozymes have a unique ROS radar that allows them to identify where large quantities are present. This capability originated from the SOD-mimicking abilities of nanozymes to convert SOD into $H_2O_2$. The therapeutic effects of nanozymes range from antioxidant, antiaging, anti-inflammatory, and several others.

An important nanozyme to consider for antioxidation purposes is nanoceria. It has been demonstrated that nanoceria could protect cardiac progenitor cells from $H_2O_2$ cytotoxicity (158). Another $H_2O_2$-scavenging nanozyme is vanadium oxide ($VO_2$), where $VO_2$ nanowires exhibited interesting GPx-mimicking activity (270).

Besides being detrimental to cells, ROS, such as $H_2O_2$ can cause inflammation. The inflammatory response can cause tissue injury. Nanoceria is used for its anti-inflammatory properties. Hirst et al. (271) showed that the $CeO_2$ NPs stopped the production of ROS and radical nitric oxide, the two primary mediators of inflammation. Nanoceria was also used as a therapeutic agent for the endovascular disease. The cells used in this experiment came from a human umbilical vein and the results demonstrated that the nanoceria improved the viability of the cell even under oxidative stress (272).

## 7.6 NANOZYMES IN BIOIMAGING

Bioimaging refers to a method of noninvasively visualizing biological processes in a body. Recent advances in imaging techniques revolve around nanozymes for robust and accurate results. Nanozymes exhibit unique physicochemical properties, such as fluorescence, super magnetism, and photothermal abilities, all of which are useful for bioimaging (273).The enzymes that are being mimicked in bioimaging include POD, CAT, and GOx. Examples of bioimaging applications of nanozymes are listed in **Table 7.8**.

### 7.6.1 EXOSOME-LIKE NANOZYMES

Exosomes are membrane-bound vesicles that can be found outside cells. Some proteins that are expressed on exosomes can be used as biomarkers for cancer diagnosis (303). Thus, nanozymes have been helpful since their characteristics make them an excellent candidate for profiling the exosomal proteins. The colorimetric abilities of nanozymes aid in the identification of exosomal proteins within three hours without the use of antibodies. The usefulness of exosome-like nanozymes goes further into cancer diagnosis through photoacoustic imaging (PAI), which is an excellent imaging technique for spatial resolution in cancer diagnosis. *In vivo* experiments illustrated that exosome-like nanozymes would accumulate in the nasopharyngeal carcinoma and trigger catalytic PAI (304). The nanozymes were able to detect increased levels of $H_2O_2$ making it possible to PAI to immediately locate the site. These exosome-like nanozymes have significantly aided the imaging process due to their enhanced circulation time, stealth ability, and improved ability to accumulate in tumors.

### 7.6.2 MOF-DERIVED NANOZYMES

MOF and its derivatives are made by joining organic and inorganic units using strong bonds. The shape, size, and functionality of MOF vary according to their need. MOF-derived nanozymes are unlike any others because of the mesoporous surface of MOF. Mesoporous is any surface that has pores that range from 2–50 nm. Because of their large surface area and mesoporous surface, MOFs are excellent for loading as many drugs as possible on the material to treat the desired site. MOFs are also widely used in bioimaging, for example, fluorescent C-dots can be made with MOF as source materials. These materials are excellent choices for bioimaging applications (305). Moreover, scaling down to a nanometer-scale would facilitate MOF in cell endocytosis progress. The ratiometric monitoring of adenosine in single cells using MOF-Lanthanide nanosheet has been reported (306). Upon the addition of target ATP, the fluorescence color in different cells changed from green to red that can be observed in different cells.

## TABLE 7.8
## List of Nanozymes Used in Bioimaging Applications

| Nanozyme | Enzyme mimic | Biomarkers* | Disease | Reference |
|---|---|---|---|---|
| Fe$_3$O$_4$ | POD | CSPG | Melanoma CTCs Tumor theranostic | (274, 275) |
| M-HFn | POD | TfR1 | Visualization of breast cancer cells Tumor tissue, high-risk plaque tissues | (276–278) |
| Fe$_3$O$_4$@Pt NPs | POD | HER2 | Point-of-care bioassay | (279) |
| Fe$_3$O$_4$/rGO | POD | Ach | Neuropsychiatric disorders | (126) |
| Co$_3$O$_4$ | POD | VEGFR | Tumor tissue | (168) |
| Fe-PDAP NFs | CAT | — | Multimodal tumor theranostic | (280) |
| CePO$_4$ : Tb, Gd nanospheres | POD | — | Multimodal imaging | (281) |
| MnO | SOD | — | Tumor theranostics | (166) |
| MnO$_2$ | — | — | Living cell BER pathway | (282) |
| MnO$_2$ nanosheet | CAT | — | UCL/PDT/RT imaging | (283) |
| CuO | POD | CEA | Tumor diagnosis | (284) |
| Gd(OH)$_3$ and Gd$_2$O$_3$ nanorods | POD | L-cysteine | Cardiovascular and neurotoxic disease | (285) |
| PB | CAT | H$_2$O$_2$ | Ultrasound imaging | (286) |
| Ag | POD | CRP | Inflammatory | (287) |
| Ag | POD | HER2 | Quantitative analysis of cancerous tissue | |
| Au | GOx | ATP | Real-time imaging of targets | (288) |
| Au | POD | Integrin GPIIb/IIIa | Quantification of membrane proteins on the cell surface | (289) |
| PtCo | OXD | — | Cancer cell imaging | (43) |
| Au NCs | OXD | Trypsin | Pancreatitis | (290) |
| Au/Ag | POD | Ach | Parkinson's and Alzheimer's disease | (291) |
| Pt@mSiO$_2$ | POD | BRCA1/2 | Breast cancer | (292) |
| PtNPs | CAT | BNP, CEA.et.al | Point-of-care diagnostics | (293) |
| Au-Fe$_3$O$_4$ | POD | — | Dual modal imaging cancer cells | (294) |
| GO-Fe$_3$O$_4$ | POD | Glucose | Diabetic | (126) |
| FA-PtNPs/GO | POD | FAR | MCF-7 cancer cell imaging | (136) |
| CoxFe$_{3-x}$O$_4$ | POD | DA | Schizophrenia | (295) |
| Fe$_3$O$_4$@ MIL-100(Fe) | POD | Cholesterol | Coronary heart, myocardial infarction, and stroke | (296) |
| Ag@Au-Fe$_3$O$_4$ | POD | Human IgG | Protein biomarker Detection | (297) |
| ZnFe$_2$O$_4$@MWNTs | POD | CEA | Tumor diagnosis | (298) |
| PB/MnO$_2$ | CAT | | Oxygen regulation of the xenografted breast cancer | (299) |

*(Continued)*

**TABLE 7.8 (Continued)**
**List of Nanozymes Used in Bioimaging Applications**

| Nanozyme | Enzyme mimic | Biomarkers* | Disease | Reference |
|---|---|---|---|---|
| V₂O₅-PDA-Au NPs | POD, GOx | Glucose | Diabetes | (300) |
| NaYF4:Yb,Er | POD | UA | Hyperuricemia, renal impairment, and liver disease | (301) |
| Fe-Co | POD | Glucose | Diabetes | (302) |

\* See Table of Symbols and Notations for some details on biomarkers

### 7.6.3 MAGNETIC RESONANCE IMAGING WITH POD MIMICS

POD-mimicking nanomaterials have been frequently reported as the most common group of nanozymes in the bioimaging field. POD nanozymes can catalyze the oxidation of substrates, such as TMB and DAB, which result in a color reaction easily detected through imaging. A specific magnetoferritin nanozyme developed by Wang et al. called M-HFn was able to recognize tumor cells through binding to overexpressed transferrin receptor1 found in tumor cells. The M-HFn nanozymes were able to identify the cancer type with a specificity of over 95% and a selectivity of 98% (273).

## 7.7 SUMMARY AND FUTURE PERSPECTIVES

In this chapter, the development and application of nanozymes in different biosensing, bioimaging, and therapeutics sectors are summarized. Various types of nanozymes and their catalytic nature and detection strategies for different analytes have been highlighted. In particular, the nanozyme-assisted sensing technologies including, electrochemical, colorimetric, fluorescence, UV–vis spectroscopy, SERS, and immunoassays have been discussed. Limitations in the existing nanozymes technologies have been identified, and the scope for further improvement are outlined. In practical clinical applications, nanozymes have existing limitations, such as poor dispersibility, easy sedimentation, limited catalytic types, and poor substrate selectivity. To improve some of these issues, researchers have recommended giving more emphasis to the morphology of the enzymes. It has been proven that nanozyme activity highly depends on its size and shape. Another unknown area is the possible toxic effects of nanozymes and their biocompatibility in the body.

   a. SERS-based sensing technique helps to develop the ultrasensitive detection of analytes. Therefore, SERS-based nanozyme applications may play a crucial role in enhancing the detection sensitivity. To date, the number of reports on nanozyme-enhanced SERS techniques in the biosensing field is very limited, and more research is needed.
   b. In general, it is evident from several scientific reports that the smaller the size of NPs, the higher their nanozymatic activity. However, there are a

limited number of reports on the shape-dependent nanozymatic activity of nanomaterials, which must be addressed and can be one of the directions of future research.

c. Moreover, the role of surface ligands on nanomaterials to enhance their nanozymatic activity is not well understood. Future research could address the effect of the surface ligands on the nanozymatic activity.

d. Nanozyme-based lateral flow assays (LFA) would be a promising biosensing technique with real-life applications. A limited number of studies on the integration of nanozymes in LFA-based biosensors have been reported.

## REFERENCES

1. Huang Y, Ren J, Qu X. 2019. *Chem. Rev.* 119(6):4357–4412
2. Wu J, Wang X, Wang Q, Lou Z, Li S, et al. 2019. *Chem. Soc. Rev.* 48, 1004–1076
3. Wang H, Wan K, Shi X. 2019. *Adv. Mater.* 31(45):1805368
4. Unnikrishnan B, Lien CW, Chu HW, Huang CC. 2021. *J. Hazard. Mater.* 401: 123397
5. Huang L, Sun DW, Pu H, Wei Q. 2019. *Comprehensive Rev. Food Sci. Food Safety* 18 (5): 1496–1513
6. Zhou Y, Liu B, Yang R, Liu J. 2017. *Bioconjug. Chem.* 28(12):2903–9
7. Singh S. 2019. *Front. Chem.* 7: e00046
8. Liang M, Yan X. 2019. *Acc. Chem. Res.* 52(8):2190–2200
9. Wang W, Gunasekaran S. 2020. *TrAC - Trends Anal. Chem.* 126: 115841
10. Wu J, Li S, Wei H. 2018. *Chem. Commun.* 54(50):6520–30
11. Jiang D, Ni D, Rosenkrans ZT, Huang P, Yan X, Cai W. 2019. *Chem. Soc. Rev.* 48: 3683–3704
12. Manea F, Houillon FB, Pasquato L, Scrimin P. 2004. *Angew. Chem. Int. Ed.* 43(45):6165–69
13. Gao, L. Zhuang, J. Nie, L. Zhang, J. Zhang, Y.Gu, N. Wang, T. Feng, J. Yang, D. Perrett, S. 2007. *Nat. Nanotechnol.* 2 (9), 577–583
14. Ahmed SR, Chand R, Kumar S, Mittal N, Srinivasan S, Rajabzadeh AR. 2020. *TrAC - Trends Anal. Chem.* 131: 116006
15. Ahmed SR, Takemeura K, Li TC, Kitamoto N, Tanaka T, et al. 2017. *Biosens. Bioelectron.* 87:558–65
16. Oh S, Kim J, Tran VT, Lee DK, Ahmed SR, et al. 2018. *ACS Appl. Mater. Interfaces* 10(15):12534–43
17. Ahmed SR, Kim J, Suzuki T, Lee J, Park EY. 2016. *Biosens. Bioelectron.* 85:503–8
18. Ahmed SR, Kim J, Tran VT, Suzuki T, Neethirajan S, et al. 2017. *Sci. Rep.* 7(1):1–11
19. Ahmed SR, Kim J, Suzuki T, Lee J, Park EY. 2016. *Biotechnol. Bioeng.* 113(10):2298–2303
20. Jv Y, Li B, Cao R. 2010. *Chem. Commun.* 46(42):8017–19
21. Zhang H, Liang X, Han L, Li F. 2018. *Small* 4(44):e1803256
22. Wang F, Ju E, Guan Y, Ren J, Qu X. 2017. *Small* 13(25): 1603051
23. Sharifi M, Faryabi K, Talaei AJ, Shekha MS, Ale-Ebrahim M, et al. 2020. *J. Mol. Liq.* 297(1):112004
24. Jiang H, Chen Z, Cao H, Huang Y. 2012. *Analyst* 137(23):5560–64
25. Song H, Li Z, Peng Y, Li X, Xu X, et al. 2019. *Analyst* 144(7):2416–22
26. Li J, Liu W, Wu X, Gao X. 2015. *Biomaterials* 48:37–44
27. Hu L, Yuan Y, Zhang L, Zhao J, Majeed S, Xu G. 2013. Anal. Chim. Acta. 762:83–86
28. Cui Y, Lai X, Liang B, Liang Y, Sun H, Wang L. 2020. *ACS Omega* 5(12):6800–6808
29. He SB, Yang L, Lin XL, Chen LM, Peng HP, et al. 2020. *Talanta* 211:120707

30. Fan J, Yin JJ, Ning B, Wu X, Hu Y, et al. 2011. *Biomaterials* 32(6):1611–18
31. Cao GJ, Jiang X, Zhang H, Croley TR, Yin JJ. 2017. *RSC Adv.* 7(82):52210–17
32. Cui M, Zhou J, Zhao Y, Song Q. 2017. *Sens. Actuators B Chem.* 243:203–10
33. Cui M, Zhao Y, Wang C, Song Q. 2017. *Microchim. Acta.* 184(9):3113–19
34. Wang Q, Hong G, Liu Y, Hao J, Liu S. 2020. *RSC Adv.* 10(42):25209–13
35. Zhou N, Zou S, Zou L, Shen R, Zhou Y, Ling L. 2019. *Can. J. Chem.* 97(4):317–23
36. Shen X, Liu W, Gao X, Lu Z, Wu X, Gao X. 2015. *J. Amer. Chem. Soc.* 137(50):15882–91
37. Ge C, Fang G, Shen X, Chong Y, Wamer WG, et al. 2016. *ACS Nano* 10(11):10436–45
38. Mohamad A, Keasberry NA, Ahmed MU. 2018. *Anal. Sci.* 34(11):1257–63
39. Gao Z, Ye H, Tang D, Tao J, Habibi S, et al. 2017. *Nano Lett.* 17(9):5572–79
40. Singh S, Tripathi P, Kumar N, Nara S. 2017. *Biosens. Bioelectron.* 92:280–86
41. Fan C, Liu J, Zhao H, Li L, Liu M, et al. 2019. *RSC Adv.* 9(58):33678–83
42. Liu C, Yan Y, Zhang X, Mao Y, Ren X, et al. 2020. *Nanoscale* 12(5):3068–75
43. Cai S, Qi C, Li Y, Han Q, Yang R, Wang C. 2016. *J. Mater. Chem. B* 4(10):1869–77
44. Xi Z, Gao W, Xia X. 2020. *Chem. Bio. chem.* 21(17):2440–44
45. Lu Y, Ye W, Yang Q, Yu J, Wang Q, et al. 2016. *Sens. Actuators B Chem.* 230:721–30
46. Qiu N, Liu Y, Guo R. 2020. *ACS Appl. Mater. Interfaces* 12(13):15553–61
47. Wang Q, Zhang L, Shang C, Zhang Z, Dong S. 2016. *Chem. Commun.* 52(31):5410–13
48. Xiong Y, Chen S, Ye F, Su L, Zhang C, et al. 2015. *Chem. Commun.* 51(22):4635–38
49. Yang H, Yang R, Zhang P, Qin Y, Chen T, Ye F. 2017. *Microchim. Acta.* 184(12):4629–35
50. Huang Y, Zhao M, Han S, Lai Z, Yang J, et al. 2017. *Adv. Mater.* 29(32): 1700102
51. Gupta AK, Gupta M. 2005. *Biomaterials* 26(18): 3995–4021
52. Chen Z, Yin JJ, Zhou YT, Zhang Y, Song L, et al. 2012. *ACS Nano* 6(5):4001–12
53. Ahmed SR, Cirone J, Chen A. 2019. *Nano Mater.* 2(4):2076–85
54. Asati A, Santra S, Kaittanis C, Nath S, Perez JM. 2009. *Angew. Chemie - Int. Ed.* 48(13):2308–12
55. Cheng H, Lin S, Muhammad F, Lin YW, Wei H. 2016. *ACS Sensors* 1(11):1336–43
56. Yang Y, Mao Z, Huang W, Liu L, Li J, et al. 2016. *Sci. Rep.* 6(1):1–7
57. Li D, Garisto SL, Huang PJJ, Yang J, Liu B, Liu J. 2019. *Inorg. Chem. Commun.* 106:38–42
58. Liu H, Liu J. 2020. *Chem. Nano Mat.* 6(6):947–52
59. Korschelt K, Schwidetzky R, Pfitzner F, Strugatchi J, Schilling C, et al. 2018. *Nanoscale* 10(27):13074–82
60. André R, Natálio F, Humanes M, Leppin J, Heinze K, et al. 2011. *Adv. Funct. Mater.* 21(3):501–9
61. Zhang L, Xia F, Song Z, Webster NAS, Luo H, Gao Y. 2015. *RSC Adv.* 5(75):61371–79
62. Nie G, Zhang L, Lei J, Yang L, Zhang Z, et al. 2014. *J. Mater. Chem. A* 2(9):2910–14
63. Sun J, Li C, Qi Y, Guo S, Liang X. 2016. *Sensors* 16(4):584
64. Song L, Zhu Y, Yang Z, Wang C, Lu X. 2018. *J. Mater. Chem. B* 6(37):5931–39
65. Gao M, Lu X, Chi M, Chen S, Wang C. 2017. *Inorg. Chem. Front.* 4(11):1862–69
66. Yan X, Song Y, Wu X, Zhu C, Su X, et al. 2017. *Nanoscale* 9(6):2317–23
67. Cheng H, Liu Y, Hu Y, Ding Y, Lin S, et al. 2017. *Anal. Chem.* 89(21):11552–59
68. Nath I, Chakraborty J, Verpoort F. 2016. *Chem. Soc. Rev.*, 45: 4127–4170
69. Li S, Liu X, Chai H, Huang Y. 2018. *TrAC - Trends in Analytical Chemistry* 105: 391–403
70. Zhao M, Huang Y, Peng Y, Huang Z, Ma Q, Zhang H. 2018. *Chem. Soc. Rev.* 47: 6267–95
71. Zhang L, Xia Z. 2011. *Phys. Chem. C.* 115(22):11170–76
72. Fan K, Xi J, Fan L, Wang P, Zhu C, et al. 2018. *Nat. Commun.* 9:1440
73. Liu S, Li Z, Wang C, Tao W, Huang M, et al. *Nat. Commun.* 11:938
74. Jiang P, Chen S, Wang C, Wang D, Diao J, et al. 2020. *Mater. Today Sustain* 9:100039
75. Wang C, Wang D, Liu S, Jiang P, Lin Z, et al. 2020. *J. Catal.* 389:150–56

76. Xu B, Wang H, Wang W, Gao L, Li S, et al. 2019. 58(15):4911–16
77. Ma W, Mao J, Yang X, Pan C, Chen W, et al. 2019. *Chem. Commun.* 55(2):159–62
78. Huo M, Wang L, Wang Y, Chen Y, Shi J. 2019. *ACS Nano* 13(2):2643–53
79. Zhang X, Wu D, Zhou X, Yu Y, Liu J, et al. 2019. *TrAC - Trends Anal. Chem.* 121: 115668
80. Li S, Shang L, Xu B, Wang S, Gu K, et al. 2019. *Angew. Chemie - Int. Ed.* 58(36): 12624–12631
81. Zhang X, Li G, Wu D, Li X, Hu N, et al. 2019. *Biosens. Bioelectron.* 137: 178–98
82. Mahmoudi T, Guardia M, Shirdel B, Mokhtarzadeh A, Baradaran B. 2019. *TrAC - Trends Anal. Chem.* 116:13–30
83. M. A, K. 2019. *Mol. Catalysis* 475:110492
84. Chaibakhsh N, Moradi-Shoeili Z. 2019. *Mater. Sci. Eng. C.* 99:1424–47
85. Song W, Zhao B, Wang C, Ozaki Y, Lu X. 2019. *J. Mater.Chem. B.* 7:850–75
86. Fu Q, Saltsburg H, Flytzani-Stephanopoulos M. 2003. *Science 301*(5635):80–
87. Guzman J, Gates BC. 2004. *J. Catal.* 226(1):111–19
88. Qiao B, Wang A, Yang X, Allard LF, Jiang Z, et al. 2011. *Nat. Chem.* 3(8):634–41
89. Wang A, Li J, Zhang T. 2018. *Nat. Rev. Chem.* 2: 65–81
90. Zhang X, Shi H, Xu BQ. 2005. *Angew. Chemie - Int. Ed.* 44(43):7132–35
91. Giannakakis G, Flytzani-Stephanopoulos M, Sykes ECH. 2019. *Acc. Chem. Res.* 52(1):237–47
92. Zhao D, Zhuang Z, Cao X, Zhang C, Peng Q, et al. 2020. *Chem. Soc. Rev.* 49:2215–64
93. Yan H, Su C, He J, Chen W. 2018. *J. Mater. Chem. A.* 6:8793–8814
94. Huang X, Groves JT. 2018. *Chem. Rev.* 118(5): 2491–2553
95. Collins TJ, Ryabov AD. 2017. *Chem. Rev.* 117(13):9140–62
96. Liu Y, Wang X, Wei H. 2020. *Analyst* 145: 4388–97
97. D'souza F, Ito O. 2012. *Chem. Soc. Rev.* 41(1):86–96
98. Zhang J, Lu X, Tang D, Wu S, Hou X, et al. 2018. *ACS Appl. Mater. Interfaces* 10(47):40808–14
99. Zhang J, Wu S, Lu X, Wu P, Liu J. 2019. *Nano Lett.* 19(5): 3214–3220
100. C. S, Y. D, Y.-Y. N, X.-G. L, J. X, X.-H. 2017. *Chem. - A Eur. J.* 23(28):6717–23
101. Sun X, Luo X, Zhang X, Xie J, Jin S, et al. 2019. *J. Am. Chem. Soc.* 141(9):3797–3801
102. Gu JW, Guo RT, Miao YF, Liu YZ, Wu GL, et al. 2021. *Appl. Surf. Sci.* 540:148316
103. Su F, Mathew SC, Lipner G, Fu X, Antonietti M, et al. 2010. *J. Am. Chem. Soc.* 132(46):16299–301
104. Neri S, Martin SG, Pezzato C, Prins LJ. 2017. *J. Am. Chem. Soc.* 139(5):1794–1997
105. Pawelek PD, Cheah J, Coulombe R, Macheroux P, Ghisla S, Vrielink A. 2000. *EMBO J.* 19(16):4204–15
106. Song Y, Qu K, Zhao C, Ren J, Qu X. 2010. *Adv. Mater.* 22(19):2206–10
107. Zaupa G, Mora C, Bonomi R, Prins LJ, Scrimin P. 2011. *Chem. - A Eur. J.* 17(17):4879–89
108. Diez-Castellnou M, Mancin F, Scrimin P. 2014. *J. Am. Chem. Soc.* 136(4):1158–61
109. Chen JL-Y, Pezzato C, Scrimin P, Prins LJ. 2016. *Chem. - A Eur. J.* 22(21):7028–32
110. Zhan P, Wang ZG, Li N, Ding B. 2015. *ACS Catal.* 5(3):1489–98
111. Sun Y, Zhao C, Gao N, Ren J, Qu X. 2017. *Chem. - A Eur. J.* 23(72):18146–50
112. Zhang H, He H, Jiang X, Xia Z, Wei W. 2018. *ACS Appl. Mater. Interfaces* 10(36):30680–88
113. Silva CS, Durão P, Fillat A, Lindley PF, Martins LO, Bento I. 2012. *Metallomics* 4(1):37–47
114. Bhagi-Damodaran A, Michael MA, Zhu Q, Reed J, Sandoval BA, et al. 2017. *Nat. Chem.* 9(3):257–63
115. Comotti M, Della Pina C, Matarrese R, Rossi M. 2004. *Angew. Chemie - Int. Ed.* 43(43):5812–15
116. Ragg R, Natalio F, Tahir MN, Janssen H, Kashyap A, et al. 2014. *ACS Nano* 8(5):5182–89

117. Guo Y, Deng L, Li J, Guo S, Wang E, Dong S. 2011. *ACS Nano* 5(2):1282–90
118. Tao Y, Lin Y, Huang Z, Ren J, Qu X. 2013. *Adv. Mater.* 25(18):2594–99
119. Qu F, Li T, Yang M. 2011. *Biosens. Bioelectron.* 26(9):3927–31
120. Song H, Ni Y, Kokot S. 2013. *Anal. Chim. Acta.* 788:24–31
121. Lin L, Song X, Chen Y, Rong M, Zhao T, et al. 2015. *Anal. Chim. Acta.* 869:89–95
122. Zhang Y, Wu C, Zhou X, Wu X, Yang Y, et al. 2013. *Nanoscale* 5(5):1816–19
123. Wang Q, Lei J, Deng S, Zhang L, Ju H. 2013. *Chem. Commun.* 49(9):916–18
124. Wang X, Qu K, Xu B, Ren J, Qu X. 2011. *Nano Res.* 4(9):908–20
125. Xie J, Cao H, Jiang H, Chen Y, Shi W, et al. 2013. *Anal. Chim. Acta.* 796:92–100
126. Qian J, Yang X, Jiang L, Zhu C, Mao H, Wang K. 2014. *Sens. Actuators B Chem.* 201:160–66
127. Zhang Z, Hao J, Yang W, Lu B, Ke X, et al. 2013. *ACS Appl. Mater. Interfaces* 5(9):3809–15
128. Nirala NR, Abraham S, Kumar V, Bansal A, Srivastava A, Saxena PS. 2015. *Sens. Actuators B Chem.* 218:42–50
129. Ragavan KV, Rastogi NK. 2016. *Sens. Actuators B Chem.* 229:570–80
130. Lin XQ, Deng HH, Wu GW, Peng HP, Liu AL, et al. 2015. *Analyst* 140(15):5251–56
131. Zhang Y, Sun X, Zhu L, Shen H, Jia N. 2011. *Electrochim. Acta.* 56(3):1239–45
132. Xing Z, Tian J, Asiri AM, Qusti AH, Al-Youbi AO, Sun X. 2014. *Biosens. Bioelectron.* 52:452–57
133. Zhang Y, Xia Z, Liu H, Yang M, Lin L, Li Q. 2013. *Sens. Actuators B Chem.* 188:496–501
134. Zhan L, Li CM, Wu WB, Huang CZ. 2014. *Chem. Commun.* 50(78):11526–28
135. Li L, Du Z, Liu S, Hao Q, Wang Y, et al. 2010. *Talanta* 82(5):1637–41
136. Zhang LN, Deng HH, Lin FL, Xu XW, Weng SH, et al. 2014. *Anal. Chem.* 86(5): 2711–18
137. Wang H, Li S, Si Y, Sun Z, Li S, Lin Y. 2014. *J. Mater. Chem. B* 2(28):4442–48
138. Chen X, Chen X, Su B, Cai Z, Oyama M. 2014. *Sens. Actuators B Chem.* 201:286–92
139. Jiao X, Song H, Zhao H, Bai W, Zhang L, Lv Y. 2012. *Anal. Methods.* 4(10):3261–67
140. Artiglia L, Agnoli S, Cristina Paganini M, Cattelan M, Granozzi G. 2014. *ACS Appl. Mater. Interfaces.* 6(22):20130–36
141. Zhao H, Dong Y, Jiang P, Wang G, Zhang J. 2015. *ACS Appl. Mater. Interfaces.* 7(12):6451–61
142. Liu Q, Ding Y, Yang Y, Zhang L, Sun L, et al. 2016. *Mater. Sci. Eng. C.* 59:445–53
143. Jampaiah D, Srinivasa Reddy T, Kandjani AE, Selvakannan PR, Sabri YM, et al. 2016. *J. Mater. Chem. B* 4(22):3874–85
144. Sun L, Ding Y, Jiang Y, Liu Q. 2017. *Sens. Actuators B Chem.* 239:848–56
145. Mu J, Wang Y, Zhao M, Zhang L. 2012. *Chem. Commun.* 48(19):2540–42
146. Qin W, Su L, Yang C, Ma Y, Zhang H, Chen X. 2014. *J. Agric. Food Chem.* 62(25):5827–34
147. Yang W, Hao J, Zhang Z, Zhang B. 2015. *New J. Chem.* 39(11):8802–6
148. Liu Q, Zhu R, Jiang Y, Zhang L, Yin H, et al. 2015. *Mater. Sci. Eng. B* 198:57–61
149. Zhang T, Cao C, Tang X, Cai Y, Yang C, Pan Y. 2017. *Nanotechnology* 28(4):45704
150. Gao Y, Wu K, Li H, Chen W, Fu M, et al. 2018. *Sens. Actuators B Chem.* 273:1635–39
151. Wang Y, Zhang X, Luo Z, Huang X, Tan C, et al. 2014. *Nanoscale* 6(21):12340–44
152. He SB, Wu GW, Deng HH, Liu AL, Lin XH, et al. 2014. *Biosens. Bioelectron.* 62:331–36
153. Gao Z, Xu M, Hou L, Chen G, Tang D. 2013. *Anal. Chim. Acta.* 776:79–86
154. Gao Z, Xu M, Lu M, Chen G, Tang D. 2015. *Biosens. Bioelectron.* 70:194–201
155. Yao J, Cheng Y, Zhou M, Zhao S, Lin S, et al. 2018. *Chem. Sci.* 9(11):2927–33
156. Chen J, Patil S, Seal S, McGinnis JF. 2006. *Nat. Nanotechnol.* 1(2):142–50
157. Kim J, Takahashi M, Shimizu T, Shirasawa T, Kajita M, et al. 2008. *Mech. Ageing Dev.* 129(6):322–31

158. Leon B, Jiuyang H, Minmin L, Wolfgang T. 2018. *Progress in Biochemistry and Biophysics* 45(2):148–68
159. Tarnuzzer RW, Colon J, Patil S, Seal S. 2005. *Nano Lett.* 5(12):2573–77
160. Zhang L, Laug L, Münchgesang W, Pippel E, Gösele U, et al. 2010. *Nano Lett.* 10(1):219–23
161. Takamiya M, Miyamoto Y, Yamashita T, Deguchi K, Ohta Y, Abe K. 2012. *Neuroscience* 221:47–55
162. Xiong B, Xu R, Zhou R, He Y, Yeung ES. 2014. *Talanta* 120:262–67
163. Wang MQ, Ye C, Bao SJ, Xu MW. 2017. *Microchim. Acta.* 184(4):1177–84
164. Shen X, Wang Q, Liu Y, Xue W, Ma L, et al. 2016. *Sci. Rep.* 6(1):1–9
165. Singh N, Savanur MA, Srivastava S, D'Silva P, Mugesh G. 2017. *Angew. Chemie - Int. Ed.* 56(45):14267–71
166. Ragg R, Schilmann AM, Korschelt K, Wieseotte C, Kluenker M, et al. 2016. *J. Mater. Chem. B* 4(46):7423–28
167. Korschelt K, Ragg R, Metzger CS, Kluenker M, Oster M, et al. 2017. *Nanoscale* 9(11):3952–60
168. Dong J, Song L, Yin JJ, He W, Wu Y, et al. 2014. *ACS Appl. Mater. Interfaces* 6(3): 1959–1970
169. Golchin J, Golchin K, Alidadian N, Ghaderi S, Eslamkhah S, et al. 2017. *Artif. Cell Nanomed. B* 45(6): 1069–1076
170. Zhao J, Gao W, Cai X, Xu J, Zou D, et al. 2019. *Theranostics* 9(10):2843–55
171. Nandi A, Yan LJ, Jana CK, Das N. *2019. Oxid. Med. Cell. Longev.* 2019: 9613090
172. Singhal A, Morris VB, Labhasetwar V, Ghorpade A. 2013. *Cell Death Dis.* 4(11): e903
173. Giordano CR, Roberts R, Krentz KA, Bissig D, Talrej D, et al. 2015. *Vis. Sci.* 56(5):3095–3102
174. Qi C, Chen Y, Huang JH, Jin QZ, Wang XG. 2012. *J. Sci. Food Agric.* 92(4):787–93
175. Baldim V, Bedioui F, Mignet N, Margaill I, Berret JF. 2018. *Nanoscale* 10(15):6971–80
176. Thakur N, Manna P, Das J. 2019. *J. of Nanobiotechnology* 17:84
177. Doskey CM, Buranasudja V, Wagner BA, Wilkes JG, Du J, et al. 2016. *Redox Biol.* 10:274–84
178. Zhang XQ, Gong SW, Zhang Y, Yang T, Wang CY, Gu N. 2010. *J. Mater. Chem.* 20(24):5110–16
179. Gao Z, Hou L, Xu M, Tang D. 2015. *Sci. Rep.* 4(1):1–8
180. Ahmed SR, Chen A. 2020. *ACS Appl. Nano Mater.* 3(9): 9462–9469
181. Ragavan KV, Ahmed SR, Weng X, Neethirajan S. 2018. *Sens. Actuators B Chem.* 272:8–13
182. Weng X, Ahmed SR, Neethirajan S. 2018. *Sens. Actuators B Chem.* 265: 242–248
183. Jang H, Ahmed SR, Neethirajan S. 2017. *Sensors* 17(5): 1079
184. R. S, Corredor JC, Nagy É, Neethirajan S. 2017. *Nanotheranostics* 1(3):338–45
185. Zhang P, Sun D, Cho A, Weon S, Lee S, et al. 2019. *Nat. Commun.* 10(1):940
186. Wei H, Wang E. 2008. *Anal. Chem.* 80(6): 2250–2254
187. Chang Q, Deng K, Zhu L, Jiang G, Yu C, Tang H. 2009. *Microchim. Acta.* 165 3–4, 299–305
188. Kim MI, Shim J, Li T, Lee J, Park HG. 2011. *Chem. - A Eur. J.* 17(38):10700–707
189. Dong YL, Zhang HG, Rahman ZU, Su L, Chen XJ, et al. 2012. *Nanoscale* 4(13):3969–76
190. Liu S, Tian J, Wang L, Luo Y, Chang G, Sun X. 2011. *Analyst* 136(23):4894–97
191. Wang W, Jiang X, Chen K. 2012. *Chem. Commun.* 48(58):7289–91
192. Malvi B, Panda C, Dhar BB, Gupta SS. 2012. *Chem. Commun.* 48(43):5289–91
193. Roy P, Lin Z-H, Liang C-T, Chang H-T. 2012. *Chem. Commun.* 48:4079–81
194. Tian J, Liu S, Luo Y, Sun X. 2012. *Catal. Sci. Technol.* 2(2):432–36
195. Liu Q, Li H, Zhao Q, Zhu R, Yang Y, et al. 2014. *Mater. Sci. Eng. C* 41:142–51
196. Wu Y, Xue P, Hui KM, Kang Y. 2014. *Biosens. Bioelectron.* 52:180–87

197. Chang Q, Tang H. 2014. *Microchim. Acta* 181(5–6):527–34
198. Zhang T, Lu Y, Luo G. 2014. *ACS Appl. Mater. Interfaces* 6(16):14433–38
199. Ai L, Li L, Zhang C, Fu J, Jiang J. 2013. *Chem. - A Eur. J.* 19(45):15105–8
200. Chen W, Chen J, Feng YB, Hong L, Chen QY, et al. 2012. *Analyst* 137(7):1706–12
201. Wang XX, Wu Q, Shan Z, Huang QM. 2011. *Biosens. Bioelectron.* 26(8):3614–19
202. Liu J, Hu X, Hou S, Wen T, Liu W, et al. 2012. *Sens. Actuators B Chem.* 166–67: 708–14
203. Wan L, Liu J, Huang XJ. 2014. *Chem. Commun.* 50(88):13589–91
204. Guo Y, Li J, Dong S. 2011. *Sens. Actuators B Chem.* 160(1):295–300
205. Shi W, Wang Q, Long Y, Cheng Z, Chen S, et al. 2011. *Chem. Commun.* 47(23):6695–97
206. Liu S, Tian J, Wang L, Luo Y, Sun X. 2012. *RSC Adv.* 2(2):411–13
207. Hu J, Wang SQ, Wang L, Li F, Pingguan-Murphy B, et al. 2014. *Biosens. Bioelectron.* 54:585–97
208. Zhang Y, Tian J, Liu S, Wang L, Qin X, et al. 2012. *Analyst* 137(6):1325–28
209. Yang W, Hao J, Zhang Z, Lu B, Zhang B, Tang J. 2014. *RSC Adv.* 4(67):35500–504
210. Liu Q, Zhu R, Du H, Li H, Yang Y, et al. 2014. *Mater. Sci. Eng. C* 43:321–29
211. Chen X, Zhou X, Hu J. 2012. *Anal. Methods* 4(7):2183–87
212. Zhang W, Ma D, Du J. 2014. *Talanta* 120:362–67
213. Wang T, Fu Y, Chai L, Chao L, Bu L, et al. 2014. *Chem. - A Eur. J.* 20(9):2623–30
214. Wang J, Han D, Wang X, Qi B, Zhao M. 2012. *Biosens. Bioelectron.* 36(1):18–21
215. Ahmed SR, Kumar S, Ortega GA, Srinivasan S, Rajabzadeh AR. 2021. *Food Chem.* 346: 128893
216. Ahmed SR, Kang SW, Oh S, Lee J, Neethirajan S. 2018. *Heliyon* 4(8): e00766
217. Ahmed SR, Neethirajan S. 2018. *Glob. Challenges* 2(4): 1700071
218. Cirone J, Ahmed SR, Wood PC, Chen A. 2019. *J. Phys. Chem. C* 123:9183–9191
219. Ahmed SR, Nagy É, Neethirajan S. 2017. *RSC Adv.* 7: 40849–40857
220. Ahmed SR, Hossain MA, Park JY, Kim SH, Lee D, et al. 2014. *Biosens. Bioelectron.* 58: 33–39
221. Ahmed SR, Hong SC, Lee J. 2011. *Front. Mater. Sci. Chin.* 5: 40–49
222. Ahmed SR, Koh K, Kang NL, Lee J. 2012. *Bull. Korean Chem. Soc.* 33(5):1608
223. Ahmed SR, Cha HR, Park JY, Park EY, Lee D, Lee J. 2012. *Nanoscale Res. Lett.* 7(1): 438
224. Lee J, Ahmed SR, Oh S, Kim J, Suzuki T, et al. 2015. *Biosens. Bioelectron.* 64: 311–317
225. Lee J, Kim J, Ahmed SR, Zhou H, Kim JM, Lee J. 2014. *ACS Appl. Mater. Interfaces* 6(23): 21380–21388
226. Wang X, Qin L, Lin M, Xing H, Wei H. 2019. *Anal. Chem.* 91(16): 10648–10656
227. Chang Y, Liu M, Liu J. 2020. *Anal. Chem.* 92(4):3118–24
228. Ahmed SR, Mogus J, Chand R, Nagy E, Neethirajan S. 2018. *Biosens. Bioelectron.* 103:45–53
229. Li Y, Zhang Y, Li F, Feng J, Li M, et al. 2017. *Biosens. Bioelectron.* 92:33–39
230. Gao ZD, Qu Y, Li T, Shrestha NK, Song YY. 2014. *Sci. Rep.* 4:6891
231. Zhang L, Xie X, Yuan Y, Chai Y, Yuan R. 2019. *Electroanalysis* 31(6):1019–25
232. Das R, Dhiman A, Kapil A, Bansal V, Sharma TK. 2019. *Anal. Bioanal. Chem.* 411(6):1229–38
233. Zhou M, Feng C, Mao D, Yang S, Ren L, et al. 2019. *Biosens. Bioelectron.*142: 111558
234. Sun D, Luo Z, Lu J, Zhang S, Che T, et al. 2019. *Biosens. Bioelectron.* 134:49–56
235. Han J, Wang Z, Wang C, Han J, Bu H. 2017. *Anal. Chim. Acta.* 962:24–31
236. Li Y, Yu C, Yang B, Liu Z, Xia P, Wang Q. 2018. *Biosens. Bioelectron.* 102:307–15
237. Tian L, Qi J, Oderinde O, Yao C, Song W, Wang Y. 2018. *Biosens. Bioelectron.* 110:110–17
238. Ling P, Lei J, Zhang L, Ju H. 2015. *Anal. Chem.* 87(7):3957–63
239. Hun X, Xie G, Luo X. 2015. *Chem. Commun.* 51(33):7100–7103

240. Zhang GY, Deng SY, Cai WR, Cosnier S, Zhang XJ, Shan DMZH. 2015. *Anal. Chem.* 87(17):9093–9100
241. Shi L, Yu Y, Chen Z, Zhang L, He S, et al. 2015. *RSC Adv.* 5(15):11541–48
242. Bhattacharjee R, Tanaka S, Moriam S, Masud MK, Lin J, et al. 2018. *J. Mater. Chem. B* 6(29):4783–91
243. Yadav S, Masud MK, Islam MN, Gopalan V, Lam AKY, et al. 2017. *Nanoscale* 9(25):8805–14
244. Masud MK, Yadav S, Islam MN, Nguyen NT, Salomon C, et al. 2017. *Anal. Chem.* 89(20):11005–13
245. Sun D, Lin X, Lu J, Wei P, Luo Z, et al. 2019. *Biosens. Bioelectron.* 142: 111578
246. Ou D, Sun D, Lin X, Liang Z, Zhong Y, Chen Z. 2019. *J. Mater. Chem. B* 7(23):3661–69
247. Jiao L, Mu Z, Miao L, Du W, Wei Q, Li H. 2017. *Microchim. Acta.* 184(2):423–29
248. Zhang T, Song Y, Xing Y, Gu Y, Yan X, et al. 2019. *Nanoscale* 11(42):20221–27
249. Wang Y, Wang Y, Pang X, Du B, Li H, et al. 2015. *Sens. Actuators B Chem.* 214:124–31
250. Ling P, Qian C, Yu J, Gao F. 2020. *Biosens. Bioelectron.* 149: 111838
251. Boriachek K, Masud MK, Palma C, Phan HP, Yamauchi Y, et al. 2019. *Anal. Chem.* 91(6):3827–34
252. Alizadeh N, Salimi A, Hallaj R, Fathi F, Soleimani F. 2019. *Mater. Sci. Eng. C* 99:1374–83
253. Xi J, Xie C, Zhang Y, Wang L, Xiao J, et al. 2016. *ACS Appl. Mater. Interfaces* 8(34):22563–73
254. Tian L, Qi J, Qian K, Oderinde O, Liu Q, et al. 2018. *J. Electroanal. Chem.* 812:1–9
255. Tian L, Qi J, Qian K, Oderinde O, Cai Y, et al. 2018. *Sens. Actuators B Chem.* 260:676–84
256. Savas S, Altintas Z. 2019. *Materials* 12(13): 2189
257. Cai X, Wang Z, Zhang H, Li Y, Chen K, et al. 2019. *J. Mater. Chem. B* 7(3):401–7
258. Chen X, Liu D, Cao G, Tang Y, Wu C. 2019. *ACS Appl. Mater. Interfaces.* 11(9):9374–84
259. Son SE, Ko E, Tran V, Hur W, Choi H, et al. 2019. *Chem. Electro. Chem.* 6(17):4666–73
260. Zhu J, Peng X, Nie W, Wang Y, Gao J, et al. 2019. *Biosens. Bioelectron.* 141: 111450
261. Wang K, Wu C, Wang F, Liao M, Jiang G. 2020. *Biosens. Bioelectron.* 150: 111869
262. Hu Y, Cheng H, Zhao X, Wu J, Muhammad F, et al. 2017. *ACS Nano* 11(6):5558–66
263. Yan M, Chen G, She Y, Ma J, Hong S, et al. 2019. *J. Agric. Food Chem.* 67(34):9658–66
264. Koo KM, Dey S, Trau M. 2018. *ACS Sensors* 3(12):2597–2603
265. Ko E, Tran VK, Son SE, Hur W, Choi H, Seong GH. 2019. *Sens. Actuators B Chem.* 294:166–76
266. Cheng H, Zhang L, He J, Guo W, Zhou Z, et al. 2016. *Anal. Chem.* 88(10):5489–97
267. Shen R, Liu P, Zhang Y, Yu Z, Chen X, et al. 2018. *Anal. Chem.* 90(7):4478–84
268. Chen GH, Chen WY, Yen YC, Wang CW, Chang HT, Chen CF. 2014. *Anal. Chem.* 86(14):6843–49
269. Ortiz-Gómez I, Salinas-Castillo A, García AG, Álvarez-Bermejo JA, Orbe-Payá I, et al. 2018. *Microchim. Acta* 185:47
270. Vernekar AA, Sinha D, Srivastava S, Paramasivam PU, D'Silva P, Mugesh G. 2014. *Nat. Commun.* 5(1):5301
271. Hirst SM, Karakoti AS, Tyler RD, Sriranganathan N, Seal S, Reilly CM. 2009. *Small* 5(24):2848–56
272. Choi SW, Kim J. 2020. *ACS Appl. Nano Mater.* 3(2):1043–62
273. Wang P, Wang T, Hong J, Yan X, Liang M. 2020. *Frontiers in Bioeng. and Biotech.* 8:15
274. Li J, Wang J, Wang Y, Trau M. 2017. *Analyst* 142(24):4788–93
275. Zhang D, Zhao YX, Gao YJ, Gao FP, Fan YS, et al. 2013. *J. Mater. Chem. B* 1(38):5100–5107
276. Fan K, Cao C, Pan Y, Lu D, Yang D, et al. 2012. *Nat. Nanotechnol.* 7(7):459–64
277. Wang T, He J, Duan D, Jiang B, Wang P, et al. 2019. *Nano Res.* 12(4):863–68

278. Cai Y, Cao C, He X, Yang C, Tian L, et al. 2015. *Int. J. Nanomedicine* 10:2619–34
279. Kim MS, Kweon SH, Cho S, An SSA, Kim MI, et al. 2017. *ACS Appl. Mater. Interfaces* 9(40):35133–40
280. Bai J, Jia X, Zhen W, Cheng W, Jiang X. 2018. *J. Am. Chem. Soc.* 140(1):106–9
281. Wang W, Jiang X, Chen K. 2012. *Chem. Commun.* 48(54):6839–41
282. Chen F, Bai M, Cao K, Zhao Y, Wei J, Zhao Y. 2017. *Adv. Funct. Mater.* 27(45): 1702748
283. Fan W, Bu W, Shen B, He Q, Cui Z, et al. 2015. *Adv. Mater.* 27(28):4155–61
284. Li J, Cao Y, Hinman SS, McKeating KS, Guan Y, et al. 2018. *Biosens. Bioelectron.* 100:304–11
285. Singh M, Weerathunge P, Liyanage PD, Mayes E, Ramanathan R, Bansal V. 2017. *Langmuir* 33(38):10006–15
286. Yang F, Hu S, Zhang Y, Cai X, Huang Y, et al. 2012. *Adv. Mater.* 24(38):5205–11
287. Sloan-Dennison S, Laing S, Shand NC, Graham D, Faulds K. 2017. *Analyst* 142(13):2484–90
288. Liu Q, Jing C, Zheng X, Gu Z, Li D, et al. 2012. *Chem. Commun.* 48(77):9574–76
289. Gao L, Liu M, Ma G, Wang Y, Zhao L, et al. 2015. *ACS Nano* 9(11):10979–90
290. Wang GL, Jin LY, Dong YM, Wu XM, Li ZJ. 2015. *Biosens. Bioelectron.* 64:523–29
291. Wang CI, Chen WT, Chang HT. 2012. *Anal. Chem.* 84(22):9706–12
292. Paul A, Paul S. 2014. *Front. Biosci. 19*: 605–18
293. Li Y, Xuan J, Song Y, Wang P, Qin L. 2015. *Lab Chip* 15(16):3300–3306
294. Lin J, Zhang W, Zhang H, Yang Z, Li T, et al. 2013. *Chem. Commun.* 49(43):4938–40
295. Niu X, Xu Y, Dong Y, Qi L, Qi S, et al. 2014. *Alloys Compd.* 587:74–81
296. Wu Y, Ma Y, Xu G, Wei F, Ma Y, et al. 2017. *Sens. Actuators B Chem.* 249:195–202
297. Zhang H, Ma L, Li P, Zheng J. 2016. *Biosens. Bioelectron.* 85:343–50
298. Liu W, Yang H, Ding Y, Ge S, Yu J, et al. 2014. *Analyst* 139(1):251–58
299. Peng J, Dong M, Ran B, Li W, Hao Y, et al. 2017. *ACS Appl. Mater. Interfaces* 9(16):13875–86
300. Qu K, Shi P, Ren J, Qu X. 2014. *Chem. - A Eur. J.* 20(24):7501–6
301. Tang Y-R, Zhang Y, Liu R, Su Y-Y, Lv Y. 2014. *Chinese J. Anal. Chem.* 41(3):330–36
302. Chen Y, Cao H, Shi W, Liu H, Huang Y. 2013. *Chem. Commun.* 49(44):5013
303. Di H, Mi Z, Sun Y, Liu X, Liu X, et al. 2020. *Theranostics* 10(20):9303–14
304. Ding H, Cai Y, Gao L, Liang M, Miao B, et al. 2019. *Nano Lett.* 19(1):203–9
305. Wang D, Jana D, Zhao Y. 2020. *Acc. Chem. Res.* 53(7):1389–1400
306. Wang HS, Li J, Li JY, Wang K, Ding Y, Xia XH. 2017. *NPG Asia Mater.* 9:e354

# 8 Gold Nanozymes in Therapeutics

*Smriti Singh and Seema Nara*[*]
Department of Biotechnology, Motilal Nehru
National Institute of Technology, Allahabad, India

## CONTENTS

## 8.1  INTRODUCTION

Various enzyme-mimetic nanomaterials, such as nanoparticles (NPs) of different metals (gold (Au) (1–10), platinum (Pt) (11, 12),bimetals (13–16)), metal oxides [iron oxide ($Fe_3O_4$) (17–20), cerium oxide ($CeO_2$) (21–25), vanadium(V) oxide ($V_2O_5$) (26, 27)], metal-organic frameworks (MOFs) (28–30), and carbon nanomaterials [single- and multi-walled carbon nanotubes (31, 32), carbon nanodots(33), graphene oxide (GO) (34), and fullerene derivatives (35)], have been identified to have remarkable catalytic properties and hence are explored for use in diverse applications. Out of these, metallic NPs, particularly, Au NPs possess remarkable properties and are ear-marked for their significant surface-to-volume ratio, tunable physical and chemical properties, good stability, facile bioconjugation chemistry, biocompatibility, and tremendous catalytic properties (36). These properties make Au an excellent metal for therapeutic applications (37–39). The commonly used Au nanostructure morphologies in therapeutics are round, sphere, rod, cone, pyramids, star, shell, cuboidal, and cluster-shaped (40–42). The enzymatic mimetic activities of Au NPs include nuclease (3, 10), esterase (1, 2), silicatein (5), glucose oxidase (GOx) (4, 8, 9), POD (7), CAT, glutathione peroxidase (GPx), and SOD (6, 43). These Au nanozyme activities (**Figure 8.1**) are explored in various fields of therapeutics. Herein, we focus

---

[*] Corresponding author: Seema Nara

DOI: 10.1201/9781003109228-8

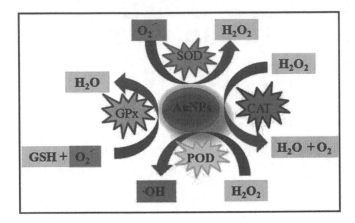

**FIGURE 8.1** Various enzyme-mimic activities of Au NPs involved in therapeutics. CAT: catalase, GPx: glutathione peroxidase, POD: peroxidase, SOD: superoxide dismutase.

on the emerging therapeutics technologies, such as antioxidants, antimicrobial, photothermal therapy (PTT), photodynamic therapy (PDT), imaging, etc., where enzyme-mimic properties of Au NPs are exploited.

Au nanozyme can modulate the generation of reactive oxygen species (ROS) (•OH and $O_2$ molecules) in biological systems, which can be used variously in therapeutics. In this section, the therapeutic applications of different Au nanozymes in imaging, antibacterial, antioxidant, neurodegenerative, and cancer therapy are presented.

## 8.2   ANTIBACTERIAL ACTIVITY

The emergence of drug resistance and abuse of antibiotics leads to the development of drug resistance in bacterial strains against many available drugs, including "ESKAPE" superbugs, which include *Enterobacter* species, methicillin-resistant *Staphylococcus aureus* (MRSA), *Klebsiella pneumoniae, Acinetobacter baumannii, Pseudomonas aeruginosa,* and vancomycin-resistant *Enterococcus faecium* (VRE) (44, 45). This is an alarming situation because most of the available antibiotics become ineffective against these bacterial strains and the bacterial virulence may turn into a major global health emergency (46, 47). Therefore, the exploration of new and safe antibacterial agents is of great significance. Researchers explored NPs as a potential antimicrobial agent, due to their extraordinary antimicrobial activity, high specific surface area, and more; and because microorganisms may not yet have developed resistance against NPs (48–51).

The intrinsic catalytic activity of Au nanozymes results in a significant amount of ROS generation, which becomes responsible for bacterial cell death. To augment this antibacterial effect of Au nanozymes, their surface has been variously modified with antimicrobial peptides (52, 53), cationic ligands (54) or they have been used in combination with other antibiotics (55, 56). Zheng et al., (57) designed small antibacterial peptide daptomycin (Dap)-conjugated Au nanocrystals (NCs) (Dap/Au

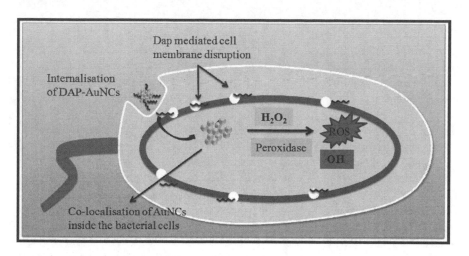

**FIGURE 8.2** Illustration of POD-mediated ROS generation and antibacterial activity of Dap-conjugated Au NCs.

NCs) as a promising candidate for future antibiotics (nanobiotics). The Dap peptide disrupted bacterial cell membranes by creating many large pores in their membrane and facilitated Dap/Au NC sentry inside the cells (**Figure 8.2**). High ROS generation by internalized Au nanozyme caused severe damage to subcellular structures and led to DNA fragmentation. Zhu et al., (58) reported antibacterial activity in protamine-conjugated 6-methyl-2-thiouracil-capped Au NCs (Prot/MTU-Au NCs) with a similar mechanism.

POD and OXD mimetic Au NPs and modified Au NPs (with mesoporous silica, aluminum-based porphyrinic MOFs, titanium oxide-graphene, and GO) displayed extraordinary antibacterial activity against *Staphylococcus aureus* and *Escherichia coli,* which were used as model microorganism from Gram-positive and Gram-negative bacteria (57, 59–63). The active mechanism behind the antimicrobial activity was reported to be intracellular ROS production, glutathione (GSH) depletion, and lipid peroxidation of bacterial cells facilitated by modified Au NPs. Intrinsic POD- and OXD-like activity of mercaptopyrimidine-conjugated Au NCswas reported possessing an excellent antibacterial activity against the superbugs *in vitro* and *in vivo* systems (64). POD- and OXD-like activity of Au NCs caused bacterial cell membrane disruption, ROS generation, and DNA damage both *in vitro* (macrophages) and *in vivo* (animal model)infections by MRSA. Wang et al., (65) integrated Au nanozymes in ultrathin graphitic carbon nitride (g-C$_3$N$_4$) and used their antibacterial activity in accelerating wound healing. These nanozymes not only showed antagonistic action against Gram-positive and Gram-negative microorganisms through •OH production but also participated in the breakdown of biofilm structures and inhibited the synthesis of new biofilms. Similar work was reported with antibiotic-conjugated Au-silver (Ag) NPs (isonicotinylhydrazide@Au-Ag NPs) which effectively combated multidrug-resistant (MDR) strain of *Mycobacterium tuberculosis* in a mice model (66).

## 8.3 CANCER THERAPY

The presence of a high level of ROS oxidizes the monomer units of lipids, nucleic acids, and protein molecules and causes irreversible cell damage. By using redox modulation, the level of ROS can be altered inside the tumor cells, and apoptosis could be activated. It has been substantiated to be an effective perspective for cancer therapy (67–73). Synchronized generation of ROS via OXD, POD, and GOx mimetic dendritic mesoporous silica-Au-iron oxide ($Fe_3O_4$) NPs (DMSN/Au/Fe NPs) resulted in mitochondrial-mediated apoptosis of tumor cells (74) (**Figure 8.3**). The cascade ROS generation was contributed by the cumulative activity of: 1) glucose catalysis by Au nanozyme;2) Fenton reactionand 3) Au nanozyme-mediated hydrogen per-oxide ($H_2O_2$) catalysis. A high level of free radicals (•OH), oxygen ($O_2$), and acidic conditions inside the endogenous environment of tumor cells, favor the efficacy of PDT, radiodynamic therapy, sonodynamic therapy, and chemodynamic therapy. This approach was explored by Liu et al. (75), where GOx and POD mimetic activity of Au NPs-doped Fe-based metal framework participated in the metabolism of glu-cose and generation of ROS inside the tumor cells. They also reported the POD-like activity in selenium (Se)-modified Au NPs (Se@Au NPs). These NPs overcame the low anticancerous activity of Au NPs by a synergistic effect of Se and Au NPs and induced a large generation of ROS inside the cells, which induced mitochondrial dysfunctioning and cellular apoptosis (76).

Available therapy for cancer-like radiotherapy and chemodynamic therapy suf-fered from the nonspecific recognition between tumor cells and healthy cells. To

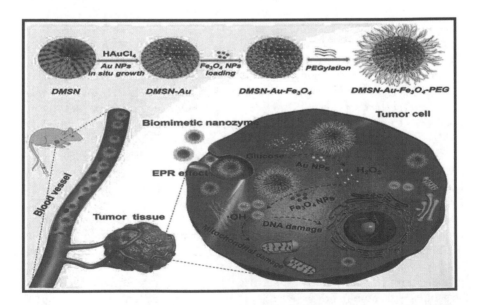

**FIGURE 8.3** Schematic representation of GOx and POD mimetic Au–$Fe_3O_4$ NPs-mediated synchronized ROS generation and tumor cell apoptosis. DMSN: dendritic mesopo-rous silica nanoparticles, EPR: enhanced permeability and retention. Adapted from Gao et al., (74).

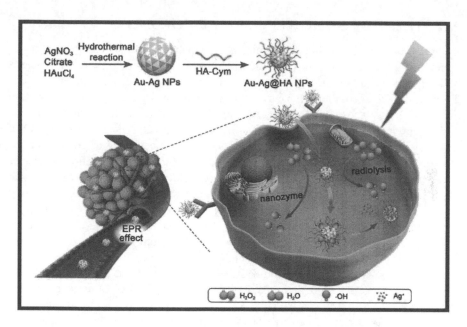

**FIGURE 8.4** Schematic of Au–Ag@HA NPs synthesis and synergistic nanozymatic activity in tumor therapy. Adapted from Chong et al., (77).

address this issue, the target/receptor-based approach is one of the best concepts, which could minimize the side effects of cancer therapy. This strategy was demonstrated by Chong et al. (77), where hyaluronic acid (HA)-modified Au–Ag bimetallic NPs (Au–Ag@HA NPs) showed effective tumor radiosensitization towards CD44, a nonkinase transmembrane glycoprotein, overexpression in breast cancer cells. The POD-like activity of Au–Ag@HA NPs catalyzed the $H_2O_2$ breakdown to hydroxyl radicals (•OH) near tumor sites, causing tumor cell death (**Figure 8.4**).

Folic acid (FA) receptors are highly expressed on the outer surface of cancerous cells, which showed affinity to FA. The POD mimetic FA-modified Au NPs, enhanced the level of ROS by decomposing $H_2O_2$ available inside the cells, causing significant cell death. Healthy cells possess antioxidant molecules, which protect them from ROS. This potential approach represents a more selective and effective treatment for cancerous cells. Au NPs loaded with IR780 iodide-loaded mesoporous carbon nanospheres modified by reduced bovine serum albumin (rBSA) and FA were used for the detection and diagnosis of the gastric tumor along with successful PTT and PDT. The POD-like activity of Au NPs embedded in the composite catalyzed $H_2O_2$ available inside tumor cells and resulted in •OH-mediated death of tumor cells (78). Similarly, Maji et al., (79) proposed a target-based therapy for cancer by using the intrinsic POD-like activity of GO-silicon-FA-Au NPs. These nanostructures were significantly capable to offer a therapeutic effect by enhancing the •OH generation from $H_2O_2$ and result in the significant death of cancerous cells.

## 8.4  THERAPY FOR NEUROLOGICAL DISORDERS

Aggregation of the amyloid-β protein, ROS generation, and copper (Cu) accumulation in the neuronal cells are the main causes of neurodegenerative diseases
(80, 81), and reduction in all these can be an effective therapy for the same. The
POD and SOD activities play an important role in regulating and controlling
the ROS levels and aggregation of the amyloid-β protein. Researchers are try-
ing to develop nanozymes, which are similar in their catalytic activity to natural
enzymes and can be used to simulate SOD and POD activities to control neurodegenerative disorders such as Alzheimer's disease (82, 83). Alzheimer's disease
can be controlled and treated by avoiding amyloid-β protein aggregation and
ROS levels in brain cells. Gao et al., (84) demonstrated this approach by using
polyoxometalate-8peptide-modified Au NPs. SOD mimetic activity of Au nanozyme complex reduced the level of ROS, whereas the protease-like activity of the
polyoxometalate prevented the aggregation of the amyloid-β protein. Au NPs also
acted like a metal chelator to extract Cu, which prevents Cu-induced aggregation
of amyloid-β oligomers and minimized the toxic effect of Cu accumulation (84).
Oxidative damage is one of the most common reasons for neuron damage, which
can be resolved by using NPs having CAT-like activity. Au NCs with various modifications were reported to catalyze $H_2O_2$ decomposition inside the neuronal cells
through their intrinsic CAT-like activity and protect from oxidative damage (85)
(**Figure 8.5**).

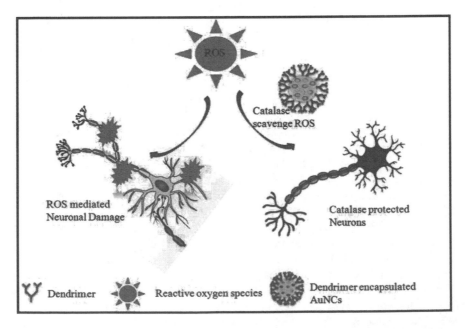

**FIGURE 8.5**  Illustration of CAT mimetic activity of dendrimer-encapsulated Au NCs. Au
NCs catalyze $H_2O_2$ and protect the neuronal cells from ROS-mediated damage.

## 8.5 PHOTOTHERMAL THERAPY (PTT) AND PHOTODYNAMIC THERAPY (PDT)

The key factor in determining the success of PDT and PTT is the availability of photosensitizers, light, and $O_2$. Conventional phototherapies suffer from flaws associated with: 1) photosensitizer's insolubility in water and easy aggregation at physiological conditions; 2) applicability of PDT for only superficial lesions; and 3) hypoxic environment inside the tumor favors PDT. To improve the therapeutic effect of PDT, nanozymes can be a superior alternative. Because of their CAT, POD, and OXD mimetic activity, they can generate high levels of free $O_2$ and •OH, which enhance the PDT effect under laser irradiation and cause apoptosis-mediated cell death. Optical properties like PTT and PDT of Au NPs can induce ROS production by their synergistic effect and results in cell death (86). This kind of nanozymatic activity was demonstrated using amine-terminated poly(amidoamine) (PAMAM) dendrimer-modified Au NCs (PAMMAM-Au NCs), Au NCs@MnO$_2$, IR780@OMCAPs@ rBSA-FA, and Au@HCNs. These NPs catalyzed the $H_2O_2$ available inside the tumor cells and resulted in the generation of a free hydroxyl group (•OH) and $O_2$, eventually leading to high tumor-cell damage due to $O_2$-boosted PDT (78, 87–89) (**Figure 8.6**).

## 8.6 ANTIOXIDANT ACTIVITY

Traditional cancer therapies, such as radio and chemotherapy, are known for their cytotoxic effects on normal cells and led to the death of healthy cells. Some NPs are also reported to have a significant cytotoxic effect on healthy cells. These treatments led to the generation of a high amount of ROS and cause neurotoxicity in the condition of ischemia/reperfusion injury (90, 91). Antioxidant enzymes, such as GPx,

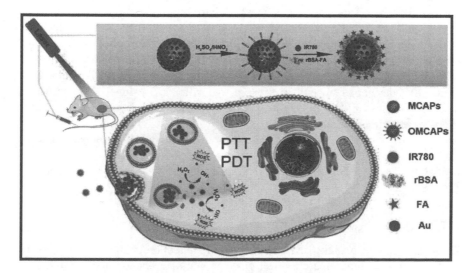

**FIGURE 8.6** Schematic of IR780@OMCAPs@rBSA-FA synthesis, its POD catalytic activity mediated target-specific therapy, and *in vivo* applications. Adapted from Zhang et al., (78).

CAT, and SOD, can neutralize these ROS and provide safety to the cells against ROS-mediated injury (92). ROS plays an important role as secondary messengers at a lower concentration in various cellular signaling pathways (93), although at high concentrations, ROS damage cells through oxidative injury and lead to apoptotic pathways (93, 94). Thus, for the maintenance of cellular equilibrium, controlling ROS levels is crucial (93, 95). Although cells produce antioxidant enzymes, oxidative stress evokes the excessive generation of ROS and highlights the significant requirement of antioxidants. For instance, natural CAT has a short life and poor uptake by the central nervous system, therefore, CAT mimetic nanozyme is a better substitute for natural CAT. Many recent studies have demonstrated the antioxidant effect of nanozymes, such as kaempferol-modified Au NPs, curcumin-capped Au NPs-conjugated reduced GO nanocomposite, 3,6-dihydroxyflavone-modified Au NPs, Au core-CeO$_2$ shell NPs, and Se-Pep@Au NPs (43, 96–100). Similarly, by using the synergistic effect of antioxidant peptide-A (Pep-A: Pro-His-Cys-Lys-Arg-Met)-conjugated Au NPs, Kalmodia et al., (101) demonstrated their antioxidant efficacy in the retinoblastoma cancer *in-vitro* model (Y79 cell line). Au NPs-Pep-A selectively targeted ROS in retinoblastoma cancer cells and decrease the ROS up to 70%. An increase in mRNA expression of antioxidant genes (GPx, SOD, and CAT) were also observed to be modulated by two-fold to three-fold.

## 8.7  IMAGING

### 8.7.1  IMAGING OF MICROBIAL BIOFILMS

Approximately, 80% of bacterial infections in humans are mainly associated with biofilm formation on living tissues (102). Biofilm is an extracellular polymeric substance secreted by microbes, which favors their growth in the form of films and secures them from exogenous agents. Therefore, these microbial biofilms are associated with chronic infections and diseases, such as endocarditis, osteomyelitis, urinary tract infections, and implant dysfunction; these are key co-morbidity threats for other diseases such as cystic fibrosis (103, 104). Imaging and tracking biofilms on medical devices and human tissues are even more challenging. Gupta et al., (105) developed an acidic pH-responsive sulfonamide-functionalized Au NPs nanozyme-based imaging system for mammalian cells (fibroblast) infected with the uropathogenic model *Pseudomonas aeruginosa* biofilms. These NPs switched the charge from zwitterionic (nonadhesive) state to cationic (adhesive) at pH of biofilms (pH 4.5–6.5), which activated pro-fluorophores (alloc-rhodamine) to fluorescent rhodamine *in situ*. This led to confocal imaging of these biofilms, as shown in **Figure 8.7**.

### 8.7.2  IMAGING OF TUMORS

To achieve high specificity and accuracy in the detection of tumor cells, it is necessary to design and prepare a novel enzyme-simulated nanoprobe specific to the target, having high catalytic and luminescent properties. The use of Au NCs and modified Au NCs with intrinsic enzymatic properties in tumor imaging is attracting

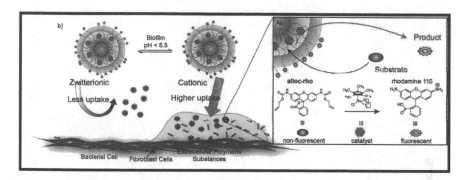

**FIGURE 8.7** Schematic of pH-switchable antibacterial activity of sulphonamide-functionalized Au NPs. The transition from zwitterionic Au NPs to cationic Au NPs activates pro-fluorophores and leads to fluorescent biofilm. Adapted from Gupta et al., (105).

research attention towards early cancer screening and diagnosis (106–109). Au NCs can be used as excellent nanoprobes in imaging and diagnosis (39). Hu et al., (110) developed a target-specific nanoprobe by employing FA-modified Au NCs (Au NCs-FA) and demonstrated *in vivo* imaging of cancerous cells in an animal model. Au NCs-FA were reported with novel luciferase and POD mimic activity, with high stability, and low cytotoxicity. Co-localization of Au NCs-FA in tumor cells was very high in comparison to normal cells. Horseradish peroxidase (HRP) cannot be applicable for *in vivo* imaging systems, due to its large size for renal clearance, non-specific degradation by proteases, reabsorbance by the tubular epithelium, and other limitations of natural enzymes. Multifunctional POD-like enzymatic activity of ultrasmall Au NCs was used as a nanoprobe for imaging colorectal cancer *in vivo* animal model (111). In comparison to HRP, the catalytic activity of Au NCs showed a 13-fold increase in colorimetric signal. Liang et al. (89) demonstrated magnetic resonance imaging of cancer cells by exploiting the CAT-like activity of Au NCs@ $MnO_2$. Au NCs participated in a high level of $O_2$ generation inside the cancerous cells and more $O_2$ levels absorb more near-infrared (NIR) irradiation. Because of this, Au provides better contrast for photoacoustic imaging, and photoacoustic signal intensity increases linearly (**Figure 8.8**).

## 8.8 SUMMARY AND FUTURE PERSPECTIVES

Au nanozymes show extremely promising and unbeatable contributions in diverse therapeutics applications, such as cancer therapy, imaging, antibacterial, antioxidant, neurodegenerative diseases, and effective photothermal, photodynamic, radiodynamic, sonodynamic, and chemodynamic therapies. Au nanozyme alone can act as a multifunctional enzyme and catalyze various enzymatic reactions under different physiological conditions. In the past decade, plenty of exciting data on the use of Au nanozymes use in therapeutics were revealed. However, very few therapeutic applications are in clinical trials. This is because the actual interaction of the NPs with the biological system is not clearly understood, such as their clearance from the human body, renal excretion, and associated cytotoxic effects. Their catalytic activity relies

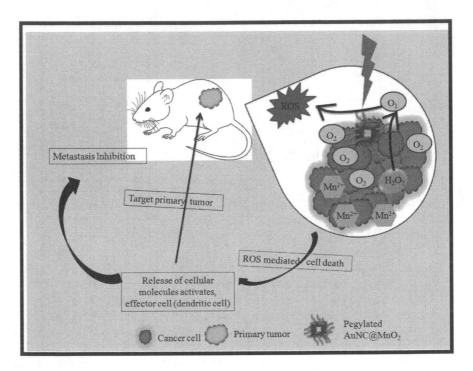

**FIGURE 8.8**    Schematic of Au NCs@MnO$_2$-mediated O$_2$-boosted cancer immunotherapy.

upon the surface accessibility of NPs and closely related to their surface properties. Once the surface of nanozymes is masked, their enzyme mimetic activity could be suppressed. A possible solution to overcome these problems is to explore a variety of functionalizations and modifications of Au NPs to enhance their physical and chemical properties.

## REFERENCES

1. Pasquato L, Rancan F, Scrimin P, Mancin F, Frigeri C. 2000. *Chemical Communications*: 2253–4
2. Pengo P, Polizzi S, Pasquato L, Scrimin P. 2005. *Journal of the American Chemical Society* 127: 1616–7
3. Manea F, Houillon FB, Pasquato L, Scrimin P. 2004. *Angewandte Chemie-International Edition* 43: 6165–9
4. Luo WJ, Zhu CF, Su S, Li D, He Y, et al. 2010. *Acs Nano* 4: 7451–8
5. Kisailus D, Najarian M, Weaver JC, Morse DE. 2005. *Advanced Materials* 17: 1234±
6. He WW, Zhou YT, Warner WG, Hu XN, Wu XC, et al. 2013. *Biomaterials* 34: 765–73
7. Jv Y, Li BX, Cao R. 2010. *Chemical Communications* 46: 8017–9
8. Comotti M, Della Pina C, Matarrese R, Rossi M. 2004. *Angewandte Chemie-International Edition* 43: 5812–5
9. Comotti M, Della Pina C, Falletta E, Rossi M. 2006. *Advanced Synthesis & Catalysis* 348: 313–6
10. Bonomi R, Selvestrel F, Lombardo V, Sissi C, Polizzi S, et al. 2008. *Journal of the American Chemical Society* 130: 15744±
11. Fan J, Yin JJ, Ning B, Wu XC, Hu Y, et al. 2011. *Biomaterials* 32: 1611–8

12. Zhang LB, Laug L, Munchgesang W, Pippel E, Gosele U, et al. 2010. *Nano Letters* 10: 219–23
13. He WW, Wu XC, Liu JB, Hu XN, Zhang K, et al. 2010. *Chemistry of Materials* 22: 2988–94
14. Slocik JM, Govorov AO, Naik RR. 2008. *Angewandte Chemie-International Edition* 47: 5335–9
15. Sun XL, Guo SJ, Chung CS, Zhu WL, Sun SH. 2013. *Advanced Materials* 25: 132–6
16. Sun XL, Guo SJ, Liu Y, Sun SH. 2012. *Nano Letters* 12: 4859–63
17. Chen Y, Hoang T, Ma SQ. 2012. *Inorganic Chemistry* 51: 12600–2
18. Gao LZ, Zhuang J, Nie L, Zhang JB, Zhang Y, et al. 2007. *Nature Nanotechnology* 2: 577–83
19. Liu SH, Lu F, Xing RM, Zhu JJ. 2011. *Chemistry-a European Journal* 17: 620–5
20. Park KS, Kim MI, Cho DY, Park HG. 2011. *Small* 7: 1521–5
21. Pirmohamed T, Dowding JM, Singh S, Wasserman B, Heckert E, et al. 2010. *Chemical Communications* 46: 2736–8
22. Kuchma MH, Komanski CB, Colon J, Teblum A, Masunov AE, et al. 2010. *Nanomedicine-Nanotechnology Biology and Medicine* 6: 738–44
23. Korsvik C, Patil S, Seal S, Self WT. 2007. *Chemical Communications*: 1056–8
24. Asati A, Kaittanis C, Santra S, Perez JM. 2011. *Analytical Chemistry* 83: 2547–53
25. Asati A, Santra S, Kaittanis C, Nath S, Perez JM. 2009. *Angewandte Chemie-International Edition* 48: 2308–12
26. Andre R, Natalio F, Humanes M, Leppin J, Heinze K, et al. 2011. *Advanced Functional Materials* 21: 501–9
27. Natalio F, Andre R, Hartog AF, Stoll B, Jochum KP, et al. 2012. *Nature Nanotechnology* 7: 530–5
28. Zheng HQ, Liu CY, Zeng XY, Chen J, Lu J, et al. 2018. *Inorganic Chemistry* 57: 9096–104
29. Feng DW, Gu ZY, Li JR, Jiang HL, Wei ZW, Zhou HC. 2012. *Angewandte Chemie-International Edition* 51: 10307–10
30. Gu ZY, Park J, Raiff A, Wei ZW, Zhou HC. 2014. *Chemcatchem* 6: 67–75
31. Song YJ, Wang XH, Zhao C, Qu KG, Ren JS, Qu XG. 2010. *Chemistry-a European Journal* 16: 3617–21
32. Cui RJ, Han ZD, Zhu JJ. 2011. *Chemistry-a European Journal* 17: 9377–84
33. Shi WB, Wang QL, Long YJ, Cheng ZL, Chen SH, et al. 2011. *Chemical Communications* 47: 6695–7
34. Song YJ, Qu KG, Zhao C, Ren JS, Qu XG. 2010. *Advanced Materials* 22: 2206–10
35. Dugan LL, Gabrielsen JK, Yu SP, Lin TS, Choi DW. 1996. *Neurobiology of Disease* 3: 129–35
36. Navyatha B, Singh S, Nara S. 2020. *Biosens Bioelect* 175: 112882
37. Byrappa K, Ohara S, Adschiri T. 2008. *Advanced Drug Delivery Reviews* 60: 299–327
38. Stark WJ. 2011. *Angewandte Chemie-International Edition* 50: 1242–58
39. Navyatha B, Nara S. 2019. *Nanomedicine* 14: 767–96
40. Li XN, Robinson SM, Gupta A, Saha K, Jiang ZW, et al. 2014. *Acs Nano* 8: 10682–6
41. Lopez-Serrano A, Olivas RM, Landaluze JS, Camara C. 2014. *Analytical Methods* 6: 38–56
42. Kumar A, Kim S, Nam JM. 2016. *Journal of the American Chemical Society* 138: 14509–25
43. Bhagat S, Vallabani NVS, Shutthanandan V, Bowden M, Karakoti AS, Singh S. 2018. *Journal of Colloid and Interface Science* 513: 831–42
44. Boucher HW, Talbot GH, Bradley JS, Edwards JE, Gilbert D, et al. 2009. *Clinical Infectious Diseases* 48: 1–12
45. Blair JMA, Webber MA, Baylay AJ, Ogbolu DO, Piddock LJV. 2015. *Nature Reviews Microbiology* 13: 42–51

46. Okano A, Isley NA, Boger DL. 2017. *Proceedings of the National Academy of Sciences of the United States of America* 114: E5052–E61
47. Zumla A, Memish ZA, Maeurer M, Bates M, Mwaba P, et al. 2014. *Lancet Infectious Diseases* 14: 1136–49
48. Zhang Y, Shareena Dasari TP, Deng H, Yu HT. 2015. *Journal of Environmental Science and Health Part C-Environmental Carcinogenesis & Ecotoxicology Reviews* 33: 286–327
49. Pelgrift RY, Friedman AJ. 2013. *Advanced Drug Delivery Reviews* 65: 1803–15
50. Miller KP, Wang L, Benicewicz BC, Decho AW. 2015. *Chemical Society Reviews* 44: 7787–807
51. Ahmed MS, Annamalai T, Li XR, Seddek A, Teng P, et al. 2018. *Bioconjugate Chemistry* 29: 1006–9
52. Chen WY, Chang HY, Lu JK, Huang YC, Harroun SG, et al. 2015. *Advanced Functional Materials* 25: 7189–99
53. Peng LH, Huang YF, Zhang CZ, Niu J, Chen Y, et al. 2016. *Biomaterials* 103: 137–49
54. Li N, Zhao PX, Astruc D. 2014. *Angewandte Chemie-International Edition* 53: 1756–89
55. Rai A, Prabhune A, Perry CC. 2010. *Journal of Materials Chemistry* 20: 6789–98
56. Yang XL, Yang JC, Wang L, Ran B, Jia YX, et al. 2017. *Acs Nano* 11: 5737–45
57. Zheng KY, Li KR, Chang TH, Xie JP, Chen PY. 2019. *Advanced Functional Materials* 29
58. Zhu HS, Li J, Wang J, Wang EK. 2019. *Acs Applied Materials & Interfaces* 11: 36831–8
59. Zhou T, Cheng Y, Zhang HY, Wang GX. 2019. *Journal of Cluster Science* 30: 985–94
60. Tao Y, Ju EG, Ren JS, Qu XG. 2015. *Advanced Materials* 27: 1097–104
61. Hu WC, Younis MR, Zhou Y, Wang C, Xia XH. 2020. *Small* 16
62. Zheng YK, Liu WW, Chen Y, Li CM, Jiang H, Wang XM. 2019. *Journal of Colloid and Interface Science* 546: 1–10
63. Zhao YY, Tian Y, Cui Y, Liu WW, Ma WS, Jiang XY. 2010. *Journal of the American Chemical Society* 132: 12349–56
64. Zheng YK, Liu WW, Qin ZJ, Chen Y, Jiang H, Wang XM. 2018. *Bioconjugate Chemistry* 29: 3094–103
65. Wang ZZ, Dong K, Liu Z, Zhang Y, Chen ZW, et al. 2017. *Biomaterials* 113: 145–57
66. Navya PN, Madhyastha H, Madhyastha R, Nakajima Y, Maruyama M, et al. 2019. *Materials Science & Engineering C-Materials for Biological Applications* 96: 286–94
67. Song XJ, Feng LZ, Liang C, Gao M, Song GS, Liu Z. 2017. *Nano Research* 10: 1200–12
68. Sun BM, Wu JR, Cui SB, Zhu HH, An W, et al. 2017. *Nano Research* 10: 37–48
69. Li ML, Xia J, Tian RS, Wang JY, Fan JL, et al. 2018. *Journal of the American Chemical Society* 140: 14851–9
70. Huang L, Chen JX, Gan LF, Wang J, Dong SJ. 2019. *Science Advances* 5
71. Yu ZZ, Zhou P, Pan W, Li N, Tang B. 2018. *Nature Communications* 9
72. Shen ZY, Liu T, Li Y, Lau J, Yang Z, et al. 2018. *Acs Nano* 12: 11355–65
73. Huang G, Chen HB, Dong Y, Luo XQ, Yu HJ, et al. 2013. *Theranostics* 3: 116–26
74. Gao SS, Lin H, Zhang HX, Yao HL, Chen Y, Shi JL. 2019. *Advanced Science* 6
75. Liu XL, Pan YC, Yang JJ, Gao YF, Huang T, et al. 2020. *Nano Research* 13: 653–60
76. Li TY, Li F, Xiang WT, Yi Y, Chen YY, et al. 2016. *Acs Applied Materials & Interfaces* 8: 22106–12
77. Chong Y, Huang J, Xu XY, Yu CG, Ning XY, et al. 2020. *Bioconjugate Chemistry* 31: 1756–65
78. Zhang AM, Pan SJ, Zhang YH, Chang J, Cheng J, et al. 2019. *Theranostics* 9: 3443–58
79. Maji SK, Mandal AK, Nguyen KT, Borah P, Zhao YL. 2015. *Acs Applied Materials & Interfaces* 7: 9807–16
80. Huang F, Wang JZ, Qu AT, Shen LL, Liu JJ, et al. 2014. *Angewandte Chemie-International Edition* 53: 8985–90

81. Geng J, Li M, Ren JS, Wang EB, Qu XG. 2011. *Angewandte Chemie-International Edition* 50: 4184–8
82. Wu JJX, Wang XY, Wang Q, Lou ZP, Li SR, et al. 2019. *Chemical Society Reviews* 48: 1004–76
83. Dashtestani F, Ghourchian H, Eskandari K, Rafiee-Pour HA. 2015. *Microchimica Acta* 182: 1045–53
84. Gao N, Dong K, Zhao AD, Sun HJ, Wang Y, et al. 2016. *Nano Research* 9: 1079–90
85. Liu CP, Wu TH, Lin YL, Liu CY, Wang S, Lin SY. 2016. *Small* 12: 4127–35
86. Zhang C, Cheng X, Chen MK, Sheng J, Ren J, et al. 2017. *Colloids and Surfaces B-Biointerfaces* 160: 345–54
87. Liu CP, Wu TH, Liu CY, Chen KC, Chen YX, et al. 2017. *Small* 13
88. Fan L, Xu XD, Zhu CH, Han J, Gao LZ, et al. 2018. *Acs Applied Materials & Interfaces* 10: 4502–11
89. Liang RJ, Liu LL, He HM, Chen ZK, Han ZQ, et al. 2018. *Biomaterials* 177: 149–60
90. Michel TM, Pulschen D, Thome J. 2012. *Current Pharmaceutical Design* 18: 5890–9
91. Sun MS, Jin H, Sun X, Huang S, Zhang FL, et al. 2018. *Oxidative Medicine and Cellular Longevity* 2018
92. Singhal A, Morris VB, Labhasetwar V, Ghorpade A. 2013. *Cell Death & Disease* 4
93. Martin KR, Barrett JC. 2002. *Human & Experimental Toxicology* 21: 71–5
94. Sharma V, Singh P, Pandey AK, Dhawan A. 2012. *Mutation Research-Genetic Toxicology and Environmental Mutagenesis* 745: 84–91
95. Wany A, Foyer CH, Gupta KJ. 2018. *Trends in Plant Science* 23: 1041–4
96. Medhe S, Bansal P, Srivastava MM. 2014. *Applied Nanoscience* 4: 153–61
97. Rajan A, Vilas V, Philip D. 2015. *Journal of Molecular Liquids* 212: 331–9
98. Al-Ani LA, Yehyei WA, Kadir FA, Hashim NM, AlSaadi MA, et al. 2019. *Plos One* 14
99. Oueslati MH, Ben Tahar L, Harrath AH. 2020. *Arabian Journal of Chemistry* 13: 3112–22
100. Zhang DC, Shen N, Zhang JR, Zhu JM, Guo Y, Xu L. 2020. *Rsc Advances* 10: 8685–91
101. Kalmodia S, Vandhana S, Rama BRT, Jayashree B, Seethalakshmi TS, et al. 2016. *Cancer Nano* 7: 1–19
102. Lewis K. 2007. *Nature Reviews Microbiology* 5: 48–56
103. Hall-Stoodley L, Costerton JW, Stoodley P. 2004. *Nature Reviews Microbiology* 2: 95–108
104. Bjarnsholt T. 2013. *Apmis* 121: 1–58
105. Gupta A, Das R, Tonga GY, Mizuhara T, Rotello VM. 2018. *Acs Nano* 12: 89–94
106. Chi XQ, Huang DT, Zhao ZH, Zhou ZJ, Yin ZY, Gao JH. 2012. *Biomaterials* 33: 189–206
107. Luo W, Zhu C, Su S, Li D, He Y, et al. 2010. *ACS Nano* 4: 7451–8
108. Wu L, Qu XG. 2015. *Chemical Society Reviews* 44: 2963–97
109. Schaller B, Graf R. 2004. *Journal of Cerebral Blood Flow and Metabolism* 24: 351–71
110. Hu DH, Sheng ZH, Fang ST, Wang YA, Gao DY, et al. 2014. *Theranostics* 4: 142–53
111. Loynachan CN, Soleimany AP, Dudani JS, Lin YY, Najer A, et al. 2019. *Nature Nanotechnology* 14: 883±

# 9 Nanozymes in Electrochemical Analysis

*Cem Erkmen, Sevinc Kurbanoglu, and Bengi Uslu*
Department of Analytical Chemistry, Faculty of
Pharmacy, Ankara University, Ankara, Turkey

## CONTENTS

## 9.1 INTRODUCTION

Enzymes, which have remarkable selectivity, are excellent biological molecules for developing biosensors (1–7). The main challenge in enzyme-based biosensing is proper preparation of the immobilization platform as it is crucial for stability, shelf life, reproducibility, and repeatability of the biosensors. Nowadays, nanozymes, nanomaterials with enzyme-like activities, are becoming potential substitutes for natural enzymes because of their excellent characteristics, such as high sensitivity, selectivity, real-time monitoring, ease of preparation and use, controllable activity, and robustness under changing environmental conditions (8–13).

Nanozymes can mimic many enzymes, such as protease, catalase (CAT), peroxidase (POD), superoxide dismutase (SOD), glucose oxidase (GOx), nicotinamide adenine dinucleotide hydrogen (NADH) POD, glutathione oxidase, etc. They can be used instead of natural enzymes in many applications, such as environmental monitoring, cancer therapy, catalysis, and the detection of pregnancy complications, diseases, and infections, hydrogen peroxide ($H_2O_2$), glucose, glutathione (GSH), various ions, cholesterol, etc. (14–24).

The enzyme-mimicking properties of nanozymes are characterized by Michaelis–Menten kinetic parameters: $K_m$, which shows the affinity toward the analyte, and $V_{max}$, which shows the reaction velocity. It is believed that nanozymes are likely to replace natural enzymes for biosensing, especially in those using electrochemical methods. Some examples include label-free immunosensors (13, 25, 26), food

DOI: 10.1201/9781003109228-9

quality and safety detection (27), environmental analysis (24), biomedical analysis (28), etc. In these and other applications, nanozymes are more preferred than natural enzymes due to their lower cost and higher stability (11, 29, 30). The short operational lifetimes and low reusability of natural enzymes have led researchers to design nonenzymatic surfaces for the detection of substrates. Since the natural enzymes are polypeptides, they are highly sensitive and selective and afford high throughput; however, they have stability problems, can be deactivated easily, and cannot be recovered under mild physiological conditions and extremely expensive. Due to these reasons, large-scale use of natural enzymes is impossible, which has led researchers to discover enzyme-mimicking materials. As shown in **Figure 9.1**, an enzyme-based immunoassay can be mimicked easily by a nanozyme-based immunoassay with a nanozyme-linked antibody (Ab) strategy with lower cost, better stability, and easier production (17).

Since Yan's research group first demonstrated the unexpected POD-mimic activity of iron oxide ($Fe_3O_4$) magnetic nanoparticles (MNPs) in 2007, various nanomaterials have been discovered to possess intrinsic enzyme-like activities. The advantages of nanomaterials not only endow nanozymes with adjustable versatility and sensitivity but also offer great potential for their future development. Nanozyme technology provides a new sensor concept to better understand the characteristics of nanozymes. It affords a systematic study of their enzymatic features, kinetics and mechanisms, and rational design of new nanozymes for practical applications. In this chapter, nanozyme-based electrochemical systems are discussed with some strategies to enhance their catalytic activity along with the factors affecting their activity.

Various electrochemical nanozyme-based applications are reviewed and summarized in tables. The current challenges and future perspectives on the development of nanozymes are also included.

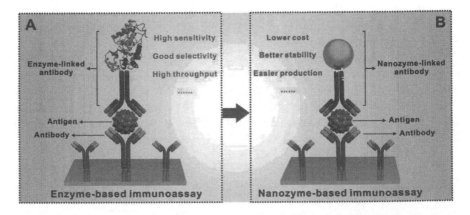

**FIGURE 9.1** Comparison of (A) natural enzyme-based immunoassays and (B) nanozyme-based immunoassays. Reprinted with permission (17).

## 9.2 FACTORS AFFECTING THE NANOZYME ACTIVITY

The primary factors that affect the nanozyme activity are its size, morphology, surface modification, doping, temperature, and pH (20). The size of nanomaterials is one of the most critical factors affecting the catalytic efficiency of nanozymes. As the size changes, the specific surface area and active sites change, directly affecting the catalytic efficiency of nanozymes (10, 31, 32). Luo et al. evaluated the catalytic efficiency of 13, 20, 30, and 50-nm size gold (Au) nanoparticles (NPs), which have GOx-like activity. Their results indicate that the catalytic activity of Au NPs tends to increase as their size became smaller (**Figure 9.2A**). The morphology of nanozymes is another critical factor affecting the catalytic performance of nanozymes. For example, the palladium (Pd) octahedra performed better than Pd nanocages in catalyzing reactive oxygen species (ROS) due to the lower surface energy (**Figure 9.2B**) (33).

Since the catalytic activity of nanozymes is influenced by pH and temperature, it is essential to establish the optimal conditions for their use (20). Some nanozymes may show POD-like properties in acidic conditions but CAT-like properties in neutral and alkaline conditions. As a good example, iron oxide NPs (both $Fe_3O_4$ and

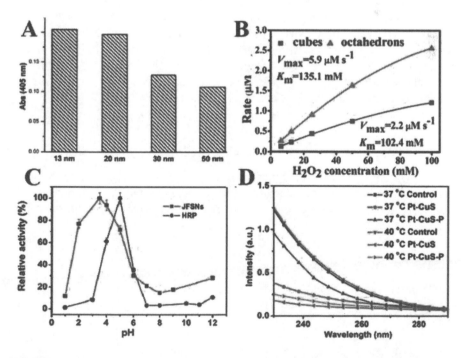

**FIGURE 9.2** (A) Factors influencing the catalytic efficiency of nanozymes. (B) Size-dependent catalytic activity of GOx-like AuNPs. (C) Morphology-dependent catalytic performance. Steady-state kinetic assay of Pd nanocubes, and Pd octahedra with $H_2O_2$. (D) pH-dependent catalytic activities of hematite–silica hybrid of Janus $\gamma$-$Fe_2O_3$/SiO2 nanostructures (JFSNs) and HRP at pH 1–12. (E) UV–vis absorption spectra of $H_2O_2$ after incubation with Pt–CuS or Pt–CuS–P at different temperatures. Reprinted with permission (20).

$\gamma$-Fe$_2$O$_3$) exhibit dual enzyme-like properties (34). The color of the 3,3',5,5' tetra-methylbenzidine (TMB)/H$_2$O$_2$ solution with iron oxide NPs turned blue after a few minutes at pH 4.8. Still, there was no color change at pH 7.4, which is a POD-like activity under acidic conditions. However, iron oxide NPs exhibit CAT-like activity in a neutral environment (34).

In another study, Liu et al. investigated the effects of pH (2 to 5) and temperature (5 to 35 °C) on POD-like properties of Fe-doped CuSn(OH)$_6$, (35). The maximum POD-like catalytic activity was obtained at 15 °C. As shown in **Figure 9.2C**, the catalytic activity of the hematite–silica ($\gamma$-Fe$_2$O$_3$/SiO$_2$) Janus nanostructure was more stable over a wider pH range (2 to 5) than that of horseradish POD (HRP) (pH ~5) (36). Liang et al. showed that elevated temperature was favorable for the activity of the Pt-CuS nanozyme (**Figure 9.2D**) (37).

Most chemical reactions occur on the surface of nanozymes. Hence, surface mod-ification affects the exposure of active sites, which will further reduce or increase the reaction efficiency. For example, when the surface of Pt-CuS Janus NPs was modi-fied with a temperature-sensitive polymer, the catalytic activity of the nanozyme decreased rapidly since the active sites of the nanozyme are blocked. However, when the temperature was increased, the catalytic activity of the nanozyme returned as the polymer confirmation was re-established (20, 37).

The catalytic activity of nanozymes can be enhanced by doping. Chen et al. investigated the catalytic activity of heparin-conjugated Fe@Fe$_3$O$_4$ NPs and Fe$_3$O$_4$@ heparin NPs by a kinetic assay. Results showed that the catalytic activity of heparin-conjugated Fe@Fe$_3$O$_4$ NPs was markedly higher than that of Fe$_3$O$_4$@heparin NPs, due to the release of Fe ions from the Fe core. It was concluded that the Fe core was crucial in enhancing the catalytic ability of the nanozyme (20, 38).

## 9.3   NANOZYME TYPES IN ELECTROCHEMICAL ANALYSIS

Generally, nanozymes are classified into two categories based on reactions of enzymes mimicked: 1) oxidoreductase-mimics (e.g., POD, OXD, CAT, SOD, nitrate reductase, etc.) and 2) hydrolase-mimics (e.g., nuclease, esterase, phosphatase, pro-tease, etc.) (10, 39).

### 9.3.1   PEROXIDASE-MIMICS

The PODs are a class of enzymes that catalyze the oxidation of substrates (S) by a peroxide [e.g., hydrogen peroxide (H$_2$O$_2$)] and yield an oxidized form of the substrate (S$_{ox}$) (40):

$$S + H_2O_2 \; S_{ox} + H_2O \; POD - like \; activity.$$

Different nanozymes with POD-like activity can be used for the direct determina-tion of H$_2$O$_2$. Moreover, indirect detection of many compounds, such as glucose, can also be achieved by POD-mimicking materials through the formation of H$_2$O$_2$. Since nearly all living-cell reactions, H$_2$O$_2$ is released or consumed, POD-mimicking nanozymes have great potential in several applications. Up to date, various nanomaterials have shown POD-like activity, such as metallic nanomaterials, metal oxides, 3-D nanomaterials, quantum dots, carbon-based nanomaterials, etc. They are summarized in **Table 9.1**, along with various sensor platforms and their $H_2O_2$ detection performance characteristics.

Fan et al. suggested a nanozyme that mimics a natural POD enzyme (41). By surface modification of $Fe_3O_4$ NPs with histidine residue, enhanced both POD-like and CAT-like activities. Their results show a nearly tenfold increase in POD-like activity toward $H_2O_2$ and a 20-fold increase in catalytic efficiency via hydrogen bond formation between the imidazole group of histidine and peroxide. This study suggests a strategy of modifying the surface of nanozymes with amino acid residues to mimic the active sites of natural enzymes. Ko et al. used the synergistic effect of bimetallic (Au and Pt) NPs and graphene oxide (GO) as a POD-like nanozyme (Au@Pt NP/GO) (42) as shown in (**Figure 9.3**). This sensing system signal was linear between 1 μM and 3 mM $H_2O_2$ concentration with a LOD of 1.62 μM. In another study, Jin et al. developed GO-Au NPs as a nanozyme on tin oxide electrode to detect $H_2O_2$ using 3,3,5,5,-tetramethylbenzidine (TMB) as a redox mediator. The peak current obtained was linear between 10 nM and 10 mM $H_2O_2$ concentration with an LOD of 1.9 nM (43). In another detection system, Lu et al. measured $H_2O_2$ released from H9C2 cardiac cells using an Au nanoflowers-encapsulated magnetic metal-organic framework ($Fe_3O_4$@ZIF-8) as a nanozymes. An ultrawide linear detection range from 5 μM to 120 mM and a low LOD of 0.9 μM was obtained (44).

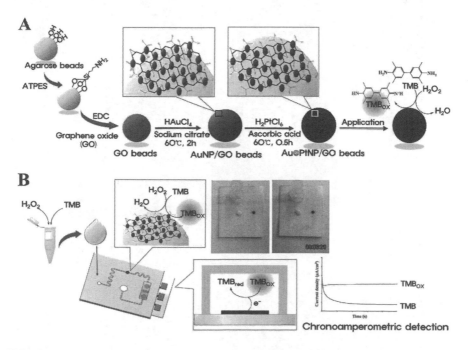

**FIGURE 9.3** The preparation of Au@PtNP/GO microbeads nanozyme (A) and $H_2O_2$ detection on an electrochemical POC device (B). Reprinted with permission (42).

# TABLE 9.1
## Some Selected POD-Like Nanozymes-Based Sensing Platforms for $H_2O_2$ Detection

| Nanozymes | Characteristics of Analytical Method | | | | | | Ref |
|---|---|---|---|---|---|---|---|
| | Method | Electrode | Medium | Linear Range | LOD | Application | |
| Au@PtNP/GO microbeads | AMP | ITO | pH 4.0 buffer solution | 1 μM–3 mM | 1.62 μM | Artificial urine | (42) |
| Nafion/GO-AuNP | DPV | ITO | mixture of potassium hydrogen phthalate, and sodium azide (pH 4.0) | $0.01 \times 10^{-3} - 10$ mM | $1.9 \times 10^{-3}$ μM | NS | (43) |
| AuNFs/Fe₃O₄@ ZIF-8-MoS₂ | AMP | GCE | 0.01 M PBS (pH 7.4) | 5 μM–120 mM | 0.9 μM | H9C2 cardiac cells | (44) |
| La₂ZnO₄/Nafion | DPV | GCE | 0.1 M PBS (pH 8.0) | 3–85 μM | 0.04 μM | Tap water, seawater, industrial effluent, well water, yogurt, milk, human urine | (45) |
| L-Cys-Ag(I) Cp/GO | AMP | GCE | 0.1 M PBS (pH 7.0) | 0.001–5 mM | 0.3 μM | Human serum, and human urine | (46) |
| AuNPs/PB/GO | AMP | GCE | 0.5 M KCl (pH 3.0) | 0.0038–5.4 mM | 1.3 μM | NS | (47) |
| 3D MoS₂/rGO | AMP | GCE | 0.01 M PBS (pH 7.4) | 2–23180 μM | 0.19 μM | Human serum | (48) |
| PdPt NCGs/SGN | AMP | GCE | 0.1 M PBS (pH 7.4) | 1–300 μM | 0.3 μM | Human serum | (49) |
| AuNPs/ZnO-NTs | AMP | GCE | 0.1 M PBS (pH 7.0) | 1–3000 μM | 0.1 μM | Commercial contact lens care solution | (50) |
| AuNPs/PSi | LSV SWV | GCE | 0.1 M PBS (pH 7.0) | 2.0–13.81 mM 0.5–6.91 mM | 14.84 μM 15.16 μM | Tap water | (51) |
| GQDs-CS/MB | AMP | GCE | 0.1 M PBS (pH 7.4) | 1–2900 μM, and 2900–11780 μM | 0.7 μM | Honey, pineapple juice, tap water, spring water | (52) |
| MoS₂/Au-Pt NPs | AMP | GCE | 0.01 M PBS (pH 7.4) | 10–19070 μM | 0.39 μM | Human serum | (53) |
| Pt/cMIL-68/MoS₂ | AMP | GCE | 0.1 M PBS (pH 7.4) | 10nM–18.3 mM | 6.26 nM | Breast cancer cells | (54) |
| MnO₂-GNSs | AMP | GCE | 0.1 M PBS (pH 7.0) | 0.0005–0.35 mM | 0.19 μM | Antiseptic solution | (55) |

(Continued)

**TABLE 9.1 (Continued)**
**Some Selected POD-Like Nanozymes-Based Sensing Platforms for $H_2O_2$ Detection**

| Nanozymes | Method | Electrode | Medium | Linear Range | LOD | Application | Ref |
|---|---|---|---|---|---|---|---|
| | | | | Characteristics of Analytical Method | | | |
| PdCo alloy NPs /CNF | AMP | CPE | 0.1 M PBS (pH 7.0) | 0.0002–23.5 mM | 0.1 μM | NS | (56) |
| PGr | AMP | GCE | 0.05 M NaOH | 2.0–37.0 μM, and 37.0–427.0 μM | 0.19 μM | NS | (57) |
| Ag NWs | AMP | Pt | 0.1 M PBS (pH 7.0) | 0.0005–30 mM | 0.2 μM | NS | (58) |
| $MnO_2$ NTs/Ag@C | AMP | GCE | 0.1 M NaOH | 0.0005–5.7 mM | 0.17 μM | Toothpaste | (59) |
| AP | AMP | SPCE | 0.1 M PBS (pH 7.4) | 200 μM–2mM | 28.9 μM | Tap water, rainwater, human urine, human serum, fetal bovine serum | (60) |
| PPy NPs/Pt NPs | AMP | GCE | 0.1 M PBS (pH 7.0) | 25–500 μM, and 500–6300 μM | 0.6 μM | Gargles | (61) |
| Au@C@Pt | AMP | GCE | 0.1 M PBS (pH 7.0) | 9.0–1860 μM, and 1860–7110 μM | 0.13 μM | NS | (62) |
| 3D NiO NSs/CF-1801 | AMP | GCE | 0.1 M PBS (pH 7.4) | 0.20–3.75 mM | 13.03 nM | Tap water, rainwater | (63) |
| Cu-BTC-MOF/ErGO | AMP | ITO | 0.1 M PBS (pH 7.0) | 4–17334 μM | 0.44 μM | Milk | (64) |
| $Pt/CeO_2$/NCNFs | AMP | GCE | PBS (pH 7.0) | 0.0005–15 mM | 0.049 μM | Cosmetics | (65) |
| $Fe_3O_4$∩MWCNTs | AMP | GCE | PBS (pH 7.4) | 0.001–0.015 μM | 0.4 nM | Milk | (66) |
| $Fe_3O_4$∩G002 | | | | 0.002–0.050 μM | 0.5 nM | | |
| $Fe_3O_4$∩G017 | | | | 0.0003–0.025 μM | 0.1 nM | | |
| Pt-DENs/CNTs | AMP | GCE | 0.1 M PBS (pH 7.0) | 0.003–0.4 mM | 0.8 μM | Living cells | (67) |
| FcAPS | AMP | GCE | 0.1 M PBS (pH 7.4) | 10 μM–10 mM | 2.07 μM | Cow's milk | (68) |
| MnTMPyP/Nafion | CV | GCE | 0.1 M PBS (pH 7.4) | 0.6–40 μM, and 40–1000 μM | 0.5 μM | Human serum | (69) |

*(Continued)*

**TABLE 9.1 (Continued)**

**Some Selected POD-Like Nanozymes-Based Sensing Platforms for $H_2O_2$ Detection**

| Nanozymes | Method | Electrode | Medium | Linear Range | LOD | Application | Ref |
|---|---|---|---|---|---|---|---|
| | | | | **Characteristics of Analytical Method** | | | |
| ERGO | AMP | GCE | 0.1 M PBS (pH 7.0) | 1–16 μM | 0.7 μM | Effluent sample | (70) |
| Nafion/Pd@CeO$_2$-NH$_2$ | AMP | GCE | 0.1 M PBS (pH 7.0) | 0.001–3.276 mM, and 3.276–17.5 mM | 0.47 μM | Milk | (71) |
| rGO-PT-Pt NPs | AMP | SPCE | PBS (pH 7.4) | 1–100 μM | 0.26 μM | Human serum | (72) |
| rGO/CS/Fc | AMP | Pt | 0.02 M PBS (pH 7.0) | 0.00002–0.003 mM, and 0.006–10 mM | 0.02 μM | Living cells | (73) |
| Co/ZnO NFs | AMP | GCE | 0.1 M NaOH | 0.25–20 mM | 1.11 × 10$^{-4}$ mM | NS | (74) |
| Nafion/Au@ SiO$_2$-APTES | AMP | GCE | 0.1 M PBS (pH 7.5) | 0.014–0.18 mM, and 0.18–7.15 mM | 4.25 μM | Contact lens cleaning solutions | (75) |
| 3D CuO/Cu NFs | AMP | GCE | 0.1 M NaOH | 2 μM–19.4 mM | 2 μM | NS | (76) |
| GL–VS$_2$ | AMP | GCE | 0.1 M NaOH | 0.1–260 μM | 26 nM | Milk, and human urine | (77) |
| CuNPs/Rutin/ MWCNTs/IL/CS | AMP | GCE | 0.1 M PBS (pH 7.4) | 0.35–2500 μM | 0.11 μM | NS | (78) |
| Gr-AuNRs | AMP | GCE | 0.1 M PBS (pH 9.0) | 30 μM–5 mM | 10 μM | Milk | (79) |
| PtAu NPs–CTAB–Gr | AMP | GCE | 0.2 M PBS (pH 7.0) | 0.005–4.8 μM | 0.0017 μM | Human serum | (80) |
| MnO$_2$/SWCNTs-Nafion | AMP | GCE | 0.1 M PBS (pH 8.0) | 5–3000 μM | 0.5 μM | Natural water samples | (81) |
| Pd/PDDA/PGR | AMP | GCE | 0.1 M PBS (pH 7.4) | 2–1672 μM | 0.9 μM | Human serum | (82) |
| GS@CeO$_2$-Pt | AMP | SPE | 0.1 M PBS (pH 7.0) | 0.001–10 mM | 0.43 μM | Contact lens cleaning solutions | (83) |
| Ag/boehmite NTs/rGO | AMP | GCE | 0.1 M PBS (pH 7.2) | 0.0005–10 mM | 0.17 μM | Disinfectant sample | (84) |
| HCLD | AMP | Au | PBS (pH 7.0) | 0.02–0.36 mM | 0.003 mM | Mouthwash liquid sample | (85) |
| Cu$_2$O/AuCu/Cu | AMP | GCE | 0.1 M PBS (pH 7.0) | 0.3–9000 μM | 0.14 μM | Gargles | (86) |
| NiMoO$_4$ NPs | AMP | GCE | 0.1 M NaOH | 0.0001–1.55 mM | 0.01 μM | Tap water, river water | (87) |

*(Continued)*

**TABLE 9.1 (Continued)**
**Some Selected POD-Like Nanozymes-Based Sensing Platforms for $H_2O_2$ Detection**

| Nanozymes | Method | Electrode | Medium | Linear Range | LOD | Application | Ref |
|---|---|---|---|---|---|---|---|
| | | | | Characteristics of Analytical Method | | | |
| AgNp@GNR | AMP | SPCE | PBS (pH 7.8) | 0.05–5 mM | 20 μM | Milk | (88) |
| $MnO_x$/CNW | AMP | Carbon rod | 0.25 M PBS (pH 7.2) | 40–10230 μM | 0.55 μM | NS | (89) |
| Na, O-$g$-$C_3N_4$ | CV LSV | GCE | PBS | 1–50 μM 1–45 μM | 0.05 μM 0.1 μM | NS | (90) |
| Ag-$Fe_2O_3$/POM/rGO | AMP | GCE | 0.1 M PBS (pH 6.8) | 0.3–3×10³ μM | 0.2 μM | Environmental water samples | (91) |
| $O_V$–$NiCo_2O_4$ | AMP | Pt | 0.05 M PBS (pH 7.0) | 0.026–6600 μM | 9 nM | Live cells | (92) |
| AuPd-PDA NTs | AMP | GCE | 0.1 M PBS (pH 7.4) | 1 μM–11.22 mM | 0.26 μM | Living cancer cells | (93) |
| rGO/PANI@Pt | AMP | GCE | 0.2 M PBS (pH 6.5) | 100–126400 μM | 1.1 μM | NS | (94) |
| rGO/PANI@PtNi | | | | | 0.5 μM | | |
| GO-PAMAM-$Fe^{2+}$ | DPV | GCE | 1 M ABS (pH 4.3) | 500 nM–2mM | 180 nM | Milk | (95) |
| $NiCo_2O_4$/$CoNiO_2$@pRGO | AMP | GCE | 0.1 M PBS (pH 7.4) | 5–3000 μM, and 3000–12000 μM | 0.41 μM | Living cancer cells | (96) |
| hollow CuO/PANI fibers | AMP | GCE | 0.1 M PBS (pH 7.4) | 0.005–9.255 mM | 0.11 μM | NS | (97) |
| Au-Pd/$MoS_2$ | DPV | GCE | 0.01 M PBS (pH 7.4) | 0.8 μM–10 mM | 0.16 μM | NS | (98) |
| 3D NHGH/$NiCo_2O_4$ NFs | AMP | GCE | 0.1 M NaOH | 1–510 μM | 0.136 μM | NS | (99) |
| $La_{0.6}Sr_{0.4}CoO_{3-\delta}$ | AMP | GCE | 0.1 M NaOH | 0.4–3350 μM | 0.12 μM | NS | (100) |
| $La_{0.6}Sr_{0.4}CoO_{3-\delta}$ / rGO | | | | 0.2–3350 μM | 0.05 μM | | |
| $LaNi_{0.6}Co_{0.4}O_3$ | | | | 6.5–3350 μM | 0.4 μM | | |
| $La_{0.6}Sr_{0.4}Co_{0.2}Fe_{0.8}O_{3-\delta}$ | | | | 2.5–3350 μM | 0.05 μM | | |
| 3D N-Co-CNT@NG | AMP | GCE | 0.1 M NaOH | 2.0–7449 μM | 2.0 μM | Human serum | (101) |

## 9.3.2 Oxidase (OXD)-Mimics

The enzymes that catalyze the oxidation of S using molecular oxygen ($O_2$) and produce $S_{ox}$ are called OXDs. In the presence of water, the yield contains $H_2O_2$. This reaction is as follows:

$$S + O_2 \; S_{ox} + H_2O \quad OXD - like \; activity$$

$$S + O_2 + H_2O \; S_{ox} + H_2O_2 \quad OXD - like \; activity.$$

OXDs are classified according to their substrate names, such as GOx, alcohol oxidase (AOx), polyphenol oxidase (PPO), lactate oxidase (LOx), cholesterol oxidase (COx), uric acid oxidase (UOx), etc. Up to date, numerous nanomaterials showed OXD-like activity by oxidizing their analytes, though PPO- and GOx-mimics are the most common. Some selected nanozyme studies related to the detection of glucose, catechol, and hydroquinone are summarized in **Tables 9.2–9.4**, respectively. As can be seen from these tables, biological samples, such as human serum and urine, were used to show the applicability of the nanozyme systems. GOx-based systems are the first examples of commercial biosensors; therefore, their nanozyme applications are crucial. Since most OXD-mimicking nanozymes cannot selectively catalyze the oxidation of specific substrates as natural enzymes, improving the selectivity of the nanozymes is still a requirement. Vennila et al. proposed Ni-Co/$Fe_3O_4$ flower-like nanocomposite for enzyme-free glucose detection (102). The enhancement in the catalytic efficiency of Ni-Co/$Fe_3O_4$ flower-like nanocomposite toward glucose can be observed in **Figure 9.4** from the cyclic voltammogram. Using the amperometric method, Ni-Co/$Fe_3O_4$ flower-like nanozyme showed GOx-mimicking properties at glassy carbon electrode toward glucose in 0.1 M NaOH solution at +0.43 V versus Ag/AgCl. The sensor response was fairly unaffected by the presence of interferents, such as ascorbic acid, uric acid, dopamine, and acetaminophen (102).

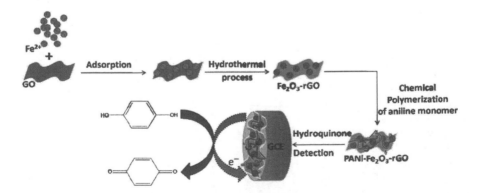

**FIGURE 9.4** Hydroquinone detection scheme using PANi–$Fe_2O_3$–rGO composite modified electrode (106).

## TABLE 9.2
## Some Selected Oxidase-Like Nanozymes-Based Platforms for Glucose Detection

| Nanozymes | Method | Electrode | Medium | Linear Range | LOD | App. | Ref |
|---|---|---|---|---|---|---|---|
| | | | | Characteristics of Analytical Method | | | |
| hollow CuO/PANI fibers | AMP | GCE | 0.1 M NaOH | 0.001–19.899 mM | 0.45 μM | NS | (97) |
| Au-Pd/MoS$_2$ | AMP | GCE | 0.1 M NaOH | 3.9–6.1 mM | 0.40 mM | NS | (98) |
| 3D NHGH/NiCo$_2$O$_4$ NFs | AMP | GCE | 0.1 M NaOH | 0.005–10.95 mM | 0.39 μM | Human serum | (99) |
| La$_{0.6}$Sr$_{0.4}$CoO$_{3-\delta}$ | AMP | GCE | 0.1 M NaOH | 5–1500 μM | 0.15 μM | NS | (100) |
| La$_{0.6}$Sr$_{0.4}$CoO$_{3-\delta}$ / rGO | | | | 2–3350 μM | 0.063 μM | | |
| LaNi$_{0.6}$Co$_{0.4}$O$_3$ | | | | 2.4–1050 μM | 0.124 μM | | |
| La$_{0.6}$Sr$_{0.4}$Co$_{0.2}$Fe$_{0.8}$O$_{3-\delta}$ | | | | 0.1–120 μM | 0.126 μM | | |
| 3D N-Co-CNT@NG | AMP | GCE | 0.1 M NaOH | 0.025–10.83 mM | 100 nM | Human serum | (101) |
| Ni-Co/Fe$_3$O$_4$ | AMP | GCE | 0.1 M NaOH | 0.001–11 mM | 0.19 μM | Human serum | (102) |
| CNF@ Ni0.66Co0.33(OH)$_2$ | AMP | GCE | 0.1 M NaOH | 1–2000 μM | 0.03 μM | Human serum | (107) |
| Cu NPs | Flow injection GPE AMP | | 100 mM NaOH + 100 mM KCl | 0.10–400 μM | 0.04 μM | Commercial human dextrose serum, Gali-dex glucose tolerance test drink, glycosyl glucose tolerance test drink | (108) |
| g-Nb-C$_3$N$_4$ | AMP | Au | 0.1 M PBS (pH 7.4) | 0.5–200 mM | 1 μM | Real blood samples | (109) |
| Cu$_2$O@CuO@NiCo$_2$O$_4$ NWs | AMP | GCE | 50 mM NaOH | 0.001–1.664 mM, and 2.164–5.664 mM | 0.6 μM | Human serum | (110) |
| PDs- NiCo$_2$O$_4$ | AMP | Ni foam | 0.1 M KOH | 5 μM–0.25 mM | 2.75 μM | NS | (111) |
| 3D Ni$_3$N/GA | AMP | GCE | 0.1 M NaOH | 0.1–7645.3 μM | 0.04 μM | Human blood serum | (112) |
| NiO | AMP | GCE | 0.1 M NaOH | 0.02–1.94 mM | 1.28 μM | Fetal bovine serum | (113) |
| 3D GWs/Cu$_2$O | AMP | CFP | 50 mM NaOH | 0.5–5166 μM | 0.21 μM | Human blood serum | (114) |
| g-C$_3$N$_4$/NiO/CuO | AMP | GCE | 0.1 M NaOH | 0.4–8500 μM | 0.1 μM | Human serum | (115) |

*(Continued)*

**TABLE 9.2 (Continued)**
**Some Selected Oxidase-Like Nanozymes-Based Platforms for Glucose Detection**

| Nanozymes | Method | Electrode | Medium | Linear Range | LOD | App. | Ref |
|---|---|---|---|---|---|---|---|
| | | | | **Characteristics of Analytical Method** | | | |
| Cu NPs | AMP | LIG | 0.1 M NaOH | 1 μM–6.0 mM | 0.39 μM | Human serum | (116) |
| CuS NSs/Cu₂O/CuO NWAs/Cu foil | AMP | HgIHgO | 0.1 M NaOH | 0.002–4.096 mM | 0.89 μM | Human serum | (117) |
| FcBA/ glucose/3APBA/4MBA/ AuNPs | DPV | ITO | 0.1 M PBS (pH 7.4) | 0.5–30 mM | 43 μM | Human urine | (118) |
| Au NPs-TiO₂/PANI | AMP | Pt plates | 0.1 M NaOH | 0.01–10 mM | 0.15 μM | NS | (119) |
| Cu@Ni organic framework | AMP | Pt | 0.1 M NaOH | 0–5 mM | 0.0004 mM | Human blood serum | (120) |
| α-Fe₂O₃ | AMP | Ni foam | 0.1 M NaOH | 0.005–0.2 mM | 0.87 μM | Commercial glucose meter | (121) |
| AuNi/NX/MWCNTs | AMP | GCE | 0.5 M NaOH | 1–1900 μM | 0.063 μM | Human serum | (122) |
| CuNWs-CNTs | AMP | GCE | 0.1 M NaOH | 0.1–2 mM | 0.00033 μM | NS | (123) |
| Ni NPs/TiO₂ NWAs | AMP | Pt | 1 M NaOH | 1 μM–7 mM | 0.18 μM | NS | (124) |
| NiO-HAC | AMP | GCE | 0.1 M NaOH | 0.01–3.3 mM | 1 μM | Human serum | (125) |
| Ni(OH)₂-PEDOT-rGO | AMP | GCE | 0.1 M NaOH | 0.002–7.1 mM | 0.6 μM | Human serum | (126) |
| HLTH | AMP | Ni foam | 0.1 M NaOH | 15 μM–2 mM | 1.49 μM | Human blood serum | (127) |
| Co@MoS₂/CNTs | AMP | GCE | 0.1 M NaOH | up to 5.2 mM | 80 nM | Human serum | (128) |
| Cu₂ZnSnS₄ QDs | AMP | FTO glass | 0.1 M NaOH | 0.5–2000 μM | 0.013 μM | Human serum | (129) |
| ZnO | EIS | ITO | 0.1 M NaOH | $10^{-9}$–$10^{-5}$ M | $10^{-9}$ M | Human blood serum | (130) |
| Cu-ZnO | | | | | | | |
| CoTe₂ NSs | AMP | Ni foam | 0.1 M NaOH | 0.01–0.250 mM | 0.59 μM | Human blood serum | (131) |
| Cu2O@Cu1.8S | AMP | GCD | 0.1 M NaOH | 0.001–1 mM | 0.0678 μM | Glucose solutions | (132) |
| Cu₂O | | | | 0.001–0.8 mM | 0.0769 μM | | |

*(Continued)*

**TABLE 9.2 (Continued)**
**Some Selected Oxidase-Like Nanozymes-Based Platforms for Glucose Detection**

| Nanozymes | Method | Electrode | Medium | Linear Range | LOD | App. | Ref |
|---|---|---|---|---|---|---|---|
| | | | | **Characteristics of Analytical Method** | | | |
| AuNP-MIPs | SWV | Au | 0.1 M KCl | 1.25 nM–2.56 μM | 1.25 nM | Human serum | (133) |
| Au/Ni/BDD | AMP | Silicon substrates | 1 M NaOH | 0.02–9 mM | 0.0026 mM | NS | (134) |
| NFG/Pd/NiAl-LDH | AMP | GSE | 0.1 M NaOH | 0.0005–10 mM | 234 nM | Human serum, and plasma | (135) |
| NiCu-OH@Cu(OH)$_2$ NRAs | AMP | Cu foam | 0.1 M NaOH | 100 nM–1.5 mM | 32 nM | Human blood serum | (136) |
| PB-AuNPs/PDA-AuNPs/ MPBA | DPV | 3DG film | 0.1 M KNO$_3$ | 5–65 μM | 1.5 μM | Human serum | (137) |
| Ag@TiO$_2$@ZIF-67 | AMP | GCE | 0.1 M NaOH | 48 μM–1 mM | 0.99 μM | NS | (138) |
| Nafion/3DOMM-TiO$_{2-x}$ | AMP | FTO | 0.1 M NaOH | 0.001–2.32 mM | 0.15 μM | NS | (139) |
| GLAD Ni GLAD NiO | AMP | Silicon substrates | 0.25 M NaOH | 0.0005–9 mM | 0.05 μM 0.007 μM | Artificial sweat, and artificial urine | (140) |
| MOF derived CoCu NRAs | AMP | Cu foam | 0.1 M NaOH | 0.001–1.07 mM | 0.72 μM | NS | (141) |
| Ni(OH)$_2$ | AMP | Pure porous PU | 0.1 M NaOH | 0.01–2.06 mM | 0.32 μM | Fetal bovine serum | (113) |
| Cu–Cu$_2$O NPs | DPV | 3DG film | NaOH | 0.8–10 mM | 16 μM | Human serum | (142) |
| NiWO$_4$ | AMP | GCE | 0.1 M KOH | 0.5 μM–0.280 mM | 0.15 μM | Human plasma | (143) |
| Ni(II)–Cp/C$_{60}$ | AMP | GCE | 0.1 M NaOH | 0.01–11 mM | 4.3 μM | Human plasma | (144) |
| AuNPs/SWCNTs | CV | Wax-printed papers. | 0.1 M NaOH | 0.5–10 mM | 148 μM | Coke | (145) |
| GNSs/GNR/Ni NPs | AMP | GCE | 0.1 M NaOH | 5 nM–5 mM | 2.5 nM | Human serum | (146) |

# TABLE 9.3
## Some Selected Oxidase-Like Nanozymes-Based Platforms for Catechol Detection

| Nanozymes | Method | Electrode | Medium | Linear Range | LOD | App. | Ref |
|---|---|---|---|---|---|---|---|
| | | | | **Characteristics of Analytical Method** | | | |
| LaCo/GNS | DPV | GCE | 0.05 M PBS (pH 7.0) | 0.009–132 μM | 1.0 nM | NS | (147) |
| $Co_3O_4$@carbon | DPV | GCE | 0.1 M PBS pH 7.0 | 0.8–127.1 μM | 0.03 μM | River water | (148) |
| ZnO | AMP | FTO | PBS (pH 7.0) | 0.1–12 ppm | 2 μM | Water | (149) |
| GR-PI film | AMP | FE | 0.1 M BRB | 0.1–10 mM | 11.3 μM | Drinking water | (150) |
| Pt-Au-OSi@CS | AMP | GCE | 0.1 M PBS | 0.06–90.98 μM | 0.02 μM | NS | (151) |
| NPG | AMP | Thin films | PBS (pH 7.2) / 0.1 M $H_2SO_4$ | 2 μM–10 mM / 5 μM–30 mM | 2 μM / 0.3 μM | NS | (152) |
| Cu-PPy | AMP | GCE | 0.1 M PBS (pH 7.0) | 0.05–1000 μM | 0.010 μM | Tap water | (153) |
| Co | AMP | ITO | 0.1 M NaOH | 1–200 μM | 1 μM | Tap water | (154) |
| Cu MOF/ZnTe/AuNPs | DPV | GCE | 0.1 M PBS pH (1.09) | $2.5\times10^{-7}$ M–$3\times10^{-4}$ M | 16 nM | Pharmaceuticals, water, tea, and human serum | (155) |
| Au/Ni(OH)$_2$/rGO | DPV | GCE | 0.1 M PBS (pH 6.0) | 0.4–33.8 μM | 0.13 μM | Lake water | (156) |
| GO@PDA–AuNPs | DPV | GCE | 0.1 M PBS (pH 7.0) | 0.3–67.55 μM | 0.015 μM | Tap water | (157) |
| EGr-TPyP | SWV | GCE | 0.1 M PBS (pH 6.0) | 1–100 μM | 0.303 μM | Commercial mineral water, and tap water | (158) |
| yolk/shell PCN-222@ZIF-8 | AMP | Silicon Wafer | NS | NS | 33 nM | Water samples | (103) |
| ZnO | CV | FTO | PBS (pH 7.0) | 2–15 μM | NS | NS | (159) |
| NiMoO$_4$ @GO | LSV | SPCE | 0.1 M PBS (pH 7.0) | 0.01–273 μM | 0.0015 μM | Industrial, domestic, and underground water | (160) |
| ZrO$_2$ NPs | AMP | Au | 0.1 M PBS (pH 7.0) | 10–90 μM | 7.68 μM | Real water | (161) |

*(Continued)*

**TABLE 9.3 (Continued)**

**Some Selected Oxidase-Like Nanozymes-Based Platforms for Catechol Detection**

| Nanozymes | Method | Electrode | Medium | Linear Range | LOD | App. | Ref |
|---|---|---|---|---|---|---|---|
| | | | | Characteristics of Analytical Method | | | |
| PM-AuNPs | DPV | GCE | PBS (pH 7.0) | 0.5–175.5 μM | 0.011 μM | Tap, and drinking water | (162) |
| CS-MIP | CV | BDD | 0.1 M PBS (pH 7.4) | 0–80 μM | $6.9 \times 10^{-7}$ M | Red wine | (163) |
| Au@NG-PPy | AMP | GCE | 0.1 M PBS (pH 7.0) | 0.1–0.9 μM | 0.0016 μM | Apple juice, green tea, and tap water | (164) |
| rGONSs@SrWO$_4$ | DPV | SPME | PBS (pH 7.0) | 0.034–672.64 μM | 7.34 nM | Drinking water, and green tea | (165) |
| GO-MF | DPAV | GCE | 0.1 M PBS (pH 7.0) | 0.01–0.1 μM | 0.00051 μM | NS | (166) |
| c-MWCNT/PDA (β-CD)/c-MWCNT | CV | GCE | PBS (pH 7.37) | 0.25–4000 μM | 0.04 μM | Tap, and lake water | (167) |
| Cu-MOF | SWV | CPE | 0.1 M PBS (pH 7.0) | $8.03 \times 10^{-7}$–$3.23 \times 10^{-5}$ M | $1 \times 10^{-7}$ M | Tap, and urban drainage water | (104) |
| CdTe QDs/Gr | DPV | GCE | PBS (pH 6.0) | 30–1000 μM | 0.09 μM | Industry, lake, and surface water | (168) |
| NH$_2$-grafted montmorillonite | DPV | GCE | 0.1 M BRB (pH 2.0) | 5–80 μM | 0.65 μM | Tap, and lake water | (169) |
| T3T | DPV | Au | BRB (pH 6.0) | 0.015–2.8 μM | 0.00188 μM | Tap, and lake water | (170) |
| PtFullerene (C$_{60}$) | DPV | PGE | 0.1 M PBS (pH 7.0) | 50.0–1500.0 μM | 2.97 μM | River water, and sanitary wastewater | (171) |
| Co$_3$O$_4$/MWCNTs | DPV | GCE | 0.2 M Na$_2$HPO$_4^-$ citrate solution (pH 8.0) | 10–700 μM | 8.5 μM | Seawater | (172) |
| PNA/Cd-ZnWO$_4$ | DPV | CPE | 0.1 M PBS (pH 7.0) | 2–35 μM | 0.03 μM | Tap water | (173) |
| P4VPBA/PPy/GO NSs | DPV | GCE | 0.05 M PBS (pH 9.0) | 7–16 μM | 0.96 μM | Tap water | (174) |
| CuO-CNF | DPV | GCE | 0.1 M ABS | 0–150 μM | 2 μM | River water | (175) |
| GCN | DPV | GCE | 0.1 M PBS (pH 7.0) | $5 \times 10^{-7}$–$5 \times 10^{-5}$ M | $5 \times 10^{-8}$ M | tap water, and Xiangjiang River water | (176) |

*(Continued)*

**TABLE 9.3 (Continued)**

**Some Selected Oxidase-Like Nanozymes-Based Platforms for Catechol Detection**

| Nanozymes | Method | Electrode | Medium | Linear Range | LOD | App. | Ref |
|---|---|---|---|---|---|---|---|
| | | | | Characteristics of Analytical Method | | | |
| AuNPs/Fe$_3$O$_4$-APTES-GO AMP | | GCE | 0.1 M PBS (pH 7.4) | 2–145 μM | 0.8 μM | Tap water | (177) |
| 3D CNNS-CNT | DPV | GCE | 0.01 M PBS (pH 7.0) | 1–200 μM | 0.09 μM | Tap water | (178) |
| TpBD-COF | DPV | CPE | PBS (pH 6.86) | 1–2000 μM | 0.46 μM | Tap, lake, and river water | (179) |
| poly (direct yellow 11) | DPV | PGE | 0.2 M PBS (pH 7.4) | 50–350 μM | 0.11 μM | Tap water | (180) |
| Au-PdNFs/rGO | DPV | GCE | 0.1 M PBS (pH 7.0) | 2.5–100 μM | 0.8 μM | Tap, lake, and river water | (181) |
| 3D NCNT@CNFs | DPV | GCE | 0.1 M PBS (pH 7.0) | 0.08–350 μM | 0.02 μM | Tap water | (182) |
| MWCNTs-PDDA-Gr | DPV | GCE | 0.2 M PBS (pH 7.0) | 0.5–400 μM | 0.018 μM | Tap water, and seawater | (183) |
| Au- gC$_3$N$_4$-MOF | DPV | CPE | 0.1 M PBS (pH 7.0) | 0.05–100 μM | 1 nM | River water | (184) |
| CDs/rGO | DPV | GCE | PBS (pH 7.0) | 1.0–950 μM | 0.28 μM | Tap, river water, and Industrial sewage | (185) |
| Tryptophan-functionalized Gr | DPV | GCE | 0.1 M PBS (pH 7.0) | 5–500 μM | 0.09 μM | Tap water | (186) |
| CdS/rGO | DPV | GCE | 0.1 M PBS (pH 7.0) | 0.5–1350 μM | 0.09 μM | Tap, well, and river water | (187) |
| PdDAN | SWV | GCE | 5.0 mM HClO$_4$ | 50–1000 μM | 0.227 nM | Natural water samples | (188) |
| PIL-MCNs/CS | DPV | GCE | 0.1 M PBS (pH 5.0) | 10–400 μM | 0.62 μM | Tap water | (189) |
| Bi$_2$WO$_6$@GNRs | DPV | SPCE | PBS (pH 7.0) | 21 nM–1550 μM | 5.31 nM | Red wine, and face cream | (190) |
| CePO$_4$ | DPV | CPE | 0.1 M PBS (pH 7.0) | 0.20–40 μM | 0.10 μM | Tap water | (191) |
| PEDOT | DPV | CFE | 0.1 M PBS (pH 7.0) | 0.52–4920 μM | 1.6 μM | Tap, and lake water | (192) |
| N, S-AGR | DPV | GCE | 0.1 M HAc–NaAc, (pH 5.0) | 1–10 μM, and 10–70 μM | 0.15 μM | Tap water | (193) |
| CuNWs-Pd- CNTs | DPV | GCE | 0.1 M PBS | 1–280 μM | 0.6 μM | City, mineral, and tap water | (194) |

**TABLE 9.4**

**Some Selected Oxidase-Like Nanozymes-Based Platforms For Hydroquinone Detection**

| Nanozymes | Method | Electrode | Medium | Linear Range | LOD | App. | Ref |
|---|---|---|---|---|---|---|---|
| | | | | Characteristics of Analytical Method | | | |
| $Bi_2WO_6$@GNRs | DPV | SPCE | PBS (pH 7.0) | 21 nM–1550 μM | 7.51 nM | Red wine, and face cream | (190) |
| $CePO_4$ | DPV | CPE | 0.1 M PBS (pH 7.0) | 0.4–50 μM | 0.27 μM | Tap water | (191) |
| PEDOT | DPV | CFE | 0.1 M PBS (pH 7.0) | 0.53–861 μM | 0.42 μM | Tap, and lake water | (192) |
| N, S-AGR | DPV | GCE | 0.1 M HAc–NaAc, (pH 5.0) | 1–10 μM, and 10–70 μM | 0.03 μM | Tap water | (193) |
| CuNWs-Pd- CNTs | DPV | GCE | 0.1 M PBS | 1–228 μM | 0.4 μM | City, mineral, and tap water | (194) |
| Pt/Fullerene ($C_{60}$) | DPV | PGE | 0.1 M PBS (pH 7.0) | 50.0–1100.0 μM | 2.19 μM | River water, and sanitary wastewater | (171) |
| $Co_3O_4$/MWCNTs | DPV | GCE | 0.2 M $Na_2HPO_4$- citrate solution (pH 8.0) | 10–800 μM | 5.6 μM | Seawater | (172) |
| PNA/Cd-$ZnWO_4$ | DPV | CPE | 0.1 M PBS (Ph 7.0) | 1–56 μM | 0.17 μM | Tap water | (173) |
| P4VPBA/PPy/GO NSs | DPV | GCE | 0.05 M PBS (pH 9.0) | 4–22 μM | 0.53 μM | Tap water | (174) |
| CuO-CNF | DPV | GCE | 0.1 M ABS | 3–80 μM | 1 μM | River water | (175) |
| GCN | DPV | GCE | 0.1 M PBS (pH 7.0) | $1×10^{-7}$–$3×10^{-5}$ M | $2×10^{-8}$ M | Tap water, and Xiangjiang River water | (176) |
| AuNPs/$Fe_3O_4$-APTES-GO AMP | DPV | GCE | 0.1 M PBS (pH 7.4) | 3–137 μM | 1.1 μM | Tap water | (177) |
| 3D CNNS-CNT | DPV | GCE | 0.01 M PBS (pH 7.0) | 1–250 μM | 0.13 μM | Tap water | (178) |
| TpBD-COF | DPV | CPE | PBS (pH 6.86) | 1–2000 μM | 0.31 μM | Tap, lake, and river water | (179) |
| poly (direct yellow 11) | DPV | PGE | 0.2 M PBS (pH 7.4) | 50–350 μM | 0.16 μM | Tap water | (180) |
| Au-PdNFs/rGO | DPV | GCE | 0.1 M PBS (pH 7.0) | 1.6–100 μM | 0.5 μM | Tap, lake, and river water | (181) |
| 3D NCNT@CNFs | DPV | GCE | 0.1 M PBS (pH 7.0) | 0.1–425 μM | 0.05 μM | Tap water | (182) |
| MWCNTs-PDDA-Gr | DPV | GCE | 0.2 M PBS (pH 7.0) | 0.5–400 μM | 0.02 μM | Tap water, and seawater | (183) |

(Continued)

**TABLE 9.4 (Continued)**
**Some Selected Oxidase-Like Nanozymes-Based Platforms For Hydroquinone Detection**

| Nanozymes | Method | Electrode | Medium | Linear Range | LOD | App. | Ref |
|---|---|---|---|---|---|---|---|
| | | | | | | Characteristics of Analytical Method | |
| Au- gC$_3$N$_4$-MOF | DPV | CPE | 0.1 M PBS (pH 7.0) | 0.005–5 μM | 1 nM | River water | (184) |
| CDs/rGO | DPV | GCE | PBS (pH 7.0) | 0.5–1000 μM | 0.17 μM | Tap, river water, and Industrial sewage | (185) |
| Tryptophan-functionalized Gr | DPV | GCE | 0.1 M PBS (pH 7.0) | 5–300 μM | 0.22 μM | Tap water | (186) |
| CdS/rGO | DPV | GCE | 0.1 M PBS (pH 7.0) | 0.2–2300 μM | 0.054 μM | Tap, well, and river water | (187) |
| PdDAN | SWV | GCE | 5.0 mM HClO$_4$ | 50–1000 μM | 0.222 nM | Natural water samples | (188) |
| PIL-MCNs/CS | DPV | GCE | 0.1 M PBS (pH 5.0) | 10–350 μM | 1.39 μM | Tap water | (189) |
| Gr-COOH | AdSV | GCE | 0.05 M H$_2$SO$_4$ in a 60:40 methanol:water mixture | 0.1–40 μM | 0.04 μM | Whitening cosmetics | (195) |
| FeWO$_4$/SnO$_2$/Nf | AMP | GCE | 0.1 M PBS (pH 7.0) | 0.01–100 μM | 0.0013 μM | Tap, lake, and river water | (196) |
| PANi–Fe$_2$O$_3$–rGO | DPV | GCE | PBS (pH 2.5) | 0.1–550 μM | 0.06 μM | Tap water | (106) |
| UiO-67 | DPV | CPE | 0.1 M PBS (pH 7.4) | 5–300 μM | 0.0036 μM | Tap, and river water | (197) |
| PN-COFs/GO | DPV | GCE | PBS (pH 6.0) | $1.0\times10^{-7}$–$1.0\times10^{-4}$ M | $9.0\times10^{-9}$ M | Whitening cream | (105) |
| Gr/Ir(III) | DPV | GCE | 1 M PBS (pH 7.2) | 0.05–100 μM | 0.0011 μM | Tap, lake, and river water | (198) |

PPO enzymes are the other type of OXDs that are mimicked by several nanozyme systems as they catalyze the oxidation of phenolic compounds related *to o*-quinonic compounds, such as catechol, hydroquinone, etc., that are mainly found in food, biological, and environmental samples, such as water, tea, pharmaceutics, human serum, etc. Their presence in a wide range of substances makes their detection critical. Gao et al. reported yolk/shell MOF@MOF heterostructure as nanozyme was more selective toward catechol (LOD = 33 nM) than other phenolic compounds, such as dopamine and L-dopa (L-3,4-dihydroxyphenylalanine). The stability of the nanozyme was relatively high; after incubation in methanol at 100 °C for 28 days, the sensor lost only 10% of the initial activity (103). In another Cu-based MOF (Cu$_3$ (BTC)$_2$(H$_2$O)$_3$]nbenzene-1,3,5-tricarboxylate) was shown to have catechol oxidase mimetic properties (104). This sensor's linear range was $8.0\times10^{-7}$ M to $3.2\times10^{-5}$ M, and the LOD was $1.0\times10^{-7}$ M catechol. Furthermore, this sensor was potentially suitable for simultaneous detection of multiple analytes, such as hydroquinone, uric acid, and catechol. Another example of nanozyme-based multianalyte detection is from Ma et al., who established a dual detection platform using a porphyrin-based covalent organic framework (PN-COF) and GO-modified electrode for the detection of hydroquinone and acetaminophen (105). This research took advantage of the synergetic effect between the electrocatalytic activity of COF and the conductivity of GO. Under optimized conditions, the linear ranges obtained were $2.0\times10^{-7}$ M to $1.5\times10^{-4}$ M for acetaminophen and $1.0\times10^{-7}$ M to $1.0\times10^{-4}$ M for hydroquinone. Reduced graphene oxide (rGO)-based nanozyme (polyaniline (PANI)-Fe$_2$O$_3$-rGO), synthesized via a simple two-step fabrication, was also used for the detection of hydroquinone (linear range = $1.0\times10^{-7}$–$5.5\times10^{-4}$ M; LOD = $6.0\times10^{-8}$) (**Figure 9.4**) (106).

### 9.3.3 OTHER NANOZYMES

Nanozymes other than POD- and OXD-mimics have also been synthesized; these include mimics of SOD (199), NADH oxidase (200), xanthine oxidase (201), cytochrome c oxidase (CcO) (202), and acetylcholinesterase (46). These nanozymes have been employed for the detection of analytes, such as xanthine, H$_2$O$_2$, different ions, norepinephrine, uric acid, tyrosine, bilirubin, etc. Selected example applications of these nanozymes are listed in **Table 9.5**.

Platinum (Pt) NPs have been widely studied for their POD- and OXD-like activities. However, Pt NPs have been shown to have NADH oxidase-like activity. Song et al. prepared a Pt NPs-deposited multiwalled carbon nanotubes (MWCNTs) as nanozyme to catalyze NADH oxidation for xylose detection over a wide detection range of 5 to 400 μM and an LOD of 1 μM in real lignocellulosic samples (200). Sun et al. prepared a hybrid nanoprobe using Fe$_3$O$_4$ magnetic NPs, cTnI-specific Tro6 aptamer (Apt), natural HRP, HRP-mimicking Au@Pt nanozymes, and G-quadruplex/hemin DNAzyme as shown in **Figure 9.5**. This Fe$_3$O$_4$/Au@Pt- HRP-DNAzyme-Tro6 nanoprobe enhanced the specificity and sensitivity of the detection of cardiac troponin I in human serum samples (LOD = 7.5 pg mL$^{-1}$), which is released into the bloodstream in the case of heart muscle damage (203).

An SOD-mimicking nanocomposite platform was devised by Dashtestani et al. based on Au NPs and a Cu(II) complex of cysteine (Cys). This nanocomposite

**TABLE 9.5**

**Some Selected Nanozymes-Based Platforms for Several Analytes**

| Nanozymes | Analyte/Substrate | Characteristics of Analytical Method | | | | | App | Ref |
|---|---|---|---|---|---|---|---|---|
| | | Method | Electrode | Medium | Linear Range | LOD | | |
| PBBA | Glycated albumin | DPV | ITO | Buffer solution (pH 4.0) | 5.0 µg mL$^{-1}$–1.0 mg mL$^{-1}$ | 3.47 µg mL$^{-1}$ | Human plasma | (211) |
| CeO$_2$ | Methyl-paraoxon | DPV | GCE | PBS (pH 6.0) | 0.1–100 µM | 0.06 µM | Herbal plant samples | (207) |
| LSG | Xanthine | DPV | Flexible electrode | 0.1 M PBS (pH 6.5) | 0.3–179.9 µM | 0.26 µM | Fish samples | (206) |
| | Hypoxanthine | | | | 0.3–159.9 µM | 0.18 µM | | |
| MIL-88 MOFs@Pt@ MIL-88 MOFs | miRNA | DPV | Au | 0.1 M PBS (pH 7.4) | 1 fM–1 nM | 0.29 fM | MCF-7 cells, MCF-10 A cells, and serums of a breast cancer patient and healthy person | (210) |
| His@AuNCs/rGO | Nitrite | DPV | GCE | 0.1 M PBS (pH 7.0) | 1–7000 µM | 0.5 µM | Sausage | (212) |
| RCA, and hemin/G-quadruplex NWs | Pb$^{2+}$ | DPV | GCE | 0.1 M PBS (pH 7.4) | 10 fM–200 nM | 3.3 fM | Tap water | (213) |
| CMC-MWCNTs/MoS$_2$ | Carbendazim | DPV | GCE | 0.1 M PBS (pH 7.0) | 0.04–100 µM | 7.4 nM | Tea and rice | (208) |
| NH$_2$-MWCNTs-BP-AgNPs | Uric acid | DPV | GCE | 0.1 M PBS (pH 7.0) | 0.1–800 µM | 0.052 µM | Bovine serum | (209) |
| | Xanthine | | | | 0.5–680 µM | 0.021 µM | | |
| | Hypoxanthine | | | | 0.7–320 µM | 0.025 µM | | |
| Fe$_3$O$_4$/PDDA/Au@ Pt-HRP-GHD-Tro6 | Cardiac troponin I | DPV | SPGE | 0.1 M PBS (pH 7.0) | 0.1 pg mL$^{-1}$–100 ng mL$^{-1}$ | 7.5 pg mL$^{-1}$ | Human serum | (203) |
| S1/CuO NPs bioconjugates MCF-7/ S1/Gr/AuNPs | Circulating tumor cells | DPV | GCE | 0.01 M PBS (pH 7.4) | 50–1×10$^4$ cells mL$^{-1}$ | 27 cells mL$^{-1}$ | Human serum | (214) |
| AuNPs/ GQDs | Quercetin | SWV | SPCE | BRB (pH 5.0) | 1.0×10$^{-10}$–1.0×10$^{-3}$ M | 3.3×10$^{-11}$ M | Human plasma | (215) |

*(Continued)*

## TABLE 9.5 (Continued)
## Some Selected Nanozymes-Based Platforms for Several Analytes

| Nanozymes | Analyte/Substrate | Method | Electrode | Medium | Linear Range | LOD | App | Ref |
|---|---|---|---|---|---|---|---|---|
| MoS₂-COOH-MWCNTs | 5-Nitroguaiacol sodium | DPV | GCE | Acetic acid buffer solution (pH 4.0) | 0.1–70 μM | 0.02 μM | Tomato | (216) |
| Yb₂O₃ | Acetaminophen | DPV | SPCE | BRB (pH 9.0) | 0.25–2000 μM | 0.055 μM | Pharmaceutical, human serum, and human urine | (217) |
| | Tramadol | | | | 0.5–5400 μM | 0.087 μM | | |
| PNC | Norepinephrine | DPV | ITO | Buffer solution (pH 6.0) | 1.0–25 μM | 863 nM | Human plasma | (218) |
| PAMTA | Adenosine | DPV | PG | 0.1 M PBS (pH 7.0) | 0.2–25.6 μM | 0.19 μM | Whole blood and urine | (219) |
| | Adenine | | | | 0.05–12.8 μM | 0.039 μM | | |
| | Uric acid | | | | 5–1200 μM | 2.74 μM | | |
| Ag/H-C₃N₄ | Carcinogenic nitrite | AMP | CC | 0.1 M PBS (pH 7.4) | 5–1000 μM | 0.216 μM | Tap water | (220) |
| Ce-HA | Norepinephrine | DPV | GCE | 0.1 M PBS (pH 7.0) | 0.1–200 μM | 0.058 μM | Human serum and human urine | (221) |
| | Uric acid | | | | 0.5–200 μM | 0.39 μM | | |
| | Tyrosine | | | | 0.1–200 μM | 0.072 μM | | |
| Ceria NCBs/CBs | Bilirubin | DPV | SPCE | 0.01 M PBS (pH 7.4) | up to 100 μM | 0.1 μM | Human serum | (222) |
| Mesoporous CuCo₂O₄ | Ascorbic acid | AMP | GCE | 0.15 M NaOH | 0.001–1 μM | 0.21 μM | Vitamin C tablets, effervescent tablets, and human urine | (223) |
| OPA/2ME | γ-Aminobutyric acid | SWV | Au | 0.01 M PBS (pH 7.4) | 250 nM –100 μM | 98 nM | Human serum, and human urine | (224) |

(Continued)

**TABLE 9.5 (Continued)**
**Some Selected Nanozymes-Based Platforms for Several Analytes**

| Nanozymes | Analyte/Substrate | Method | Electrode | Medium | Characteristics of Analytical Method | | App | Ref |
|---|---|---|---|---|---|---|---|---|
| | | | | | Linear Range | LOD | | |
| NiO NPs | Glucose | AMP | GCE | 0.1 M NaOH | 1.25–600 μM | 0.38 μM | Orange juice, peach juice, pear-pineapple juice, and coke soda | (225) |
| | Fructose | | | | 1.28–600 μM | 0.39 μM | | |
| | Sucrose | | | | 1.35–600 μM | 0.41 μM | | |
| | Lactose | | | | 1.35–600 μM | 0.40 μM | | |
| | Total sugars | | | | 1.31–600 μM | 0.39 μM | | |
| NiCo$_2$S$_4$ porous sphere | Hydrazine | AMP | GCE | 0.2 M NaOH | 0.0017–7.8 mM | 0.6 μM | Tap water | (226) |
| CuOx@mC | Glyphosate | DPV | GCE | 0.1 M PBS (pH 5.5) | 10−15–10−4 M | 7.69×10−7 nM | Apple | (227) |
| TyrH/PdPt NPs/CS-IL/Gr-MWCNTs-IL | Tyrosine | DPV | GCE | 0.05 M PBS (pH 2.0) | 0.01×10−9 − 8×10−9 M, and 8×10−9−160×10−9 M | 0.009×10−9 M | Yogurt, egg, and cheese | (228) |
| CuO-NPs/3D Gr | Malathion | DPV | GCE | CBS (pH 5.0) | 0.03–1.5 nM | 0.01 nM | Lake water | (229) |
| Pd/N-rGO | Estradiol | DPV | GCE | PBS (pH 7.0) | 0.1–400 μM | 1.8 nM | Human urine and milk | (230) |
| NiS/GO | Urea | DPV | GCE | 1 M KOH | 0.1–1.0 mM | 3.79 μM | Milk | (231) |
| NiAl-LDH/CD | Acetylcholine | AMP | GCE | 0.1 M KOH | 5–6885 μM | 1.7 μM | NS | (232) |
| PEDOT/TA | Cholesterol | AMP | SPE | 0.1 M PBS (pH 7.0) | 3 μM −1 mM | 0.95 μM | Egg yolk sample | (233) |
| CuO/CeO$_2$ | Dopamine | DPV | SPCE | PBS (pH 7.0) | 0.025–98.5 μM | 0.016 μM | Pharmaceutical and human serum | (234) |
| rGO-MOS$_2$-PEDOT | Nitrite | DPV | GCE | 0.1 M PBS (pH 4.0) | 1–1000 μM | 0.059 μM | Tap water, pond water, packaged drinking water, and milk | (235) |

(Continued)

**TABLE 9.5 (Continued)**
**Some Selected Nanozymes-Based Platforms for Several Analytes**

| Nanozymes | Analyte/Substrate | Method | Electrode | Medium | Linear Range | LOD | App | Ref |
|---|---|---|---|---|---|---|---|---|
| | | | | | Characteristics of Analytical Method | | | |
| Pd@UiO-66 MOFs | miRNA | DPV | Au | 0.1 M PBS (pH 7.4) | 20 fM–600 pM | 0.713 fM | Human serum | (236) |
| WS$_2$ | Uric acid Quercetin | DPV | GCE | 0.1 M PBS (pH 7.2) | 5–1000 μM 0.010–50 μM | 1.2 μM 0.002 μM | Human serum | (237) |
| NiO@Au | Lactic acid | LSV | GCE | 1 M KOH | 100.0 μM, and 0.5 M | 11.6 μM | Human serum and human urine | (238) |
| CSHj-Ab$_2$/BSA/CEA/Ab$_1$/MoS$_2$-Au | Carcinoembryonic antigen | DPV | GCE | 0.1 M PBS (pH 7.0) | 0.0001–80 ng mL$^{-1}$ | 0.03 pg mL$^{-1}$ | Human serum | (239) |
| MOF-CS/Ab$_1$/PSA/Ab$_2$-QDs | Prostate specific antigen | DPV | GCE | PBS (pH 7.0) | 1 pg mL$^{-1}$–100 ng mL$^{-1}$ | 0.45 pg mL$^{-1}$ | Human serum | (240) |
| Ab$_2$-SWCNTs-GQDs/CEA/Ab$_1$/rGO-AuNPs | Carcinoembryonic antigen | SWV | GCE | PBS (pH 8.5) | 0.05–0.65 ng mL$^{-1}$ | 5.3 pg mL$^{-1}$ | Human serum | (241) |
| Apt/ AuPd NPs@ rGO/MWCNTs | Oxaliplatin | DPV | GCE | PBS (pH 7.0) | 0.18–170 nM | 0.06 nM | Pharmaceutical injection, human serum, and human urine | (242) |
| N-HMCS | Superoxide anion (O$_2^-$) | AMP | SPCE | 0.1 M PBS (pH 7.4) | 20–480 μM | 2.2 μM | Living cells | (243) |
| CuS@Pd/N–rGO | Xanthine | DPV | GCE | 0.1 M PBS (pH 3.7) | 0.7–200 μM | 0.028 μM | Chicken serum and human urine | (244) |
| β-Cyclodextrin/Fe$_3$O$_4$ | Cholesterol | AMP | SPCE | 50 mM PBS (pH 7.4) | 2.88–150 μM | 2.88 μM | Cream milk | (245) |
| Cu$_2$O@g-C$_3$N$_4$ NSTs | 8-Hydroxy-2′-deoxyguanosine | AMP | RDE | 0.1 M PBS (pH 7.0) | 0.025–910 μM | 0.045 μM | Human serum and urine | (246) |
| MnO$_2$/Gr | Cholesterol | DPV | PG | PBS (pH 7.0) | 1.2–24 nM | 0.42 nM | Human serum | (247) |

*(Continued)*

**TABLE 9.5 (Continued)**
**Some Selected Nanozymes-Based Platforms for Several Analytes**

| Nanozymes | Analyte/Substrate | Method | Electrode | Medium | Linear Range | LOD | App | Ref |
|---|---|---|---|---|---|---|---|---|
| | | | | | Characteristics of Analytical Method | | | |
| S(O) MWCNT | 6-Mercaptopurine | AMP | CPE | 0.1 M PBS (pH 7.0) | 1.0–100 μM | 0.24 μM | Human plasma, human urine | (248) |
| PdPt NCRs | Oxalic acid | AMP | GCE | 0.1 M HClO$_4$ | 10–4700 μM, and 4700–11800 μM | 1 μM | Spinach, swiss chard | (249) |
| HZC | Pentachlorophenol | AMP | SPCE | 0.1 M PBS (pH 6.0) | $3.75\times10^{-8}$–$1.006\times10^{-4}$ M | $2.05\times10^{-9}$ M | Packaging extract | (250) |
| NiS$_2$-rGO/ Curcumin NPs | Methyl parathion 4-Nitrophenol | DPV | GCE | 0.1 M PBS (pH 7.4) | 0.25–80 μM | 8.7 nM 6.9 nM | Tomato, apple juices, and river water | (251) |
| Au@Pt-PEI-rGO | Chicoric acid | DPV | GCE | Na$_2$HPO$_4$-citric acid solution (pH 3.0) | 0.3 μM–0.03 mM | 4.8 nM | NS | (252) |
| Pd@NCF | Uric acid Dopamine | DPV | GCE | PBS (pH 7.0) | 0.5–100 μM 0.5–230 μM | 76 nM 107 nM | Human serum | (253) |
| MoNPs@ f-MWCNTs | Dopamine | AMP | SPCE | 0.1 M PBS (pH 7.0) | 0.01–1609 μM | 0.00126 μM | Human serum, rat brain serum, and dopamine injection | (254) |
| MIL(Fe)- 101 MOFs@ GO | Carbofuran Carbaryl | DPV | GCE | BRB (pH 4.0) | 5–200 nM 1–300 nM | 1.2 nM 0.5 nM | Cucumber, oranges, tomatoes, and cabbage | (255) |
| RuS$_2$ NPs | Dopamine | AMP | GCE | 0.1 M PBS (pH 7.0) | 0.1–80 μM | 0.0738 μM | NS | (256) |
| Co$_3$O$_4$-CuNi-rGO | Ascorbic acid | AMP | GCE | 0.1 M PBS (pH 7.0) | 2.5–100 μM | 0.34 μM | Vitamin C tablets, orange, and vitamin water | (257) |
| NiNWs | Ethanol | AMP | CPE | 0.1 M NaOH | $(0.1–1.1)\ 10^{-4}$ M | 0.31 μM | Vodka and cane brandy | (258) |
| PET-AC | Carbofuran hydrolysate | AMP | GCE | 0.1 M PBS (pH 7.0) | 1–10 μM | 0.03 μM | Agricultural fields | (259) |

**TABLE 9.5 (Continued)**
**Some Selected Nanozymes-Based Platforms for Several Analytes**

| Nanozymes | Analyte/Substrate | Method | Electrode | Medium | Characteristics of Analytical Method | | App | Ref |
|---|---|---|---|---|---|---|---|---|
| | | | | | Linear Range | LOD | | |
| CS-Fe$_3$O$_4$ | Parathion | SWV | GCE | McIlvaine buffer solution (pH 5.0) | $3.43 \times 10^{-7}$–$4.46 \times 10^{-6}$ M | $1.87 \times 10^{-7}$ M | Carrot, lettuce, tomato, rice, orange | (260) |
| β-Cyclodextrin–GQD | L-Tyrosine | DPV | GCE | 0.1 M PBS (pH 7.4) | 0.1–1.5 µM | NS | NS | (261) |
| FPBA-DA/TCPP-GO | Sialic acid | DPV | GCE | PBS (pH 7.4) | 0.1–7.5 mM | 28.5 µM | Human blood and urine | (262) |
| AgNPs-PANI-Nano-ZSM-5 | Lindane | DPV | GCE | 0.1 M KCl | 0.01–900 µM | 5 nM | Tap water, Sutlej river water | (263) |
| Ag/BSA/ PCT Ab/NiFe PBA NCs@TB | Procalcitonin | DPV | GCE | PBS (pH 7.0) | 0.001–25 ng mL$^{-1}$ | $3 \times 10$–4 ng mL$^{-1}$ | Human serum | (264) |
| MIP/ MWCNTs | Pyruvic acid | DPV | CPE | Ammonium acetate solution (pH 7.0) | 0.1–200 µM | 0.048 µM | Human plasma and urine | (265) |
| PdNPs/ PNIPAM-CS microgel | Paraoxon-ethyl | DPV | GCE | 0.1 M PBS (pH 7.0) | 0.01 µM–1.3 mM | 0.7 nM | Bok choy, and water | (266) |
| MWCNTs-Pt NPs | Homovanillic acid Vanillylmandelic acid | DPV | GCE | 0.1 M PBS (pH 7.0) | $2 \times 10^{-7}$–$8 \times 10^{-5}$ M; $5 \times 10^{-7}$–$8 \times 10^{-5}$ M | $8 \times 10^{-8}$ M; $1.73 \times 10^{-7}$ M | Human urine | (267) |
| Au NPs | Kanamycin | DPV | Au | ABS (pH 4.0) | $1.0 \times 10^{-10}$–$6.0 \times 10^{-8}$ M | $6.0 \times 10^{-11}$ M | Honey | (204) |
| mC-PdNST | Brevetoxin B | DPV | GCE | ABS (pH 6.5) | 0.01–10 ng mL$^{-1}$ | 5.0 pg mL$^{-1}$ | Seafood samples | (268) |
| Cu(II)-PLH- COOH-MWCNTs | Salvianic acid A | DPV | Pt | PBS (pH 3.0) | 0.4–1000 µM | 0.037 µM | Salvia miltiorrhiza, and medicinal liquids | (269) |
| Fe(II)-BTC | Nitric oxide (NO) | DPV | GCE | PBS (pH 7.4) | 18–$9 \times 10^3$ nM | 7.2 nM | Sodium nitroprusside | (270) |

*(Continued)*

**TABLE 9.5 (Continued)**

**Some Selected Nanozymes-Based Platforms for Several Analytes**

| Nanozymes | Analyte/Substrate | Method | Electrode | Medium | Linear Range | LOD | App | Ref |
|---|---|---|---|---|---|---|---|---|
| | | | | | Characteristics of Analytical Method | | | |
| Au@Pd/MoS$_2$@ MWCNTs | Hepatitis B e antigen | AMP | GCE | PBS (pH 7.38) | 0.1–500 pg mL$^{-1}$ | 26 fg mL$^{-1}$ | Human serum | (271) |
| Co$_3$O$_4$@CeO$_2$-Au@ Pt-Ab$_2$ | Squamous cell carcinoma antigen | AMP | GCE | PBS (pH 6.98) | 100 fg mL$^{-1}$ –80 ng mL$^{-1}$ | 33 fg mL$^{-1}$ | Human serum | (272) |
| PtNPs@ MWCNTs | Xylose | AMP | GCE | 0.1 M PBS (pH 7.0) | 5–400 μM | 1 μM | Lignocellulosic samples | (200) |
| Au/Co@ HNCF | Uric acid | DPV | GCE | 0.1 M PBS (pH 7.4) | 0.1–25 μM | 0.023 μM | Human serum | (205) |
| AuNPs/Cu-Cys/CP | Superoxide anion (O$_2^-$) | AMP | CPE | 0.02 M PBS (pH 7.4) | 3.1–326 μM | 0.25 μM | NS | (199) |
| Fe$_3$O$_4$ NPs/MMIPs | Acetylthiocholine chloride | CV | GCE | 0.2 M PBS (pH 7.0) | 2.85–160 μM | 0.86 μM | NS | (273) |
| | Acetylcholinesterase | | | | 0.53–20000 ng mL$^{-1}$ | 0.16 ng mL$^{-1}$ | | |
| | Choline oxidase | | | | 22.76–400 ng mL$^{-1}$ | 6.83 ng mL$^{-1}$ | | |

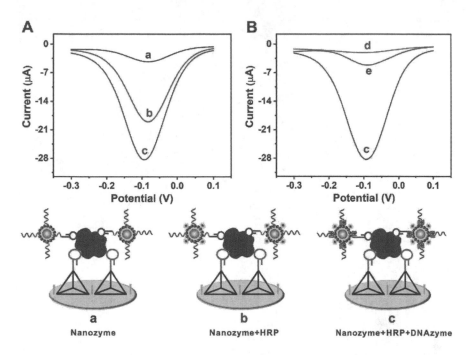

**FIGURE 9.5** Top: (A) Differential pulse voltammetry (DPV) responses of: (a) SPGE/NTHTro4/MCH/cTnI with $Fe_3O_4$/PDDA/Au@Pt-Tro6 nanoprobe; (b) $Fe_3O_4$/PDDA/Au@Pt-HRP-Tro6 nanoprobe; and (c) $Fe_3O_4$/PDDA/Au@Pt-HRP- GHD-Tro6 nanoprobe. (B) DPV responses of the SPGE/NTH-Tro4/MCH: (d) background DPV (modified electrode without target cTnI); (e) blank signal (the modified electrode after incubation in $Fe_3O_4$/PDDA/Au@Pt-HRP-GHD-Tro6 nanoprobe without target cTnI). (c) SPGE/NTH-Tro4/MCH/cTnI/$Fe_3O_4$/PDDA/Au@Pt- HRP-GHD-Tro6. The DPV measurements were performed in the 100-mM PBS (pH 7.0) solution with 3-mM HQ and 2-mM $H_2O_2$ (amplitude 50 mV, incubation time 60 min, cTnI concentration 10 ng.mL$^{-1}$). Bottom: Schematics of (a) nanozyme, (b) nanozyme+HRP, and (c) nanozyme+HRP+DNAzyme. Reprinted with permission (203).

was immobilized onto a carbon paste electrode (CPE) and used for the detection of superoxide anions. They prepared three different electrodes: 1) Au NPs/CPE; 2) Cu-Cys/CPE; and 3) Au NPs/Cu-Cys/CPE. The best performance (linear range = 3.1 to 326 µM; LOD = 0.2 µM) was obtained with Au NPs/Cu-Cys/CPE. The sensor was resistant to interference from dimethyl sulfoxide (DMSO), citric acid, uric acid, and $H_2O_2$. (199). Moreover, using Au NPs, Wang et al. developed an enzyme-free platform for kanamycin detection based on the target-induced replacement of an Apt and recovered the catalytic activity of Au NPs (**Figure 9.6**). The AuNPs exhibited POD-like activity for catalyzing the reaction of TMB and thionine in the presence of $H_2O_2$. Nonspecific binding between Au NPs and kanamycin-specific Apt, and the Apt was responsible for kanamycin detection in standard solutions and honey samples with LODs of 0.06 nM, and 0.73 nM, respectively (204).

Bimetallic NPs-decorated carbon-based materials also provide enzyme-like features for the determination of different analytes. Wang et al. published one of the

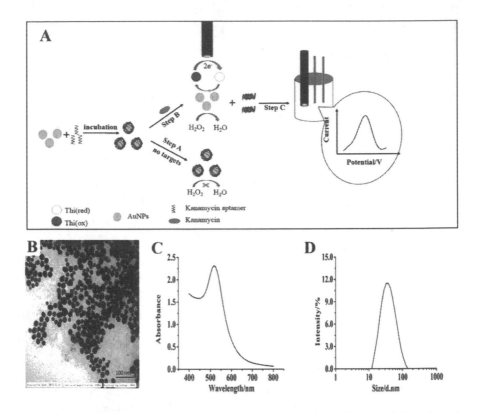

**FIGURE 9.6** (A) Illustration of the electrochemical detection of kanamycin based on the Apt and nanozyme. (B) Characterization of Au NPs. TEM image of Au NPs, (C) UV–vis spectra of Au NPs, and (D) Zeta size measurement of Au NPs. Reprinted with permission (204).

best examples of this nanozyme (205). They synthesized Au/cobalt (Co) bimetallic NPs-decorated hollow nanoporous carbon framework (HNCF) as a nanozyme for sensitive electrochemical determination of uric acid (LOD = 0.023 μM). The synthesis of Au/Co@HNCF has achieved the specific binding between kanamycin and by pyrolysis of the Au (III)-etched ZIF-67. The results of structural and morphological characterizations can be seen in **Figure 9.7**.

As a different enzyme application of nanozyme-based platforms, CcO catalyzes the reduction of $O_2$ to water using a heme/Cu hetero-binuclear active site in mitochondria. Kitagishi et al. fixed tridentate Cu(II) complex onto 5,10,15,20-tetrakis(4-sulfonatophenyl)porphinatoiron(III) (FeIIITPPS) through supramolecular complexation between FeIIITPPS and a per-O-methylated β-cyclodextrin dimer linked by a (2,2′:6′,2″-terpyridyl)Cu(II) complex (CuIITerpyCD2) to form a superoxotype FeIII–$O_2$–/CuI complex like CcO (202). The reduced FeIITPPS/CuITerpyCD2 complex reacted with $O_2$ in an aqueous solution at pH 7.0 and 25 °C. They examined the electrocatalytic $O_2$ reduction reaction to demonstrate the CcO-like function of this system. The results suggested that the FeTPPS/CuTerpyCD2 hetero-binuclear structure was effective for electrochemical analysis of the $O_2$ reduction. Zhu et al.

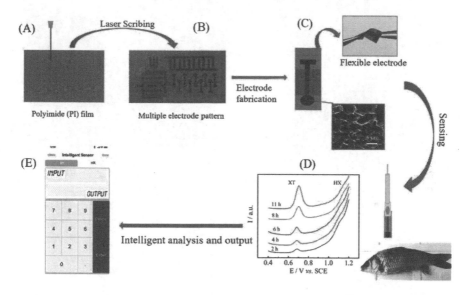

**FIGURE 9.7** Schematic representation of the LSG flexible electrode. Inset: the SEM Image of LSG. Reprinted with permission (206).

developed a facile and rapid one-step mass production of flexible 3-D porous graphene nanozyme platform as shown in **Figure 9.7** (206).

This flexible electrode as nanozyme was used for simultaneous determination of xanthine and hypoxanthine for evaluation of fish freshness. The authors calculated the $K_m$, $V_{max}$ values for the two analytes and concluded that, due to the very close peak-to-peak distance between xanthine and hypoxanthine, both $K_m$ and $V_{max}$ affected by each other. The $K_m$ value of the flexible 3-D porous graphene nanozyme toward xanthine was found lower than the native enzyme, indicating that the nanozyme shows better affinity toward xanthine and hypoxanthine. The linear ranges of detection were from 0.3 to 179.9 µM for xanthine (LOD = 0.26 µM) and from 0.3 to 159.9 µM for hypoxanthine (LOD = 0.18 µM) (206).

Sun et al. reported a cerium oxide ($CeO_2$)-based nanozyme platform for the detection of methyl-paraoxon, in which the phosphatase-like activity of $CeO_2$ degraded methyl-paraoxon into para-nitrophenol. On the other hand, $CeO_2$ exhibited the organophosphorus hydrolase-like activity, which can catalyze the decomposition of methyl-paraoxon to generate para-nitrophenol. Moreover, the electrochemical signal of para-nitrophenol was amplified after coating the nanozyme on the electrode surface. The experimental results suggested that this nanozyme-assisted electrochemical method is simple, rapid, and sensitive for methyl-paraoxon determination (207). Nanozymes, which are advantageous for pesticide determination, have also been pursued (208). Researchers developed electrochemical nanozyme sensors using graphene-like molybdenum disulfide ($MoS_2$)/MWCNTs for the analysis of carbendazim residues in tea and rice samples (**Figure 9.8**). The nanozyme platform provided low electron transfer resistance, high effective surface area, good film electrode stability, and excellent electrocatalytic capacity. Moreover, it

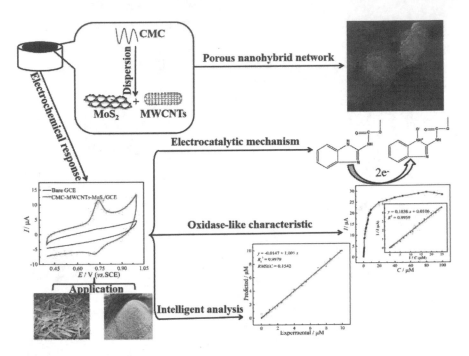

**FIGURE 9.8** The fabrication of MoS$_2$/MWCNTs porous nanohybrid network with OXD-like characteristic as electrochemical nanozyme sensor coupled with machine learning for intelligent analysis of carbendazim in tea and rice samples. Reprinted with permission (208).

exhibited unique OXD-like activity with a range was 0.04 μM–100 μM, and LOD was 7.4 nM carbendazim (208). Another nanozyme platform constructed with MWCNT was reported by Xue et al. (209). They developed *in-situ* reduction and deposition of silver (Ag) NPs on the black phosphorene (BP) surface and its amino-functionalized MWCNT (NH$_2$-MWCNT) nanocomposite for simultaneous determination of uric acid, xanthine, and hypoxanthine (209). The reciprocal of peak response current was proportional to the reciprocal of analyte concentration. Therefore, it was suggested that NH$_2$-MWCNT-BP-AgNPs exhibited the OXD-like nanozyme characteristic. Moreover, the developed nanozyme showed exceptional a $K_m$ of 36.63 μA and an $I_{max}$ of 6.08 μM. The sensor's working stability and repeatability combined with acceptable recoveries in real sample tests (209).

Several studies have shown that exosomal micro RNA (miRNA) can promote the development and progression of tumors by mediating the translation of messenger RNA (mRNA), such as ovarian, breast, and lung cancers. Therefore, exosomal miRNAs have been discovered as important and reliable biomarkers for the early diagnosis of tumors (210). Li et al. reported an electrochemical sensor based on the cascade primer exchange reaction with MOF@Pt@MOF nanozyme for ultrasensitive determination of exosomal miRNA. The multilayered nanozyme platform consisted of a layer of Pt NPs encapsulated between two layers of MIL-88. This platform exhibited an excellent POD-like activity toward H$_2$O$_2$ decomposition. The LOD was

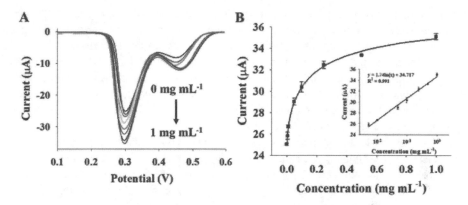

**FIGURE 9.9** (A) DPV responses of 0.5 mM TMBox (pH 4.0) with different GA concentrations (0, 0.005, 0.01, 0.05, 0.1, 0.25, 0.5, 1.0 mg mL$^{-1}$) at a potential range from 0.1 to 0.6 V on an ITO electrode. (B) A plot of reduction currents at 0.30 V versus different concentrations of GA. The inset shows a log-scale linear plot. Reprinted with permission (211).

0.29 fM for miRNA, and different miRNAs included single-base mismatch, double-base mismatch, noncomplementary sequence, miRNA-122, and miRNA-155 were used for the selectivity studies of the nanozyme. The analytical performance of the nanozyme indicated that it could be used as an alternative sensing platform for the early diagnosis of cancer (210). Son et al. synthesized PB NPs for the determination of glycated albumin in human plasma samples (211). They reported that PB NPs exhibited excellent POD-like activity, catalyzing the oxidation of TMB in the presence of H$_2$O$_2$ within 1 min. When the TMB and H$_2$O$_2$ solutions were introduced to the sandwich complex, the PB NPs nanozyme of the complex displayed a strong catalytic performance for TMB oxidation, generating TMBox. The TMBox molecules were subsequently reduced on the indium tin oxide electrode surfaces. While the K$_m$ value of the PBNPs for TMB was slightly higher than those obtained with other NPs, PB NPs exhibited the smallest K$_m$ value for H$_2$O$_2$, establishing that its affinity toward H$_2$O$_2$ is high. Studies showed that to achieve the maximum activity, PB NPs require the lowest concentration of H$_2$O$_2$. As a POD mimic, the PB NPs were used to determine glycated albumin levels by exploiting boronate affinity. The linear range of detection was 10 μg mL$^{-1}$ to 2 mg mL$^{-1}$, and the LOD was 7.3 μg mL$^{-1}$ (**Figure 9.9**) (211).

## 9.4 SOME CHALLENGES AND OVERCOMES

Although nanozymes have been widely used in sensing platforms of pharmaceuticals, pesticides, H$_2$O$_2$, glucose, catechol, proteins, metal ions, anions, cancer cells, and pathogens, several challenges remain. The natural-enzyme-based platforms are more sensitive compared to many nanozyme platforms for the detection of various compounds. Different factors, such as the size, shape, composition, surface modification of nanozymes, and single-atom strategy may be efficient methods to improve the desired catalytic efficiency of nanozymes. It is believed that single-atom nanozymes will become increasingly used in the platform design as they can provide more active sites for reactions. The surface of nanozymes platforms is the primary factor of catalytic activity of nanozymes. Inappropriate nanozyme platforms cause blocking of the active surface by biomolecules due to nonspecific binding. Therefore, a decrease in catalytic activity and interference problems may occur during the detection of target compounds. To eliminate these problems, functionalizing the nanozymes with suitable ligands or proteins are essential. Moreover, efforts must be made to ensure that the surface modification does not change the nature of the interaction between nanozymes and substrates (9–11, 23, 24).

Another challenge is their aggregation. Nanozymes easily aggregate in high ionic strength samples. As a result of this, the catalytic activity of nanozymes can decrease, and interference effects may occur. Protection of the nanozymes with different molecules, such as proteins or organic ligands, could help prevent aggregation. Therefore, more reliable results could be provided (18, 274).

Even though nanozymes show a low specificity toward target molecules, the development of new substrates and oxidants can further improve the selectivity and sensitivity of nanozyme-based sensors. Different metal ions, such as Au, Pt, Ag, Fe, Co, Cu, and Ce, can be used to prepare nanozymes. Moreover, nanozymes can be modified with amino acids and organosulfur compounds to improve specific interaction with target metal ions. The modified nanozyme may have an affinity toward its metal ion species in the sample. The adsorption or chemisorption of the same metal ions on the surfaces of nanozymes will change the surface oxidation states, changing the enzyme-mimic activity or selectivity of the probes (9, 11, 18, 21, 22).

Despite advances in nanozyme-based platforms and extensive applications of nanozymes, a general weakness for all analyses is their poor reproducibility. Nowadays, NPs that show enzyme-like activities can be synthesized in very small scales in laboratories. Therefore, the nanozymes synthesized from different batches are not as good in reproducibility as expected. Furthermore, developments in industrial production due to the development of nanotechnology will standardize the production of nanomaterials in commercial and long-term applications of nanozymes. Moreover, many researchers have demonstrated the therapeutic effects of nanozyme platforms through cell or animal experiments. However, the *in vivo* explanation of the mechanism of nanozyme systems in biological experiments is still unclear. The processes in the human body are not known precisely. Therefore, to advance nanozymes in therapeutic applications, all of their potential benefits and risks about cellular processes, clinical toxicity, immunogenicity, pharmacokinetics, and so on should be investigated. In recent years, nanozymes platforms have been widely used for the detection of concentration and distribution of specific biochemical compounds in the biological environment. In the future, evidence for the distribution and mechanism of action of biochemical compounds in living organisms can be provided with the development of multifunctional nanozymes and combining their enzyme-like properties for diagnostic purposes. Furthermore, it is crucial to explore the probability of using nanozymes in multipurpose activities due to the multifunctional use of NPs in biosensing and therapeutic applications. Therefore, the simultaneous utilization of magnetic, thermal, and optical properties of nanozymes can optimize their biosensing and biomedical applications (9–11, 18, 23, 24, 274).

## 9.5 SUMMARY AND FUTURE PERSPECTIVES

Conventional methods for the detection of different analytes, such as high-performance liquid chromatography (HPLC), ultraviolet-visible (UV–vis) spectroscopy, etc., are time-consuming, costly, and not applicable for on-site monitoring. Therefore, there is a need for rapid, precise, sensitive, portable, and cost-effective methods to detect and measure analytes, such as pharmaceuticals, pesticides, ions, hormones, biomarkers, etc. Since its discovery in 2007 that $Fe_3O_4$ NPs exhibit POD-like activity, nanozymes have attracted much attention from many researchers for enzyme-like detection applications. The high sensitivity of enzyme-based platforms is due to the catalytic signal amplification from enzyme labels. Therefore, the continual development of nanozyme platforms, which have the desired catalytic activity and efficiency, will be an essential mission in the near future. An emerging trend is a need for on-site analyses using quantitative platforms for different practical applications such as monitoring human health or pests in environmental samples with personalized equipment. As an effective strategy, integrating assay platforms with portable devices, e.g., smartphones, can realize this goal. Researchers may be combined nanozyme-based assay platforms with smartphones to achieve the in-field, fast, and convenient monitoring of target compounds in food safety, environmental analysis, and clinical practice will occur. Moreover, it is believed that combined nanozyme-based assay platforms with portable devices and other advanced technologies will be an exciting direction in the analytical field. However, as mentioned above, many interdisciplinary activities are required to be well-developed to achieve a potential nanozyme-based detection system. In general, nanozymes-based platforms are divided into two: 1) oxidoreductase mimics and 2) hydrolase mimics. Oxidase mimics are generally found in the application, and researchers primarily utilized the oxidase-like family-based nanozymes, such as POD-like, superoxide dismutase-like, glucose oxidase-like, NADH POD-like, CAT-like, and glutathione oxidase-like nanozymes. At the same time, hydrolase-like nanozymes are less synthesized and studied. Therefore, new types of nanozymes that can mimic different kinds of enzymes still need to be discovered.

## REFERENCES

1. Pumera M, Sánchez S, Ichinose I, Tang J. 2007. *Sensors Actuators, B Chem.* 123(2):1195–1205
2. Singh T, Singh AK. 2019. *Adv. Enzym. Technol.*: 225–71
3. Scheller FW, Yarman A, Bachmann T, Hirsch T, Kubick S, et al. 2014. *Adv. Biochem. Eng. Biotechnol.* 140:1–28
4. Prodromidis MII, Karayannis MII. 2002. *Electroanalysis.* 14(4):241–61
5. Mehrotra P. 2016. *J. Oral Biol. Craniofacial. Res.* 6(2):153–59
6. Scheller FW, Schubert F, Renneberg R, Müller HG, Jänchen M, Weise H. 1985. *Biosensors.* 1(2):135–60
7. Bollella P, Gorton L. 2018. *Curr. Opin. Electrochem.* 10:157–73
8. Chang Y, Gao S, Liu M, Liu J. 2020. *Anal. Methods* 12(39):4708–23
9. Liang M, Yan X. 2019. *Acc. Chem. Res.* 52(8):2190–2200
10. Huang Y, Ren J, Qu X. 2019. *Chem. Rev.* 119(6):4357–4412
11. Wei H, Wang E. 2013. *Chem. Soc. Rev.* 42(14):6060–93

12. Gao L, Fan K, Yan X. 2020. *In Nanozymology*. pp. 105–40. Springer, Singapore
13. Attar F, Shahpar MG, Rasti B, Sharifi M, Saboury AA, et al. 2019. *J. Mol. Liq.* 278:130–44
14. Tang X-N, Liu C-Z, Chen X-R, Deng Y-Q, Chen X-H, et al. 2019. *Carbon N. Y.* 146:147–54
15. Golchin J, Golchin K, Alidadian N, Ghaderi S, Eslamkhah S, et al. 2017. *Nanomed. Biotechnol.*: 1069–76
16. Li S, Liu X, Chai H, Huang Y. 2018. *TrAC Trends Anal. Chem.* 105:391–403
17. Niu X, Cheng N, Ruan X, Du D, Lin Y. 2020. *J. Electrochem. Soc.* 167(3):037508
18. Unnikrishnan B, Lien CW, Chu HW, Huang CC. 2021. *J. Hazard Mater.* 401:123397
19. Wang Q, Wei H, Zhang Z, Wang E, Dong S. 2018. *TrAC Trends Anal. Chem.* 105:218–224
20. Yu Z, Lou R, Pan W, Li N, Tang B. 2020. *Chem. Commun.* 56(99):15513–24
21. Zhang R, Fan K, Yan X. 2020. *Sci. China Life Sci.* 63(8):1183–1200
22. Hasan A, Nanakali NMQ, Salihi A, Rasti B, Sharifi M, et al. 2020. *Talanta.* 215:120939
23. Sharifi M, Hosseinali SH, Yousefvand P, Salihi A, Shekha MS, et al. 2020. *Mater. Sci. Eng. C* 108:110422
24. Meng Y, Li W, Pan X, Gadd GM. 2020. *Environ. Sci. Nano.* 7(5):1305–18
25. Dong H, Fan Y, Zhang W, Gu N, Zhang Y. 2019. *Bioconjug. Chem.* 30(5):1273–1296
26. Tan Z, Dong H, Liu Q, Liu H, Zhao P, et al. 2019. *Biosens. Bioelectron.* 142:111556
27. Huang L, Sun DW, Pu H, Wei Q. 2019. *Compr. Rev. Food Sci. Food Saf.* 18(5):1496–1513
28. Jiang D, Ni D, Rosenkrans ZT, Huang P, Yan X, Cai W. 2019. *Chem. Soc. Rev.* 48(14):3683–3704
29. Wu J, Wang X, Wang Q, Lou Z, Li S, et al. 2019. *Chem. Soc. Rev.* 48(4):1004–76
30. Dong W, Zhuang Y, Li S, Zhang X, Chai H, Huang Y. 2018. *Sensors Actuators, B Chem.* 255:2050–57
31. Gao L, Zhuang J, Nie L, Zhang J, Zhang Y, et al. 2007. *Nat. Nanotechnol.* 2(9): 577–83
32. Luo W, Zhu C, Su S, Li D, He Y, et al. 2010. *ACS Nano.* 4(12):7451–58
33. Ge C, Fang G, Shen X, Chong Y, Wamer WG, et al. 2016. *ACS Nano.* 10(11):10436–45
34. Chen Z, Yin JJ, Zhou YT, Zhang Y, Song L, et al. 2012. *ACS Nano.* 6(5):4001–12
35. Liu H, Ding YN, Yang B, Liu Z, Zhang X, Liu Q. 2018. *ACS Sustain. Chem. Eng.* 6(11):14383–93
36. Lu C, Liu X, Li Y, Yu F, Tang L, et al. 2015. *ACS Appl. Mater. Interfaces* 7(28):15395–402
37. Liang S, Deng X, Chang Y, Sun C, Shao S, et al. 2019. *Nano Lett.* 19(6):4134–45
38. Chen M, Deng G, He Y, Li X, Liu W, et al. 2020. *ACS Appl. Bio Mater.* 3(1):639–47
39. Chang Y, Gao S, Liu M, Liu J, Nisnevitch M, et al. 2020. *Sensors.* 22(39):4708–23
40. Pundir C, Deswal R, Narwal V. 2018. *Bioprocess. Biosyst. Eng.* 41(3):313–329.
41. Fan K, Wang H, Xi J, Liu Q, Meng X, et al. 2017. *Chem. Commun.* 53(2):424–27
42. Ko E, Tran VK, Son SE, Hur W, Choi H, Seong GH. 2019. *Sensors Actuators, B Chem.* 294:166–76
43. Jin GH, Ko E, Kim MK, Tran VK, Son SE, et al. 2018. *Sensors Actuators, B Chem.* 274:201–9
44. Lu J, Hu Y, Wang P, Liu P, Chen Z, Sun D. 2020. *Sensors Actuators, B Chem.* 311:127909
45. Rahman MM, Adeosun WA, Asiri AM. 2020. *Microchem. J.* 159:105536
46. Zhang Q, Hu Y, Wu D, Ma S, Wang J, et al. 2018. *Talanta.* 183:258–67
47. Liu X, Zhang X, Zheng J. 2021. *Microchem. J.* 160:105595
48. Yang H, Zhou J, Bao J, Ma Y, Zhou J, et al. 2021. *Microchem. J.* 162:2–9
49. Fu Y, Huang D, Li C, Zou L, Ye B. 2018. *Anal. Chim. Acta.* 1014:10–18
50. Chen L, Xu X, Cui F, Qiu Q, Chen X, Xu J. 2018. *Anal. Biochem.* 554:1–8
51. Rashed MA, Harraz FA, Faisal M, El-Toni AM, Alsaiari M, Al-Assiri MS. 2021. *Anal. Biochem.* 615:114065

52. Mollarasouli F, Asadpour-Zeynali K, Campuzano S, Yáñez-Sedeño P, Pingarrón JM. 2017. *Electrochim. Acta.* 246:303–14
53. Zhou J, Zhao Y, Bao J, Huo D, Fa H, et al. 2017. *Electrochim. Acta.* 250:152–58
54. Wei P, Sun D, Niu Y, Lu X, Zhai H. 2020. *Electrochim. Acta.* 359:136962
55. Guan JF, Huang ZN, Zou J, Jiang XY, Peng DM, Yu JG. 2020. *Ecotoxicol. Environ. Saf.* 190:110123
56. Liu D, Guo Q, Zhang X, Hou H, You T. 2015. *J. Colloid Interface Sci.* 450:168–73
57. Hou B, Liu H, Qi S, Zhu Y, Zhou B, et al. 2018. *J. Colloid Interface Sci.* 510:103–10
58. Qin X, Wang H, Miao Z, Li J, Chen Q. 2015. *Talanta.* 139:56–61
59. Zhang S, Zheng J. 2016. *Talanta.* 159:231–37
60. Thiruppathi M, Lin PY, Chou YT, Ho HY, Wu LC, Ho J A. 2019. *Talanta.* 200:450–57
61. Xing L, Rong Q, Ma Z. 2015. *Sensors Actuators, B Chem.* 221:242–47
62. Zhang Y, Li Y, Jiang Y, Li Y, Li S. 2016. *Appl. Surf. Sci.* 378:375–83
63. Liu M, An M, Xu J, Liu T, Wang L, et al. 2021. *Appl. Surf. Sci.* 542:148699
64. Golsheikh AM, Yeap GY, Yam FK, Lim HS. 2020. *Synth. Met.* 260:116272
65. Guan H, Zhao Y, Cheng J, Zhang Y, Yang Q, Zhang B. 2020. *Synth. Met.* 270:116604
66. Venosta L, Bracamonte M V., Rodríguez MC, Jacobo SE, Bercoff PG. 2017. *Sensors Actuators, B Chem.* 248:460–69
67. Liu JX, Ding SN. 2017. *Sensors Actuators, B Chem.* 251:200–207
68. Mattoussi M, Matoussi F, Raouafi N. 2018. *Sensors Actuators, B Chem.* 274:412–18
69. Peng R, Offenhäusser A, Ermolenko Y, Mourzina Y. 2020. *Sensors Actuators, B Chem.* 321:128437
70. Mutyala S, Mathiyarasu J. 2016. *Mater. Sci. Eng. C* 69:398–406
71. Guler M, Turkoglu V, Kivrak A, Karahan F. 2018. *Mater. Sci. Eng. C* 90:454–60
72. Huang Y, Xue Y, Zeng J, Li S, Wang Z, et al. 2018. *Mater. Sci. Eng. C* 92:590–98
73. Bai Z, Li G, Liang J, Su J, Zhang Y, et al. 2016. *Biosens. Bioelectron.* 82:185–94
74. Wang L, Wu T, Wu H, Zhong J, Wang N, Wang R. 2018. *Prog. Nat. Sci. Mater. Int.* 28(1):24–27
75. Bayram L, Guler M. 2019. *Prog. Nat. Sci. Mater. Int.* 29(4):390–96
76. Yuan R, Li H, Yin X, Zhang L, Lu J. 2018. *J. Mater. Sci. Technol.* 34(9):1692–98
77. Karthik R, Vinoth Kumar J, Chen SM, Sundaresan P, Mutharani B, et al. 2018. *Ultrason Sonochem.* 48:473–81
78. Roushani M, Dizajdizi BZ. 2015. *Catal Commun.* 69:133–37
79. Pang P, Yang Z, Xiao S, Xie J, Zhang Y, Gao Y. 2014. *J. Electroanal. Chem.* 727:27–33
80. Liu P, Li J, Liu X, Li M, Lu X. 2015. *J. Electroanal. Chem.* 751:1–6
81. Zakaria ABM, Leszczynska D. 2016. *J. Electroanal. Chem.* 766:30–36
82. Xue W, Bo X, Zhou M, Guo L. 2016. *J. Electroanal. Chem.* 781:204–11
83. Yang X, Ouyang Y, Wu F, Hu Y, Zhang H, Wu Z. 2016. *J. Electroanal. Chem.* 777:85–91
84. Zhao C, Zhang H, Zheng J. 2017. *J. Electroanal. Chem.* 784:55–61
85. Sukeri A, Bertotti M. 2017. *J. Electroanal. Chem.* 805:18–23
86. Liang X, Li W, Han H, Ma Z. 2019. *J. Electroanal. Chem.* 834:43–48
87. Karami C, Taher MA. 2019. *J. Electroanal. Chem.* 847:113219
88. Stanković V, Đurđić S, Ognjanović M, Mutić J, Kalcher K, Stanković DM. 2020. *J. Electroanal. Chem.* 876:2–7
89. Bohlooli F, Yamatogi A, Mori S. 2021. *Sens. Bio-Sens. Res.* 31:100392
90. Mohammad A, Khan ME, Yoon T, Hwan Cho M. 2020. *Appl. Surf. Sci.* 525:146353
91. Ross N, Civilized Nqakala N. 2020. *Anal. Lett.* 53(15):2445–64
92. Balasubramanian P, He S Bin, Jansirani A, Deng HH, Peng HP, et al. 2020. *New J Chem* 44(33):14050–59
93. He G, Gao F, Li W, Li P, Zhang X, et al. 2019. *Anal. Methods.* 11(12):1651–56
94. He F-G, Yin J-Y, Sharma G, Kumar A, Stadler FJ, Du B. 2019. *Nanomaterials.* 9(8):1109
95. Tang J, Huang L, Cheng Y, Zhuang J, Li P, Tang D. 2018. *Microchim. Acta.* 185(12):569

96. Wang M, Wang C, Liu Y, Hu B, He L, et al. 2020. *Microchim. Acta.* 187(8):436
97. Liu T, Guo Y, Zhang Z, Miao Z, Zhang X, Su Z. 2019. *Sensors Actuators B, Chem.* 286:370–76
98. Li X, Du X. 2017. *Sensors Actuators B, Chem.* 239:536–43
99. Lu Z, Wu L, Zhang J, Dai W, Mo G, Ye J. 2019. *Mater. Sci. Eng. C* 102:708–17
100. He J, Sunarso J, Zhu Y, Zhong Y, Miao J, et al. 2017. *Sensors Actuators, B Chem.* 244:482–91
101. Balamurugan J, Thanh TD, Karthikeyan G, Kim NH, Lee JH. 2017. *Biosens. Bioelectron.* 89:970–77
102. Vennila P, Yoo DJ, Kim AR, Kumar GG. 2017. *J. Alloys Compd.* 703:633–42
103. Cao Q, Xiao Y, Liu N, Huang R, Ye C, et al. 2020. *Sensors Actuators B, Chem.* 329:129133
104. Brondani D, Zapp E, da Silva Heying R, de Souza B, Cruz Vieira I. 2017. *Electroanalysis.* 29(12):2810–17
105. Ma B, Guo H, Wang M, Wang Q, Yang W, et al. 2020. *Microchem. J.* 155:104776
106. Radhakrishnan S, Krishnamoorthy K, Sekar C, Wilson J, Kim SJ. 2015. *Chem. Eng. J.* 259:594–602
107. Fu R, Lu Y, Ding Y, Li L, Ren Z, et al. 2019. *Microchem. J.* 150:104106
108. Ayaz S, Karakaya S, Emir G, Dilgin DG, Dilgin Y. 2020. *Microchem. J.* 154:104586
109. Imran H, Manikandan PN, Dharuman V. 2021. *Microchem. J.* 160:105774
110. Zhang RX, Yang P, Zhang YX. 2020. *Mater. Lett.* 272:127850
111. Jo HJ, Shit A, Jhon HS, Park SY. 2020. *J. Ind. Eng. Chem.* 89:485–93
112. Yin D, Bo X, Liu J, Guo L. 2018. *Anal. Chim. Acta.* 1038:11–20
113. Guo S, Zhang C, Yang M, Zhou Y, Bi C, et al. 2020. *Anal. Chim. Acta.* 1109:130–39
114. Yang H, Bao J, Qi Y, Zhao JY, Hu Y, et al. 2020. *Anal. Chim. Acta.* 1135:12–19
115. Lotfi Z, Gholivand MB, Shamsipur M. 2020. *Anal. Biochem.:* 114062
116. Zhang Y, Li N, Xiang Y, Wang D, Zhang P, et al. 2020. *Carbon N. Y.* 156:506–13
117. Wei C, Zou X, Liu Q, Li S, Kang C, Xiang W. 2020. *Electrochim. Acta.* 334:135630
118. Chen M, Cao X, Chang K, Xiang H, Wang R. 2021. *Electrochim. Acta.* 368:137603
119. Chiu WT, Chang TFM, Sone M, Tixier-Mita A, Toshiyoshi H. 2020. *Talanta.* 212(2019):120780
120. Kim S eun, Muthurasu A. 2020. *J. Electroanal. Chem.* 873:114356
121. Liu Y, Zhao W, Li X, Liu J, Han Y, et al. 2020. *Appl. Surf. Sci.* 512:145710
122. Amiripour F, Ghasemi S, Azizi SN. 2021. *Appl. Surf. Sci.* 537:147827
123. Palve YP, Jha N. 2020. *Mater. Chem. Phys.* 240:122086
124. Huo K, Fu J, Zhang X, Xu P, Gao B, et al. 2017. *Sensors Actuators, B Chem.* 244:38–46
125. Ni Y, Xu J, Liang Q, Shao S. 2017. *Sensors Actuators B, Chem.* 250:491–98
126. Sheng L, Li Z, Meng A, Xu Q. 2018. *Sensors Actuators B, Chem.* 254:1206–15
127. Chandrasekaran NI, Manickam M. 2019. *Sensors Actuators B, Chem.* 288:188–94
128. Li X, Ren K, Zhang M, Sang W, Sun D, et al. 2019. *Sensors Actuators B, Chem.* 293:122–28
129. Zhou X, Gu X, Chen Z, Wu Y, Xu W, Bao J. 2020. *Sensors Actuators B, Chem:* 129117
130. Mahmoud A, Echabaane M, Omri K, El Mir L, Ben Chaabane R. 2019. *J. Alloys Compd.* 786:960–68
131. Farid A, Pan L, Usman M, Khan IA, Khan AS, et al. 2021. *J. Alloys Compd.* 861:158642
132. Cao M, Wang H, Ji S, Zhao Q, Pollet BG, Wang R. 2019. *Mater. Sci. Eng. C* 95:174–82
133. Sehit E, Drzazgowska J, Buchenau D, Yesildag C, Lensen M, Altintas Z. 2020. *Biosens. Bioelectron.* 165:112432
134. Yao K, Dai B, Tan X, Ralchenko V, Yang L, et al. 2020. *J. Electroanal. Chem.* 871:114264
135. Shishegari N, Sabahi A, Manteghi F, Ghaffarinejad A, Tehrani Z. 2020. *J. Electroanal. Chem.* 871:114285

136. Zhou F, You C, Wang Q, Chen Y, Wang Z, et al. 2020. *J. Electroanal. Chem.* 876:114477
137. Liu Q, Zhong H, Chen M, Zhao C, Liu Y, et al. 2020. *RSC Adv.* 10(56):33739–46
138. Arif D, Hussain Z, Sohail M, Liaqat MA, Khan MA, Noor T. 2020. *Front. Chem.* 8:1–8
139. Li Q, Chen L, Guo C, Liu X, Han D, Wang W. 2021. *J. Mater. Sci.* 56(4):3414–29
140. Singer N, Pillai RG, Johnson AID, Harris KD, *Microchim. Acta.* 187(4):15–20
141. Wei C, Li X, Xiang W, Yu Z, Liu Q. 2020. *Sensors Actuators, B Chem.* 324:128773
142. Khosroshahi Z, Karimzadeh F, Kharaziha M, Allafchian A. 2020. *Mater. Sci. Eng. C* 108:110216
143. Mollarasouli F, Majidi MR, Asadpour-Zeynali K. 2021. *J. Taiwan Inst. Chem. Eng.* 000:1–8
144. Shahhoseini L, Mohammadi R, Ghanbari B, Shahrokhian S. 2019. *Appl. Surf. Sci.* 478:361–72
145. Tran VK, Ko E, Geng Y, Kim MK, Jin GH, et al. 2018. *J. Electroanal. Chem.* 826:29–37
146. Jothi L, Jayakumar N, Jaganathan SK, Nageswaran G. 2018. *Mater. Res. Bull.* 98:300–307
147. Suvina V, Kokulnathan T, Wang TJ, Balakrishna RG. 2020. *Microchim. Acta.* 187(3):189
148. Zhou T, Gao W, Gao Y, Wang Q. 2019. *J. Electrochem. Soc.* 166(12):B1069–78
149. Maikap A, Mukherjee K, Mondal B, Mandal N, Meikap AK. 2019. *Biosens. Bioelectron.* 128:32–36
150. Zhao H, Wang Y, Qian S, Xu CF, Li W, et al. 2019. *Int. J. Electrochem. Sci.* 14(2):1997–2003
151. Yuan D, Chen S, Hu F, Wang C, Yuan R. 2012. *Sensors Actuators, B Chem.* 168:193–99
152. Quynh BTP, Byun JY, Kim SH. 2015. *Sensors Actuators B, Chem.* 221:191–200
153. Aravindan N, Preethi S, Sangaranarayanan M V. 2017. *J. Electrochem. Soc.* 164(6):B274–84
154. Premlatha S, Bapu GNKR. 2018. *J. Alloys. Compd.* 767:622–31
155. Mollarasouli F, Kurbanoglu S, Asadpour-Zeynali K, Ozkan SA. 2020. *J. Electroanal. Chem.* 856:113672
156. Wang H, Wang Y, Li S, Qu J. 2017. *Anal. Methods.* 9(2):338–44
157. Palanisamy S, Thangavelu K, Chen SM, Thirumalraj B, Liu XH. 2016. *Sensors Actuators B, Chem.* 233:298–306
158. Coroş M, Pogăcean F, Măgeruşan L, Roşu MC, Porav AS, et al. 2018. *Sensors Actuators B, Chem.* 256:665–73
159. Maikap A, Mukherjee K, Mondal B, Mandal N. 2016. *RSC Adv.* 6(69):64611–16
160. Boopathy G, Keerthi M, Chen SM, Umapathy MJ, Kumar BN. 2020. *Mater. Chem. Phys.* 239:121982
161. Bansal P, Bhanjana G, Prabhakar N, Dhau JS, Chaudhary GR. 2017. *J. Mol. Liq.* 248:651–57
162. Palanisamy S, Ramaraj SK, Chen SM, Chiu TW, Velusamy V, et al. 2017. *J. Colloid. Interface Sci.* 496:364–70
163. Salvo-Comino C, Rassas I, Minot S, Bessueille F, Rodriguez-Mendez ML, et al. 2020. *Mater. Sci. Eng. C.* 110:1–6
164. Vellaichamy B, Ponniah SK, Prakash P. 2017. *Sensors Actuators B, Chem.* 253:392–99
165. Manavalan S, Govindasamy M, Chen SM, Rajaji U, Chen TW, et al. 2018. *J. Taiwan Inst. Chem. Eng.* 89:215–23
166. Luo H, Zhao YY, Jin XY, Yang JM, Cong H, et al. 2020. *Electroanalysis.* 32(7):1449–58
167. Wang Y, Liu X, Liu S, Zhang Y, Chang FX. 2020. *Anal. Lett.* 53(7):1061–74
168. Gao Z-Y, Gao Y-L, Wang E, Xu S, Chen W. 2016. *J. Electrochem. Soc.* 163(7):H528–33
169. Dongmo LM, Jiokeng SLZ, Pecheu CN, Walcarius A, Tonle IK. 2020. *Appl. Clay Sci.* 191:105602
170. Tabanlıgil Calam T. 2019. *Int. J. Environ. Anal. Chem.* 99(13):1298–1312
171. Zhu Y, Huai S, Jiao J, Xu Q, Wu H, Zhang H. 2020. *J. Electroanal. Chem.* 878:114726

172. Song Y, Zhao M, Wang X, Qu H, Liu Y, Chen S. 2019. *Mater. Chem. Phys.* 234:217–23
173. Dang Y, Wang X, Cui R, Chen S, Zhou Y. 2019. *J. Electroanal. Chem.* 834:196–205
174. Mao H, Liu M, Cao Z, Ji C, Sun Y, et al. 2017. *Appl. Surf. Sci.* 420:594–605
175. Alshahrani LA, Liu L, Sathishkumar P, Nan J, Gu FL. 2018. *J. Electroanal. Chem.* 815:68–75
176. Jiang H, Wang S, Deng W, Zhang Y, Tan Y, et al. 2017. *Talanta.* 164:300–306
177. Erogul S, Bas SZ, Ozmen M, Yildiz S. 2015. *Electrochim. Acta.* 186:302–13
178. Zhang H, Huang Y, Hu S, Huang Q, Wei C, et al. 2015. *Electrochim. Acta.* 176:28–35
179. Xin Y, Wang N, Wang C, Gao W, Chen M, et al. 2020. *J. Electroanal. Chem.* 877:114530
180. Chetankumar K, Kumara Swamy BE, Sharma SC. 2020. *Microchem. J.* 156:104979
181. Chen Y, Liu X, Zhang S, Yang L, Liu M, et al. 2017. *Electrochim. Acta.* 231:677–85
182. Guo Q, Zhang M, Zhou G, Zhu L, Feng Y, et al. 2016. *J. Electroanal. Chem.* 760:15–23
183. Song D, Xia J, Zhang F, Bi S, Xiang W, et al. 2015. *Sensors Actuators B, Chem.* 206:111–18
184. Mashhadizadeh MH, Kalantarian SM, Azhdeh A. 2020. *Electroanalysis*: 160–69
185. Zhang W, Zheng J, Lin Z, Zhong L, Shi J, et al. 2015. *Anal. Methods.* 7(15):6089–94
186. Jiang H, Zhang D, He Z, Lian Q, Xue Z, et al. 2015. *Anal. Lett.* 48(9):1426–36
187. Hu S, Zhang W, Zheng J, Shi J, Lin Z, et al. 2015. *RSC Adv.* 5(24):18615–21
188. Khalifa Z, Hassan K, Abo Oura MF, Hathoot A, Azzem MA. 2020. *ACS Omega.* 5(30):18950–57
189. Song Y, Zhang Y, Li J, Tan C, Li Y. 2020. *P. J. Electroanal. Chem.* 865:114157
190. Rajaji U, Govindasamy M, Chen SM, Chen TW, Liu X, Chinnapaiyan S. 2018. *Compos. Part. B Eng.* 152:220–30
191. Dang Y, Zhai Y, Yang L, Peng Z, Cheng N, Zhou Y. 2016. *RSC Adv.* 6(87):83994–2
192. Song Y, Yang T, Zhou X, Zheng H, Suye SI. 2016. *Anal. Methods.* 8(4):886–92
193. Xiao L, Yin J, Li Y, Yuan Q, Shen H, et al. 2016. *Analyst.* 141(19):5555–62
194. Sabbaghi N, Noroozifar M, Tohidinia M, Farsadrooh M. 2017. *Int. J. Electrochem. Sci.* 12(9):8777–92
195. Cotchim S, Promsuwan K, Dueramae M, Duerama S, Dueraning A, et al. 2020. *J. Electrochem. Soc.* 167(15):155528
196. Karthika A, Ramasamy Raja V, Karuppasamy P, Suganthi A, Rajarajan M. 2020. *Arab. J. Chem.* 13(2):4065–81
197. Zhang T, Wei JZ, Sun XJ, Zhao XJ, Tang HL, et al. 2020. *Inorg. Chem.* 59(13):8827–35
198. Mohd Yazid SNA, Md Isa I, Ali NM, Hashim N, Saidin MI, et al. 2020. *Int. J. Environ. Anal. Chem.* 00(00):1–18
199. Dashtestani F, Ghourchian H, Eskandari K, Rafiee-Pour HA. 2015. *Microchim. Acta.* 182(5–6):1045–53
200. Song H, Ma C, Wang L, Zhu Z. 2020. *Nanoscale.* 12(37):19284–92
201. Wang Y, Zhao H, Song H, Dong J, Xu J. 2020. *Microchim. Acta.* 187(10):1–9
202. Kitagishi H, Shimoji D, Ohta T, Kamiya R, Kudo Y, et al. 2018. *Chem. Sci.* 9(7):1989–95
203. Sun D, Lin X, Lu J, Wei P, Luo Z, et al. 2019. *Biosens. Bioelectron.* 142:111578
204. Wang C, Liu C, Luo J, Tian Y, Zhou N. 2016. *Anal. Chim. Acta.* 936:75–82
205. Wang K, Wu C, Wang F, Liao M, Jiang G. 2020. *Biosens. Bioelectron.* 150:111869
206. Zhu Y, Liu P, Xue T, Xu J, Qiu D, et al. 2021. *Microchem. J.* 162:105855
207. Sun Y, Wei J, Zou J, Cheng Z, Huang Z, et al. 2020. *J. Pharm. Anal.* In Press:
208. Zhu X, Liu P, Ge Y, Wu R, Xue T, et al. 2020. *J. Electroanal. Chem.* 862:113940
209. Xue T, Sheng Y, Xu J, Li Y, Lu X, et al. 2019. *Biosens. Bioelectron.* 145:111716
210. Li X, Li X, Li D, Zhao M, Wu H, et al. 2020. *Biosens. Bioelectron.* 168:112554
211. Son SE, Gupta PK, Hur W, Choi H, Lee HB, et al. 2020. *Anal. Chim. Acta.* 1134:41–49
212. Liu L, Du J, Liu W e., Guo Y, Wu G, et al. 2019. *Anal. Bioanal. Chem.* 411(10):2189–2200
213. Qing M, Yuan Y, Cai W, Xie S, Tang Y, et al. 2018. *Sensors Actuators, B Chem* 263:469–75

214. Tian L, Qi J, Qian K, Oderinde O, Liu Q, et al. 2018. *J. Electroanal. Chem.* 812:1–9
215. Stefanov C, Negut CC, Gugoasa LAD, van Staden J (Koos) F. 2020. *Microchim. Acta.* 187(11):611 (1-10)
216. Lu X, Liu G, Di P, Li Y, Xue T, et al. 2020. *Food Anal. Methods.* 13(11):2028–38
217. Khairy M, Banks CE. 2020. *Microchim. Acta.* 187(2):126 (1–10)
218. Son SE, Ko E, Tran VK, Hur W, Choi H, et al. 2019. *ChemElectroChem.* 6(17):4666–73
219. Krishnan RG, Rejithamol R, Saraswathyamma B. 2020. *Microchem. J.* 155:104745
220. Shen Y, Ma C, Zhang S, Li P, Zhu W, et al. 2020. *Sci. Total Environ.* 742:140622
221. Kanchana P, Navaneethan M, Sekar C. 2017. *Mater. Sci. Eng. B Solid-State Mater. Adv. Technol.* 226:132–40
222. Lu ZJ, Cheng Y, Zhang Y, Wang X, Xu P, et al. 2021. *Sensors Actuators, B Chem.* 329:129224
223. Xiao X, Zhang Z, Nan F, Zhao Y, Wang P, et al. 2021. *J. Alloys Compd.* 852:157045
224. Alamry KA, Hussein MA, Choi J woo, El-Said WA. 2020. *J. Electroanal. Chem.* 879:114789
225. Fernández I, González-Mora JL, Lorenzo-Luis P, Villalonga R, Salazar-Carballo PA. 2020. *Microchem. J.* 159:105538 (1–9)
226. Duan C, Dong Y, Sheng Q, Zheng J. 2019. *Talanta.* 198:23–29
227. Gu C, Wang Q, Zhang L, Yang P, Xie Y, Fei J. 2020. *Sensors Actuators B, Chem.* 305:127478
228. Varmira K, Mohammadi G, Mahmoudi M, Khodarahmi R, Rashidi K, et al. 2018. *Talanta.* 183:1–10
229. Xie Y, Yu Y, Lu L, Ma X, Gong L, et al. 2018. *J. Electroanal. Chem.* 812:82–89
230. Li J, Jiang J, Zhao D, Xu Z, Liu M, et al. 2018. *J. Alloys Compd.* 769:566–75
231. Sunil Kumar Naik TS, Saravanan S, Sri Saravana KN, Pratiush U, Ramamurthy PC. 2020. *Mater. Chem. Phys.* 245:122798
232. Wang L, Chen X, Liu C, Yang W. 2016. *Sensors Actuators, B Chem.* 233:199–205
233. Thivya P, Ramya R, Wilson J. 2020. *Microchem. J.* 157:105037
234. Chen TW, Chinnapaiyan S, Chen SM, Ali MA, Elshikh MS, Mahmoud AH. 2020. *Ultrason Sonochem.* 63:104903
235. Madhuvilakku R, Alagar S, Mariappan R, Piraman S. 2020. *Anal. Chim. Acta.* 1093:93–105
236. Meng T, Shang N, Nsabimana A, Ye H, Wang H, et al. 2020. *Anal. Chim. Acta.* 1138:59–68
237. Durai L, Kong CY, Badhulika S. 2020. *Mater. Sci. Eng. C.* 107:110217
238. Maduraiveeran G, Chen A. 2021. *Electrochim. Acta.* 368:137612
239. Song Y, Li W, Ma C, Sun Y, Qiao J, et al. 2020. *Sensors Actuators, B Chem.* 319:128311
240. Ehzari H, Amiri M, Safari M. 2020. *Talanta.* 210:120641
241. Luo Y, Wang Y, Yan H, Wu Y, Zhu C, et al. 2018. *Anal. Chim. Acta.* 1042:44–51
242. El-Wekil MM, Darweesh M, Shaykoon MSA, Ali R. 2020. *Talanta.* 217:121084
243. Liu L, Zhao H, Shi L, Lan M, Zhang H, Yu C. 2017. *Electrochim. Acta.* 227:69–76
244. Cui Y, Li J, Liu M, Tong H, Liu Z, et al. 2020. *Microchim. Acta.* 187(11):589 (1–11)
245. Willyam SJ, Saepudin E, Ivandini TA. 2020. *Anal. Methods.* 12(27):3454–61
246. Rajaji U, Selvi SV, Chen SM, Chinnapaiyan S, Chen TW, Govindasamy M. 2020. *Microchim. Acta.* 187(8):1–10
247. Rison S, Akshaya KB, Bhat VS, Shanker G, Maiyalagan T, et al. 2020. *MnO_2 Electroanalysis.* 32(10):2128–36
248. Manasa G, Raj C, Satpati AK, Mascarenhas RJ. 2020. *Electroanalysis.* 32(11):2431–41
249. Dodevska T, Shterev I. 2020. *Monatshefte fur Chemie.* 151(4):495–504
250. Zhu X, Zhao H, Shen J, Chen H, Cai X, et al. 2020. *Microchim. Acta.* 187(4):224 (1–8)
251. Mejri A, Mars A, Elfil H, Hamzaoui AH. 2019. *Microchim. Acta.* 186(11):1–9
252. Jiao J, Pan M, Liu X, Liu J, Li B, Chen Q. 2020. *Nanomaterials.* 10(3):499 (1–13)

253. Yao Y, Zhong J, Lu Z, Liu X, Wang Y, et al. 2019. *Microchim. Acta.* 186(12):795 (1–10)
254. Keerthi M, Boopathy G, Chen SM, Chen TW, Lou BS. 2019. *Sci. Rep.* 9(1):1–12
255. Soltani-Shahrivar M, Karimian N, Fakhri H, Hajian A, Afkhami A, Bagheri H. 2019. *Electroanalysis.* 31(12):2455–65
256. Deepika J, Sha R, Badhulika S. 2019. *Microchim. Acta.* 186(7):480–10
257. Du J, Tao Y, Zhang J, Xiong Z, Xie A, et al. 2019. *Mater. Technol.* 34(11):665–73
258. Tettamanti CS, Ramírez ML, Gutierrez FA, Bercoff PG, Rivas GA, Rodríguez MC. 2018. *Microchem. J.* 142:159–66
259. Ayyalusamy S, Mishra S, Suryanarayanan V. 2018. *Sci. Rep.* 8(1):1–9
260. Piovesan J V., Haddad VF, Pereira DF, Spinelli A. 2018. *J. Electroanal. Chem.* 823:617–23
261. Shadjou N, Hasanzadeh M, Talebi F. 2018. *J. Anal. Chem.* 73(6):602–12
262. Liu T, Fu B, Chen J, Yan Z, Li K. 2018. *Electrochim. Acta.* 269:136–43
263. Kaur B, Srivastava R, Satpati B. 2015. *RSC Adv.* 5(71):57657–65
264. Gao Z, Li Y, Zhang C, Zhang S, Jia Y, Dong Y. 2020. *Anal. Chim. Acta.* 1097:169–75
265. Alizadeh T, Nayeri S. 2020. *Anal. Bioanal. Chem.* 412(3):657–67
266. Mutharani B, Ranganathan P, Chen SM, Karuppiah C. 2019. *Microchim. Acta.* 186(3):167–11
267. Fu B, Chen H, Yan Z, Zhang Z, Chen J, et al. 2020. *J. Electroanal. Chem.* 866:1141165–67
268. Lin Y, Zhou Q, Lin Y, Lu M, Tang D. 2015. *Anal. Chim. Acta.* 887:67–74
269. Wang Z, Chen Y, Dong W, Zhou J, Han B, et al. 2018. *Biosens. Bioelectron.* 121:257–64
270. Huang P, Zhang B, Dang X, Chen H, Zheng D. 2020. *J. Electroanal. Chem.* 860:113890
271. Gao Z, Li Y, Zhang X, Feng J, Kong L, et al. 2018. *Biosens. Bioelectron.* 102:189–95
272. Li Y, Zhang Y, Li F, Feng J, Li M, et al. 2017. *Biosens. Bioelectron.* 92:33–39
273. Wang L, Miao L, Yang H, Yu J, Xie Y, et al. 2017. *Sensors Actuators B, Chem.* 253:108–14
274. Zhang Y, Li S, Liu H, Long W, Zhang XD. 2020. *Front. Chem.* 8:1–13

# 10 Nanozymes as Photothermal-Catalytic Agents

*Xianwen Wang[1,2]\*, Xiaoyan Zhong[3],*
*Haisheng Qian[2], and Zhengbao Zha[1]\**
[1]School of Food and Biological Engineering,
Hefei University of Technology, Hefei,
P. R. China
[2]School of Biomedical Engineering, Research
and Engineering Center of Biomedical Materials,
Anhui Medical University, Hefei, P. R. China
[3]Department of Toxicology, School of Public
Health, Jiangsu Key Laboratory of Preventive
and Translational Medicine for Geriatric Diseases,
Medical College of Soochow University, Suzhou,
P. R. China

## CONTENTS

---

\* Corresponding authors: Xianwen Wang and Zhengbao Zha

DOI: 10.1201/9781003109228-10

## 10.1  INTRODUCTION

Nanozymes can mimic the catalytic process of natural enzymes and regulate cell redox levels, especially reactive oxygen species (ROS) (1). ROS as intermediate products generated in the process of oxygen metabolism mainly include hydroxyl radical (•OH), superoxide anion (•$O_2^-$), and hydrogen peroxide ($H_2O_2$). Abnormally elevated levels of ROS can destroy the homeostasis of redox in the body and cause oxidative stress. Nanozymes with peroxidase (POD)-like or oxidase (OXD)-like activity can convert $H_2O_2$ or $O_2$ into high concentrations of ROS to kill tumor cells or bacteria, respectively, thereby obtaining good therapeutic effects (2). Although the generation of ROS by nanozymes is a promising strategy for the construction and preparation of antimicrobial agents/tumor therapeutic agents, nanozymes still have the problems of low therapeutic effects and potential side effects due to the high reactivity, limited diffusion distance, and lifetime of ROS in biological systems. In addition, the high expression of reductive glutathione (GSH) in tumors or infected sites would weaken the therapeutic effect of ROS generated by nanozymes with POD-like or superoxide dismutase (SOD)-like activity (3). Therefore, it is very important to further improve the catalytic efficiency of nanozymes (4).

The catalytic activity of nanozymes is proportional to the temperature according to the Arrhenius equation. Photothermal therapy (PTT) is a noninvasive therapy that employs photothermal reagents to convert NIR light energy into hyperthermia to kill tumor cells or bacteria (5). Therefore, the combination of PTT and nanozymes-based catalytic therapy can improve the ROS generation efficiency while reducing the indirect damage caused by PTT, thus achieving significant synergistic effects (6–8). Various types of nanozymes used in biomedical applications have been comprehensively reviewed (9–11). However, the use of nanozymes as photothermal-catalytic agents for tumor/antibacterial treatments has not yet been summarized. In this chapter, nanozymes as photothermal-catalytic agents for tumor/antibacterial therapy were systematically summarized. We start with a brief introduction of the mechanism of light-responsive nanozymes, especially the relationship between catalytic activity and photothermal performance. The synergistic effect of catalytic therapy based on the nanozymes and PTT in cancer/antibacterial therapy is emphatically discussed. The problems, challenges, and future perspectives of nanozymes as photothermal-catalytic agents for biomedical applications are also addressed.

## 10.2  NANOZYMES AS PHOTOTHERMAL-CATALYTIC AGENTS FOR CANCER/ANTIBACTERIAL THERAPY

Nanozymes as photothermal catalytic agents are mainly divided into the following categories based on different metal elements: 1) iron (Fe)-based nanozymes; 2) copper (Cu)-based nanozymes; 3) molybdenum (Mo)-based nanozymes; 4) tungsten (W)-based nanozymes; 5) cobalt/nickel/vanadium (Co/Ni/V)-based nanozymes; 6) multiple metals-based nanozymes; and 7) others. These nanozymes and their applications are summarized in **Table 10.1** and are discussed in more detail below.

## TABLE 10.1
## Nanozymes as Photothermal-Catalytic Agents for Cancer/Antibacterial Therapy

| Materials | Applications | Ref. |
|---|---|---|
| **Fe-Based Nanozymes** | | |
| $FeS_2$ | Cancer therapy/MRI | (12) |
| $Fe_2P$ | Cancer therapy, MRI, PA imaging | (13) |
| TOPY-PEG | Cancer therapy, MRI | (14) |
| $FePPOP_{BFPB}$ | Antibacterial therapy | (15) |
| $Fe_3O_4$-C | Antibacterial therapy | (16) |
| FeS | Antibacterial therapy | (17) |
| $Fe_3S_4$ | Cancer therapy, MRI | (18) |
| $FePS_3$ | Cancer therapy | (19) |
| $Fe_3O_4$@PPy@GOx | Cancer therapy, MRI, PA imaging | (20) |
| Fe-ABTS | Cancer therapy, PA imaging | (21) |
| **Cu-Based Nanozymes** | | |
| Hollow $Cu_2Se$ | Cancer therapy, PA imaging | (22) |
| $Cu_{2-x}Se$-GOx | Cancer therapy, imaging | (23) |
| $Cu_3P$ | Cancer therapy, MRI, PA imaging | (24) |
| $Cu_{2-x}Te$ | Cancer therapy | (22) |
| $Cu_{2-x}S$ | Cancer therapy, PA imaging | (25) |
| Cu-PTT | Cancer therapy | (26) |
| CuS/G5-GOx | Cancer therapy | (27) |
| BP@Cu@PEG-RGD | Cancer therapy, PET imaging | (28) |
| $SrCuSi_4O_{10}$ | Cancer therapy, PA imaging | (29) |
| Hollow $Cu_9S_8$ | Cancer therapy, PA imaging | (30) |
| $SiO_2$@CuO | Cancer therapy | (31) |
| Cu SASs/NPC | Antibacterial therapy | (32) |
| LS-CuS | Antibacterial therapy | (33) |
| $Cu_2MoS_4$ | Antibacterial therapy | (34) |
| **Mo-Based Nanozymes** | | |
| $MoS_2$ | Antibacterial therapy | (35) |
| $MoO_{3-x}$ | Antibacterial therapy | (36) |
| Mo-POM | Cancer therapy, PA imaging | (37) |
| $MoS_2$-hydrogel | Antibacterial therapy | (38) |
| 3D-$MoS_2$ | Cancer therapy | (39) |
| **W-Based Nanozymes** | | |
| $W_{18}O_{49}$ | Cancer therapy, PA imaging | (40) |
| $WO_{3-x}$@HA | Cancer therapy, PA imaging | (41) |
| $WO_{3-x}$@$\gamma$-PGA | Cancer therapy, PA imaging | (42) |
| $WS_2QDs$-Van@lipo | Antibacterial therapy | (43) |

(*Continued*)

**TABLE 10.1 (Continued)**

**Nanozymes as Photothermal-Catalytic Agents for Cancer/Antibacterial Therapy**

| Materials | Applications | Ref. |
|---|---|---|
| **Co/Ni/V-Based Nanozymes** | | |
| $CoS_2$ | Cancer therapy, PA imaging | (44) |
| $NiS_2$ | Antibacterial therapy | (45) |
| $TA@VO_x$ | Cancer therapy | (46) |
| $Ti_3C_2$/CoNWs | Antibacterial therapy | (47) |
| $Co_3O_4$ | Cancer therapy, MRI, PA imaging | (48) |
| **Multiple Metals-Based Nanozymes** | | |
| $MoSe_2$/$CoSe_2$ | Cancer therapy, MRI | (49) |
| $CuFe_2O_4$ | Antibacterial therapy | (50) |
| $Co_2Fe_{0.75}Mn_{0.25}S_6$ | Cancer therapy | (51) |
| $CuS$-$MnO_2$ | Cancer therapy, MRI | (52) |
| FePtMn-Ce6/FA | Cancer therapy, MRI, FL imaging | (53) |
| $FeO$/$MoS_2$ | Cancer therapy, MRI | (54) |
| W/Mo-POM | Antibacterial therapy | (55) |
| $Au@MnO_2$ | Cancer therapy, MRI, PA imaging | (56) |
| TRF-mCuGd | Cancer therapy, MRI | (57) |
| Fe-MoOx | Cancer therapy, MRI | (58) |
| ICG/CAC-LDH | Cancer therapy | (59) |
| **Other Nanozymes** | | |
| MnGdOP@PDA | Cancer therapy, MRI | (60) |
| $rGO@MnO_2$ | Cancer therapy, MRI | (61) |
| Au | Antibacterial therapy | (62) |
| C | Antibacterial therapy | (63) |

## 10.2.1 FE-BASED NANOZYMES

Fe-based nanozymes often exhibit POD-like catalytic activity, which can convert $H_2O_2$ into highly toxic •OH through Fenton reaction, which can effectively kill tumor cells or bacteria (37, 64, 65). Therefore, Fe-based nanozymes are the most common Fenton agents used for chemodynamic therapy (CDT) (66,67). For example, Tang *et al.* proposed a new tumor microenvironment (TME)-mediated POD-like nanozymes of antiferropyrite ($FeS_2$) nanocubes (NCBs), which used the excessively generated $H_2O_2$ in the tumors for self-enhanced magnetic resonance imaging (MRI) and PTT/CDT (**Figure 10.1a**) (12). $FeS_2$ NCBs could activate peroxides in the TME, which led to *in situ* surface oxidation, thereby producing lots of •OH to kill tumor cells. The increase of surface Fe valence significantly promoted the MRI manifestations with CDT. In addition, the local hyperthermia of PTT could accelerate the Fenton process in tumors and realize a synergistic PTT/CDT. This was the first time to use the pyrite-based TME-response price variable strategy to develop collaborative

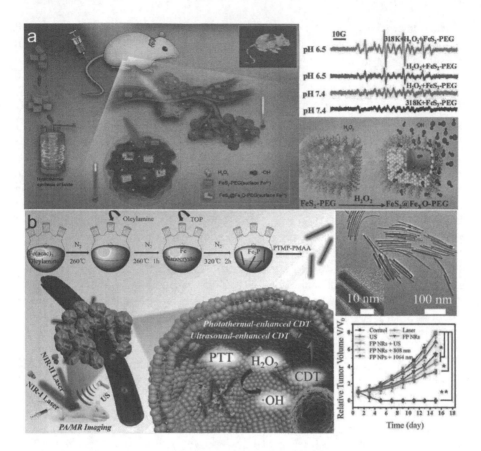

**FIGURE 10.1** Fe-based nanozymes for cancer therapy. (a) $FeS_2$ NCs were prepared for self-enhanced MRI and combined PTT/CDT (12). (b) 1D $Fe_2P$ NRs with ultrasound/NIR light-enhanced Fenton effects and satisfactory PTCE were synthesized for combined PTT-CDT of cancer, obtaining remarkable therapeutic effect (13). Adapted from (12) with permission from Wiley-VCH, copyright 2017; adapted from (13) with permission from Wiley-VCH, copyright 2018.

nano-cancer prevention research, which would open up new dimensions for the design of other TME-based anti-cancer strategies.

The strict reaction conditions (pH: 3–5) of POD-like nanozymes impede its application in tumor treatment. Thus, how to enhance the Fenton or Fenton-like reaction efficiency of nanozymes at tumor sites has always been a major obstacle to CDT (68). To this end, Zhang *et al.* successfully prepared biocompatible $Fe_2P$ nanorods (NRs) with the ultrasound/NIR light-enhanced Fenton effect and satisfactory photothermal conversion efficiency (PTCE, 56.6%), obtaining a remarkable therapeutic effect (**Figure 10.1b**) (13). More importantly, $Fe_2P$ NRs acted as POD-like nanozymes, which could produce a large amount of •OH in the presence of $H_2O_2$, the ultrasound and mild photothermal effect could further improve the catalytic performance of $Fe_2P$ NRs. In addition, the strong traverse relaxivity and high photothermal conversion efficiency (PTCE) of $Fe_2P$ NRs meant that they were excellent MRI and photoacoustic (PA) imaging agents. This was the first report on the use of metal phosphides to respond to second NIR (NIR-II) laser and ultrasound to enhance the CDT effect with satisfactory therapeutic efficiency.

The Z-type heterojunction with high separation efficiency of electron ($e^-$)-hole ($h^+$) pair and enhanced redox potential shows a great potential in the photonic theory, but it has not yet been explored and challenged. Recently, Pan *et al.* successfully prepared a new type of two-dimensional (2D) thermally oxidized pyrite nanosheets (TOPY NSs) with $FeS_2$ core and iron oxide ($Fe_2O_3$) shell for combined photothermal-photodynamic-chemodynamic therapy (PTT-PDT-CDT) of tumors (14). Both the $Fe_2O_3$ shell and $Fe^{3+}/Fe^{2+}$ inside TOPY NSs could respond to TME by consuming GSH and producing $O_2$ and •OH through Fenton reaction. The production of •OH from $OH^-$ and •$O_2$ from $O_2$ on the valence band of $Fe_2O_3$ and conduction band of $FeS_2$, respectively, was significantly improved under 650 nm irradiation. Moreover, TOPY NSs could act as photothermal nanomaterials for PTT to produce local hyperthermia, which enhanced the therapeutic efficacy of POD-like nanozymes. Thus, such unprecedented nanocomposites with Z-scheme heterojunctions successfully integrated PTT/PDT/CDT with multiple imaging functions, opening up a new way for tumor treatment with the good therapeutic performance and low side effects.

Bacterial infections pose a major threat to human health, mainly owing to the evolution of mutant strains that are resistant to antibiotic therapy. As a feasible alternative, Fe-based nanozymes have become attractive antibacterial agents (69). Recently, Agnihotri *et al.* reported that iron sulfide (FeS) nanoparticles (NPs) have excellent photothermal performance and POD-like catalytic activity for efficient antibacterial treatment (**Figure 10.2a**) (17). The time-dependent release of $Fe^{2+}$ ions was observed from these FeS NPs. Their dual-mode antibacterial effects were observed in both Gram-negative and Gram-positive bacterial strains due to the high concentration of ROS and light-induced heat based on FeS NPs. The photothermal performance of FeS NPs could further enhance their catalytic activity, leading to the gradual increase of ROS content inside bacteria, which is considered the main antibacterial mechanism. The results showed that FeS NPs are powerful antibacterial agents that could be used to replace traditional antibiotic-based antibacterial strategies.

Nanozymes with more active defect-rich edge sites and a rough surface can trap bacteria, showing higher bacteria binding ability and improving antibacterial activity (70). For instance, Liu *et al.* successfully prepared carbon-iron oxide nano-hybrid with rough surface (rough C-$Fe_3O_4$, RCF) for NIR-II photo-responsive synergistic antibacterial treatment (**Figure 10.2b**) (16). RCF with good photothermal effect and POD-like activity could achieve synergistic PTT/CDT in the NIR-II biological window. More interestingly, RCF with a rough surface showed enhanced bacterial adhesion, thereby benefiting PTT and CDT via effective interaction between bacteria and RCF. *In vitro* antibacterial experiments showed that RCF had a broad-spectrum synergistic antibacterial performance on different types of bacteria. It is worth noting that the rat wound model with methicillin-resistant *Staphylococcus aureus* (MRSA) infection also achieved synergistic antibacterial activity *in vivo*. This work proposed a simple strategy for constructing antibacterial agents for practical antimicrobial applications by rationally designing morphology and composition. RCF

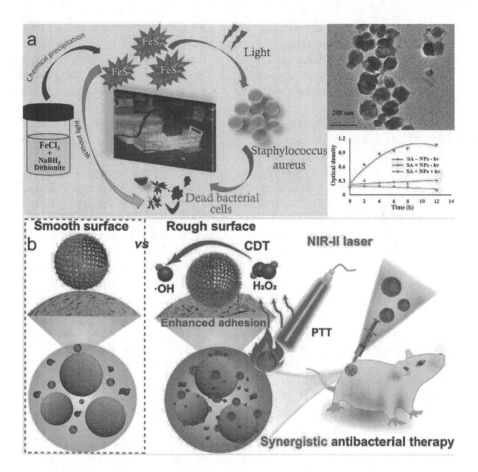

**FIGURE 10.2** Fe-based nanozymes for antibacterial therapy. (a) FeS NPs with excellent photothermal performance and POD-like catalytic activity were synthesized for efficient antibacterial treatment (17). (b) Carbon-iron oxide nano-hybrids with RCF were fabricated for NIR-II photo-responsive synergistic antibacterial therapy (16). Adapted from (17) with permission from American Chemical Society, copyright 2020; adapted from (16) with permission from American Chemical Society, copyright 2021.

with good photothermal effect and POD-like catalytic activity had huge potential in the effective treatment of multidrug resistance (MDR) bacterial infections. Thus, Fe-based nanozymes are currently the most extensively studied nanozymes, showing strong catalytic activity. The combination of catalytic therapy and PTT based on the Fe-based nanozymes can produce a significant synergistic effect and have broad application potential in tumor therapy and antibacterial therapy.

## 10.2.2 Cu-Based Nanozymes

Cu-based nanomaterials not only possess excellent photothermal property (71) but also undergo a Fenton-like reaction in a wide pH range, showing catalytic effects similar to Fe-based nanozymes. $Cu^+$ can effectively catalyze $H_2O_2$ to generate •OH, and its catalytic efficiency ($1 \times 10^4$ $M^{-1}s^{-1}$) is significantly stronger than $Fe^{2+}$ (76 M $M^{-1}s^{-1}$) (72). Therefore, the use of Cu-based nanozymes for biomedical applications has received extensive attention (62). For example, Wu *et al.* reported the intrinsic ability of Cu-based nanozymes to catalyze the generation of OH from $H_2O_2$ in a wide pH range, and its performance was comparable to or even better than most Fe-based nanozymes (25). In particular, ultra-small PEGylated $Cu_{2-x}S$ ($Cu_{2-x}S$-PEG) nanodots (~5 nm) were prepared, which could be used as POD-like nanozymes for combined PTT-CDT against cancer (**Figure 10.3a**). More importantly, $Cu_{2-x}S$-PEG nanodots could be used for PA imaging and PTT in the NIR-II biological window due to its excellent NIR-II absorption and photothermal performance. Both *in vitro* and *in vivo* experiments systematically proved the high efficacy of PTT-CDT based on $Cu_{2-x}S$-PEG nanodots. This work not only reported the use of Cu-based nanomaterials for combined PTT-CDT but also enriched new nano-catalysts based on the Fenton-like reaction for catalytic tumor therapy. Compared with other Cu-based nanomaterials, copper selenides ($Cu_2Se$) are very promising not only because they possess similar NIR absorption and excellent photothermal effect but also since Se and Cu are crucial trace elements in the human body (73). To this end, Wang *et al.* synthesized $Cu_2Se$ hollow nanocubes (HNCBs) with good POD-like catalytic performance and excellent NIR-II absorbance for photothermal-enhanced CDT against cancer (**Figure 10.3b**) (22). $Cu_2Se$ HNCBs were successfully prepared using $Cu_2O$ NCBs as templates by the sacrificial template method. During the conversion of $Cu_2O$ NCBs to $Cu_2Se$ HNCBs, the NIR-II absorption of the samples gradually increased, while the Fenton-like catalytic properties gradually decreased. The optimal reaction time selected in the experiment was 1.5 h to obtain $Cu_2Se$ HNCBs with strong Fenton-like catalytic property and good photothermal performance. The obtained PEG-$Cu_2Se$ HNCBs modified by sulfhydryl polyethylene glycol (SH-PEG) had satisfactory physiological stability. *In vitro* and *in vivo* experiments displayed that PEG-$Cu_2Se$ HNCBs generated lots of •OH through the Fenton-like reaction, thereby effectively destroying cancer cells and tumor tissues. The gentle photothermal performance produced by PEG-$Cu_2Se$ HNCBs under 1064-nm laser irradiation further accelerated the catalytic rate of the Fenton-like reaction, which significantly improved the efficiency of tumor treatment. Cancer cells and tumor tissues were completely eradicated under laser irradiation by combining PTT and CDT *in vitro* and *in vivo*.

The kinetics of the Fenton or Fenton-like reaction has a significant impact on the therapeutic effect of cancer. It is important to improve the reaction kinetics at the maximum concentration of $H_2O_2$ to rapidly produce a large amount of ROS to achieve a satisfactory therapeutic effect. Therefore, the combination of PTT, CDT, and starvation therapy can obtain significant synergistic effects. For example, Wang *et al.* prepared biomimetic nano-catalysts (CS-GOx@CM) for synergistic PTT-CDT-starvation therapy by combining the tumor cell membrane (CM), ultra-small $Cu_{2-x}Se$ (CS) NPs, and glucose oxidase (GOx) (**Figure 10.3c**) (23).

CS NPs with strong NIR-II absorbance were coupled with GOx to effectively convert glucose *in situ* to increase the concentration of $H_2O_2$ to promote the Fenton-like reaction, and then the NPs were coated with cancer CM to enhance their accumulation and retention at the tumor sites. The experimental results revealed that the obtained CS-GOx@CM NPs triggered the cascade reaction *in vitro* and *in vivo*, and

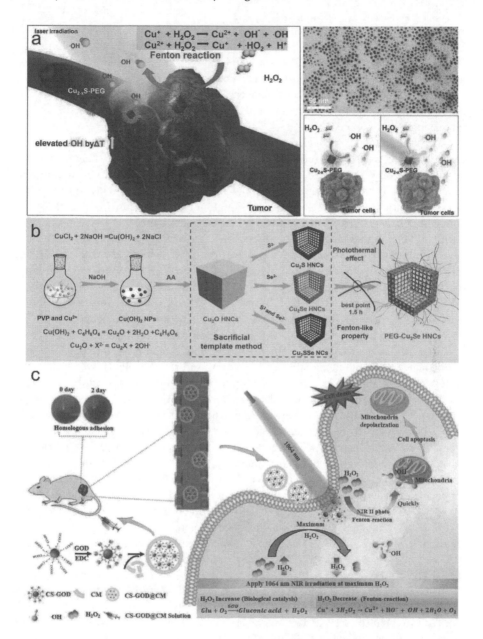

**FIGURE 10.3** Cu-based nanozymes for cancer therapy. (a) Ultra-small $Cu_{2-x}$S-PEG nanodots (25). (b) $Cu_2$Se HNCBs (22). (c) $Cu_{2-x}$Se-GOx@CM NPs were reported for combined PTT-CDT of cancer.(23). Adapted from (25) with permission from Elsevier, copyright 2019; adapted from Ref. (22) with permission from American Chemical Society, copyright 2019; adapted from (23) with permission from Wiley-VCH, copyright 2020.

converted glucose into $H_2O_2$ and gluconic acid, thereby significantly increasing the Fenton-like reaction rate of CS NPs. CS-GOx@CM NPs could further enhance the Fenton-like catalytic rate of CS NPs under 1064-nm laser irradiation, which could generate a large amount of •OH and other types of ROS in a short time, thus obtaining an excellent therapeutic effect of cancer. This work guided the rational design of high-performance biomimetic nano-catalysts for PTT-CDT from the perspective of increasing reaction kinetics.

Cu-based nanozymes are also used significantly in antibacterial therapy (74). For example, Xie *et al.* synthesized lignosulfonate lignin-copper sulfide (LS-CuS) nanocomposites using lignin (LS) as growth templates and stabilizers, which could be used as a new type of antibacterial agent (**Figure 10.4a**) (33). Owing to the monodispersed CuS NPs in the three-dimensional network structure of LS, LS-CuS nanocomposites exhibited stronger photothermal effect and POD-like activity than pure CuS NPs. In addition, the local heat produced by PTT further enhanced the POD-like activity of nanozymes, thereby effectively destroying bacteria through PTT-CDT, which provided a promising strategy to kill MDR bacteria. Finally, the LS-CuS nanocomposites were incorporated into the waterborne polyurethane (WPU) film. Owing to the uniform dispersion of LS-CuS nanocomposite in WPU film, the bactericidal effect of LS-CuS@WPU composite film reached more than 90%, which had huge potential for WPU-based antibacterial coatings.

Due to the recent huge achievements in the field of catalysis, the high catalytic performance of single-atom catalysts has been used in other fields, where the separated metal atoms are located on the support (75). Single-atom catalysts exhibit good catalytic activity and can make maximum use of metals, which is particularly vital for antibacterial/cancer treatment to obtain effective disease treatment with relatively low metal concentrations (76). Very recently, our group reported Cu single-atom sites/N-doped porous carbon (Cu SASs/NPC) prepared by fabricated through the pyrolysis-etching-adsorption-pyrolysis strategy for photothermal-catalytic antibacterial therapy (**Figure 10.4b**) (32). Cu SASs/NPC exhibited a stronger photothermal effect, catalytic activity, and GSH-depleting function compared with NPC. Interestingly, Cu SASs/NPC could act as POD-like nanozymes to effectively catalyze $H_2O_2$ to generate •OH, thereby killing different types of bacteria. The good photothermal performance remarkably enhanced the POD-like catalytic activity of Cu SASs/NPC, thereby producing more ROS and obtaining better antibacterial properties *in vitro*. More importantly, *in vivo* experiments exhibited that Cu SASs/NPC could effectively destroy internal bacterial infections spread by MRSA pathogens on wounds, which achieved better wound healing. In general, this work highlighted the satisfactory antibacterial effect of Cu SASs/NPC, and further expanded the bioapplications of Cu SASs.

Cu-based nanomaterials have unparalleled enzyme-like catalytic properties and versatility and are peculiarly attractive in the therapy of bacterial infections, especially against MDR bacteria. However, their inherent unsatisfactory catalytic activity greatly limits their antibacterial properties. To solve related problems, Shan *et al.* successfully developed new NIR-II light-responsive nanozymes ($Cu_2MoS_4$ nanoplates) to effectively eradicate MDR bacteria (**Figure 10.4c**) (34). $Cu_2MoS_4$ nanoplates exhibited inherent dual enzyme-like properties, which could generate

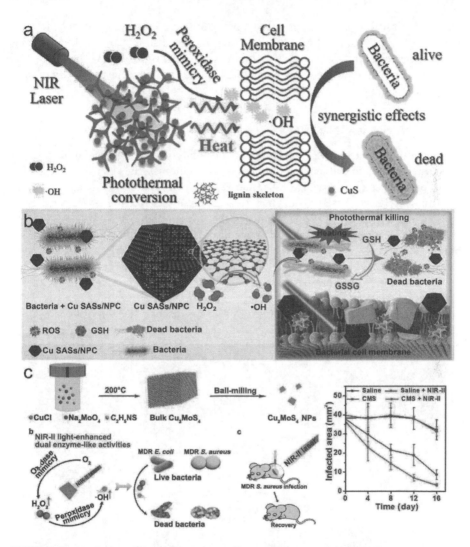

**FIGURE 10.4** Cu-based nanozymes for antibacterial therapy. (a) LS-CuS nanocomposites (33). (b) Cu SASs/NPC was synthesized for photothermal-catalytic antibacterial therapy (32). (c) $Cu_2MoS_4$ nanoplates with NIR-II light-enhanced dual enzyme-like activities were prepared to effectively eradicate MDR bacteria (34). Adapted from (33) with permission from American Chemical Society, copyright 2021; adapted from (32) with permission from Elsevier, copyright 2021; adapted from (34) with permission from Wiley-VCH, copyright 2020.

ROS by Fenton-like reaction. Importantly, $Cu_2MoS_4$ nanoplates possessed NIR-II light-enhanced OXD and POD-like catalytic activity to increase the production of ROS, thereby effectively killing bacteria. Moreover, $Cu_2MoS_4$ nanoplates exhibited good therapeutic performance of MDR *S. aureus* infection *in vivo* as well as negligible toxicity to cells and mice, showing that they had potential antibacterial applications. These results proved that a combination of the catalytic treatment and

PTT of $Cu_2MoS_4$ nanozymes provided a new antibacterial strategy for the effective therapy of MDR bacterial-related infections. In short, most Cu-based nanozymes with strong catalytic activity and photothermal performance have been used as photothermal-catalytic agents for biomedical applications, especially for tumor/antimicrobial therapy.

### 10.2.3 MO-BASED NANOZYMES

Using Mo-based nanomaterials to simulate the catalytic function of natural enzymes is an interesting and challenging task. Mo-based nanomaterials can simulate a variety of enzyme activities, such as OXD and POD. However, it is still a huge challenge to manufacture Mo-based nanozymes that accurately perform enzyme activity in TME without causing off-target toxicity to the surrounding normal tissues (77). For this reason, Ling *et al.* successfully synthesized biodegradable molybdenum oxide nano-bulbs ($MoO_{3-x}$ NUs) with good enzymatic activity, which selectively performed therapeutic activity in the TME through a cascade of catalytic reactions, while maintaining normal tissues harmless due to the responsive biodegradation of $MoO_{3-x}$ NUs in the physiological environment (**Figure 10.5a**) (78). Specifically, $MoO_{3-x}$ NUs firstly induced catalase (CAT)-type reactive decomposition of $H_2O_2$

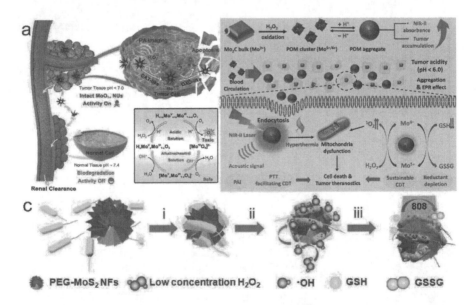

**FIGURE 10.5** Mo-based nanozymes for cancer/antibacterial therapy. (a) Biodegradable $MoO_{3-x}$ NUs with good enzymatic activity were constructed for catalytic therapy against cancer (78). (b) Mo-POM was reported as Fenton-like and photothermal agents for combined PTT-CDT of tumors (37). (c) PEG-$MoS_2$ nanoflowers were reported as biocompatible antibacterial agents for convenient, rapid, and effective wound disinfection (35). Adapted from (78) with permission from American Chemical Society, copyright 2020; adapted from (37) with permission from Wiley-VCH, copyright 2019; adapted from (35) with permission from American Chemical Society, copyright 2016.

in the TME, generating a large amount of $O_2$ for subsequent OXD-type reactivity of $MoO_{3-x}$ NUs, then, lots of cytotoxic $\bullet O_2^-$ were produced for cancer cell apoptosis. Interestingly, once exposed to normal tissues or neutral blood, $MoO_{3-x}$ NUs could quickly lose enzyme activity through pH-responsive biodegradation, and then removed from the body through urine, thereby ultimately ensuring safety. The current study demonstrated the concept of biodegradation *in vivo* catalytic activity tunable nanozymes for cancer-specific cascade catalytic treatment with minimal off-target toxicity.

On the strength of Mo (V)-induced internal charge transfer under NIR laser irradiation and their tunable electronic structure, Mo-based nanostructures are very sensitive to redox and pH conditions, providing a promising method for the combination of PTT/CDT (79). For example, $Mo_2C$-derived polyoxometalate (Mo-POM) was reported as Fenton-like agents and photothermal nanomaterials for combined PTT-CDT of tumors (**Figure 10.5b**) (37). Mo-POM exhibited good optical absorption in the NIR II region and POD-like catalytic activity. POM aggregated in the acidic TME could achieve specific tumor targeting. In addition to the powerful ability of Mo-POM to produce $^1O_2$ through the Russell mechanism, and excellent photothermal performance of Mo-POM enhanced their CDT effect, provided additional tumor ablation methods, and allowed NIR-II PA imaging. Thanks to the reversible redox properties of Mo, POM-based therapies could evade the antioxidant defense system. In addition, combined with the specific response to TME and local laser irradiation, side effects would be avoided to a large extent.

Infections caused by MDR bacteria are still a serious threat to human health. It is of great significance to explore effective alternative antibacterial methods. For example, Zhao *et al.* successfully prepared PEG-functionalized $MoS_2$ (PEG-$MoS_2$) nanoflowers, which could be used as biocompatible antibacterial agents for rapid, convenient, and effective wound disinfection (**Figure 10.5c**) (35). PEG-$MoS_2$ nanoflowers exhibited strong POD-like activity and NIR absorption, which could effectively catalyze the decomposition of $H_2O_2$ to generate $\bullet OH$. A mechanism based on the exogenous $\bullet OH$-enhanced PTT against bacteria was proposed. First, the bacteria were exposed to PEG-$MoS_2$ nanoflowers before adding $H_2O_2$. PEG-$MoS_2$ nanoflowers captured by bacteria not only greatly reduced the concentration of $H_2O_2$ but also effectively catalyzed the decomposition of $H_2O_2$ to generate $\bullet OH$. Then, the exogenous $\bullet OH$ interacted with the bacteria, which caused membrane stress and destroyed the cell wall to damage the integrity of the membrane, thereby making the bacteria more vulnerable to heat. PEG-$MoS_2$ nanoflowers could generate overheating under 808 nm laser irradiation, which further increased the catalytic rate of PEG-$MoS_2$ nanozymes. The combination of catalytic therapy and PTT provided rapid and significant antibacterial effects for skin wounds. Importantly, PEG-$MoS_2$ nanoflowers effectively consumed GSH, which destroyed the intercellular protective system of bacteria, thereby effectively improving the antibacterial efficiency.

## 10.2.4  W-BASED NANOZYMES

W-based nanozymes have shown good POD-like or OXD-like catalytic activity due to the existence of different valence states of W (80). Among them, tungsten oxide

(WO$_{3-x}$) has excellent local surface plasmon resonance absorption capacity and the resulting significant photothermal conversion performance (81). In addition, WO$_{3-x}$ is a common type of photocatalyst used to degrade organic dyes, indicating that it has great application potential as Fenton-like agents for CDT due to the co-existence of W$^{6+}$ and W$^{5+}$ valence states in WO$_{3-x}$ (82). For example, Yang et al. successfully synthesized ultra-small WO$_{3-x}$@γ-poly-L-glutamic acid (WO$_{3-x}$@γ-PGA) NPs with excellent photothermal effect and catalytic activity for combined PTT-CDT of cancer (42). Interestingly, WO$_{3-x}$@γ-PGA NPs could act as POD-like nanozymes to generate a large amount of •OH in the presence of H$_2$O$_2$ through Fenton-like reaction, thus giving WO$_{3-x}$@γ-PGA NPs excellent catalytic performance. The mild photothermal effect came from WO$_{3-x}$@γ-PGA NPs which could further enhance its catalytic performance. More importantly, in vitro and in vivo experiments showed that the synergistic therapeutic effect of PTT-CDT based on WO$_{3-x}$@γ-PGA NPs was far superior to that of CDT or PTT alone. Therefore, this work extended the application of W-based nanozymes in tumor treatment. Similarly, Yang et al. prepared W$_{18}$O$_{49}$ NRs by a one-step pyrolysis method, which has strong NIR absorption capacity and excellent Fenton-like reaction performance and explored their use in combined PTT-CDT of cancer under the guidance of PA imaging (40). This study provided low-cost and easily prepared therapeutic agents (W$_{18}$O$_{49}$ NRs) for combined PTT-CDT.

Targeted PTT-CDT can further improve the treatment efficiency of tumors while reducing their damage to normal tissues (83). To this end, Ding et al. prepared multifunctional WO$_{3-x}$ theranostic agents to realize the combined PTT-PDT-CDT guided by NIR-II PA imaging (**Figure 10.6a**) (41). During the preparation process, oxygen vacancies were formed in WO$_{3-x}$, which narrowed the bandgap and enabled WO$_{3-x}$ NPs to have good optical absorption in the full spectrum range. The surface of WO$_{3-x}$ NPs was modified by hyaluronic acid (HA) to enhance physiologic dispersibility and tumor targeting efficiency. After activation by NIR-II irradiation, WO$_{3-x}$@HA NPs possessed excellent PTCE, ROS generation, and PA imaging capabilities under NIR laser irradiation. Meanwhile, WO$_{3-x}$@HA NPs also showed good Fenton-like catalytic rate and GSH depletion performance. The effective photothermal performance of WO$_{3-x}$@HA NPs accelerated the Fenton-like process, thereby achieving enhanced PTT/PDT/CDT. The formation of oxygen vacancies was found to be the key to the catalytic, photodynamic, and photothermal properties of WO$_{3-x}$@HA NPs, and the corresponding possible mechanism was proposed. In vitro and in vivo experiments proved that WO$_{3-x}$@HA NPs achieved highly efficient synergistic treatment by combing PTT, PDT, and CDT under the guidance of real-time NIR-II PA imaging.

The high concentration of GSH in the infected tissues severely limits the catalytic performance of nanozymes (84). To this end, Xu et al. reported a smart antibacterial nano-platform (WS$_2$ QDs-Van@lipo) based on the encapsulating tungsten sulfide quantum dots (WS$_2$ QDs) and antibiotic vancomycin in thermosensitive liposomes (Van@lipo) for efficient antibacterial through PTT-CDT-chemotherapy (**Figure 10.6b**) (43). The system used the photothermal sensitivity of WS$_2$ QDs to achieve selective liposome rupture for targeted drug delivery. WS$_2$ QDs showed strong POD-like and OXD-like activity under physiological conditions, which could oxidize GSH to further enhance CDT efficacy. In addition, it was found that the mild photothermal effect generated by PTT promoted multiple enzyme-mimicking

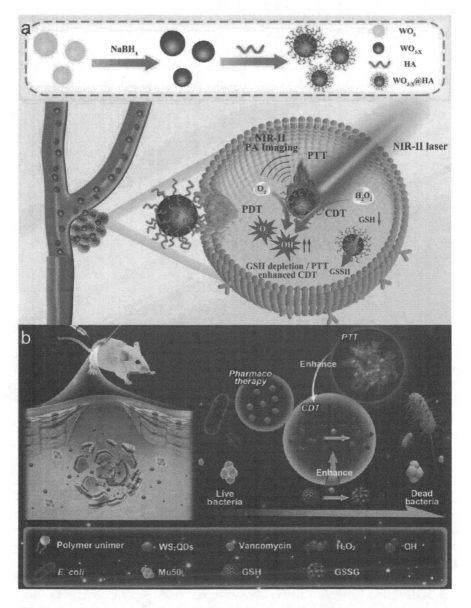

**FIGURE 10.6** W-based nanozymes for cancer/antibacterial therapy. (a) $WO_{3-x}$ NPs were fabricated to realize the combined PTT-PDT-CDT guided by PA imaging (41). (b) A smart antibacterial nano-platform ($WS_2QDs$-Van@lipo) based on encapsulating $WS_2$ QDs and antibiotic vancomycin in thermosensitive liposomes were successfully synthesized for efficient antibacterial through PTT-CDT-chemotherapy (43). Adapted from (41) with permission from Royal Society of Chemistry, copyright 2021; adapted from (43) with permission from American Chemical Society, copyright 2020.

activities of WS$_2$ QDs. WS$_2$QDs-Van@lipo exerted antibacterial effects on Gram-positive Mu50 and Gram-negative *E. coli*, and destroyed the biofilm, thereby increasing the permeability of the therapeutic agent inside the biofilm. *In vivo* studies on mice with skin abscesses caused by Mu50 showed that WS$_2$QDs-Van@lipo could provide effective antibacterial activity without significant toxicity. Taken together, the antibacterial platform enabled NIR light-mediated drug release to support synergistic PTT-PDT-chemotherapy, thereby elucidating a new strategy for antibacterial therapy.

## 10.2.5   Co/Ni/V-Based Nanozymes

Co/Ni/V-based nanozymes usually exhibit catalytic activity similar to that of Fe-based nanozymes and are also widely used in tumor/antibacterial treatments (74). Among them, Co-based nanozymes have also been reported for combined PTT catalytic therapy against cancer in recent years (48, 85). For example, our research group successfully prepared monodisperse cobalt disulfide nanoclusters (CoS$_2$ NCs) for combined PTT-CDT against cancer (**Figure 10.7a**) (44). In the presence of suitable solvents and surfactants, monodisperse CoS$_2$ NCs were formed through the oligomerization of ultra-small nanocrystals by the La Mer scheme. The obtained CoS$_2$ NCs showed good catalytic performance, satisfactory NIR absorption, high PTCE, and achieved photothermal-enhanced CDT both *in vitro* and *in vivo*. Interestingly, CoS$_2$ NCs decomposed into small particles, most of which were easily oxidized, gradually turning them into ions, and then rapidly excreted via feces and urine by the reticuloendothelial system. In addition, no obvious toxicity of these NCs was found, indicating that CoS$_2$ NCs possessed excellent biosafety. Therefore, our work emphasized a powerful theranostic agent (CoS$_2$ NCs) to achieve high-efficiency, low-toxicity cancer therapy by combing PTT and CDT.

Ni-based nanomaterials are extensively used in biomedicine due to their excellent biocompatibility, outstanding photothermal effect, and biodegradability (86, 87). It is worth noting that Ni-based nanomaterials are excellent nanozymes similar to POD, which can detect glucose and H$_2$O$_2$ by colorimetry (88). Ni-based nanomaterials with POD-like catalytic activity and photothermal performance can be used for antibacterial treatment (45). For instance, our group prepared monodisperse nickel disulfide (NiS$_2$) nanozymes for PTT-catalytic antibacterial treatment by a simple solvothermal method (**Figure 10.7b**) (45). The obtained NiS$_2$ nanozymes have excellent NIR absorption, high PTCE (43.8%), and satisfactory hydrogen peroxide (HRP)-like catalytic activity. The as-prepared NiS$_2$ nanozymes could generate •OH through a Fenton-like reaction in the presence of H$_2$O$_2$. Moreover, a mild photothermal effect could improve the catalytic activity of NiS$_2$ nanozymes, thereby achieving the results of photothermal-enhanced catalytic antibacterial treatment. Interestingly, NiS$_2$ nanozymes could also act as another nanozyme (glutathione peroxidase, GPx), which accelerated the consumption of GSH, thereby enhancing the bactericidal effect. More importantly, the experimental results of wound healing exhibited that the synergistic antibacterial nano-platform could be easily used for wound disinfection. Most importantly, NiS$_2$ nanozymes are biodegradable, which could be quickly excreted from the body through feces and urine, without causing

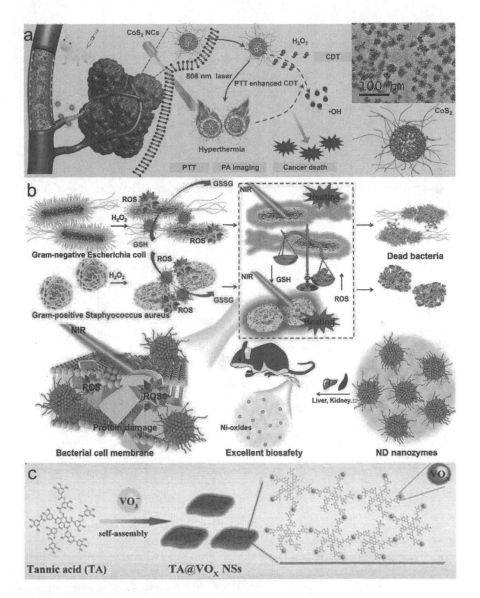

**FIGURE 10.7** Co/Ni/V-based nanozymes for cancer/antibacterial therapy. (a) Bio-degradable CoS$_2$ nanoclusters were designed for combined PTT-CDT against cancer (44). (b) Monodisperse NiS$_2$ nanozymes were prepared for PTT-catalytic antibacterial treatment by a simple solvothermal method (45). (c) TA@VO$_x$ NSs were fabricated for combined PTT-CDT of cancer (46). Adapted from (44) with permission from Elsevier, copyright 2020; adapted from (45) with permission from Elsevier, copyright 2020; adapted from (46) with permission from Wiley-VCH, copyright 2020.

any obvious toxicity through systematic evaluation. In general, $NiS_2$ nanozymes as multifunctional antibacterial agents had broad prospects in biomedicine.

V-based nanozymes also showed satisfactory POD-like and OXD-like catalytic activity (89), but the selection of suitable V-based nanozymes with easy synthesis, multifunction, tumor specificity, and good therapeutic properties is of significance for cancer therapy (90). For example, Jiang *et al.* successfully prepared a new type of natural polyphenol tannic acid (TA) hybrid with mixed-valence vanadium oxide nanosheets ($TA@VO_x$ NSs) for combined PTT-CDT of cancer (**Figure 10.7c**) (46). In this system, $VO_x$ was assembled with TA through the coordination inter- action of metal phenols, and the reduction of vanadium from $V^{5+}$ to $V^{4+}$ partially introduced high NIR absorption and POD-like activity. The existence of mixed- valence vanadium oxides in $TA@VO_x$ NSs was proved to be the key for the catalytic reaction of $H_2O_2$ to •OH. Thanks to the POD-like activity of $TA@VO_x$ NSs, the overproduction of $H_2O_2$ in the TME could achieve tumor-specific CDT. As an effective supplement to CDT, NIR absorption enabled $TA@VO_x$ NSs to have NIR light-mediated conversion capabilities for PTT of cancer. In addition, *in vitro,* and *in vivo* experiments proved that $TA@VO_x$ NSs could effectively inhibit tumor growth by synergistic CDT/PTT. These results provided a promising way to develop novel V-based nanozymes for enhanced synergistic cancer-specific treatments. Thus, Co/ Ni/V-based nanozymes have been reported for PTT-catalytic therapy owing to their strong photothermal performance and good catalytic effect.

## 10.2.6 MULTIPLE METALS-BASED NANOZYMES

In general, nanozymes containing multiple metals can produce better catalytic effects due to the synergy of different elements. In addition, due to the presence of different elements, this type of nanozymes can also exhibit other excellent physico- chemical properties (55). With the complicated internal environment of solid tumors and bacteria, the more functional metallic elements in the nanozymes, the more intelligent roles in modulating $H_2O_2$ and GSH for ideal anti-tumor/anti-bacterial effects. In various multimetal nanozymes, CoFeMn dichalcogenide, which was $Co_2Fe_{0.75}Mn_{0.25}S_6$ nanosheets (CFMS NSs) were reported as effective nanozymes for synergetic PTT-CDT of tumors (**Figure 10.8a**) (51). In this study, CFMS NSs were obtained by vulcanizing a lamellar CoFeMn-layered double hydroxide. After polyvinyl pyrrolidone (PVP) covering, CFMS-PVP NSs showed enhanced disper- sion stability and biocompatibility. To maximize the photothermal performance, the ratio of Co, Fe, and Mn ions was optimized. It was revealed that $Co_2Fe_{0.75}Mn_{0.25}S_6$- PVP had the greatest absorbance at 808 nm and possessed the best photothermal performance under laser irradiation (808 nm, 1.0 $Wcm^{-2}$), with a PTCE value of 89.0%, the highest PTCE among the 2-D transition metal dichalcogenides materi- als. Besides the outstanding photothermal ability, due to the existence of Fenton and Fenton-like element Fe and Co, CFMS-PVP NSs could be used for CDT by generating •OH upon adding $H_2O_2$ in the weak acidic condition of pH 6.5. By cal- culating the reduced Michaelis-Menten constant ($K_m$) from $0.46 \times 10^{-3}$ M to $0.26 \times 10^{-3}$ M, and increased maximum reaction velocity ($V_{max}$) from $2.74 \times 10^{-8}$ M $s^{-1}$ to $3.77 \times 10^{-8}$ M $s^{-1}$, after applying laser, it was confirmed that heat could accelerate

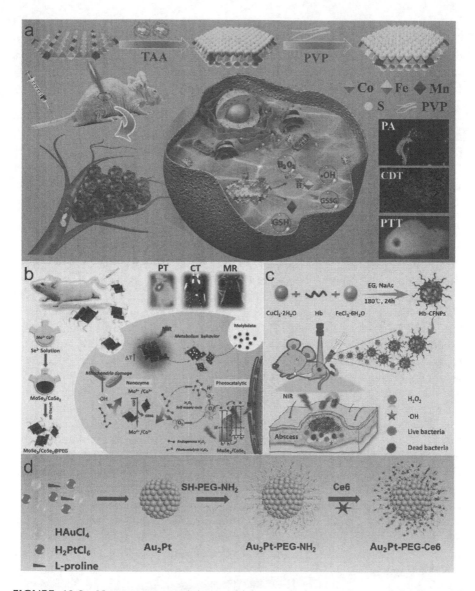

**FIGURE 10.8** Nanozymes containing multiple metal elements for cancer/antibacterial therapy. (a) $Co_2Fe_{0.75}Mn_{0.25}S_6$ nanosheets were reported as effective nanozymes with POD-like activity for PTT-CDT of tumors.(51). (b) $MoSe_2/CoSe_2$@PEG NSs were designed for in-situ $H_2O_2$ production enhanced PTT/CDT of cancer.(49). (c) Hb-CFNPs were synthesized as photothermal/Fenton agents for antimicrobial treatment (50). (d) $Au_2Pt$-PEG-Ce6 nanocomposites were designed for synergistic PTT/PDT/CDT of cancer (66). Adapted from (51) with permission from Wiley-VCH, copyright 2020; adapted from (49) with permission from Wiley-VCH, copyright 2020; adapted from (50) with permission from American Chemical Society, copyright 2019; adapted from (66) with permission from Elsevier, copyright 2020.

the generation of ROS, thereby enhancing CDT. Since the reductive GSH was not detrimental to ROS accumulation, the GSH depletion by CFMS-PVP NSs was investigated. It was found that after incubation with GSH, most of $Mn^{3+}$ and $Mn^{4+}$ ions were reduced to $Mn^{2+}$ ions, indicating that the redox reaction contributed to the GSH consumption. Both *in vitro* and *in vivo* studies showed the synergistic PTT/CDT by CFMS-PVP NSs.

Although the concentration of $H_2O_2$ in tumors and bacteria are relatively high, the absolute content (~100 µM) is still far from sufficient to guarantee the production of lethal doses of •OH, thus limiting the efficacy of CDT (91). To supply extra $H_2O_2$ inside tumors, Li *et al.* synthesized $MoSe_2/CoSe_2$@PEG (MC@PEG) NSs for *in situ* $H_2O_2$ production enhanced PTT/CDT of cancer (**Figure 10.8b**) (49). Owing to the narrow bandgap, and high NIR harvest, MC@PEG exhibited a high (62.5%) PTCE for PTT. Routinely, the ions with high valence states of $Mo^{6+}$ and $Co^{3+}$ reduced to $Mo^{4+}$ and $Co^{2+}$, not only functioned as POD-mimic nanozymes for CDT, with three times the POD-like activity of $MoSe_2$@PEG alone but also eliminated GSH. Interestingly, different from all of the previously reported methods for $H_2O_2$ supplementation, including directly transporting $H_2O_2$, GOx-based enzymes, and some peroxides (*e.g.,* $CuO_2$, $CaO_2$, and $MgO_2$) based strategies, this work achieved photocatalytic $H_2O_2$ generation by MC@PEG under 808-nm laser irradiation. To discover the formation mechanism of $H_2O_2$, both energy band measurement and density functional theory (DFT) calculation were conducted, these results revealed that the typical-II heterostructure of $MoSe_2/CoSe_2$ possessed the effective charge separation, leading to the photo-excited electrons aggregation in the conduction band of $MoSe_2$ and then, the holes gathered to the valence band of $CoSe_2$. This single-electron transfer process to the dissolved $O_2$ determined $H_2O_2$ production, showing nearly four times $H_2O_2$ generation than $MoSe_2$@PEG alone. In addition, the CAT-like activity of MC@PEG would further supply $O_2$ supplement for $H_2O_2$ generation. Moreover, this nanocomposite could be eliminated via urine and feces within two weeks, which was beneficial for the biosafety. Hence, the multinanozymes ability, photothermal performance, and GSH-depleting property with biodegradation make MC@PEG very useful in clinical applications.

As another fatal healthcare issue with high morbidity and mortality, the better synergistic strategies with magnified therapeutic effects and less adverse effects for bacterial infection have also gained considerable attention than antibiotics-based monotherapy worldwide. Thanks to the similar internal environment of bacteria with a high concentration of $H_2O_2$ and GSH, Liu *et al.* developed hemoglobin-functionalized and magnetic spinel-structured copper ferrite NPs (Hb-CF NPs) as photothermal/Fenton agents for antimicrobial treatment (**Figure 10.8c**) (50). In the presence of limited $H_2O_2$, the excellent Fenton and Fenton-like reactions of $Fe^{2+}$ and $Cu^+$ ions in Hb-CF NPs could effectively generate •OH for CDT, which could increase the permeability of the bacterial cell membrane that was sensitive to heat, showing a broad-spectrum antibacterial property against different types of bacteria. Due to a certain degree of oxidation, the surface $Fe^{3+}$ and $Cu^{2+}$ ions depleted GSH to reduce the reducibility of bacteria and further improved CDT. The damaged bacteria would be killed nearly completely under 808-nm laser irradiation. The Hb modification could enhance the catalytic activity of CF NPs via Fenton reaction between

Hb $Fe^{2+}$ and $H_2O_2$. Accordingly, this Hb-CF NPs-based multifunctional therapeutic system was highly efficient against bacterial infection.

In addition to the combined duplex PTT-CDT of cancer and bacterial infection mentioned above, triple therapy might be more efficient in controlling the progression of tumors (92). For this purpose, Wang *et al.* covalently linked chlorin e6 (Ce6) to $Au_2Pt$ nanozymes ($Au_2Pt$-PEG-Ce6) for synergistic PTT/PDT/CDT of cancer (**Figure 10.8d**) (66). As the production of $^1O_2$ by Ce6 was highly dependent on $O_2$, $Au_2Pt$ nanozymes with the CAT-like activity were investigated. It was shown that the generation of $O_2$ by $Au_2Pt$ was maintained over a broad pH range, with a $K_m$ of 7.71 mM, which was much lower than that of CAT ($K_m$ =71.6 mM), suggesting a higher affinity of $Au_2Pt$ to $H_2O_2$. Besides converting $H_2O_2$ into $O_2$ to relieve hypoxia for PDT, $Au_2Pt$ could also convert it into •OH for CDT. In addition, the high PTCE of $Au_2Pt$-PEG (31.5%) could work for PTT and the heat could also increase the CAT-like activity of the nanozyme. Therefore, both *in vitro* and *in vivo* studies confirmed remarkable delay in the tumor growth tumor via $Au_2Pt$-PEG-Ce6 mediated synergistic PTT/PDT/CDT.

## 10.2.7 OTHER NANOZYMES

In addition to the single or multiple metal elements-based nanozymes, other metals- or nonmetal elements-based nanozymes have also been reported for PTT-CDT of cancer and bacterial infection (64, 93). Among these nanozymes, manganese (Mn) ions have been widely studied for CDT via Fenton-like reaction (94). For example, Zhao *et al.* fabricated polydopamine (PDA)-coated gadolinium oxide ($Gd_2O_3$) nanoplate with Mn doping to form MnGdOP@PDA-PEG for MRI-guided synergetic PTT-CDT of cancer (**Figure 10.9a**) (60). Originally, $Gd_2O_3$ nanoplates were characterized with high performance in $T_1$-weighted MRI. By covering with PDA, this system could also be used for PTT. Due to the doping of paramagnetic Mn ions, the MRI performance was significantly enhanced by the exposed Mn and Gd cluster, showing a higher $r_1$ value of 5.3 $mM^{-1}s^{-1}$ than nondoped GdOP (3.3 $mM^{-1}s^{-1}$) at 1.5 T, which was consistent with the results at 0.5 T. Moreover, the Fenton-like reaction between Mn ions and $H_2O_2$ could also achieve high-efficiency CDT, and could be further enhanced by PTT as revealed by the decreased absorption peak of methylene blue. Based on this work, MnGdOP@PDA-PEG is a nanozyme with POD-like activity useful for synergetic PTT-CDT of cancer. Besides the doping method, Mn ions in the form of $MnO_2$ could also function as POD-like nanozymes for CDT by GSH activation. For example, Ma *et al.* anchored $MnO_2$ NPs onto the surface of reduced graphene oxide (rGO) NSs to design rGO@$MnO_2$ nanocomposites for efficient PTT-CDT against cancer (**Figure 10.9b**) (61). Different from PDA as photothermal agents, reduced graphene oxide (rGO) as one of the most popular graphene-based materials had high absorbance in the NIR region for PTT. $Mn^{4+}$ ions in $MnO_2$ could first react with GSH to form $Mn^{2+}$ ions, followed by reacting with $H_2O_2$ to generate •OH for CDT. These sequential reactions achieved GSH depletion and triggered CDT. Similarly, the heat effect of rGO under NIR light irradiation also elevated the efficacy of a Fenton-like reaction, showing PTT-enhanced CDT of cancer.

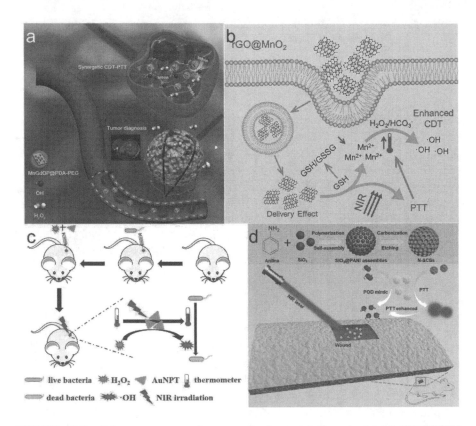

**FIGURE 10.9** Other nanozymes for cancer/antibacterial therapy. (a) MnGdOP@PDA-PEG NPs were prepared for MRI-guided synergetic PTT-CDT of cancer (60). (b) rGO@MnO$_2$ nanocomposites were reported for efficient PTT-CDT of cancer (61). (c) AuNPTs were fabricated as effective Fenton-like agents for PTT-CDT of MRSA-infected wounds (62). (d) N-SCS were reported to mimic multiple enzymes, including POD, CAT, OXD, and SOD for light-enhanced synergetic anti-bacterial therapy (63). Adapted from (60) with permission from Elsevier, copyright 2019; adapted from (61) with permission from Elsevier, copyright 2021; adapted from (62) with permission from Royal Society of Chemistry, copyright 2021; adapted from (63) with permission from Royal Society of Chemistry, copyright 2020.

Gold (Au), in the form of Au nanoplates, could be used as effective Fenton-like agents for PTT-CDT of MRSA-infected wounds (**Figure 10.9c**) (62). Besides the traditional photothermal property of Au nanoplates, they could function as nanozymes that mimic POD for •OH generation. With the co-existence of Au nanoplates, H$_2$O$_2$, and NIR irradiation, 99.98% of MRSA and *E. coli* were killed *in vitro*, and *in vivo* wound healing was further achieved by combined PTT and CDT.

For nonmetal elements-based nanozymes, N-doped sponge-like carbon spheres (N-SCSs) were first reported by Xi *et al.* to mimic multiple enzymes, including POD, CAT, OXD, and SOD for light-enhanced synergetic anti-bacterial therapy (**Figure 10.9d**) (63). Compared with their previously reported carbon materials, the N doping endowed N-SCSs with the function of carbon nanozymes. First, the POD and OXD-like activity of the N-SCSs was studied. With the co-existence of N-SCSs and $H_2O_2$, the color of 3,3′,5,5′ tetramethylbenzidine (TMB) turned to dark blue, indicating the efficient generation of •OH. It is widely recognized that the catalytic ability of enzymes is highly dependent on pH and temperature. As a consequence, the catalytic abilities of N-SCSs mimicking POD and OXD were tested at different temperatures (20°C –60°C) and pH (2.6–10). The optimal conditions for the POD and OXD-like reactions were 40°C and pH 4.5. The mechanism behind the good performance of N-SCSs as nanozymes was much due to the large surface area- up to 842.9 $m^2$ $g^{-1}$, which allowed active sites to be exposed to $H_2O_2$. Moreover, the addition of laser not only elevated the Fenton-like reaction rate but further increased active surfaces on the N-SCSs by increasing the donating or accepting electrons capacity of carbon materials to improve POD-like performance. Second, N-SCSs also exhibited CAT and SOD-like activities under neutral conditions. Encouraged by the outstanding behaviors in heat and ROS generations, N-SCSs effectively killed Gram-negative bacteria (*E. coli*), Gram-positive bacteria (*S. aureus*), and MDR bacteria for wound healing. Thus, this synergetic anti-infection strategy expanded the application of carbon-based nanozymes in biomedicine.

## 10.3   SUMMARY AND FUTURE PERSPECTIVES

The combination of PTT and nanozymes-based catalytic therapy can produce a significant synergistic effect, which can overcome the shortcomings of monotherapy, thereby improving the killing effect on tumors or bacteria. This chapter systematically summarized the latest application progress of nanozymes as photothermal-catalytic agents for cancer/antibacterial therapy. The relationship between the photothermal performance and the catalytic activity of nanozymes was emphasized. Although there has been much progress made in nanozymes as photothermal-catalytic agents, there are still many challenges and key problems to be solved.

First, most nanozymes not only catalyze a specific substrate like natural enzymes. Although having multiple enzyme-like activities may be beneficial, in some cases, poor substrate selectivity may lead to undesirable side reactions in a biological environment (95). Therefore, it is a great challenge to improve the selectivity of nanozymes.

Second, lots of catalytic mechanism of nanozymes are still unclear and need to be fully elucidated. A better understanding of the catalytic mechanism can reveal its structure-activity relationship and better regulate the substrate selectivity and catalytic efficiency (8). Collaborative efforts of different disciplines, such as artificial intelligence technologies, machine learning, and computational research, can be combined to clarify the catalytic mechanism of nanozymes.

Third, it is necessary to recognize that the catalytic activity of most nanozymes is still lower than the corresponding natural enzymes, and sometimes nanozymes cannot meet the requirements of practical applications. Although these limitations can be overcome by adjusting the concentration of nanozymes, this may lead to toxicity problems with concentration-dependent effects. Therefore, it is very important to construct nanozymes with satisfactory catalytic efficiency.

Finally, the application of nanozymes in the disease diagnosis and treatment is still in its infancy. In addition, the relationship between the therapeutic effect and safety of nanozymes needs to be balanced. Therefore, it is essential to systematically evaluate the safety of nanozymes. These problems are both challenges and opportunities for nanozymes. In short, nanozymes as photothermal-catalytic agents for cancer/antibacterial therapy have very broad application prospects.

## ACKNOWLEDGMENTS

This work was supported by the National Natural Science Foundation of China (21574035), the University Synergy Innovation Program of Anhui Province (GXXT-2019-045), and the Fundamental Research Funds for the Central Universities (JZ2018HGPA0273).

## REFERENCES

1. Dai Y, Ding Y, Li L. 2021. *Chinese Chemical Letters*: DOI: org/10.1016/j.cclet.2021.03.036.
2. Zhang Y, Jin Y, Cui H, Yan X, Fan K. 2020. *RSC Advances* 10: 10–20
3. Zhong X, Wang X, Cheng L, Tang Ya, Zhan G, et al. 2020. *Advanced Functional Materials* 30: 1907954
4. Wang Z, Zhang R, Yan X, Fan K. 2020. *Materials Today* 40: 81–119
5. Liu Y, Bhattarai P, Dai Z, Chen X. 2019. *Chemical Society Reviews* 48: 2053–108
6. Wang X, Cheng L. 2019. *Nanoscale* 11: 15685–708
7. Wang C, Wang H, Xu B, Liu H. 2021. *View* 2: 20200045
8. Yao J, Zheng F, Yao C, Xu X, Akakuru OU, et al. 2020. *Wiley Interdisciplinary Reviews: Nanomedicine and Nanobiotechnology*: e1682
9. Huang Y, Ren J, Qu X. 2019. *Chemical Reviews* 119: 4357–412
10. Wei H, Wang E. 2013. *Chemical Society Reviews* 42: 6060–93
11. Wu J, Wang X, Wang Q, Lou Z, Li S, et al. 2019. *Chemical Society Reviews* 48: 1004–76
12. Tang Z, Zhang H, Liu Y, Ni D, Zhang H, et al. 2017. *Advanced Materials* 29: 1701683
13. Liu Y, Zhen W, Wang Y, Liu J, Jin L, et al. 2019. *Angewandte Chemie International Edition* 58: 2407–12
14. Meng Y, Li W, Pan X, Gadd GM. 2020. *Environmental Science: Nano* 7: 1305–18
15. Li D, Fang Y, Zhang X. 2020. *ACS Applied Materials & Interfaces* 12: 8989–99
16. Liu Z, Zhao X, Yu B, Zhao N, Zhang C, Xu F-J. 2021. *ACS Nano* 15: 7482–90
17. Agnihotri S, Mohan T, Jha D, Gautam HK, Roy I. 2020. *ACS Omega* 5: 597–602
18. Guan G, Wang X, Li B, Zhang W, Cui Z, et al. 2018. *Nanoscale* 10: 17902–11
19. Zhang Q, Guo Q, Chen Q, Zhao X, Pennycook SJ, Chen H. 2020. *Advanced Science* 7: 1902576
20. Feng W, Han X, Wang R, Gao X, Hu P, et al. 2019. *Advanced Materials* 31: 1805919
21. Liu F, Lin L, Sheng S, Xu C, Wang Y, et al. 2020. *Nanoscale* 12: 1349–55
22. Wang X, Zhong X, Lei H, Geng Y, Zhao Q, et al. 2019. *Chemistry of Materials* 31: 6174–86
23. Wang T, Zhang H, Liu H, Yuan Q, Ren F, et al. 2020. *Advanced Functional Materials* 30: 1906128
24. Liu Y, Wu J, Jin Y, Zhen W, Wang Y, et al. 2019. *Advanced Functional Materials* 29: 1904678
25. Wang H, Wan K, Shi X. 2019. *Advanced Materials* 31: 1805368
26. Hu C, Cai L, Liu S, Liu Y, Zhou Y, Pang M. 2020. *Bioconjugate Chemistry* 31: 1661–70
27. Kong L, Yuan F, Huang P, Yan L, Cai Z, et al. 2020. *Small* 16: 2004161

28. Hu K, Xie L, Zhang Y, Hanyu M, Yang Z, et al. 2020. *Nature Communications* 11: 2778
29. Yang C, Younis MR, Zhang J, Qu J, Lin J, Huang P. 2020. *Small* 16: 2001518
30. Wang Y, An L, Lin J, Tian Q, Yang S. 2020. *Chemical Engineering Journal* 385: 123925
31. Sun M, Yang D, Sun Q, Jia T, Kuang Y, et al. 2020. *Journal of Materials Chemistry B* 8: 10559–76
32. Wang X, Shi Q, Zha Z, Zhu D, Zheng L, et al. 2021. *Bioactive Materials* 6: 4389–401
33. Xie Y, Qian Y, Li Z, Liang Z, Liu W, et al. 2021. *ACS Sustainable Chemistry & Engineering*: DOI: org/10.1021/acssuschemeng.1c01589
34. Shan J, Yang K, Xiu W, Qiu Q, Dai S, et al. 2020. *Small* 16: 2001099
35. Yin W, Yu J, Lv F, Yan L, Zheng LR, et al. 2016. *ACS Nano* 10: 11000–11
36. Zhang Y, Li D, Tan J, Chang Z, Liu X, et al. 2021. *Small* 17: 2005739
37. Zhao P, Tang Z, Chen X, He Z, He X, et al. 2019. *Materials Horizons* 6: 369–74
38. Sang Y, Li W, Liu H, Zhang L, Wang H, et al. 2019. *Advanced Functional Materials* 29: 1900518
39. Jiang H, Du Y, Chen L, Qian M, Yang Y, et al. 2020. *International Journal of Pharmaceutics* 586
40. Guo Q, Wang D, Yang G. 2019. *Journal of Biomedical Nanotechnology* 15: 2090–9
41. Ding Y, Huang R, Luo L, Guo W, Zhu C, Shen X-C. 2021. *Inorganic Chemistry Frontiers* 8: 636–46
42. Liu P, Wang Y, An L, Tian Q, Lin J, Yang S. 2018. *ACS Applied Materials & Interfaces* 10: 38833–44
43. Xu M, Hu Y, Xiao Y, Zhang Y, Sun K, et al. 2020. *ACS Applied Materials & Interfaces* 12: 50260–74
44. Wang X, Zhong X, Zha Z, He G, Miao Z, et al. 2020. *Applied Materials Today* 18: 100464
45. Wang X, Fan L, Cheng L, Sun Y, Wang X, et al. 2020. *iScience* 23: 101281
46. Pan C, Ou M, Cheng Q, Zhou Y, Yu Y, et al. 2020. *Advanced Functional Materials* 30: 1906466
47. Liu Y, Tian Y, Han Q, Yin J, Zhang J, et al. 2021. *Chemical Engineering Journal* 410: 128209
48. Liu Y, Jia Q, Guo Q, Wei W, Zhou J. 2018. *Biomaterials* 180: 104–16
49. Li Y, Jia R, Lin H, Sun X, Qu F. 2021. *Advanced Functional Materials* 31: 2008420
50. Liu Y, Guo Z, Li F, Xiao Y, Zhang Y, et al. 2019. *ACS Applied Materials & Interfaces* 11: 31649–60
51. Zhu Y, Wang Y, Williams GR, Fu L, Wu J, et al. 2020. *Advanced Science* 7: 2000272
52. Sun H, Zhang Y, Chen S, Wang R, Chen Q, et al. 2020. *ACS Applied Materials & Interfaces* 12: 30145–54
53. Yang B, Dai Z, Zhang G, Hu Z, Yao X, et al. 2020. *Advanced Healthcare Materials* 9: 1901634
54. Zhang S, Jin L, Liu J, Liu Y, Zhang T, et al. 2020. *Nano-Micro Letters* 12: 180
55. Shi Y, Yin J, Peng Q, Lv X, Li Q, et al. 2020. *Biomaterials Science* 8: 6093–9
56. Wang H, An L, Tao C, Ling Z, Lin J, et al. 2020. *Nanoscale* 12: 5139–50
57. Zhang G, Xie W, Xu Z, Si Y, Li Q, et al. 2021. *Materials Horizons* 8: 1017–28
58. Chen Y, Gao M, Zhang L, Ha E, Hu X, et al. 2021. *Advanced Healthcare Materials* 10: 2001665
59. Wang Z, Fu L, Zhu Y, Wang S, Shen G, et al. 2021. *Journal of Materials Chemistry B* 9: 710–8
60. Zhao Z, Xu K, Fu C, Liu H, Lei M, et al. 2019. *Biomaterials* 219: 119379
61. Ma B, Nishina Y, Bianco A. 2021. *Carbon* 178: 783–91

62. Hao Y-N, Zhang W-X, Gao Y-R, Wei Y-N, Shu Y, Wang J-H. 2021. *Journal of Materials Chemistry B* 9: 250–66
63. Xi J, Wei G, Wu Q, Xu Z, Liu Y, et al. 2019. *Biomaterials Science* 7: 4131–41
64. Chen M, Zhou H, Liu X, Yuan T, Wang W, et al. 2020. *Small* 16: e2002343
65. Liu X, Jin Y, Liu T, Yang S, Zhou M, et al. 2020. *ACS Biomaterials Science & Engineering* 6: 4834–45
66. Wang M, Chang M, Chen Q, Wang D, Li C, et al. 2020. *Biomaterials* 252: 120093
67. Tang Z, Liu Y, He M, Bu W. 2019. *Angewandte Chemie-International Edition* 58: 946–56
68. Tang Z, Zhao P, Wang H, Liu Y, Bu W. 2021. *Chemical Reviews* 121: 1981–2019
69. Su L, Cai Y, Wang L, Dong W, Mao G, et al. 2020. *Microchimica Acta* 187: 132
70. Cao F, Zhang L, Wang H, You Y, Wang Y, et al. 2019. *Angewandte Chemie International Edition* 58: 16236–42
71. Liu K, Liu K, Liu J, Ren Q, Zhao Z, et al. 2020. *Nanoscale* 12: 2902–13
72. Ma B, Wang S, Liu F, Zhang S, Duan J, et al. 2019. *Journal of the American Chemical Society* 141: 849–57
73. Zhang S, Sun C, Zeng J, Sun Q, Wang G, et al. 2016. *Advanced Materials* 28: 8927–36
74. Liang M, Yan X. 2019. *Accounts of Chemical Research* 52: 2190–200
75. Huo M, Wang L, Wang Y, Chen Y, Shi J. 2019. *ACS Nano* 13: 2643–53
76. Lu X, Gao S, Lin H, Yu L, Han Y, et al. 2020. *Advanced Materials* 32: 2002246
77. Zu Y, Yao H, Wang Y, Yan L, Gu Z, et al. 2021. *View*: 20200188
78. Hu X, Li F, Xia F, Guo X, Wang N, et al. 2019. *Journal of the American Chemical Society* 142: 1636–44
79. Bao T, Yin W, Zheng X, Zhang X, Yu J, et al. 2016. *Biomaterials* 76: 11–24
80. Wu C, Wang S, Zhao J, Liu Y, Zheng Y, et al. 2019. *Advanced Functional Materials* 29: 1901722
81. Wen L, Chen L, Zheng S, Zeng J, Duan G, et al. 2016. *Advanced Materials* 28: 5072–9
82. Boruah PJ, Khanikar RR, Bailung H. 2020. *Plasma Chemistry and Plasma Processing*: 1–18
83. Hu Z, Wang S, Dai Z, Zhang H, Zheng X. 2020. *Journal of Materials Chemistry B* 8: 5351–60
84. Klare W, Das T, Ibugo A, Buckle E, Manefield M, Manos J. 2016. *Antimicrobial agents and chemotherapy* 60: 4539–51
85. Iqbal S, Fakhar-e-Alam M, Atif M, Amin N, Ali A, et al. 2020. *Journal of Photochemistry and Photobiology A: Chemistry* 386: 112130
86. Wen M, Ouyang J, Wei C, Li H, Chen W, Liu YN. 2019. *Angewandte Chemie International Edition* 58: 17425–32
87. Lei Z, Zhang W, Li B, Guan G, Huang X, et al. 2019. *Nanoscale* 11: 20161–70
88. Alizadeh N, Salimi A, Hallaj R, Fathi F, Soleimani F. 2018. *Journal of Nanobiotechnology* 16: 1–14
89. Lei H, Wang X, Bai S, Gong F, Yang N, et al. 2020. *ACS Applied Materials & Interfaces* 12: 52370–82
90. Wang X, Wang X, Zhong X, Li G, Yang Z, et al. 2020. *Applied Physics Reviews* 7: 041411
91. Li SL, Jiang P, Jiang FL, Liu Y. 2021. *Advanced Functional Materials*: 2100243
92. Meng X, Zhang X, Liu M, Cai B, He N, Wang Z. 2020. *Applied Materials Today* 21: 100864
93. Sun H, Zhou Y, Ren J, Qu X. 2018. *Angewandte Chemie International Edition* 57: 9224–37
94. Lin LS, Song J, Song L, Ke K, Liu Y, et al. 2018. *Angewandte Chemie* 130: 4996–5000
95. Liu X, Gao Y, Chandrawati R, Hosta-Rigau L. 2019. *Nanoscale* 11: 21046–60

# 11 Nanozymes in Detecting Environmental Pollutants

*Xin Li,[a,b] Peng Liu,[a] Mengzhu Wang,[a] and Xiangheng Niu[a,*]*
[a]School of Chemistry and Chemical Engineering, Jiangsu University, Zhenjiang, PR China
[b]School of Environment and Safety Engineering, Jiangsu University, Zhenjiang, PR China

## CONTENTS

## 11.1 INTRODUCTION

Inorganic ions are highly related to the environmental security of surface water. Pollutant ions in water, especially in drinking water, are easily absorbed by organisms, and they can interact with some biomolecules and further inhibit their functions, resulting in huge damage to living organisms. Therefore, monitoring pollutant ions is always a major focus of environmental analysis. Traditional methods, such as inductively coupled plasma (ICP)-mass spectrometry (MS), ICP-optical emission

* Corresponding author: Xiangheng Niu

DOI: 10.1201/9781003109228-11

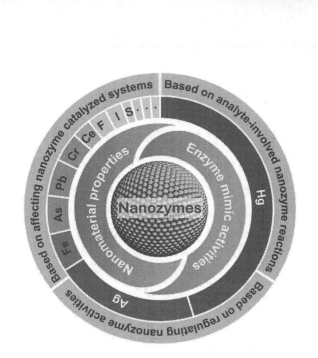

**FIGURE 11.1** Principles and strategies based on nanozyme catalysis for the determination of various environmental pollutant ions.

spectroscopy (OES), atomic absorption spectroscopy (AAS), atomic fluorescence spectrometry (AFS), ion chromatography, etc., for the detection of inorganic pollutant ions, usually need tedious pretreatment, expensive instruments, and skillful operators (1, 2). As a consequence, it is urgent to explore accurate and rapid methods for pollution ion in-field analysis. As an emerging tool, nanozymes are finding increasing use in the field of pollutant ion detection (3). This is mainly because nanozyme activities or/and nanozyme-catalyzed systems can be impacted by these ions. For instance, some ions can involve themselves in reaction systems as an enzyme mimic, and some of them can regulate the catalytic activity by interacting with nanozymes. By using these principles, several facile methods have been established to detect various Pollutant ions.

In this chapter, the state-of-the-art progress of nanozymes applied in environmental ion analysis is summarized (**Figure 11.1** and **Table 11.1**). The general detection strategies based on nanozyme catalysis for environmental pollutant ions are classified and discussed, including target-involved catalytic reactions, regulating the activity of nanozymes, and affecting nanozyme-catalyzed systems. Typical examples of inorganic ion analysis using nanozyme catalysis are discussed and commented on. The opportunities and trends of nanozymes in the toxic ion detection field are also included.

## 11.2   ANALYTE-INVOLVED NANOZYME REACTIONS

Some metal ions, including chromium ($Cr^{3+}\leftrightarrow Cr^{6+}$), iron ($Fe^{2+}\leftrightarrow Fe^{3+}$), copper ($Cu^{+}\leftrightarrow Cu^{2+}$), and cerium ($Ce^{3+}\leftrightarrow Ce^{4+}$), often exist in the environment in various forms, and they are toxic at high concentrations, threatening the health of living

**TABLE 11.1**

**Detection of Various Ions Based on Nanozyme Catalysis**

| Nanozyme | Analyte | Sensing Principle | Detection Mode | Linear Range | LOD | Ref. |
|---|---|---|---|---|---|---|
| *Based on analyte-involved nanozyme reactions* | | | | | | |
| Au@Hg | $Cr^{6+}$ | Au@Hg acts as an oxidoreductase to catalyze the redox reaction of $Cr^{6+}$ and TMB | Colorimetric | 0.001–2 µM | 0.71 nM | (4) |
| PEI-Ag NCs | $Cr^{6+}$ | PEI-AgNCs act as an oxidoreductase nanozyme to catalyze the redox reaction between TMB and $Cr^{6+}$ | Colorimetric | 5–100 µM | 1.1 µM | (5) |
| PtRu NPs | $Fe^{2+}$ | $Fe^{2+}$ acts as a reactant and PtRu NPs show the ability to catalyze the oxidation of $Fe^{2+}$ to $Fe^{3+}$ in the presence of dissolved oxygen | Colorimetric | 0.2–6 mM | 0.05 µM | (6) |
| $Ce^{4+}$ | $Ce^{4+}$ | By intentionally hydrolyzing $Ce^{4+}$ into its hydrolysate, the hydrolysate acts as an enzyme mimic with enhanced activity with the assistance of $F^-$ to catalyze a color reaction | Colorimetric | 0–200 µM | 3.8 µM | (7) |
| $Cu^{2+}$ | $Cu^{2+}$ | $Cu^{2+}$ directly triggers the oxidation of TMB, and the $Cu^{2+}$-catalyzed oxidation reaction can be effectively improved by nucleotides or nucleobases | Colorimetric | 0–150 nM | 3.3 nM | (8) |
| *Based on regulating nanozyme activities* | | | | | | |
| Pt NPs | $Hg^{2+}$ | $Hg^{2+}$ directly covers the POD activity of Pt NPs via the specific interaction between $Hg^{2+}$ and Pt | Colorimetric | 0–120 nM | 7.2 nM | (9) |
| CuS | $Hg^{2+}$ | The catalytic activity of CuS is dramatically inhibited because of the formation of HgS on the CuS surface | Colorimetric | 3–40 µM | 0.22 µM | (10) |
| BSA-AgNCs | $Hg^{2+}$ | $Hg^{2+}$ can improve the OXD-like activity of BSA-AgNCs through the direct interaction between $Hg^{2+}$ and AgNCs | Colorimetric | 30–225 nM | 10 nM | (11) |
| Ch-PtNPs | $Ag^+$ | The Pt species endows Ch-PtNPs with excellent OXD activity, but the activity is inhibited by $Ag^+$ due to the strong metallophilic interaction between $Pt^{2+}$ and $Ag^+$ | Colorimetric | 5–1000 nM | 4 nM | (12) |

*(Continued)*

**TABLE 11.1 (Continued)**
**Detection of Various Ions Based on Nanozyme Catalysis**

| Nanozyme | Analyte | Sensing Principle | Detection Mode | Linear Range | LOD | Ref. |
|---|---|---|---|---|---|---|
| CoOOH | $As^{5+}$ | CoOOH nanoflakes with intrinsic POD-like activity are used to generate signals by catalyzing the oxidation of ABTS; when $As^{5+}$ is added, the CoOOH nanoflakes will specifically bind with $As^{5+}$ through the electrostatic attraction and As–O bond, and such that active sites on CoOOH are masked, resulting in the decrease of nanozyme activity | Colorimetric, electrochemical | 4–500 ppb; 0.1–200 ppb | 3.7 ppb; 56.1 ppt | (13) |
| $Fe_3O_4$ NPs | $As^{5+}$ | When $As^{5+}$ is added to the catalytic system containing $Fe_3O_4$ NPs, MB, and $H_2O_2$, $As^{5+}$ will rapidly adsorb onto the surface of $Fe_3O_4$ NPs due to strong electrostatic attraction, thus leading to the block of the active sites on $Fe_3O_4$ NPs | Colorimetric | 0–4 nM | 0.358 nM | (14) |
| GNPs | $Ce^{3+}$ | $Ce^{3+}$ can significantly activate the activity of Au NPs via its electron-donating capability and redox recycling ability | Colorimetric | 10–160 nM | 2.2 nM | (15) |
| $CeO_2$ | $Al^{3+}$ | The coordination between $Al^{3+}$ and $CeO_2$ leads to the aggregation of $CeO_2$, thus regulating down the activity of the nanozyme | Chemiluminescence | 0.03–3.5 μM | 10 nM | (16) |
| $WS_2$ nanosheets | $Pb^{2+}$ | Pb(II) can be specifically adsorbed onto the surface of layered $WS_2$ nanosheets through the stronger binding with oxygen atoms in hydroxyl or carbonyl, and it will further block the electron transfer between $WS_2$ nanosheets and $H_2O_2$, leading to the inhibition of the POD-mimic activity | Colorimetric | 5–80 μg/L | 4 μg/L | (17) |
| $MoS_2$ | $Fe^{2+}$ | $Fe^{2+}$ remarkably enhances the catalytic activity of $MoS_2$ nanosheets toward the oxidation of OPD to form a fluorescent substance called DAPN, and the $MoS_2$/OPD/$H_2O_2$ sensor displays substantial fluorescence enhancement after the addition of $Fe^{2+}$ | Fluorescence | 0.005–0.2 μM | 3.5 nM | (18) |
| Ni/Al-Fe(CN)$_6$ LDH | $Cr^{6+}$ | $Cr^{6+}$ promotes the POD-like activity of Ni/Al-Fe(CN)$_6$ LDH | Colorimetric | 0.067–10 μM | 0.039 μM | (19) |

(Continued)

**TABLE 11.1 (Continued)**
**Detection of Various Ions Based on Nanozyme Catalysis**

| Nanozyme | Analyte | Sensing Principle | Detection Mode | Linear Range | LOD | Ref. |
|---|---|---|---|---|---|---|
| $CeO_2$ | $F^-$ | The OXD activity of nanoceria is increased by the capping of $F^-$ | Colorimetric | $0$–$100\ \mu M$ | $0.64\ \mu M$ | (20) |
| $VO_x$ | $I^-$ | The poor POD activity of $VO_x$ can be significantly boosted by a small amount of $I^-$, which can modulate the surface charge of $VO_x$ and change its electronic structure | Colorimetric | $0.0033$–$33.3\ \mu M$ | $74\ pM$ | (21) |
| $Fe_3O_4$ MNPs | $PO_4^{3-}$ | Phosphate ion inhibits the POD activity of $Fe_3O_4$ MNPs through its adsorption onto the surface of $Fe_3O_4$ MNPs via the strong interaction between phosphate ion and $Fe^{3+}$, inducing a reduced colorimetric signal | Colorimetric | $0.2$–$200\ \mu M$ | $0.11\ \mu M$ | (22) |
| $Ce_xZr_{1-x}O_2$ | $PO_4^{3-}$ | Phosphate ion greatly promotes the POD-like activity of $Ce_xZr_{1-x}O_2$ toward positively charged TMB via surface charge modulation | Colorimetric | $0.33$–$266.7\ \mu M$ | $0.09\ \mu M$ | (23) |
| Oxidized UiO-66(Ce/Zr) | $PO_4^{3-}$ | When oxidized UiO-66(Ce/Zr) is incubated with phosphate ions, the surface charge of oxidized UiO-66(Ce/Zr) is changed due to the newly formed Zr–O–P bond, greatly affecting the affinities between the nanozyme and different chromogenic substrates | Dual-channel ratiometric colorimetric | $0.066$–$666.7\ \mu M$ | $14\ nM$ | (24) |
| UiO-66(Ce/Zr)-NH$_2$ | $PO_4^{3-}$ | When phosphate ions are introduced, the POD-mimetic activity of UiO-66(Fe/Zr)-NH$_2$ is suppressed because of the good affinity between Zr–O nodes and phosphate ions | Ratiometric fluorescence | $0.2$–$266.7\ \mu M$ | $85\ nM$ | (25) |
| Cu NCs | $S^{2-}$ | $S^{2-}$ may be attached to the surface of CuNCs due to the strong interaction of $Cu^+$ and $S^{2-}$, greatly impeding the conversion of $H_2O_2$ to OH$^-$ | Colorimetric | $0.5$–$20\ \mu M$ | $0.5\ \mu M$ | (26) |
| Citrate-capped Pt NPs | $Hg^{2+}$ | $Hg^{2+}$ is reduced to $Hg^0$ by citrate under the catalysis of Pt NPs to form an amalgam, which significantly inhibits the POD activity of Pt NPs | Colorimetric | $0.01$–$4\ nM$ | $8.5\ pM$ | (27) |
| Au@AgPt NPs | $Hg^{2+}$ | The presence of $Hg^{2+}$ induces the POD activity depression of Au@AgPt NPs and leads to color and SERS signal changes | Colorimetric, SERS | $1$–$100\ \mu M$; $0.001$–$10\ \mu M$ | $0.52\ \mu M$; $0.28\ nM$ | (28) |

*(Continued)*

**TABLE 11.1 (Continued)**

**Detection of Various Ions Based on Nanozyme Catalysis**

| Nanozyme | Analyte | Sensing Principle | Detection Mode | Linear Range | LOD | Ref. |
|---|---|---|---|---|---|---|
| Au NPs | $Hg^{2+}$ | $Hg^{2+}$ ions are reduced by citrate to form $Hg^0$ on the surface of Au NPs, changing the properties of Au NPs and stimulating the Au NP catalyzed oxidation of TMB | Visual | 1–600 nM | 0.3 nM | (29) |
| $g\text{-}C_3N_4\text{-}Au$ | $Hg^{2+}$ | The catalytic activity of $g\text{-}C_3N_4\text{-}Au$ is dramatically stimulated by $Hg^{2+}$ as a result of the deposition of metallic Hg on the material surface | Colorimetric | 5–500 nM | 3.0 nM | (30) |
| $Au/Fe_3O_4/GO$ | $Hg^{2+}$ | $Hg^{2+}$ is first reduced by citrate to form $Hg^0$, and then $Hg^0$ disperses on the surface of Au NPs, improving the POD activity of $Au/Fe_3O_4/GO$ | Colorimetric | 1–50 nM | 0.15 nM | (31) |
| Cu NPs | $Hg^{2+}$ | Cu NPs have a reducing effect on $Hg^{2+}$ and lead to the formation of CuHg alloy, which can increase the POD activity of Cu NPs by improving the affinity between Cu NPs and substrates | Dual-wavelength colorimetric | 0.05–10 μM; 0.1–6 μM | 0.185 μM; 0.052 μM | (32) |
| $CS\text{-}MoSe_2$ | $Hg^{2+}$ | The promotion effect of $Hg^{2+}$ on $CS\text{-}MoSe_2$ activity is generated from the in situ reduction of chitosan-captured $Hg^{2+}$ on $MoSe_2$ surface | Colorimetric | 0.025–2.5 μM | 3.5 nM | (33) |
| $g\text{-}C_3N_4\text{-}PtNPs$ | $Ag^+$ | $Ag^+$ is reduced to $Ag^0$ by citric acid under the catalysis of Pt NPs, and metallic $Ag^0$ is further adsorbed onto the surface of $g\text{-}C_3N_4\text{-}Pt$ NPs, significantly inhibiting the POD activity of the nanozyme | Colorimetric | 0.05–5 nM | 22 pM | (34) |
| BSA@AuNCs | $Ag^+$ | $Ag^+$ selectively reacts with $Au^0$ through a redox reaction, which induces an apparent inhibition of the POD-like activity of BSA@Au NCs | Colorimetric | 0.5–10 μM | 0.204 μM | (35) |
| $Cys\text{-}Fe_3O_4$ | $Hg^{2+}$ | The POD activity of $Fe_3O_4$ is first inhibited by surface modification, and in the presence of $Hg^{2+}$, Cys on $Fe_3O_4$ surface will fall off due to the stronger coordination between Cys and $Hg^{2+}$, and such that active sites are exposed again and the catalytic ability is restored | Colorimetric | 0.02–90 nM | 5.9 pM | (36) |
| His-Pd | $Ag^+$ | The POD-like activity of bare Pd NPs is boosted after the modification of Cys, but the ability is significantly covered resulting from the stronger interaction between $Ag^+$ and Cys | Colorimetric | 30–300 nM | 4.7 nM | (37) |

*(Continued)*

**TABLE 11.1 (Continued)**
**Detection of Various Ions Based on Nanozyme Catalysis**

| Nanozyme | Analyte | Sensing Principle | Detection Mode | Linear Range | LOD | Ref. |
|---|---|---|---|---|---|---|
| Pd-DTT | $As^{3+}$ | With the addition of $As^{3+}$, the OXD activity of Pd-DTT is significantly suppressed because it can strongly chelate with the sulphydryl groups in DTT | Colorimetric | 0.033–333.3 μg/L | 35 ng/L | (38) |
| AuNCs | $Pb^{2+}$ | The POD activity of GSH-capped Au NCs is enhanced when $Pb^{2+}$ is added, which is triggered by the aggregation of Au NCs due to the GSH-$Pb^{2+}$ interaction | Colorimetric | 2–250 μM | 2 μM | (39) |
| BSA-AuNCs | $UO_2^{2+}$ | In the absence of $UO_2^{2+}$, BSA-Au NCs show intrinsic POD activity, but this ability is significantly restrained by $UO_2^{2+}$ via its interaction with the hydroxyl groups in BSA | Colorimetric | 12–160 μM | 1.86 μM | (40) |
| $Fe_3O_4$-DHCA | $PO_4^{3-}$ | $Zr^{4+}$ is first adsorbed onto the surface of the nanozyme through electrostatic interaction, and then it can capture phosphate ions through specific interaction, thereby reducing the exposed active sites and inhibiting the catalytic activity of $Fe_3O_4$-DHCA | Colorimetric | 0.066–33.3 μM | 49.8 nM | (41) |
| FeCo-LDH | $P_2O_7^{4-}$ | The fluorescence signal of PDA generated under the catalysis of FeCo-LDH can be quenched/recovered upon consequently adding $Fe^{3+}$ and PPi | Fluorescence | 33–500 μM | 54 μM | (42) |
| $MoS_2$ QDs | $P_2O_7^{4-}$ | The peroxide-like activity of $MoS_2$ quantum dots can be manipulated by aggregation/dispersion induced by $Fe^{3+}$ and PPi | Colorimetric | 2.0–7.0 μM | 1.82 μM | (43) |
| $Fe_3O_4$ MNPs | $Hg^{2+}$ | The POD activity of MNPs is blocked by ssDNA, and the catalytic ability is recovered by $Hg^{2+}$ due to the specific interaction between $Hg^{2+}$ and ssDNA | Colorimetric | 5–75 μM | 5 μM | (44) |
| MVC-MOF | $Hg^{2+}$ | MVC-MOF exhibits instinct OXD activity, which can be inhibited by ssDNA, and in the presence of $Hg^{2+}$, ssDNA prefers bonding with $Hg^{2+}$ | Colorimetric | 0.05–6 μM | 10.5 nM | (45) |

(Continued)

**TABLE 11.1 (Continued)**
**Detection of Various Ions Based on Nanozyme Catalysis**

| Nanozyme | Analyte | Sensing Principle | Detection Mode | Linear Range | LOD | Ref. |
|---|---|---|---|---|---|---|
| $Mn_3O_4$ NPs | $Hg^{2+}$ | Some oligonucleotides can reduce the OXD activity of $Mn_3O_4$, and the inhibition effect is canceled by heavy metals like $Hg^{2+}$ | Colorimetric | 10–200 µg/L | 3.8 µg/L | (46) |
| Au NPs | $K^+$ | The inherent POD activity is inhibited by some target-specific aptamers, and when $K^+$ exists, the aptamers leave the surface of Au NPs to bond with $K^+$, leading to the catalytic ability recovery of Au NPs | Colorimetric | 0.1–1000 nM | 0.06 nM | (47) |
| Fe-Co LDH | $As^{3+}$ | As(III) is firmly anchored onto the Fe* sites of 3-MPA-modified Fe-Co-LDH via forming a stable Fe–As(III)–3-MPA–As(III)–Fe structure, masking the active sites and interlayer channels of the nanozyme | Colorimetric | 0.1–8.33 µM | 35 nM | (48) |
| *Based on affecting nanozyme catalyzed systems* | | | | | | |
| C-dots/$Mn_3O_4$ | $Fe^{2+}$ | Both TMB and $Fe^{2+}$ can be oxidized under the catalysis of C-dots/$Mn_3O_4$, and such that the presence of $Fe^{2+}$ can competitively affect the nanozyme catalyzed oxidation of TMB | Colorimetric | 0.03–0.83 µM | 0.03 µM | (49) |
| $MoS_2$/g-$C_3N_4$ | $S^{2-}$ | $S^{2-}$ may involve the competitive oxidation between $S^{2-}$ and chromogenic TMB and the re-reduction of oxidized TMB | Colorimetric | 0.1–10 µM | 37 nM | (50) |

beings. Therefore, strict monitoring is required. However, the detection of these polyvalent ions is difficult because they are easy to convert, hydrolyze, and coordinate. Thus, they are not suitable for long-distance transport to the laboratory for analysis. Recently, visual methods based on nanozyme catalysis have been reported for infield rapid sensing of these polyvalent ions. In these cases, polyvalent metal ions directly involve in nanozyme catalyzed systems as reactants or as enzyme mimics.

## 11.2.1 ANALYTES ACTING AS REACTANTS

It is known that $Cr^{6+}$ is more toxic than $Cr^{3+}$. Yet, quantitative detection of $Cr^{6+}$ is more challenging because $Cr^{6+}$ and $Cr^{3+}$ easily convert to each other due to their redox properties. Therefore, naked eyes or colorimetric sensors based on nanozyme catalysis are suitable for rapid and *in situ* detection of toxic $Cr^{6+}$. In a typical nanozyme-catalyzed system (taking POD as an example), $H_2O_2$ is decomposed to produce hydroxyl radicals under the catalysis of a POD mimic, and these radicals can further oxidize a substrate (e.g., TMB) to its colorful product (TMBox), providing colorimetric signals for sensing. Based on this, Lu et al. considered whether $Cr^{6+}$ could replace $H_2O_2$ to participate in the chromogenic reaction (4). They proved that Au@Hg could act as an oxidoreductase to catalyze the redox reaction between $Cr^{6+}$ and TMB (**Figure 11.2A**). With the signal amplification effect contributed to Au@Hg, a highly sensitive and selective strategy was established for $Cr^{6+}$ detection. This concept is attractive because the type of nanozymes is enriched and expanded to ion analysis. However, two points remain to be further considered: 1) the use of toxic Hg in the nanozyme inevitably causes secondary pollution to the environment and 2) the detection cost may be potentially reduced by replacing Au with other cheaper metals.

With the above considerations, our group proposed a green and cost-efficient photometric method for $Cr^{6+}$ sensing by using polyethylenimine-stabilized silver nanoclusters (PEI-AgNCs) as a catalyst (**Figure 11.2B**) (5), and the real role of PEI-AgNCs in the catalytic system was uncovered in detail (**Figure 11.2C**). It was proved that PEI-AgNCs acted as neither an oxidant nor an OXD mimic. Instead, the material worked as an oxidoreductase mimic to catalyze the redox reaction between TMB and $Cr^{6+}$. In detail, electrons tended to flow from TMB to PEI-AgNCs and then delivered to $Cr^{6+}$. Therefore, the PEI-AgNCs material could be regarded as an electron mediator to accelerate the redox process due to easier electron transfer. Besides, the PEI species modified on the Ag surface not only stabilized the formation of small-sized Ag clusters but also benefited the adsorption of $Cr^{6+}$. The proposed nanozyme is attractive in terms of material cost and reduced secondary pollution to the environment. With the above-mentioned advantages, the use of PEI-AgNCs for $Cr^{6+}$ detection in real practice is greatly promising. Nonetheless, the detection efficiency of this assay still needs to be improved, because the sensitivity and limit of detection (LOD) are not enough for low-content sample measurement. Similar to $Cr^{6+}$ and $Cr^{3+}$, $Fe^{2+}$, and $Fe^{3+}$ can also convert each other in the presence of dissolved oxygen. Yin et al. found that PtRu NPs can catalyze the oxidation of $Fe^{2+}$ to $Fe^{3+}$ in the presence of dissolved oxygen, just as a ferroxidase (6). Thereby, they proposed PtRu NPs as a ferroxidase mimic and further developed a $Fe^{2+}$ detection method by employing the ferroxidase-like activity of PtRu NPs.

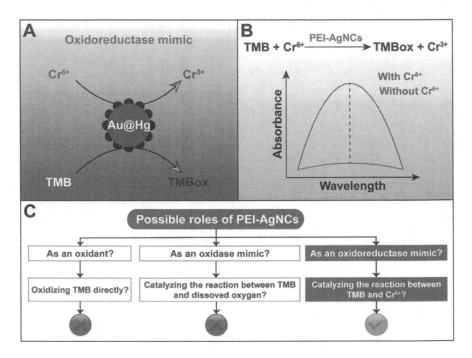

**FIGURE 11.2** (**A**) The concept of Au@Hg as an oxidoreductase mimic catalyzing the redox reaction between TMB and $Cr^{6+}$ [reproduced with permission from (4)]. (**B**) A green and cost-efficient photometric method for $Cr^{6+}$ determination by using PEI-AgNCs to promote the reaction of TMB and $Cr^{6+}$, and (**C**) Possible roles of PEI-AgNCs in the color reaction [reproduced with permission from (5)].

## 11.2.2 ANALYTES ACTING AS NANOZYMES

Some ions, including $Ce^{4+}$ and $Cu^{2+}$, are believed to exhibit some enzyme-like activities due to their redox properties. Thus, the detection of these ions can be realized by using their catalytic ability to trigger colorimetric reactions. To obtain better detection results, the catalytic performance of these ions can be adjusted and optimized through a series of methods. For example, Liu's group proposed a concept of intentionally hydrolyzing $Ce^{4+}$ to achieve a stable response (7). It was difficult to detect $Ce^{4+}$ due to its easy hydrolysis. However, after fully hydrolyzing the target through heating, the resulting hydrolysate, similar to $CeO_2$, exhibited enhanced enzyme-mimetic activity with the assistance of $F^-$ to catalyze the ABTS color reaction (**Figure 11.3A**). Based on this concept, they developed a colorimetric sensor for $Ce^{4+}$, obtaining an LOD of 3.8 μM. Similarly, they found that the $Cu^{2+}$-catalyzed TMB oxidation reaction could be effectively improved by the addition of nucleotides or nucleobases (**Figure 11.3B**) (8). Thus, a colorimetric strategy for $Cu^{2+}$ determination was achieved. Compared to previous reports, detection of these ions does not require additional catalysts, because these ions themselves can act as enzyme mimics to generate color signals. However, the catalytic ability of these ions is often

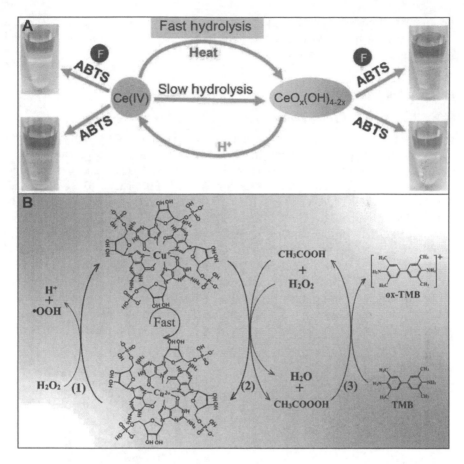

**FIGURE 11.3** (**A**) Heat-promoted hydrolysis of $Ce^{4+}$ and its enzyme-like activity boosted by $F^-$ [reproduced with permission from (7)]. (**B**) $Cu^{2+}$-catalyzed oxidation of TMB in the presence of guanosine 5'-monophosphate [reproduced with permission from (8)].

weak, and the detection requires the assistance of other substances. Therefore, the detection sensitivity and stability need to be further improved in this strategy.

## 11.3   REGULATING NANOZYME ACTIVITY

Since nanozymes are heterogeneous catalysts, their catalytic ability is closely related to material structure and surface property. Some ions can inhibit or improve the activity of nanozymes by direct or indirect adsorption, coordination, and precipitation. With target ions inducing some enzymatic activity changes, the signal outputs originating from nanozyme catalysis change with the level of target ions. Thus, these ions can be determined based on regulating nanozyme activities. According to the interactions between nanozymes and target ions, the sensing strategies can further be divided into: 1) directly regulating the activity of nanozymes (direct interaction between ions and nanozymes, *in situ* reduction of toxic ions on nanozyme surface, the interaction between ions and modifiers on nanozyme surface, etc.) and 2) indirectly regulating the activity of nanozymes (with the assistance of ions, chemical molecules, or biological species).

## 11.3.1 DIRECTLY REGULATING THE ACTIVITY OF NANOZYMES

### 11.3.1.1 Interactions Between Analytes and Active Nanozymes

Mercury ($Hg^{2+}$) ions pose a huge threat to the environment and human health. Nanozyme-based sensors are promising candidates to determine $Hg^{2+}$ due to their stability, convenience, and cost-effectiveness. Recently, lots of nanozyme studies have been reported for the effective detection of $Hg^{2+}$. For instance, Fu et al. found that $Hg^{2+}$ can inhibit the enzymatic activity of Pt NPsNPs by absorbing on the nanozyme surface (**Figure 11.4A**) (9). It was the first report of utilizing the POD mimic activity of Pt NPs for the colorimetric detection of $Hg^{2+}$. The results showed that with the presence of other common interfering ions, the nanozyme could selectively respond to the target $Hg^{2+}$, meanwhile providing a low LOD of 7.2 nM in the linear range of 0–120 nM. The proposed strategy has great value in environmental $Hg^{2+}$ monitoring. However, it is worth noting that the high cost of noble metals will restrict their widespread use. Another selective detection of $Hg^{2+}$ is based on the strong affinity between $Hg^{2+}$ and S-containing species. In this regard, nanozymes

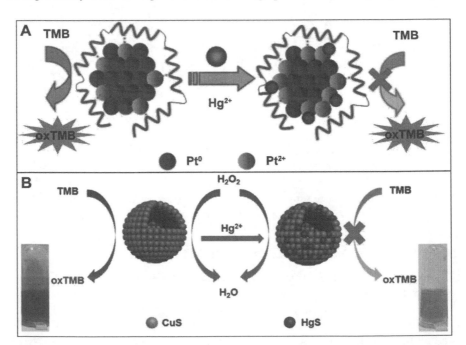

**FIGURE 11.4** (**A**) $Hg^{2+}$ ions can down-regulate the enzymatic activity of Pt NPsNPs [reproduced with permission from (9)]. (**B**) The addition of $Hg^{2+}$ leads to the production of HgS on the CuS surface and further reduces the enzymatic activity of the latter (reproduced with permission from (51)).

containing S species, such as copper sulfide (CuS) (10, 51), were employed for $Hg^{2+}$ detection. The CuS material not only exhibited excellent POD mimic activity but also presented selectivity and rapid uptake toward $Hg^{2+}$. As shown in **Figure 11.4B**, $Hg^{2+}$ significantly inhibited the POD activity of CuS via forming a layer of HgS on the nanozyme surface, and such that a colorimetric platform was developed for $Hg^{2+}$ sensing. Furthermore, by integrating this strategy with a red–green–blue (RGB) color sensor, a portable $Hg^{2+}$ nanosensor with a highly sensitive, selective, and rapid response was obtained. This method, based on the specific interaction between $Hg^{2+}$ and S-containing species, benefits the selective adsorption of $Hg^{2+}$ and enriches the target ion before detection. However, in this sensor nanozymes gradually become poisoned and lose activity, and hence are not suitable for long-term reuse.

On the contrary, a few studies have demonstrated that $Hg^{2+}$ can accelerate the catalytic efficiency of some nanozymes (11, 52, 53). Wang et al. reported that $Hg^{2+}$ could improve the OXD-like activity of bovine serum albumin (BSA)-AgNCs and fabricated a facile $Hg^{2+}$ colorimetric sensor (11). Lu et al. proposed a colorimetric method for $Hg^{2+}$ detection by employing $MoS_2$ as a nanozyme (52). They described that $Hg^{2+}$ could accelerate the electron transfer from $MoS_2$ nanosheets to $H_2O_2$, thereby triggering the POD-like activity of the material. Recently, Lu's group proposed a colorimetric monitoring strategy of $Hg^{2+}$ by triggering the POD activity of Au NPs-decorated carbon dots (Au NPs@C-dots) (53). They explained that, after the addition of $Hg^{2+}$, the electrostatic attraction between Au NPs@C-dots and the TMB substrate was changed, resulting in more substrates binding to the nanozyme surface and increasing its activity. This study provides new insight into the interactions between nanozymes, substrates, and target ions. Though there are lots of examples of detecting $Hg^{2+}$ using nanozyme catalysis, the underlying mechanisms remain to be further uncovered.

In addition to $Hg^{2+}$, $Ag^+$ (12), $Ce^{3+}$ (15), $Cr^{6+}$ (19), $Fe^{2+}$ (18, 54), arsenic ($As^{5+}$) (13, 14), lead ($Pb^{2+}$) (17, 55), aluminum ($Al^{3+}$) (16), fluorine ($F^-$) (20, 56), iodine ($I^-$) (21, 57), sulfur ($S^{2-}$) (26), and phosphate ($PO_4^{3-}$) (22–25, 58) can also directly interact with the active moieties in nanozymes, thus inhibiting or stimulating the catalytic activity of the latter. For example, Deng et al. developed a colorimetric detection method for $Ag^+$ based on inhibiting the OXD activity of chitosan (Ch)-Pt NPs (**Figure 11.5A**) (12). The results showed that the Pt species endowed Ch-Pt NPs with excellent OXD activity, but the activity would be inhibited by $Ag^+$ due to the strong metallophilic interaction between $Pt^{2+}$ and $Ag^+$. As a consequence, the proposed method provided good selectivity against other ions, and the linear range for $Ag^+$ was 5–1000 nM with an LOD of 4 nM. Recently, Qiu's group developed a dual-mode (colorimetric and electrochemical) sensor for $As^{5+}$ monitoring by using nanozyme activity modulation (13). In their work, cobalt oxyhydroxide (CoOOH) nanoflakes were prepared with intrinsic POD-like activity to produce color signals by catalyzing the oxidation of ABTS in the presence of $H_2O_2$. When $As^{5+}$ was introduced into the catalytic system, CoOOH nanoflakes would specifically bind with $As^{5+}$ through the electrostatic attraction and As–O bond. As a result, the active sites on CoOOH were masked, thus decreasing the nanozyme activity. Based on the enzymatic activity turn-down effect induced by $As^{5+}$, a switch-off colorimetric sensor for $As^{5+}$ was explored with an LOD of 3.72 ppb. In addition to the color change, the oxidation process of ABTS could

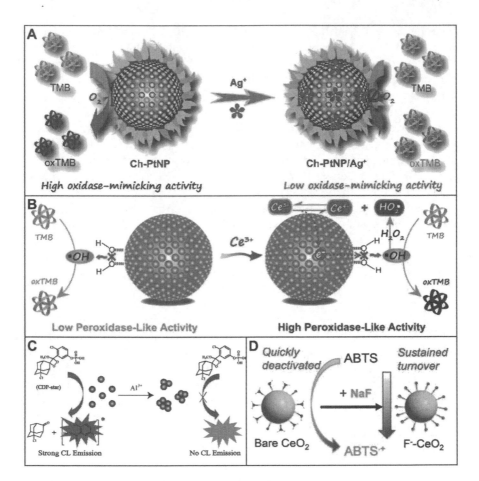

**FIGURE 11.5** **(A)** A colorimetric method for Ag⁺ sensing based on inhibiting the OXD-like activity of chitosan (Ch)-PtNPs (reproduced with permission from (12)). **(B)** $Ce^{3+}$-stimulated POD mimetic activity of Au NPs (reproduced with permission from (15)). **(C)** $Al^{3+}$-induced aggregation of nanoceria leading to the decrease of its phosphatase mimetic activity (reproduced with permission from (16)). **(D)** shows the capping of F⁻ on the $CeO_2$ surface, which can significantly improve the OXD activity of the latter (reproduced with permission from (20)).

also provide electrochemical signal outputs. Therefore, electrochemical sensing of the target $As^{5+}$ with higher sensitivity was further obtained. This dual-mode strategy provides a variety of options for $As^{5+}$ detection, where colorimetry can be used to achieve rapid on-site monitoring and electrochemical measurement for higher sensitivity and accuracy.

Deng et al. investigated the effect of $Ce^{3+}$, a rare-earth ion, on the POD-like activity of bare Au NPs (15). Surprisingly, $Ce^{3+}$ could significantly activate the enzyme-like activity of Au NPs with no interferences from other common ions (**Figure 11.5B**). They further found that the enzymatic activity enhancement promoted by $Ce^{3+}$ was highly related to its electron-donating capability and redox recycling ability.

According to this phenomenon, a $Ce^{3+}$ colorimetric sensing method was developed with an LOD of 2.2 nM. In addition to colorimetric and electrochemical analyses, the chemiluminescent mode has also been utilized for target ion determination based on nanozyme catalysis. Tian et al. reported a highly sensitive chemiluminescent strategy for $Al^{3+}$ sensing based on the phosphatase mimetic activity of nanoceria (**Figure 11.5C**) (16). The coordination between $Al^{3+}$ and nanoceria could lead to the aggregation of nanoceria, thus down-regulating its catalytic activity toward the hydrolysis of a substrate.

Apart from metal cations, inorganic anions can also directly regulate the catalytic activity of nanozymes, among which the influences of halide ions on some nanozymes have been intensively explored (20, 21, 56, 57, 59). For instance, Liu's group found that the OXD activity of nanoceria increased by more than 100 times after capping of $F^-$ (**Figure 11.6D**) (20). Further experiments verified that the surface charge of nanoceria could be modulated by $F^-$, accelerating the electron transfer. Based on this, an ultrasensitive and selective method of $F^-$ sensing was achieved with an LOD of 0.64 μM. Practical applications of the method were also demonstrated by employing it to monitoring $F^-$ in water and toothpaste. Additionally, our group found that $I^-$ could boost the activity of $VO_x$ via the synergetic modulation of surface charge and electronic structure (21). The $VO_x$ nanozyme showed quite low catalytic efficiency toward the TMB chromogenic reaction when trace $VO_x$ was utilized. It was surprisingly found that a small amount of $I^-$ (3.3 μM) could greatly promote the nanozyme activity and efficiency. Zeta potential and X-ray photoelectron spectroscopy (XPS) measurements revealed that $I^-$ could modulate the surface charge of the $VO_x$ material and change its electronic structure. Given the positive effect of $I^-$, we achieved the highly sensitive determination of the target with an LOD down to 74 pM. For other halide ions, Liu et al. investigated the impacts of various halide ions ($F^-$, $I^-$, chlorine, ($Cl^-$), and bromine ($Br^-$)) on Au NPs (59). They found that $F^-$ and $Cl^-$ could not influence the activity of Au NPs because the two species had no or very weak interactions with Au. However, $Br^-$ and $I^-$ could effectively inhibit the POD activity of Au NPs due to their strong affinities toward Au NPs. Their work systematically revealed the charge rule of anion-mediated Au nanozyme activity, which will be of great significance in discriminating these halide ions in complicated matrices.

Given that the level of phosphate ions is a significant indicator of eutrophication in environmental waters, it becomes quite important to develop efficient methods for phosphate ion monitoring (22–25, 58, 60). Recently, our group developed a smartphone-assisted on-off photometric approach for phosphate ion analysis based on the analyte-promoted POD-mimicking catalytic activity of porous $Ce_xZr_{1-x}O_2$ (x≥0.5) (23). The $Ce^{4+}/Ce^{3+}$ redox pair in $Ce_xZr_{1-x}O_2$ endowed it with certain activity to catalyze the TMB color reaction with the participation of $H_2O_2$, and both the existing zirconium ($Zr^{4+}$) and $Ce^{4+}$ species enabled the nanozyme to specifically recognize phosphate ion. It was observed that the bonded phosphate ion could greatly promote the POD-like activity of the $Ce_xZr_{1-x}O_2$ nanocomposite toward positively charged TMB. According to this new finding, high-performance sensing of phosphate ion with a wide detection range, high sensitivity, and good selectivity was realized, with an LOD down to 0.09 μM. Further, a 3D-printed smartphone-based system was designed and coupled with the sensing method, enabling a rapid, convenient, in-field, and instrument-free analysis of phosphate ions. To improve the stability and repeatability of detection, we further proposed a high-performance dual-channel ratiometric colorimetric method for phosphate ion sensing based on the analyte-triggered differential OXD-mimicking activity changes of oxidized Ce-Zr metal-organic frameworks (MOFs) (oxidized UiO-66(Ce/Zr)) (24). By integrating two active metal sites into the MOF, the prepared nanomaterial not only exhibited excellent OXD-like activity to catalyze the oxidation of TMB and ABTS but also improved the recognition ability toward phosphate ion, where the enzymatic ability came from Ce sites and the specific capability was mainly assigned to the existence of Zr sites. When oxidized UiO-66(Ce/Zr) was pretreated with phosphate ions, the surface state of oxidized UiO-66(Ce/Zr) changed due to the newly formed Zr–O–P with negative charges (**Figure 11.6A**). The changes in electronegativity greatly affected the affinities between the nanozyme and different chromogenic substrates, leading to target-induced differential OXD-like activity toward TMB and ABTS. With the above phenomenon, a dual-channel ratiometric colorimetric method was established for phosphate ion monitoring. Compared to other single-signal colorimetric methods, this work achieved a wider detection range from 66 nM to 666.7 µM and an LOD of 14 nM. Moreover, practical analysis in tap and river water was also conducted, indicating its potential for practical use. Furthermore, a Fe-Zr bi-MOF (UiO-66(Fe/Zr)-NH$_2$) with triple functions of self-fluorescence, POD-mimic activity, and specific recognition of Pi was designed and developed for the high-performance ratiometric fluorescent sensing of phosphate ion (**Figure 11.6B**) (25). The sensor was built by coordinating a fluorescent organic ligand (BDC-NH$_2$) with two types of inorganic metal ions (Zr$^{4+}$ and Ce$^{4+}$). The inherent fluorescence of UiO-66(Fe/Zr)-NH$_2$ was observed at 435 nm. In the presence of H$_2$O$_2$ and OPD, the UiO-66(Fe/Zr)-NH$_2$ nanozyme could catalyze the oxidation of OPD to its fluorescent product OPDox, which exhibited a fluorescence signal at 555 nm. Interestingly, the generated OPDox could effectively quench the self-fluorescence of UiO-66(Fe/Zr)-NH$_2$ via the inner filter effect. When phosphate ion was introduced, the POD-mimetic activity of UiO-66(Fe/Zr)-NH$_2$ was significantly suppressed because of the good affinity between Zr–O nodes and phosphate ion. The turn-down POD-mimic activity reduced the generation of OPDox in the catalytic system, thus weakening the fluorescence signal at 555 nm. Meanwhile, the inner filter effect was inhibited due to less OPDox, and such that the self-fluorescence of UiO-66(Fe/Zr)-NH$_2$ at 435 nm was recovered again. As a result, the fluorescence ratio of I$_{555}$/I$_{435}$ gradually changed with the addition of phosphate ion. The LOD of this method was 85 nM and the linear range was 0.2–266.7 µM, and it was competent for an accurate analysis of phosphate ion in various water matrices.

### 11.3.1.2 Interactions Between Analytes and Inactive Modifiers on Nanozyme Surface

Some nanozyme-based assays face several problems, including the low enzymatic activity, poor selectivity, and easy agglomeration of NPs. Fortunately, these problems can be alleviated by modifying the surface of nanozymes. Because the surface states of particles directly determine the activity of nanozymes, the catalytic ability and detection efficiency of nanozymes can be effectively tuned by affecting the

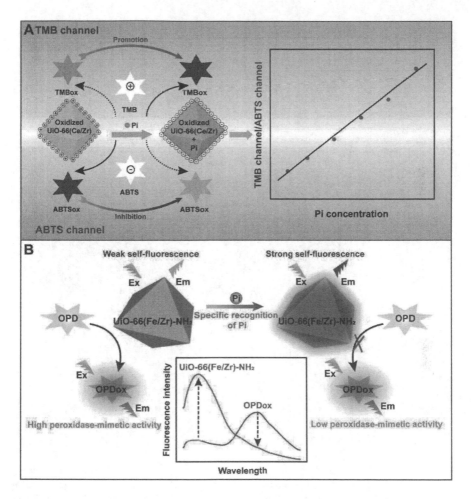

**FIGURE 11.6** (**A**) Dual-channel ratiometric colorimetric sensing of phosphate ions based on target-induced differential OXD-like activity changes of oxidized UiO-66(Ce/Zr) (reproduced with permission from (24)). (**B**) High-performance ratiometric fluorescent phosphate ion sensing based on UiO-66(Fe/Zr)-NH$_2$ with three functions (reproduced with permission from (25)).

electronic structure, adjusting surface acidity, changing site exposure, enhancing target adsorption, etc. Up to now, species, including inorganic ions, citrate, amino acids, chitosan, β-cyclodextrin (β-CD), and proteins, are popular coating agents to modify the surface of nanozymes, providing potential functional groups for selective recognition of targets.

In this regard, our group proposed a novel strategy for ultrasensitive Hg$^{2+}$ detection based on the Hg$^{2+}$-triggered POD-mimicking activity of cysteine-decorated ferromagnetic particles (Cys-Fe$_3$O$_4$) (36). As depicted in **Figure 11.7A**, the POD activity of Fe$_3$O$_4$ was first inhibited by surface modification due to the blocking effect caused by the coordination of Cys on the Fe$_3$O$_4$ surface. In the presence of

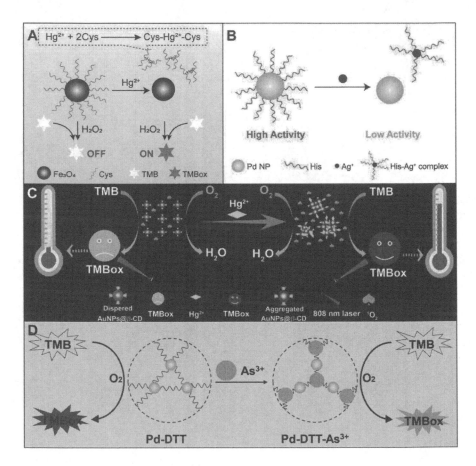

**FIGURE 11.7** **(A)** The detection principle of $Hg^{2+}$ based on target-triggered POD activity of Cys-$Fe_3O_4$ [reproduced with permission from (36)]. **(B)** $Ag^+$ sensing principle based on inhibiting the POD activity of His-Pd NPs via losing the surface modifier His (reproduced with permission from (37)). **(C)** Photothermometric detection of $Hg^{2+}$ based on aggregation-enhanced OXD-like activity of Au NPs@β-CD [reproduced with permission from (61)]. **(D)** Reassembly-induced OXD-mimicking activity inhibition of Pd-DTT by $As^{3+}$ (reproduced with permission from (38)).

$Hg^{2+}$, the stronger coordination between Cys and $Hg^{2+}$ resulted in the exfoliation of Cys from the $Fe_3O_4$ surface, and thus the catalytic sites on $Fe_3O_4$ were exposed again and the catalytic ability was also restored to generate an obvious color signal. By using the $Hg^{2+}$-triggered POD activity of Cys-$Fe_3O_4$, an enzyme-mimicking biosensor was fabricated to determine $Hg^{2+}$ in the linear range of 0.02–90 nM, presenting an LOD down to 5.9 pM. This sensor also exhibited excellent selectivity attributed to the strong coordination interaction between Cys and $Hg^{2+}$. On the contrary, the POD activity of Pd NPs could be dramatically boosted after modifying them with histidine (His) (37). However, the ability was significantly inhibited when $Ag^+$ was added, due to the stronger interaction between $Ag^+$ and His (**Figure 11.7B**). Based on the target-suppressed POD-mimicking activity principle, a highly sensitive determination of $Ag^+$ (linear range = 30–300 nM; LOD = 4.7 nM). The proposed sensor exhibits advantages of simple fabrication, high detection sensitivity, outstanding selectivity, and visual readout.

Apart from the above-mentioned principles, aggregation and dispersion of nanozymes can also be utilized to detect pollutant ions. For example, Hu et al. found that the POD activity of glutathione (GSH)-capped Au NCs was enhanced when $Pb^{2+}$ was introduced. The results explained that the stimulated activity was triggered by the aggregation of Au NCs due to the GSH-$Pb^{2+}$ interaction (39). Based on this finding, a simple and reliable colorimetric method for $Pb^{2+}$ detection was developed. Recently, Xue et al. reported a novel $Hg^{2+}$ detection method based on the aggregation-activated OXD-like activity of Au NPs (61). As displayed in **Figure 11.7C**, β-CD-capped Au NPs had poor ability to catalyze the oxidation of TMB to its product TMBox. Thus, no temperature change could be measured under laser irradiation. However, due to the specific interaction between $Hg^{2+}$ and β-CD modified on AuNPs surface, the OXD activity was significantly boosted by the $Hg^{2+}$-induced aggregation of AuNPs, resulting in the rapid production of TMBox. As a result, under the laser irradiation, the generated TMBox provided a temperature response due to the photothermal effect. With the principle, the concentration of $Hg^{2+}$ could be colorimetrically detected (linear range = 0.4–15 μM; LOD = 0.035 μM), and it could also be detected simply through a thermometer reader, with an LOD of 0.06 μM. Similarly, we proposed a colorimetric sensing strategy of $As^{3+}$ based on the reassembly-induced OXD-like activity inhibition of dithiothreitol (DTT)-capped Pd NPs (38). The Pd-DTT nanozyme had a strong catalytic ability to convert TMB into blue TMBox. By the addition of $As^{3+}$, the OXD activity of Pd-DTT was significantly suppressed because it could strongly chelate with the sulphydryl groups in DTT (**Figure 11.7D**), resulting in a recombination of the Pd-DTT nanozyme. With this principle, detection of $As^{3+}$ in a wide linear range was achieved.

### 11.3.1.3 *In Situ* Reduction of Analytes Onto Nanozyme Surface

Some ions, especially $Hg^{2+}$ and $Ag^+$, can be easily *in situ* reduced and deposited onto the surface of nanozymes, which can dramatically affect the catalytic activity of nanozymes by changing their surface chemistry properties. According to the principle regulating the activity of nanozymes by *in situ* reduction, several methods for $Hg^{2+}$ and $Ag^+$ detection have been reported, including colorimetric, fluorescence, SERS, and smartphone-assisted readout. Invariably, the *in situ* reduction of metal ions significantly changes the catalytic activity of nanozymes, providing the basis for ion sensing. The intrinsic POD activity of Pt-based nanomaterials, such as Pt NPs (62–64), citrate-capped Pt NPs (27), Pt NPs@UiO-66-NH$_2$ (65), and Au@AgPt NPs (28), can be selectively suppressed by $Hg^{2+}$ due to the specific interaction between Pt NPs and $Hg^{2+}$. Wei et al. demonstrated that citrate-capped Pt NPs had a strong ability to catalyze the colorimetric system of TMB and $H_2O_2$, but this ability was inhibited once $Hg^{2+}$ was added because $Hg^{2+}$ was reduced into $Hg^0$ by citrate under the catalysis of Pt NPs to form an amalgam (27). To improve the detection performance, Ma et al. chose OPD as a fluorescent and colorimetric probe to make the response to the inhibition effect of $Hg^{2+}$ on the POD activity of Pt NPs, and this dual-readout measurement effectively improved the accuracy of $Hg^{2+}$ detection (63). Further, Chen et al.

realized the simple in-field measurement of $Hg^{2+}$ by constructing a paper-based colorimetric device via pre-loading Pt NPs and TMB on test strips (64).

Recently, a novel colorimetric/SERS dual-mode detection method of $Hg^{2+}$ was proposed by using SERS-active POD-like Au@AgPt NPs (28). As shown in **Figure 11.8A**, the Au@AgPt NPs integrated the SERS activity of Au and POD activity of Pt, which not only catalyzed the reaction between TMB and $H_2O_2$ but also acted as a colorimetric/SERS dual-mode probe to signal the reaction. Experiments demonstrated that the presence of $Hg^{2+}$ could affect the catalytic and SERS properties of Au@AgPt NPs, generating less TMBox due to the degenerated POD activity. Thus, the colorimetric and SERS signals originating from TMBox were correspondingly weakened. Based on this principle, a linear range from 1 to 100 μM with an LOD of 0.52 μM was obtained for $Hg^{2+}$ sensing by UV-vis measurement, and more sensitive SERS sensing of the target was achieved with an LOD as low as 0.28 nM.

Cao's group investigated how $Hg^{2+}$ regulated the POD activity of Au NPs in different electrolyte environments (66). Their results showed that the ability of bare Au NPs to catalyze the oxidation of TMB by $H_2O_2$ was greatly inhibited under a high salt concentration inducing severe agglomeration of Au NPs (**Figure 11.8B**). When $Hg^{2+}$ was further added, the reaction system had no response at all. Instead, they functionalized Au NPs with oligo-ethylene glycol (OEG) to keep their stability in high ionic strength environments. Although these OEG-modified Au NPs were effectively protected from agglomeration at high salt concentrations, their enzyme activity was still inhibited due to surface coating. Interestingly, it was found that the catalytic activity of OEG-Au NPs could be selectively recovered in the presence of $Hg^{2+}$, where the Au-Hg amalgam was formed on the nanozyme surface. As a result, they proposed a highly sensitive and selective assay for $Hg^{2+}$ sensing. Also, the proposed assay was very suitable for the detection of $Hg^{2+}$ ions in real samples, especially in seawater.

Similarly, $Ag^+$ can also stimulate the enzymatic activity of some nanozymes, and these nanozymes include graphitic carbon nitride $(g\text{-}C_3N_4)$-Pt NPs (34), BSA@ AuNCs (35), β-Casein-AuNPs (67), and ZIF-8/GO (68). Typically, Tang et al.

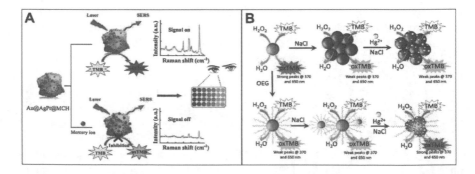

**FIGURE 11.8** (**A**) Colorimetric/SERS dual-mode detection of $Hg^{2+}$ based on Au@AgPt NPs (reproduced with permission from Ref. (28)). (**B**) The detection principle of $Hg^{2+}$ via the enzyme-like activity of Au NPs in different electrolyte environments (reproduced with permission from Ref. (66)).

prepared a g-$C_3N_4$-Pt NPs hybrid, which showed outstanding performance in catalyzing the oxidation of TMB to produce colored products (34). When $Ag^+$ was reduced by citric acid and deposited on the surface of g-$C_3N_4$-Pt NPs, the POD-mimic ability of g-$C_3N_4$-Pt NPs would be inhibited efficiently. Based on this mechanism, a rapid and economical colorimetric assay was developed for ultrasensitive detection of $Ag^+$ with an LOD down to the pM level.

## 11.3.2 INDIRECTLY REGULATING THE ACTIVITY OF NANOZYMES

The catalytic activity of nanozymes is not only influenced by their surface properties but also related to the systems where they exist. Some specific interactions between additional molecules and targets (e.g., $Hg^{2+}$ and T-rich ssDNA) can be employed to adjust the nanozyme-involved systems for ion sensing.

### 11.3.2.1 With the Assistance of Ions

Xia's group fabricated a colorimetric sensor based on the aggregation/dispersion-mediated POD-like activity of $MoS_2$ QDs (15). It is commonly regarded that the enzyme-mimetic activity of NPs is closely related to their aggregation state. They found that the original, highly dispersive $MoS_2$ QDs showed poor POD-like activity in an aqueous solution, but the addition of $Fe^{3+}$ would induce the aggregation of $MoS_2$ QDs as verified by atomic force microscopy (AFM), thus enhancing the catalytic activity toward TMB oxidation with the presence of $H_2O_2$. However, the aggregation state would be broken by the introduction of PPi due to the strong interaction between $Fe^{3+}$ and PPi, and such that the activity dropped down again. Based on this principle, the determination of PPi based on the aggregation/dispersion-mediated POD-like activity of $MoS_2$ QDs had been well established with good analytical performance. However, the reasons for $Fe^{3+}$ inducing the aggregation of $MoS_2$ QDs and the stimulated POD-like activity of the aggregated QDs are still unclear. It is believed that once these underlying mechanisms are fully uncovered, the controllable aggregation and dispersion of QDs acting as potential nanozymes will be a general strategy for more sensing applications. Besides, our group developed a sensor for PPi detection according to the formation of fluorescent polydopamine (PDA) catalyzed by POD-like FeCo-layered double hydroxide (LDH) (**Figure 11.9A**) (42). The fluorescent signal of PDA could be significantly quenched by the addition of $Fe^{3+}$ due to the generation of the PDA-$Fe^{3+}$ complex, but the quenching effect was canceled as soon as the addition of PPi, which had a strong affinity to bond with $Fe^{3+}$, resulting in the fluorescence recovery of PDA.

Recently, our group fabricated a naked-eye visible colorimetric sensor for the specific detection of $PO_4^{3-}$ based on the $Zr^{4+}$-mediated active surface masking of carboxylated $Fe_3O_4$ nanozyme, as shown in **Figure 11.9B** (41). Compared to bare $Fe_3O_4$ NPs, the modification of 3,4-dihydroxyhydrocinnamic acid (DHCA) on the surface of $Fe_3O_4$ NPs made the $Fe_3O_4$-DHCA material have a stronger ability to trigger the color reaction of TMB in the presence of $H_2O_2$. Based on the prominent affinity of $Zr^{4+}$ toward phosphate ions, the color reaction could be inhibited by $PO_4^{3-}$ with the participation of $Zr^{4+}$, which could further be used to the sensitive and selective determination of $PO_4^{3-}$ with excellent performance. This method needs multiple

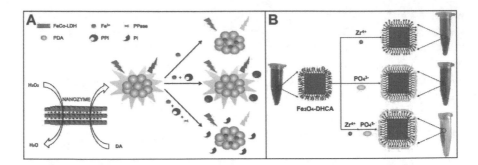

**FIGURE 11.9** **(A)** *In situ* formation of fluorescent PDA catalyzed by POD-mimicking FeCo-LDH and its use for pyrophosphate (PPi) and phosphatase (PPase) activity sensing (reproduced with permission from (42)). **(B)** $Zr^{4+}$-assisted POD-mimicking activity inhibition of DHCA-modified $Fe_3O_4$ nanocubes for $PO_4^{3-}$ sensing (reproduced with permission from (41)).

additions of $Zr^{4+}$ and the analyte. To simplify the operation, the development of new nanozymes integrating the enzyme-like catalytic function with the strong $Zr^{4+}$ recognition sites is highly desired.

### 11.3.2.2 With the Assistance of DNA or Aptamers

DNA or RNA with target-binding affinities, namely aptamers, have emerged as attractive bioreceptors due to their characteristics, such as relatively high and specific affinities to small molecules, easy synthesis and modification, and high flexibility and thermal stability. Many reports have introduced simple colorimetric assays for the detection of metal ions based on the catalytic activity of nanozymes, which is varied depending on the interactions between nanozymes, targets, and specific ssDNA (69). Specifically, ssDNA can be adsorbed onto the surface of these nanomaterials and cover the catalytic activity. Due to the specific interaction between $Hg^{2+}$ and thymine (T)-rich ssDNA, the ssDNA can easily coordinate with $Hg^{2+}$ to form the T–Hg–T structure, thus releasing the activity of nanozymes again. By this approach, some interesting studies have been reported for $Hg^{2+}$ sensing (44, 46). For instance, as depicted in **Figure 11.10A**, a mixed-valence state Ce-based MOF (MVC-MOF) was prepared by the partial oxidation of Ce(III). The synthesized MOF contained a mixed state of $Ce^{3+}/Ce^{4+}$, generating instinct OXD activity. By the addition of ssDNA, the catalytic ability of MVC-MOF was inhibited because the adsorbed ssDNA shielded its active sites. However, in the presence of $Hg^{2+}$, ssDNA preferred to bond with $Hg^{2+}$ and thus released MVC-MOF from inhibition. Based on this principle, colorimetric determination of $Hg^{2+}$ was developed via the OXD-like activity inhibition of MVC-MOF by ssDNA. The content of $Hg^{2+}$ could be linearly detected in the range of 0.05–6 μM with an LOD of 10.5 nM. Apart from $Hg^{2+}$, highly selective detection of other ions, like potassium ($K^+$) (47) and $Pb^{2+}$ (70), has also been achieved via a similar method. Although this kind of strategy makes use of the specific interaction between ions and DNA, providing outstanding selectivity during detection, the instability of DNA is still a problem.

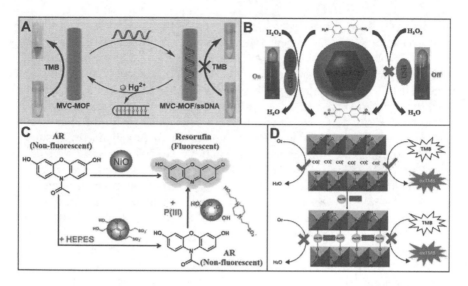

**FIGURE 11.10**  (A) The colorimetric detection method of $Hg^{2+}$ is based on the inhibition effect of DNA on the OXD-like activity of MVC-MOF [reproduced with permission from (45)]. (B) The principle of $Hg^{2+}$ detection based on GSH-involved nanozyme catalysis [reproduced with permission from (71)]. (C) The fluorescence turn-on strategy for phosphite detection [reproduced with permission from (72)]. (D) $As^{3+}$ sensing mechanism based on the 3-MPA-assisted active site and interlayer channel dual-masking of OXD-like Fe-Co-LDH [reproduced with permission from (48)].

### 11.3.2.3   With the Assistance of Biothiols

Biothiols are a class of important biomolecules. More importantly, these species offer extremely strong affinities toward $Hg^{2+}$ ions. Therefore, they are usually used to provide specific recognition sites for $Hg^{2+}$ detection. Generally, if sulfhydryl-containing compounds are added to nanozyme catalyzed systems, it will greatly suppress these chromogenic reactions due to their competitive oxidation with substrates. However, the inhibition effect can be canceled as the addition of $Hg^{2+}$, because biothiols prefer to bond with $Hg^{2+}$ due to the strong affinity between biothiols and $Hg^{2+}$. Thereby, an "off–on" colorimetric sensor for $Hg^{2+}$ detection can be fabricated with excellent sensitivity and selectivity. As shown in **Figure 11.10B**, a colorimetric sensor based on $Fe_3O_4$@ZIF-67 as a POD mimic was fabricated for the selective determination of $Hg^{2+}$ under the mediation of GSH (71). Originally, the POD activity of $Fe_3O_4$@ZIF-67 could catalyze the oxidation reaction of TMB to TMBox, resulting in an obvious color change in the solution. But with the presence of GSH, the strong reducibility of the thiol would contribute to a competition effect with TMB or directly reduce TMBox into TMB again, leading to a color fading phenomenon. Interestingly, the color signal would be recovered after the addition of $Hg^{2+}$ due to the specific interaction between $Hg^{2+}$ and GSH. With this strategy, other nanozymes, such as $MnO_2$ nanorods (73), C-dots (74), and Au@$NH_2$-MIL-125(Ti) (75), have also been explored for the detection of $Hg^{2+}$ with the assistance of biothiols.

#### 11.3.2.4  With the Assistance of Other Molecules

Liu's group presented a fluorescent "turn-on" sensor for the quantitative and highly selective analysis of phosphite based on the different coordination strengths of N and P lone-pair electrons toward NiO (72). In their work, an N-containing compound, HEPES, was employed as an inhibitor for the OXD activity of NiO NPs toward the oxidation of Amplex red (**Figure 11.10C**). Among various phosphorus (P)-, selenium (Se)-, As-, and S-containing species, along with different cations, phosphite was the only one that could restore the activity, likely due to its stronger affinity with the nanozyme surface. Under optimal conditions, the sensor detected phosphite ions up to 1 mM with an LOD of 1.46 μM. Besides, our group proposed a colorimetric method for $As^{3+}$ detection based on the 3-mercaptopropionic acid (3-MPA)-assisted active site and interlayer channel dual-masking of OXD-like FeCo-LDH (**Figure 11.10D**). The FeCo-LDH showed high OXD-mimicking activity to catalyze the oxidation of colorless TMB to blue TMBox. With the presence of 3-MPA, $As^{3+}$could anchor onto the Fe* sites in FeCo-LDH by forming a robust Fe- $As^{3+}$-3-3-MPA- $As^{3+}$-Fe structure, masking both the active sites and interlayer channels of FeCo-LDH for catalysis. Based on this rule, an LOD as low as 0.035 μM was achieved for the determination of $As^{3+}$. Also, the 3-MPA-assisted method could effectively exclude the possible interferences from $As^{5+}$, Hg(II), and Pb(II).

### 11.4  BASED ON AFFECTING NANOZYME CATALYZED SYSTEMS

When there is competitive oxidation between ions, such as $Fe^{2+}$ (49, 76) and $S^{2-}$ (50), and chromogenic substrates, the color evolution of the chromogenic substrate can be affected. With this principle, the inhibition degree of nanozyme catalyzed systems can be used for the detection of these ions. For instance, C-dots/$Mn_3O_4$ as an instinct OXD mimic can accelerate the oxidation of $Fe^{2+}$ to $Fe^{3+}$ (**Figure 11.11**),

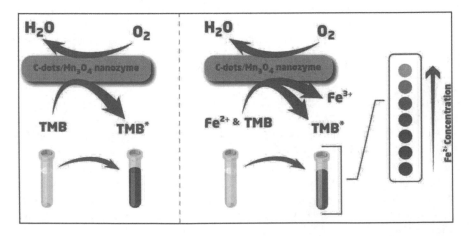

**FIGURE 11.11**   $Fe^{2+}$ affecting the C-dots/$Mn_3O_4$ catalyzed TMB color reaction for $Fe^{2+}$ sensing (49).

which inevitably affects the oxidation of TMB catalyzed by the nanozyme. The competitive interaction between TMB and $Fe^{2+}$ can further be employed to determine $Fe^{2+}$ ions. As a result, based on the competitive oxidation of TMB and $Fe^{2+}$, selective detection of the latter was achieved (linear range= 0.03–0.83 μM; LOD = 0.03 μM). Besides, $S^{2-}$ can also be detected in a similar method (50), and the underlying mechanism of $S^{2-}$ detection may involve the competitive oxidation between the targeted $S^{2-}$ and chromogenic TMB with $H_2O_2$, as well as the re-reduction of oxidized TMB by $S^{2-}$ ions. However, some reducing anions such as ascorbate potentially disturb the sensing system, which will be a major limitation of the proposed method.

## 11.5  SUMMARY AND FUTURE PERSPECTIVES

With the merits of easy mass production, low cost, and excellent robustness against harsh environments, nanozymes are attractive candidates in enzyme-based sensor development. A tremendous progress has been made in utilizing the instinct physicochemical properties of nanozymes to overcome the high cost and instability of natural commercial enzyme-based biosensors. In this chapter, some basic strategies of nanozyme-based detection for various pollutant ions were summarized.

Although the field using nanozyme catalysis to detect pollutant ions is booming, it is still in its infancy. There are several difficulties to overcome: (a) at present, the type of targets that nanozyme-based sensors can detect is still very limited. Although some effective detection strategies for different pollutant ions have been successfully proposed, toxic pollutants in the environment are far more than these species. As a result, their application is still quite limited in the environmental analytical field. In this respect, establishing new nanozyme-based sensing principles and strategies to deal with more pollutants will be actively pursued. (b) another challenge for nanozyme-based sensors is their selectivity toward targets. For some extremely toxic pollutants, the presence of trace amounts may seriously affect the ecological environment and human health. However, as for some nanozyme-based assays, the selective detection of certain ions is still insufficient, which cannot meet the requirements for practical detection. Therefore, endowing nanozymes with reliable and specific recognition sites and improving the detection selectivity is necessary. (c) currently, most nanozyme-based assays for pollutant ions rely on colorimetric detection. Although the colorimetric mode is convenient for signal reading, its relatively poor sensitivity limits wider application. Fortunately, thanks to the features of photoelectric, thermal, and magnetic properties of nanomaterials, nanozyme-based sensors can also realize multimode detection. Therefore, expanding different sensing modes to meet various needs will bring better prospects for nanozymes in the environmental monitoring field.

## ACKNOWLEDGMENTS

X. Niu appreciates the support from the National Natural Science Foundation of China (No. 21605061) and the Cultivation Project for Excellent Young Teachers in Jiangsu University (No. 4111310004).

# REFERENCES

1. Aragay G, Pons J, Merkoci A. 2011. *Chem Rev* 111: 3433–58
2. Quang DT, Kim JS. 2010. *Chem Rev* 110: 6280–301
3. Sun H, Cai S, Wang C, Chen Y, Yang R. 2020. *ChemBioChem* 21: 2572–84
4. Zhang X, Liu W, Li X, Zhang Z, Shan D, et al. 2018. *Anal Chem* 90: 14309–15
5. Xue Q, Li X, Peng Y, Liu P, Peng H, Niu X. 2020. *Microchimica Acta* 187: 263
6. Liu C, Yan Y, Zhang X, Mao Y, Ren X, et al. 2020. *Nanoscale* 12: 3068–75
7. Wang Y, Yang J, Zhao Y, Liu J. 2019. *Chem Commun* 55: 13434–7
8. Peng D, Liang R-P, Qiu J-D, Liu J. 2019. *J Anal Test* 3: 260–8
9. Li W, Bin C, Zhang HX, Sun YH, Wang J, et al. 2015. *Biosens Bioelectron* 66: 251–8
10. Xiong Y, Su L, Yang H, Zhang P, Ye F. 2015. *New J Chem* 39: 9221–7
11. Wang GL, Jin LY, Wu XM, Dong YM, Li ZJ. 2015. *Anal Chim Acta* 871: 1–8
12. Deng H, He S, Lin X, Yang L, Lin Z, et al. 2019. *Chin Chem Lett*
13. Wen SH, Zhong XL, Wu YD, Liang RP, Zhang L, Qiu JD. 2019. *Anal Chem* 91: 6487–97
14. Babu Christus AA, Panneerselvam P, Ravikumar A. 2018. *Anal Methods* 10: 4378–86
15. Deng H-H, Luo B-Y, He S-B, Chen R-T, Lin Z, et al. 2019. *Anal Chem* 91: 4039–46
16. Tian X, Liao H, Wang M, Feng L, Fu W, Hu L. 2020. *Biosens Bioelectron* 152: 112027
17. Tang Y, Hu Y, Yang Y, Liu B, Wu Y. 2020. *Analytica Chimica Acta* 1106: 115–25
18. Wang Y, Hu J, Zhuang Q, Ni Y. 2016. *Biosens Bioelectron* 80: 111–7
19. Amini R, Rahimpour E, Jouyban A. 2020. *Analytica Chimica Acta* 1117: 9–17
20. Liu B, Huang Z, Liu J. 2016. *Nanoscale* 8: 13562–7
21. Niu X, He Y, Li X, Song H, Zhang W, et al. 2017. *ChemistrySelect* 2: 10854–9
22. Chen C, Lu L, Zheng Y, Zhao D, Yang F, Yang X. 2015. *Analytical Methods* 7: 161–7
23. Li X, Liu B, Hu Z, Liu P, Ye K, et al. 2020. *Environ Res* 189: 109921
24. Li X, Niu X, Liu P, Xu X, Du D, Lin Y. 2020. *Sens Actuators B Chem* 321: 128546
25. Gökçal B, Kip Ç, Tuncel A. 2020. *J Alloys Compounds* 843: 156012
26. Liao H, Hu L, Zhang Y, Yu X, Liu Y, Li R. 2018. *Mikrochim Acta* 185: 143
27. Wu G-W, He S-B, Peng H-P, Deng H-H, Liu A-L, et al. 2014. *Anal Chem* 86: 10955–60
28. Song C, Li J, Sun Y, Jiang X, Zhang J, et al. 2020. *Sens Actuators B Chem* 310: 127849
29. Long YJ, Li YF, Liu Y, Zheng JJ, Tang J, Huang CZ. 2011. *Chem Commun (Camb)* 47: 11939–41
30. Wu X, Chen T, Wang J, Yang G. 2018. *J Mater Chem B* 6: 105–11
31. Zhang S, Li H, Wang Z, Liu J, Zhang H, et al. 2015. *Nanoscale* 7: 8495–502
32. Li Q, Wu F, Mao M, Ji X, Wei L, et al. 2019. *Anal Methods* 11: 4014–21
33. Huang L, Zhu Q, Zhu J, Luo L, Pu S, et al. 2019. *Inorg Chem* 58: 1638-46
34. Tang S, Wang M, Li G, Li X, Chen W, Zhang L. 2018. *Mikrochim Acta* 185: 273
35. Chang Y, Zhang Z, Hao J, Yang W, Tang J. 2016. *Sens Actuators B Chem* 232: 692–7
36. Niu X, He Y, Li X, Zhao H, Pan J, et al. 2019. *Sens Actuators B Chem* 281: 445–52
37. Zhang W, Niu X, Meng S, Li X, He Y, et al. 2018. *Sens Actuators B Chem* 273: 400–7
38. Jin R, Xing Z, Kong D, Yan X, Liu F, et al. 2019. *J Mater Chem B* 7: 1230–7
39. Liao H, Liu G, Liu Y, Li R, Fu W, Hu L. 2017. *Chem Commun (Camb)* 53: 10160–3
40. Zhang D, Chen Z, Omar H, Deng L, Khashab NM. 2015. *ACS Appl Mater Interfaces* 7: 4589–94
41. Li X, Liu B, Ye K, Ni L, Xu X, et al. 2019. *Sens Actuators B Chem* 297: 126822
42. Xu X, Zou X, Wu S, Wang L, Niu X, et al. 2019. *Analytica Chimica Acta* 1053: 89–97
43. Xia W, Zhang P, Fu W, Hu L, Wang Y. 2019. *Chem Commun* 55: 2039–42
44. Kim YS, Jurng J. 2013. *Sens Actuators B Chem* 176: 253–7
45. Wang C, Tang G, Tan H. 2018. *Mikrochim Acta* 185: 475
46. Wang J, Wang J, Zhou P, Tao H, Wang X, Wu Y. 2020. *Microchimica Acta* 187: 99
47. Chen Z, Tan L, Wang S, Zhang Y, Li Y. 2016. *Biosens Bioelectron* 79: 749–57

48. Xu X, Zou X, Wu S, Wang L, Pan J, et al. 2019. *Microchimica Acta* 186: 815
49. Honarasa F, Peyravi F, Amirian H. 2020. *J Iranian Chem Soc* 17: 507–12
50. Liu X, Huang L, Wang Y, Sun J, Yue T, et al. 2020. *Sens Actuators B Chem* 306: 127565
51. Fang Y, Zhang Y, Cao L, Yang J, Hu M, et al. 2020. *ACS Appl Mater Interfaces* 12: 11761–8
52. Lu Y, Yu J, Ye W, Yao X, Zhou P, et al. 2016. *Microchimica Acta* 183: 2481–9
53. Liu W, Tian L, Du J, Wu J, Liu Y, et al. 2020. *Analyst* 145: 5500–7
54. Hu J, Zhuang Q, Wang Y, Ni Y. 2016. *Analyst* 141: 1822–9
55. Sun K, Li S-Y, Chen H-L, Huang Q-G, Si Y. 2019. *Int J Environ Anal Chem* 99: 501–14
56. Yu R, Wang R, He X, Liu T, Shen J, Dai Z. 2019. *Chem Commun* 55: 11543–6
57. He S-B, Chen F-Q, Xiu L-F, Peng H-P, Deng H-H, et al. 2020. *Anal Bioanal Chem* 412: 499–506
58. Wang X, Qin L, Lin M, Xing H, Wei H. 2019. *Anal Chem*
59. Liu Y, Xiang Y, Zhen Y, Guo R. 2017. *Langmuir* 33: 6372–81
60. Zhao Y, Li H, Lopez A, Su H, Liu J. 2020. *ChemBioChem* n/a
61. An P, Rao H, Gao M, Xue X, Liu X, et al. 2020. *Chem Commun* 56: 9799–802
62. Kora AJ, Rastogi L. 2018. *Sens Actuators B Chem* 254: 690–700
63. Zhou Y, Ma Z. 2017. *Sens Actuators B Chem* 249: 53–8
64. Chen W, Fang X, Li H, Cao H, Kong J. 2016. *Sci Rep* 6: 31948
65. Li H, Liu H, Zhang J, Cheng Y, Zhang C, et al. 2017. *ACS Appl Mater Interfaces* 9: 40716–25
66. Logan N, McVey C, Elliott C, Cao C. 2020. *Nano Res* 13: 989–98
67. Liu Y, Xiang Y, Ding D, Guo R. 2016. *RSC Adv* 6: 112435–44
68. Li C-r, Hai J, Fan L, Li S-l, Wang B-d, Yang Z-y. 2019. *Sens Actuators B Chem* 284: 213–9
69. Chatterjee B, Das SJ, Anand A, Sharma TK. 2020. *Mater Sci Energy Technol* 3: 127–35
70. Tao Z, Zhou Y, Duan N, Wang Z. 2020. *Catalysts* 10: 600
71. Christus AAB, Panneerselvam P, Ravikumar A, Morad N, Sivanesan S. 2018. *J Photochem Photobiol Chem* 364: 715–24
72. Chang Y, Liu M, Liu J. 2020. *Anal Chem* 92: 3118–24
73. Yang H, Xiong Y, Zhang P, Su L, Ye F. 2015. *Anal Methods* 7: 4596–601
74. Mohammadpour Z, Safavi A, Shamsipur M. 2014. *Chem Eng J* 255: 1–7
75. Zhang Y, Song J, Pan Q, Zhang X, Shao W, et al. 2020. *J Mater Chem B* 8: 114–24
76. Zhang K, Hu X, Liu J, Yin J-J, Hou S, et al. 2011. *Langmuir* 27: 2796–803

# 12 Nanozymes in Pesticides Detection

*Mai Luo[a], Ting Wang[a], Ling Chen[a], Zehua Cheng[a], Sundaram Gunasekaran[b,*], Jinchao Wei[a,*] and Peng Li[a,*]*

[a]State Key Laboratory of Quality Research in Chinese Medicine, Institute of Chinese Medical Sciences, University of Macau, Macau, China

[b]Department of Biological Systems Engineering and Department of Materials Science and Engineering, University of Wisconsin–Madison, Madison, WI, USA

## CONTENTS

## 12.1 INTRODUCTION

Pesticide is a general term that can include plant growth regulators, herbicides, fungicides, repellents, and insecticides. Due to the low cost-to-productivity ratio, pesticides are used excessively and inappropriately (1, 2). Therefore, the excess pesticides

---

* Corresponding authors: Sundaram Gunasekaran, Jinchao Wei, and Peng Li

DOI: 10.1201/9781003109228-12

end up in soils, plants, fruits, cereals, and animal foods. This has already caused long-term damage to the ecosystem and has become a severe threat to our planet (3). The herbicides, triazine, and choroacetamides, were, respectively, detected in the water and soil samples (4). The organochloride pesticides have been forbidden to use due to their high toxicity and durability, but still can be found in the natural environment (5, 6). Pesticides, such as dichlorodiphenyltrichloroethane (DDT), aldrin, mirex, etc., have already become persistent organic pollutants (POPs), which could bioaccumulate in the food chain (7–9). The organophosphorus pesticides (OPs) are known to irreversibly inhibit acetylcholinesterase (AChE) (10, 11) and cause disorders of the nervous and reproductive systems (12–15). Continuous exposure to OPs increases the risk of Alzheimer's disease, Parkinson's disease, and other neurological diseases (16, 17). Faced with these severe threats, it is increasingly important to routinely monitor the presence and distribution of pesticide residues in foods and the environment.

The standard methods of pesticide detection rely on large-scale precise instruments, such as liquid chromatography-mass spectrometry (LC-MS), micellar electrokinetic chromatography (MEKC), gas chromatography-mass spectrometry (GC-MS), etc. (18–21). These instruments are highly sensitive, reliable, and stable for pesticide detection. But they are costly, requiring tedious sample preparation, and professionally trained operators. Therefore, these analytical techniques are unable to quickly and accurately quantify pesticides outside the laboratory. To overcome these drawbacks, novel approaches that are simple, easy-to-operate, and can be used on-site are being developed. Some of these new approaches include colorimetric, fluorescent, electrochemical, and chemiluminescence (22, 23).

Since pesticides inhibit enzyme activity, the concentration of pesticide present in a sample is inversely proportional to the enzyme activity. This is the basis for the ability of natural enzymes for pesticide residue sensing. Based on this principle, various approaches for the detection of OPs, carbamates, and other pesticides have been developed (24–26). According to different detection needs, various enzymes, such as AChE, butyrylcholinesterase (BChE), and organophosphorus hydrolase, could be applied individually or in combination in analyzing hazardous pesticides due to their high selectivity and sensitivity (27–30). However, the enzymatic sensors are limited by the inherent problems of natural enzymes, including weak adaptability, low stability, high cost, etc. (31). These seriously affected the detection systems application and hindered the further development of rapid pesticide analysis.

Therefore, nanozymes are extensively explored in various methods to detect pesticides. Also, the concept of dual-mode detection is increasingly being adopted. All these prove the powerful potential of nanozymes in pesticide detection. The leading materials for nanozymes synthesis are iron (Fe), gold (Au), carbon, and cerium (Ce), and a few nanozymes are synthesized from manganese (Mn), copper (Cu), and other materials. Some reported nanozymes, like Fe-based magnetic nanomaterials (NMs), could be reused multiple times with stable catalyzing activity to save cost and prevent secondary damage to the environment. Carbon-based oxide and other materials were also used to prepare the nanozyme with peroxidase (POD), oxidase (OXD), laccase, or other enzyme-like activities (32–34). Nanozyme-based different sensing modalities, such as colorimetric, fluorescent, electrochemical, chemiluminescent, surface-enhanced Raman scattering (SERS), etc., have proven to be highly sensitive, stable, and applicable in real samples.

## 12.2 APPLICATIONS

### 12.2.1 COLORIMETRIC METHODS

The colorimetric method is a detection strategy in which a color change signal is obtained upon target detection. Most nanozymes do not possess a specific recognition capacity for pesticides. Therefore, the enzymes or other recognition elements, collectively known as molecular recognition elements (MREs), are commonly found in detection systems. With the development of nanozymes, they are used to replace horseradish peroxidase (HRP) and other enzymes in colorimetric detection. Many nanozymes exhibit excellent enzyme-like catalytic performance, which could catalyze chromogenic substrates, such as 3',5,5'-tetramethylbenzidine (TMB), 2,'-azino-bis(3-ethylbenzothiazoline-6-sulfonic acid) diammonium salt (ABTS), o-phenylenediamine (OPD), etc., to produce colorimetric output signals. Many colorimetric methods that use NMs or nanocomposites of noble metals, Fe, carbon, etc., are summarized in **Table 12.1**.

#### 12.2.1.1 Noble Metal Nanomaterials

Noble metals, platinum (Pt), palladium (Pd), silver (Ag), and Au, are transition metals and possess multiple advantages, such as stability, biocompatibility, and easy functionalization. Hence, they are useful for synthesizing nanozymes with high catalytic activity. Au NMs, because of their surface plasmon resonance property and ease of functionalization, are widely employed as a sensitive and selective multifunctional element in colorimetric detection (35). Pesticides, such as malathion, methyl-paraoxon, and dimethoate, represent direct inhibition of nanozyme activity by covering the active site, hindering electron transfer, and preventing ion conversion by a ternary complex (36–38). Singh et al. synthesized Pd-Au bimetal nanozyme and successfully applied it for malathion quantification. Their detection mechanism relied on the interaction between the functional group of Au nanorods (NRs) and the sulfanyl group of malathion. By combining the properties of both metals, the Pd@Au NRs provided high catalytic activity while maintaining the selectivity for malathion (39). In another work, three-dimensional (3D) graphene foam (GF) was selected to load the Pt nanoclusters (NCs). The prepared nanohybrid showed high activity, reusability, and stability in the reaction. As shown in **Figure 12.1A**, the nanozyme, Pt NC/3D GF, could catalyze the dihydroxybenzene isomer (catechol or hydroquinone), TMB, and other substrates by its multifunctional enzyme-mimicking activity. This method could also distinguish catechol and hydroquinone colorimetrically (40).

Relying only on recognition and catalyzation of nanozymes, the detection system could have low selectivity and poor sensitivity. To improve such limitations, aptamers, antibodies, enzymes, and other MREs are employed in the detection. As an autonomous recognizer, an aptamer can be RNA and single-stranded or double-stranded DNA (ssDNA or dsDNA). Using Au NPs as nanozymes for catalyzing TMB oxidation, the aptamers S-18 exhibited unique inhibitory properties for Au NPs, which was applied to detect acetamiprid (41). As shown in **Figure 12.1B**, the inhibition mechanism relied on that the bases of aptamer were attracted by the

## TABLE 12.1
## Nanozyme-Assisted Colorimetric Detection for Pesticides

| Nanozyme | Mimic Aactivity | MREs | Color Material | Pesticide | LOD | Reference |
|---|---|---|---|---|---|---|
| **Noble Metal-Based Manomaterials** | | | | | | |
| GNPs | POD | S-18 | TMB | Acetamiprid | 0.1 ppm | (42) |
| GNRs | POD | GNPs | TMB | Malathion | 1.78 µg/mL | (38) |
| AuNPs | POD | GNPs | TMB | Methyl Parathion | 78.95 nmol/L | (37) |
| AuNPs | POD | S-18 | ABTS | Acetamiprid | 1.02 µg/L | (41) |
| AuNPs | POD | GNPs | OPD | Dimethoate | 4.7 µg/L | (36) |
| Au NRs | - | Au NRs | Au NRs | Malathion Chlorpyrifos | 0.15 ppt | (67) |
| Pd@Au NRs | POD | GNPs | TMB/OPD | Malathion | 60 ng/mL | (39) |
| Au@Pt | POD | antibody-mab | TMB | Parathion | $2.13 \times 10{-}3$ µg/L | (68) |
| Pt NPs | POD | antibody-mab | TMB | Parathion | $2.0 \times 10{-}3$ µg/L | (69) |
| Pt NPs | POD | AChE | TMB | Carbofuran Dichlorvos | 2.3 µg/L 1.4 µg/L | (47) |
| PtPd NPs | POD | AChE | Catechol | Ethyl-paraoxon | 1 nmol/L | (46) |
| Pt–Ni(OH)$_2$ | POD | Antibody modified Pt–Ni(OH)2 NSs | TMB | Acetochlor Fenpropathrin | 0.63 ng/mL 0.24 ng/mL | (44) |
| Pt NC/s3D GF | Oxidase | Pt NC / 3D GF | TMB | Catechol Hydroquinone | $5.0 \times 10{-}8$ mol/L $1.0 \times 10{-}8$ mol/L | (40) |
| AgNPs | POD | *Chl* aptamer | TMB | Chlorpyrifos | 11.3 ppm | (43) |
| Ag$_3$PO$_4$NPs | Oxidase | Ag3PO4 NPs | TMB | Chlorpyrifos | 9.97 ppm | (70) |
| **Iron-Based Nanomaterials** | | | | | | |
| Fe$_3$O$_4$ MNPs | POD | AChE | TMB | Sarin Methyl-paraoxon Acephate | 1 nmol/L 10 nmol/L 5 µmol/L | (50) |
| Fe$^{3+}$ | POD | AChE | TMB | Paraoxon DDVP Dimethoate DDT | 0.15 nmol/L 0.35 nmol/L 11 nmol/L 0.85 nmol/L | (54) |
| Fe-N-C | POD | AChE | TMB | Paraoxon-ethyl | 2.19 ng/mL | (53) |
| Fe-N-C | Oxidase | AChE | TMB | Paraoxon-ethyl | 0.97 ng/mL | (71) |
| 3D GF/m-Fe$_3$O$_4$ | POD | 3D GF/m-Fe$_3$O$_4$ | TMB | PNP | 0.045 µmol/L | (51) |
| Fe$_3$O$_4$ | POD | 4-AAP | 4-AAP/H$_2$O$_2$ | Phenol | 3.79 µmol/L | (72) |
| Fe$_3$O$_4$@MnOx | Oxidase | 4-AAP | 4-AAP | Chlorophenols | 0.85 µmol/L | (52) |
| Fe$_3$O$_4$-TiO$_2$/rGO | POD | TMB | TMB | Atrazine | 2.98 µg/L | (73) |
| MIL-101(Fe) | POD | AChE | TMB | Paraoxon-ethyl | 1 ng/mL | (74) |
| Cu-MOF(Fe$_3$O$_4$) NPs | POD | Aptasensor | TMB | Chlorpyrifos | 4.4 ng/mL | (75) |

*(Continued)*

## TABLE 12.1 (Continued)
## Nanozyme-Assisted Colorimetric Detection for Pesticides

| Nanozyme | Mimic Aactivity | MREs | Color Material | Pesticide | LOD | Reference |
|---|---|---|---|---|---|---|
| **Carbon-Based Nanomaterials** | | | | | | |
| Hemin-rGO | POD | Aptamer | TMB | Acetamiprid | 40 nmol/L | (57) |
| NG, NSG, GO | POD | NG, NSG, GO | TMB | Lactofen, Fluoroxypyr-meptyl, Bensulfuron-methyl, Fomesafen, Diafenthiuron | 5 µmol/L | (56) |
| 3DRGO-NiFe$_2$O$_4$/NiO | POD | AChE | TMB | Dichlorvos | 10 µg/mL | (76) |
| GO | POD | AChE | TMB | Dimethoate, Methyl-paraoxon Chlorpyrifos | 2 ppb 1 ppb 2 ppb | (58) |
| **Other Nanomaterials** | | | | | | |
| PAA-CeO$_2$ | Oxidase | AChE | TMB | Dichlorvos Methyl-paraoxon | 8.62 ppb 26.73 ppb | (60) |
| CeO$_2$ NPs | Oxidase | AChE | TMB | Chlorpyrifos | 7.6 ng/mL | (77) |
| CeGO NRs | POD | AChE | TMB | Chlorpyrifos | 3.43 ng/mL | (78) |
| MnO$_2$ NSs | Oxidase | AChE | TMB | Paraoxon | 1.0 ng/mL | (61) |
| MnO$_2$ NSs | Oxidase | GAPD | TMB | Chlorothalonil | 0.024 ng/mL | (79) |
| MnO$_2$ NSs | Oxidase | ACP | ABTS | Parathion-methyl | 0.028 µg/mL | (80) |
| γ-MnOOH | Oxidase | AChE | TMB | Omethoate Dichlorvos | 10 ng/mL1 3 ng/mL | (62) |
| CH-Cu | Laccase | CH-Cu | Epinephrine | Epinephrine | 0.31 µg/mL | (65) |
| ssDNA-Hemin | POD | ssDNA | TMB | Isocarbophos | 0.6 µg/L | (66) |
| GeO$_2$ | POD | AChE | TMB | Paraoxon | 14 fmol/L | (63) |
| Cu–N–C | POD | AChE | TMB | Paraoxon-ethyl | 0.60 ng/mL | (64) |

charged electrons on the surface of NPs. After acetamiprid was added, it competed with the aptamer for binding, and the nanozyme is released (42). Further, by screening the aptamer, chlorpyrifos was successfully detected by the chlorpyrifos aptamer-modified Ag NPs with a limit of detection (LOD) of 11.3 ppm (43).

Lateral flow immunoassay (LFIA) uses the antigen–antibody (Ab) reaction. Recently, nanozyme-assisted immunoassay showed potential in pesticide detection for their high catalytic activity and stability (45). As shown in **Figure 12.1C**, the Pt NPs-anchored two-dimensional (2D) Ni(OH)$_2$ nanosheets (NSs) were synthesized for naked-eye colorimetric detection of acetochlor and fenpropathrin. In the presence of these pesticides, a certain amount of the Ab-modified nanozymes could precisely recognize the targets and across the test line without interaction with

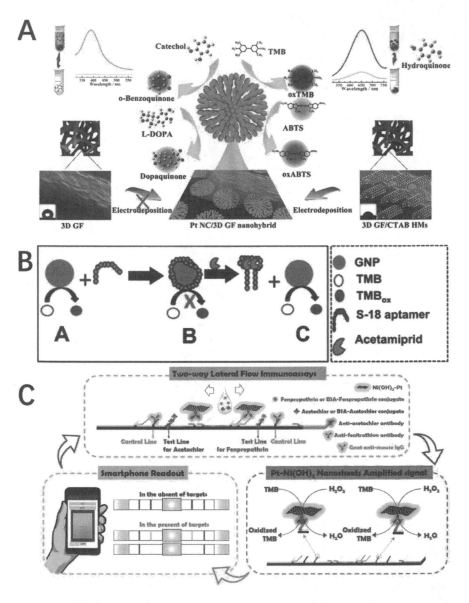

**FIGURE 12.1** Different recognition elements for pesticide detection: (**A**) graphic abstract of Pt NC/3D GF nanohybrid nanozyme-assisted detection system for dihydroxybenzene isomers quantification. Reprinted with permission from (40). Copyright from 2020 American Chemical Society. (**B**) diagram of acetamiprid determination by S-18 aptamer modified gold nanoparticles. Reprinted with permission from (42). Copyright from 2014 American Chemical Society. (**C**) schematic diagram of fenpropathrin and acetochlor detection based on Pt-Ni(OH)$_2$ nanosheets together with antibody recognition. Reprinted with permission from (44). Copyright from 2018 Elsevier.

the bovine serum albumin (BSA)-pesticide conjugates for substrate oxidation. The uncombined Pt-Ni(OH)$_2$NSs could catalyze TMB to amplify the signal. This method was developed as a smartphone-based application with LODs of 0.63 and 0.24 ng/mL, respectively, for acetochlor and fenpropathrin detection (44). The nanozyme represented an effective signal amplifier in enzyme-linked immunosorbent assay (ELISA), which was used for ethyl-paraoxon detection (46). With the help of AChE, the nanozymes constructed of platinum NPs have been successfully applied in the rapid quantification of dichlorvos and carbofuran (47).

### 12.2.1.2 Iron-Based Nanomaterials

Iron oxide (Fe$_3$O$_4$) can form magnetic nanoparticles (MNPs, i.e., m-Fe$_3$O$_4$), which possess OXD- or POD-mimicking activity. An external magnet could easily aggregate MNPs in a suspension, which can be retrieved and reused. When optimized, the MNPs can maintain good catalytic activity over multiple uses. This ability to be recycled is a significant advantage of MNPs compared to other nanozymes.

The MNPs are generally used to catalyze a redox reaction, and the major catalytic pathway is either generating reactive oxygen species (ROS) or an electron transfer process (48, 49). By coupling with different MREs, the MNPs can be used in various pesticide analyses (50). The simple Fe$_3$O$_4$ NPs exhibit some instability, such as easy aggregation due to the strong dipole–dipole attraction and large surface-area-to-volume ratio. For better adaptive detection, researchers have designed various Fe-based nanozyme schemes. For example, 3D GF was used to couple with mesoporous Fe$_3$O$_4$ nanohybrid. The 3D GF provided a large surface area for catalyzing, which greatly reduced the aggregation tendency and possessed a higher affinity to TMB. Also, the rich $\pi$-stacking or hydrophobicity on the surface of 3D GF could effectively help to recognize certain small molecules (**Figure 12.2A**). The research has revealed that p-nitrophenol (p-NP) inhibited the POD-mimicking activity of the nanozyme by masking the active site (51). In another research, the manganese oxide (MnOx) decorated iron-based nanozyme was used to detected chlorophenols (CPs). Through a simple hydrothermal method, the MnO$_x$ was successfully grown on the Fe$_3$O$_4$ surface. This core-shell Fe$_3$O$_4$@MnO$_x$ exhibited high oxidase-mimicking activity, which could oxidize the 4-aminoantipyrine (4-AAP) and CPs complex to produce differently colored products (**Figure 12.2B**). Due to the various number of chlorine atoms and substitution position existed in different CPs, the CPs could be quantified via interaction with the Fe$_3$O$_4$@MnO$_x$ for different affinity (52). Furthermore, both boron-doped Fe-N-C single-atom catalyst and ferric ions (Fe$^{3+}$) alone were reported to exhibit POD-like activity and then applied for the sensitive detection of several pesticides (53, 54).

### 12.2.1.3 Carbon-Based Nanomaterials

Carbon-based NMs exhibit high biocompatibility, high catalytic activity, and unique electronic property (55). For example, graphene oxide (GO) is a multifunctional carbon material with the merits of being green, cost-effective, readily available, and easily combined. The undecorated GO could catalyze oxidation reactions as other POD- and OXD-mimicking nanozymes. Besides, GO possesses a stereochemical

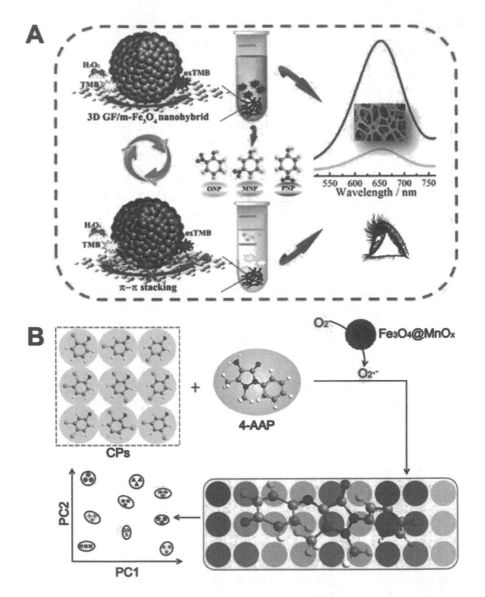

**FIGURE 12.2** (**A**) The schematic abstract of 3D GF/m-Fe$_3$O4-assisted detection system. Reprinted with permission from (51). Copyright 2018 Elsevier. (**B**) The principle of Fe$_3$O$_4$@ MnOx-based colorimetric method. Reprinted with permission from (52). Copyright 2020 Elsevier.

structure with a large surface area for reaction. Thus, GO is easily modified with other functional materials depending on different needs.

Wei et al. prepared three different heteroatom-doped GO (e.g., nitrogen (N)-doped graphene (NG), N, and sulfur (S) co-doped graphene (NSG)), which could simultaneously detect multiple pesticides substrates (**Figure 12.3A**). Due to different affinities

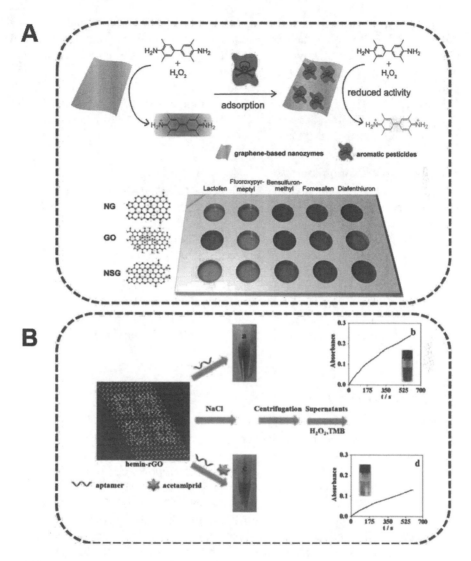

**FIGURE 12.3** **(A)** Schematic of carbon-based nanozyme for colorimetric detection of pesticides. Reprinted with permission from (56). Copyright 2020 American Chemical Society. **(B)** The principle of acetamiprid detection by using hemin-rGO nanozyme. Reprinted with permission from (57). Copyright 2015 Elsevier.

between the nanozyme and pesticide, the NG, NSG, and GO were inhibited to various extents, which led to different blue colors. The pesticide could mask active sites of NG and NSG by conjugation stacking (π-π). However, GO could form a hydrogen bond with herbicide fomesafen for stronger affinity. To increase accuracy, 2D canonical score plots were used to transform the colorimetric response of the three nanozymes (56). This analytical strategy provided a way to use rapid and straightforward nanozymes to determine multiple targets, not just a single pesticide molecule.

Hemin is a metal complex with POD-mimicking activity, which contains proto-porphyrin IX, $Fe^{3+}$ ion, and helium (He) atom. After coupling hemin with reduced GO (rGO), the catalytic activity of the hemin-rGO composite could be inhibited by the acetamiprid aptamer. In the presence of acetamiprid, the aptamer was attracted to form an aptamer-target complex, which restored the oxidation of TMB (**Figure 12.3B**). This system can detect acetamiprid from 0.1 to 10 μmol/L with LOD 40 nmol/L (57). In other studies, GO was applied to detect dimethoate, methyl paraoxon, and chlorpyrifos (58).

### 12.2.1.4  Other Nanomaterials

In addition to NMs mentioned above, Ce-, Mn-, Cu-, and germanium (Ge)-based NMs have also been used to prepare nanozymes with OXD, POD, laccase, and other catalytic activities (59–66).

The nanoceria (Ce NPs), decorated by polyacrylic acid, exhibited OXD-mimicking activity and was used for colorimetric detection of dichlorvos and methyl-paraoxon (60). With the help of AChE and acetylcholine (ACh), Mn-based nanozyme was used for detection and quantification of paraoxon and omethoate (61, 62). Liang et al. synthesized germanium dioxide ($GeO_2$) nanozyme for paraoxon detection (63). Cu-based NMs as nanozymes have proven to possess multiple applications and were successfully applied in ethyl-paraoxon detection and chlorophenols or bisphenols degradation (64, 65).

### 12.2.2  Fluorescent Methods

Due to the high sensitivity and quick response, fluorescent detection is usually con-sidered one of the most common methods for pesticide detection. For example, the carbon quantum dot (CQD) has been developed as a stable fluorescent probe for vari-ous applications. It affords high fluorescent intensity, good biocapacity, and simple preparation, which are conducive to improving pesticide detection ability. Taking the CQDs as the optical source, the p-nitrophenol (p-NP) was successfully detected. The p-NP could be decomposed from methyl-paraoxon by nanoceria (**Figure 12.4A**). Due to the inner filter effect, the UV absorption of p-NP can decrease the fluorescent intensity of CQDs. The concentration of p-NP appears to be inversely proportional to the fluorescence intensity of CQDs. The designed analytical method was verified by *Panax quinquefolius* and tap water substrate. The recovery rates of this detec-tion system ranged from 85 to 103% (81). With high fluorescent intensity, the CQDs were also used in the visual detection for methyl-paraoxon under a 365 nm UV lamp (82). In other work, the substrate, amplex red, could be catalyzed into resorufin by nanozyme catalysis with high fluorescent intensity, which was used in glyphosate quantification (**Figure 12.4B**) (83). In the fluorescent method development, single signal fluorescent probes were easily affected by the fluctuation from the fluorescent probe and the light source. To solve these issues, the ratiometric detection system was developed. The Ce-based fluorescent polymer was synthesized and applied in methyl-paraoxon detection (84).

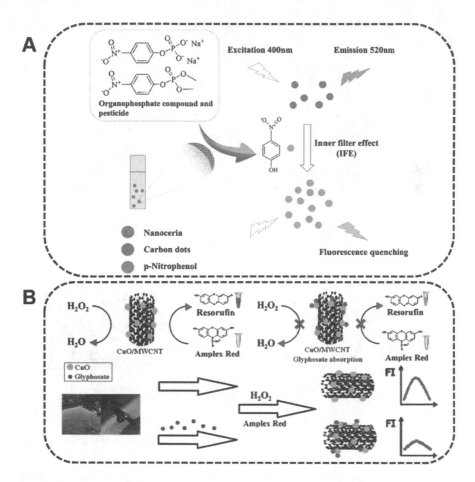

**FIGURE 12.4** **(A)** Illustration of the fluorescent detection system for methyl-paraoxon. Reprinted with permission from (81). Copyright 2019 Springer. **(B)** Graphic abstract of nanozyme-assisted fluorescent detection for glyphosate. Reprinted with permission from (83). Copyright 2016 Elsevier.

## 12.2.3 ELECTROCHEMICAL METHODS

Nanozymes are widely used to catalyze redox reactions to achieve signal amplification in electrochemical detection (85). With the development of nanozyme, the sensitivity and selectivity were greatly improved in electrochemical detention (86, 87). Through a facile hydrothermal method, a bifunctional nanozyme was successfully prepared by cerium oxide, which could be used to modify the glassy carbon electrode. The nanozyme could decompose the methyl-paraoxon and amplify the signal of p-NP by promoting the electron transfer (**Figure 12.5A**). The proposed detection system showed high sensitivity and selectivity. The LOD was 0.06 μmol/L, and the system was verified by *Coix lacryma-jobi, Adenophora stricta,* and *Semen nelumbinis* samples with recoveries from 80.9 to 116.8% (85). Simultaneously, the amino

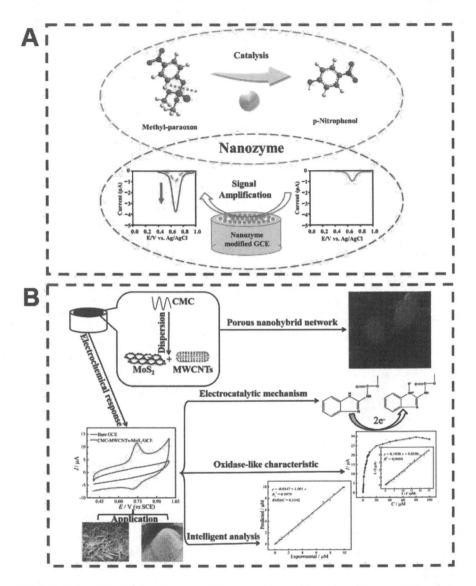

**FIGURE 12.5** (A) Graphic abstract of the electrochemical detection for methyl-paraoxon. Reprinted with permission from (85). (B) Schematic of CBZ detection by MoS2/MWCNTs porous nanohybrid. Reprinted with permission from (88). Copyright from 2020 Elsevier.

acids conjugated nanozyme, prepared by Qiu's research group, proved that the catalytic mechanism imitates the proton transfer relay in natural hydrolase, which was already used in methyl paraoxon, methyl parathion, and ethyl paraoxon detection (LOD: 0.2 μmol/L) (87). Further, in recent years, machine learning has attracted the researchers' attention due to its quick computation and easy application. Zhu et al. developed an intelligent analysis for carbendazim (CBZ) based on electrochemical analysis and machine learning technology (**Figure 12.5B**). Before the detection, the electrode was modified by a molybdenum disulfide (MoS$_2$)/multiwalled carbon nanotubes (MWCNTs) porous nanohybrid network. After the CBZ was added, the nanozyme exhibited a direct electron transfer effect similar to natural oxidase, which helped realize the CBZ quantification. Through the artificial neural networks for intelligent analysis by machine learning, the parameters (e.g., $R^2$, RMSE, and RPD) of the detection system were better than the traditional regression model. Based on the purposed method, the detection system could sensitively detect the CBZ from 0.04 to 100 μM with LOD 7.4 nmol/L (88).

## 12.2.4 CHEMILUMINESCENCE METHOD

CL is a chemical reaction phenomenon in that a substrate is oxidized to a product with the energy released by the emission of luminescence, which is widely applied in biological assays, chemical molecule analyses, environmental monitoring, and clinical diagnoses (89–91). Most CL detection methods rely on luminol as the luminophore; other commonly used luminophores are peroxyoxalate, lucigenin, and acridinium esters derivatives (92–95). However, the conventional luminescence mechanism needs H$_2$O$_2$ to be the oxidizing agent, which would reduce the repeatability and selectivity in the CL detection. Natural enzymes have been used to oxidize CL compounds in commercial ELISA. However, due to its expensive preparation method, unrecyclable and unstable factors, the application of natural enzyme has seriously hindered CL analysis. Therefore, the POD-like activity of nanozymes was used to replace the biological catalyst and H$_2$O$_2$ in CL detection, and various CL detection methods for pesticides detection have been developed (32, 96, 97).

Iron oxide (Fe$_3$O$_4$) could oxidize dissolved oxygen into superoxide anions at the surface of NPs (**Figure 12.6A**) (96, 98). The ethoprophos could protect superoxide anions from free-radical scavengers such as ethanol. After adding luminol, the superoxide anions could oxidize the solution with strong CL intensity (96). To improve the detection sensitivity, synthesizing nanozymes of higher catalytic activity is seen as the first choice. The Au NPs/metal-organic gels (Au NPs/MOGs (Fe)) hybrid was synthesized through an *in situ* method and was used to catalyze luminol oxidation for CL detection. This composite, which promoted the production of

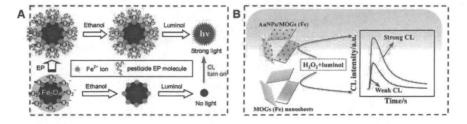

**FIGURE 12.6** (A) Fe$_3$O$_4$ NPs as POD-mimicking nanozyme for ethoprophos detection by CL method. Reprinted with permission from (96). Copyright 2012 American Chemical Society. (B) Schematic of CL detection system using AuNPs/metal-organic gels composite. Reprinted with permission from (97). Copyright from 2018 American Chemical Society.

ROS, had a higher POD-mimicking activity and higher CL emission than MOGs (Fe) nanosheets (**Figure 12.6B**). This was applied in ethoprophos detection with LOD of 1 nmol/L (97). Other pesticides, dimethoate, dipterex, carbaryl, chlorpyrifos, and carbofuran, were also sensitively detected by CL analysis (32). **Table 12.2** is a summary of various fluorescent, electrochemical, and chemiluminescent methods of pesticides detection.

**TABLE 12.2**

**Nanozymes-Assisted Fluorescent, Electrochemical, and Chemiluminescent Methods in Pesticides Detection**

| Nanozyme | Enzyme-Mimicking Activity | MREs | Pesticide(s) | LOD | Reference |
|---|---|---|---|---|---|
| **Fluorescent Methods** | | | | | |
| CuO/MWCNTs. | POD | CuO/MWCNTs. | Glyphosate | 0.67 ppb | (83) |
| $CeO_2$ | Phosphatase | $CeO_2$ | Methyl-paraoxon | 0.375 µmol/L | (81) |
| $Sm-CeO_2$ | Phosphatase | $Sm-CeO_2$ | Methyl-paraoxon | 1 µmol/L | (84) |
| $CeO_2$ ˙ | Phosphatase | $CeO_2$ | Methyl-paraoxon | 0.1 µmol/L | (82) |
| CuS NPs | POD | CuS NPs | DDVP | 0.1 ng/mL | (99) |
| $Fe-MIL-88NH_2$ | POD | $Fe-MIL-88NH_2$ | Catechol | 0.0913 µmol/L | (100) |
| **Electrochemical Methods** | | | | | |
| NiO NPs | - | NiO NPs | Parathion | 0.024 µmol/L | (86) |
| $TiO_2$@ DA@S/H/E | Phosphohydrolase | $TiO_2$ NPs-AAs | Methyl paraoxon Methyl parathion Ethyl paraoxon | 0.2 µmol/L | (87) |
| $MoS_2$/MWCNTs | Oxidase | $MoS_2$/MWCNTs | Carbendazim | 7.4 nmol/L | (88) |
| $CeO_2$ | Phosphohydrolase | $CeO_2$ | Methyl-paraoxon | 0.06 µmol/L | (85) |
| $MoS_2$-COOH-MWCNT | Oxidase | $MoS_2$-COOH-MWCNT | 5-nitroguaiacol sodium | 0.02 µmol/L | (101) |
| AuNPs/FcDr/ rGO | - | AuNPs/FcDr/ rGO | Dichlorvos | 0.21 µmol/L | (102) |
| PB @ $Ti_3C_2Tx$ | Oxidase | AChE | Malathion | $1.3 \times 10^{-16}$ mol/L | (103) |
| Fc-TED/g-C3N4/GO | - | Fc-TED/g-C3N4/GO | Metolcarb | 8.3 nmol/L | (104) |
| **Chemiluminescent Methods** | | | | | |
| Lum-AgNP | POD | Lum-AgNP | Dimethoate Dipterex Carbaryl Chlorpyrifos Carbofuran | 24 µg/mL 24 µg/mL 24 µg/mL 24 µg/mL 24 µg/mL | (32) |
| $Fe_3O_4$ | POD | $Fe_3O_4$ | Ethoprophos | 0.1 nmol/L | (96) |
| AuNPs/MOGs (Fe) hybrids | POD | AuNPs/MOGs (Fe) hybrids | Ethoprophos | 7.4 nmol/L | (97) |

## 12.2.5 DUAL-MODE ANALYTICAL METHOD

Dual-mode detection systems commonly rely on the catalytic product property in optical, electrochemical, and other characteristics. The major strategies of dual-mode pesticide detection could be divided into two areas. The first is dual-mode detection based on pesticide decomposition. The nanoceria-assisted detection method already proved the detection effectiveness. The nanoceria decomposed the methyl-paraoxon to yellow p-NP with the characteristic peak of UV absorption at 400 nm (**Figure 12.7A**). To improve the accuracy of colorimetric detection, the analytical

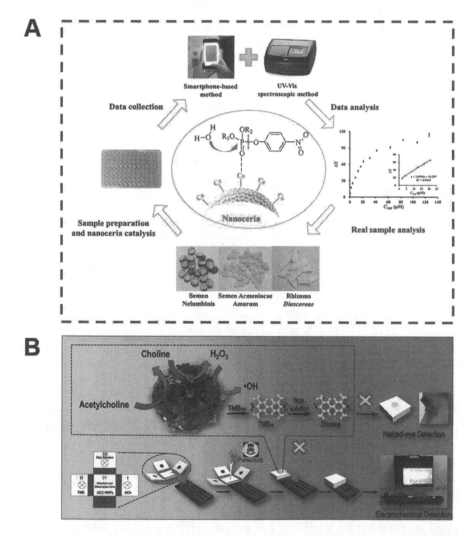

**FIGURE 12.7** (**A**) Schematic of the UV and colorimetric dual-mode detection method. Reprinted with permission from (105). Copyright from 2019 Elsevier. (**B**) Schematic of the electrochemical and colorimetric dual-mode detection method. Reprinted with permission from (106). Copyright 2019 Elsevier.

**TABLE 12.3**

**Nanozyme-Based Dual-Mode Detection System for Pesticide Detection**

| Nanozyme | Analytical Techniques | Mimicking Activity | MREs | Pesticide | LOD | Reference |
|---|---|---|---|---|---|---|
| CeO$_2$ | UV-vis and colorimetric | Phosphohydrolase | CeO$_2$ | Methyl-paraoxon | 0.42 μmol/L | (105) |
| ACC-HNFs | electrochemical and colorimetric | POD | AChE | Paraoxon | Electrochemistry: 6 fg/mL Colorimetry: 10 pg/mL | (106) |
| AuNCs-MnO$_2$ | Fluorometric and colorimetric | POD | AChE | Carbaryl | 0.125 μg/L | (107) |
| Pt NPs | Colorimetric and SERS | POD | MIPs Pt@BSA-hapten | Triazophos | 1 ng/mL | (110) |
| Fe$_3$O$_4$ NPs@ ZIF-8 | Colorimetric and fluorometric | POD | AChE | Diazinon | 0.2 nmol/L | (108) |
| Cu$^{2+}$-gC3N4 | Fluorometric and colorimetric | POD | AChE | Malathion | Florescence: 6.798 nmol/L Colorimetry: 1.497 nmol/L | (109) |

system used a smartphone to read the color information. Based on this strategy, the methyl-paraoxon concentration was measured by colorimetric and UV absorption signals (105). The second is based on substrate oxidation by nanozyme catalysis. As shown in **Figure 12.7B**, Jin et al. used the Cu-based hybrid nanoflowers (HNFs) to absorb the AChE and choline oxidase (ChO) for all-in-one enzyme-inorganic HNFs (ACC-HNFs). The strong enzyme loading capacity of ACC-HNFs came from the fact that it provides many active sites and can adsorb enzymes into internal crevices. Hence, screen-printed carbon electrodes (SPCE) that can produce both electrochemical and colorimetric signals were successfully prepared. When paraoxon was added to the SPCE, its content eventually reduced diimide production by inhibiting the catalytic activity of AChE in the ACC-HNFs (106). Based on the oxidation of substrates, the SERS and fluorescent techniques were, respectively, used to couple with the colorimetric detection for pesticide determination (107–110). Several dual-mode and miscellaneous systems for pesticides detection are, respectively, listed in **Tables 12.3 and 12.4**.

## 12.3   SUMMARY AND FUTURE PERSPECTIVES

In this chapter, we focused on the latest progress in pesticide detection by nanozyme-assisted analytical methods. The catalytic activity of nanozyme greatly influences the sensitivity of the detection system. To achieve lower LOD, there is a continual need

**TABLE 12.4**

**Other Reported Potential Applications for Nanozymes in Pesticide Detection**

| Nanozyme | Analytical Techniques | Mimicking Activity | Target | Application | Reference |
|---|---|---|---|---|---|
| Fe-SAs/NC | FL | POD | AChE | Detection | (111) |
| CeO$_2$ | Colorimetric | Oxidase | AChE Esterase Urease | Detection | (112) |
| CoOOH NFs | Colorimetric | POD | AChE | Detection | (113) |
| UiO-66(Ce / Zr) | Colorimetric | Oxidase | Phosphate ion | Detection | (114) |
| CeO$_2$ | Immunoassays | Oxidase | Fenitrothion | Detection | (115) |
| Au-Pt | SERS | Oxidase | glyphosate | Detection | (116) |
| Cerium oxide | - | Phosphodiesterase | Parathion Methyl paraoxon | Degradation | (117) |
| Zr-doped CeO$_2$ | - | Phosphohydrolase | Methyl paraoxon | Degradation | (118) |
| Zr-incorporated CeO2 | - | Phosphotriesterase | Paraoxon Parathion Methyl paraoxon Methyl parathion | Degradation | (119) |
| Fe$_3$O$_4$ NPs | - | Laccase | phenolic pollutants | Degradation | (53) |
| CuS @ rGO | - | – | Atrazine | Degradation | (120) |
| CNT | - | - | Paraoxon | Degradation | (121) |

for developing highly active nanozymes. The sensitivity and specificity of detection can also be improved by introducing other MREs, such as antibodies, aptamers, polymeric ligands, and even natural enzymes into the detection system.

Depending on the material and its catalytic properties, different nanozymes afford different advantages. Nanozymes of noble metals, Fe, and Mn possess the catalytic activity of POD. These metal-based nanozymes can be used alone or combined in different ways to enhance their catalytic activity. Fe-based MNPs as nanozymes can not only catalyze the oxidation reaction but also can be reused. Nanozymes are mostly heterogeneous catalysts, and they often formed a signal transduction pathway for pesticides together with homogeneous catalysts (for example, natural enzymes). Among them, Mn-based nanozymes are widely used to work with AChE and ACh systems. The TCH could induce the decomposition of Mn-based nanozyme, followed by the changes in catalytic activity. Cerium ions show unique degradation activity in pesticide detection and high catalytic activity for specific OPs. Its catalytic activity mainly comes from the interaction between trivalent and tetravalent Ce ions in CeO$_2$. As a nonmetallic multifunctional material, GO is often used to synthesize nanozyme with other NMs and widely applied in analytical areas to optimize the water solubility and increase the enzyme-like activities (122–124). The GO represented the unique carrying capacity in pesticide detection for promoting the nanomaterial loading and nanozyme-substrate interaction, which derived from the effective π-π stacking effect and large specific surface area (73, 125).

Unlike conventional analytical methods, most novel methods could only detect one or a few pesticides in one test. Moreover, compared with all pesticides, the types of pesticides that could be tested are still very few. However, nanozyme-based methods show unique advantages in real-time detection on-site monitoring of some specific pesticides. The huge potential of nanozymes will attract more attention and cover more pesticide species. The limited catalytic activity has been the major obstacle of nanozyme development. Therefore, in the future, the nanozymes with a higher enzyme-like activity that can catalyze more reactions will emerge as a breakthrough development and help overcome the existing limitations and challenges for multiple pesticide determination.

## ACKNOWLEDGMENTS

We gratefully acknowledge the financial support from Macau Science and Technology Development Fund (147/2019/A3) and Guangxi Innovation-driven Development Special Foundation Project (GuiKe AA18118049).

## REFERENCES

1. Dasgupta S, Meisner C, Huq M. 2007. *Journal of agricultural economics* 58: 91–114
2. Jallow MF, Awadh DG, Albaho MS, Devi VY, Thomas BM. 2017. *Science of the total environment* 574: 490–8
3. Bajwa U, Sandhu KS. 2014. *Journal of food science and technology* 51: 201–20
4. Bonansea RI, Amé MV, Wunderlin DA. 2013. *Chemosphere* 90: 1860–9
5. Dong C, Zeng Z, Li X. 2005. *Talanta* 66: 721–7
6. Ivdra N, Herrero-Martín S, Fischer A. 2014. *Journal of chromatography A* 1355: 36–45
7. Jahnke A, MacLeod M, Wickström Hk, Mayer P. 2014. *Environmental science & technology* 48: 11352–9
8. Daley JM, Paterson G, Drouillard KG. 2014. *In Reviews of Environmental Contamination and Toxicology, Volume 227*, pp. 107–55: Springer
9. Van Ael E, Covaci A, Blust R, Bervoets L. 2012. *Environment international* 48: 17–27
10. Colovic MB, Krstic DZ, Lazarevic-Pasti TD, Bondzic AM, Vasic VM. 2013. *Current neuropharmacology* 11: 315–35
11. Assis CRD, Linhares AG, Oliveira VM, França RCP, Carvalho EVMM, et al. 2012. *Science of the total environment* 441: 141–50
12. Franco R, Li S, Rodriguez-Rocha H, Burns M, Panayiotidis MI. 2010. *Chemico-biological interactions* 188: 289–300
13. Fry DM. 1995. *Environmental health perspectives* 103: 165–71
14. Koifman S, Koifman RJ, Meyer A. 2002. *Cadernos de Saúde Pública* 18: 435–45
15. Bretveld RW, Thomas CM, Scheepers PT, Zielhuis GA, Roeleveld N. 2006. *Reproductive biology and endocrinology* 4: 30
16. Parrón T, Requena M, Hernández AF, Alarcón R. 2011. *Toxicology and applied pharmacology* 256: 379–85
17. Yan D, Zhang Y, Liu L, Yan H. 2016. *Scientific reports* 6: 1–9
18. Wei J, Cao J, Tian K, Hu Y, Su H, et al. 2015. *Analytical methods* 7: 5801–7
19. Wei J-C, Hu J, Cao J-L, Wan J-B, He C-W, et al. 2016. *Journal of agricultural and food chemistry* 64: 932–40

20. Bernardi G, Kemmerich M, Ribeiro LC, Adaime MB, Zanella R, Prestes OD. 2016. *Talanta* 161: 40–7
21. Machado I, Gérez N, Pistón M, Heinzen H, Cesio MV. 2017. *Food chemistry* 227: 227–36
22. Wang W, Gunasekaran S. 2020. *TrAC trends in analytical chemistry* 126: 115841
23. Kalyani N, Goel S, Jaiswal S. 2020. *Environmental chemistry letters*
24. Montes R, Céspedes F, Gabriel D, Baeza M. 2018. *Journal of nanomaterials* 2018: 7093606
25. Cui H-F, Wu W-W, Li M-M, Song X, Lv Y, Zhang T-T. 2018. *Biosensors and bioelectronics* 99: 223–9
26. Wang P, Li H, Hassan MM, Guo Z, Zhang Z-Z, Chen Q. 2019. *Journal of agricultural and food chemistry* 67: 4071–9
27. Wang Y, Zhang S, Du D, Shao Y, Li Z, et al. 2011. *Journal of materials chemistry* 21: 5319–25
28. Arduini F, Neagu D, Scognamiglio V, Patarino S, Moscone D, Palleschi G. 2015. *Chemosensors* 3: 129–45
29. Du D, Chen W, Zhang W, Liu D, Li H, Lin Y. 2010. *Biosensors and bioelectronics* 25: 1370–5
30. Zhang P, Sun T, Rong S, Zeng D, Yu H, et al. 2019. *Bioelectrochemistry* 127: 163–70
31. Lin Y, Ren J, Qu X. 2014. *Accounts of chemical research* 47: 1097–105
32. He Y, Xu B, Li W, Yu H. 2015. *Journal of agricultural and food chemistry* 63: 2930–4
33. Liu J, Meng L, Fei Z, Dyson PJ, Zhang L. 2018. *Biosensors and bioelectronics* 121: 159–65
34. Liang H, Lin F, Zhang Z, Liu B, Jiang S, et al. 2017. *ACS applied materials & interfaces* 9: 1352–60
35. Priyadarshini E, Pradhan N. 2017. *Sensors and actuators B: chemical* 238: 888–902
36. Hu Y, Wang J, Wu Y. 2019. *Analytical methods* 11: 5337–47
37. Pandey A, Srivastava S, Gayatri, Rai P, Pandey A. 2020. *Advanced science, engineering and medicine* 12: 232–41
38. Biswas S, Tripathi P, Kumar N, Nara S. 2016. *Sensors and actuators B: chemical* 231: 584–92
39. Singh S, Tripathi P, Kumar N, Nara S. 2017. *Biosensors and bioelectronics* 92: 280–6
40. Qiu N, Liu Y, Guo R. 2020. *ACS applied materials & interfaces* 12: 15553–61
41. Yang W, Wu Y, Tao H, Zhao J, Chen H, Qiu S. 2017. *Analytical methods* 9: 5484–93
42. Weerathunge P, Ramanathan R, Shukla R, Sharma TK, Bansal V. 2014. *Analytical chemistry* 86: 11937–41
43. Weerathunge P, Behera BK, Zihara S, Singh M, Prasad SN, et al. 2019. *Analytica chimica acta* 1083: 157–65
44. Cheng N, Shi Q, Zhu C, Li S, Lin Y, Du D. 2019. *Biosensors and bioelectronics* 142: 111498
45. Jiang D, Ni D, Rosenkrans ZT, Huang P, Yan X, Cai W. 2019. *Chemical society reviews* 48: 3683–704
46. Zhao Y, Yang M, Fu Q, Ouyang H, Wen W, et al. 2018. *Analytical chemistry* 90: 7391–8
47. Cao J, Wang M, She Y, Abd El-Aty AM, Hacımüftüoğlu A, et al. 2019. *Microchimica acta* 186: 390
48. Su H, Liu D-D, Zhao M, Hu W-L, Xue S-S, et al. 2015. *ACS applied materials & interfaces* 7: 8233–42
49. Chen T, Wu X, Wang J, Yang G. 2017. *Nanoscale* 9: 11806–13
50. Liang M, Fan K, Pan Y, Jiang H, Wang F, et al. 2012. *Analytical chemistry* 85: 308–12
51. Qiu N, Liu Y, Xiang M, Lu X, Yang Q, Guo R. 2018. *Sensors and actuators B: chemical* 266: 86–94
52. Xu X, Wu S, Guo D, Niu X. 2020. *Analytica chimica acta* 1107: 203–12

53. Jiao L, Xu W, Zhang Y, Wu Y, Gu W, et al. 2020. *Nano Today* 35: 100971
54. Xu Y, Yu T, Wu X-Q, Shen J-S, Zhang H-W. 2015. *RSC Advances* 5: 101879–86
55. Sun A, Mu L, Hu X. 2017. *ACS applied materials & interfaces* 9: 12241–52
56. Zhu Y, Wu J, Han L, Wang X, Li W, et al. 2020. *Analytical chemistry* 92: 7444–52
57. Yang Z, Qian J, Yang X, Jiang D, Du X, et al. 2015. *Biosensors and bioelectronics* 65: 39–46
58. Chu S, Huang W, Shen F, Li T, Li S, et al. 2020. *Nanoscale* 12: 5829–33
59. Abnous K, Danesh NM, Ramezani M, Alibolandi M, Emrani AS, et al. 2018. *Microchimica acta* 185: 216
60. Zhang S-X, Xue S-F, Deng J, Zhang M, Shi G, Zhou T. 2016. *Biosensors and bioelectronics* 85: 457–63
61. Yan X, Song Y, Wu X, Zhu C, Su X, et al. 2017. *Nanoscale* 9: 2317–23
62. Huang L, Sun D-W, Pu H, Wei Q, Luo L, Wang J. 2019. *Sensors and actuators B: chemical* 290: 573–80
63. Liang X, Han L. 2020. *Advanced functional materials* 30: 2001933
64. Wu Y, Wu J, Jiao L, Xu W, Wang H, et al. 2020. *Analytical chemistry* 92: 3373–9
65. Wu J, Wang X, Wang Q, Lou Z, Li S, et al. 2019. *Chemical society reviews* 48: 1004–76
66. Luo D, Chen H, Zhou P, Tao H, Wu Y. 2019. *Analytical and bioanalytical chemistry* 411: 7857–68
67. MB B, Manippady SR, Saxena M, John NS, Balakrishna RG, Samal AK. 2020. *Langmuir*
68. Liu Y, Bhattarai P, Dai Z, Chen X. 2019. *Chemical society reviews* 48: 2053–108
69. Chen G, Jin M, Yan M, Cui X, Wang Y, et al. 2019. *Microchimica acta* 186: 339
70. Kushwaha A, Singh G, Sharma M. 2020. *RSC Advances* 10: 13050–65
71. Wu Y, Jiao L, Luo X, Xu W, Wei X, et al. 2019. *Small* 15: 1903108
72. Wu S, Guo D, Xu X, Pan J, Niu X. 2020. *Sensors and actuators B: chemical* 303: 127225
73. Boruah PK, Das MR. 2020. *Journal of hazardous materials* 385: 121516
74. Xu W, Kang Y, Jiao L, Wu Y, Yan H, et al. 2020. *Nano-micro letters* 12: 1–12
75. Liu Q, He Z, Wang H, Feng X, Han P. 2020. *Microchimica acta* 187: 1–9
76. Wei Z, Li H, Wu J, Dong Y, Zhang H, et al. 2020. *Chinese chemical letters* 31: 177–80
77. Chen Z, Wang Y, Mo Y, Long X, Zhao H, et al. 2020. *Sensors and actuators B: chemical* 323: 128625
78. Lin L, Ma H, Yang C, Chen W, Zeng S, Hu Y. 2020. *Materials advances* 1: 2789–96
79. Sheng E, Lu Y, Tan Y, Xiao Y, Li Z, Dai Z. 2020. *Food chemistry* 331: 127090
80. Wang J, Lu Q, Weng C, Li X, Yan X, et al. 2020. *ACS biomaterials science & engineering* 6: 3132–8
81. Wei J, Yang Y, Dong J, Wang S, Li P. 2019. *Microchimica acta* 186: 66
82. Luo M, Wei J, Zhao Y, Sun Y, Liang H, et al. 2020. *Microchemical journal* 154: 104547
83. Chang Y, Lin Y, Xiao G, Chiu T, Hu C. 2016. *Talanta* 161: 94–8
84. Wei J, Xue Y, Dong J, Wang S, Hu H, et al. 2020. *Chinese medicine* 15: 22
85. Sun Y, Wei J, Zou J, Cheng Z, Huang Z, et al. 2020. *Journal of pharmaceutical analysis*
86. Khairy M, Ayoub HA, Banks CE. 2018. *Food chemistry* 255: 104–11
87. Qiu L, Lv P, Zhao C, Feng X, Fang G, et al. 2019. *Sensors and actuators B: chemical* 286: 386–93
88. Zhu X, Liu P, Ge Y, Wu R, Xue T, et al. 2020. *Journal of electroanalytical chemistry* 862: 113940
89. Tang C, Vaze A, Rusling J. 2017. *Lab on a chip* 17: 484–9
90. Qi Y, Xiu F-R, Yu G, Huang L, Li B. 2017. *Biosensors and bioelectronics* 87: 439–46
91. Zhong Y, Tang X, Li J, Lan Q, Min L, et al. 2018. *Chemical communications* 54: 13813–6
92. Lan Y, Yuan F, Fereja TH, Wang C, Lou B, et al. 2018. *Analytical chemistry* 91: 2135–9

93. Nakazono M, Nanbu S. 2018. *Luminescence* 33: 345–8
94. Zargoosh K, javad Chaichi M, Shamsipur M, Hossienkhani S, Asghari S, Qandalee M. 2012. *Talanta* 93: 37–43
95. Tian X, Liao H, Wang M, Feng L, Fu W, Hu L. 2020. *Biosensors and bioelectronics* 152: 112027
96. Guan G, Yang L, Mei Q, Zhang K, Zhang Z, Han M-Y. 2012. *Analytical chemistry* 84: 9492–7
97. He L, Jiang ZW, Li W, Li CM, Huang CZ, Li YF. 2018. *ACS applied materials & interfaces* 10: 28868–76
98. Gao L, Zhuang J, Nie L, Zhang J, Zhang Y, et al. 2007. *Nature nanotechnology* 2: 577–83
99. Liu Y, Lin X, Ji X, Hao Z, Tao Z. 2020. *Microchimica acta* 187: 1–8
100. Hou L, Qin Y, Lin T, Sun Y, Ye F, Zhao S. 2020. *Sensors and actuators B: chemical* 321: 128547
101. Lu X, Liu G, Di P, Li Y, Xue T, et al. 2020. *Food analytical methods* 13: 2028–38
102. Yan L, Yan X, Li H, Zhang X, Wang M, et al. 2020. *Microchemical journal*: 105016
103. He Y, Zhou X, Zhou L, Zhang X, Ma L, et al. 2020. *Industrial & engineering chemistry research* 59: 15556–64
104. Xiao F, Li H, Yan X, Yan L, Zhang X, et al. 2020. *Analytica chimica acta* 1103: 84–96
105. Wei J, Yang L, Luo M, Wang Y, Li P. 2019. *Ecotoxicology and environmental safety* 179: 17–23
106. Jin R, Kong D, Zhao X, Li H, Yan X, et al. 2019. *Biosensors and bioelectronics* 141
107. Yan X, Kong D, Jin R, Zhao X, Li H, et al. 2019. *Sensors and actuators B: chemical* 290: 640–7
108. Bagheri N, Khataee A, Hassanzadeh J, Habibi B. 2019. *Spectrochimica acta part A: molecular and biomolecular spectroscopy* 209: 118–25
109. Chen Y, Zhu Y, Zhao Y, Wang J, Li M. 2020. *Food chemistry*: 128560
110. Yan M, Chen G, She Y, Ma J, Hong S, et al. 2019. *Journal of agricultural and food chemistry* 67: 9658–66
111. Wang M, Liu L, Xie X, Zhou X, Lin Z, Su X. 2020. *Sensors and actuators B: chemical*: 128023
112. Cheng H, Lin S, Muhammad F, Lin Y-W, Wei H. 2016. *ACS sensors* 1: 1336–43
113. Jin R, Xing Z, Kong D, Yan X, Liu F, et al. 2019. *Journal of materials chemistry B* 7: 1230–7
114. Li X, Niu X, Liu P, Xu X, Du D, Lin Y. 2020. *Sensors and actuators B: chemical* 321: 128546
115. Chen Z-J, Huang Z, Huang S, Zhao J-L, Sun Y, et al. 2020. *Analyst*
116. Ma J, Feng G, Ying Y, Shao Y, She Y, et al. 2020. *Analyst*
117. Janoš P, Ederer J, Došek M, Štojdl J, Henych J, et al. 2019. *Environmental science: nano* 6: 3684–98
118. Khulbe K, Roy P, Radhakrishnan A, Mugesh G. 2018. *ChemCatChem* 10: 4826–31
119. Khulbe K, Mugesh G. 2019. *Polyhedron* 172: 198–204
120. Alhaddad M, Shawky A. 2020. *Journal of molecular liquids* 318: 114377
121. Blaskievicz SF, Endo WG, Zarbin AJ, Orth ES. 2020. *Applied catalysis B: environmental* 264: 118496
122. Ruan X, Liu D, Niu X, Wang Y, Simpson CD, et al. 2019. *Analytical chemistry* 91: 13847–54
123. Wang Q, Zhang X, Huang L, Zhang Z, Dong S. 2017. *ACS applied materials & interfaces* 9: 7465–71
124. Adegoke O, Zolotovskaya S, Abdolvand A, Daeid NN. 2020. *Talanta* 216: 120990
125. Boruah PK, Darabdhara G, Das MR. 2021. *Chemosphere* 268: 129328

# 13 DNAzymes in Food and Environmental Contaminants Detection

*Kaiyu He, Liu Wang, and Xiahong Xu**
State Key Laboratory for Managing Biotic and Chemical
Threats to the Quality and Safety of Agro-products; Institute
of Agro-product Safety and Nutrition, Zhejiang Academy of
Agricultural Sciences, Hangzhou, China

## CONTENTS

## 13.1  INTRODUCTION

For a considerable time, nucleic acids were merely regarded as the means for the storage of genetic information, but this view was updated with the discovery of catalytic RNAs (ribozymes) by Cech et al. (1) To date, various ribozymes and deoxyribozymes (DNAzyme) have emerged through *in vivo* discovery and *in vitro* selection. Among them, one interesting example is horseradish peroxidase (HRP)-mimicking DNAzyme, which was first reported to show POD-mimic activity by Sen et al. (2) Typically, base pairing occurs between guanine (G) and cytosine (C) or adenine (A) and thymine (T) through hydrogen bonds, which is the basis of duplex formation. However, DNA can fold into a variety of alternative structures other than the canonical Watson-Crick duplex. Among the non-canonical DNA nanostructures, a four-stranded topology known as G-quadruplex (G4) can associate with hemin (iron (III)-protoporphyrin IX) to form POD-mimicking DNAzymes (3–8). Compared with natural protein enzymes, G4-hemin DNAzymes have several advantages, including ease of preparation, cost-effectiveness, and more stable activity. Due to their POD activity and DNA sequence designability, G4-hemin DNAzymes have

* Corresponding author: Xiahong Xu

DOI: 10.1201/9781003109228-13

been employed as versatile signal generators in numerous colorimetric, fluorescent, and electrochemical biosensors for rapid sensing of various target analytes (9–11).

DNA G4 structures are formed by specific repetitive G-rich DNA sequences (12). As shown in **Figure 13.1**, in these G-rich DNA sequences, four G bases form a G-quartet *via* Hoogsteen base pairings, then two or more G-quartets stack upon each other to form a G4 structure, and the intervening sequences are extruded as single-stranded loops. G4 structures can be formed by one, two, or four single-stranded DNA (ssDNA) molecules, which makes them flexible in biosensing applications. G4 structures are formed by ssDNA that engage in more complex conformations, of which folding topologies, the orientation of loops, and capping structures play important roles. One sequence may form several conformations that exhibit different stabilities and are influenced by environmental conditions. G4 structures exhibit diverse topologies as presented in **Figure 13.1**. Depending on the DNA strand direction, parallel, antiparallel, and mixed antiparallel-parallel conformations are distinguished (13). Circular dichroism (CD) spectra are frequently applied to characterize different topologies of G4 structures. Parallel G4 structures have a dominant positive CD peak at 260 nm, and a negative peak at 240 nm; whereas, antiparallel G4 structures have a negative peak at 260 nm and a positive peak at 290 nm. The topologies of G4 affect the catalytic activity of DNAzymes, which results from their ability

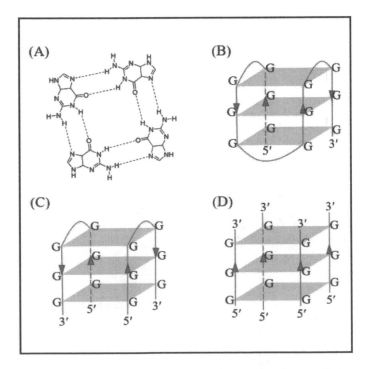

**FIGURE 13.1**  G-tetrad and G-quadruplexes. **(A)** G-tetrad structure, **(B)** monomolecular folded G-quadruplex (antiparallel structure), **(C)** bimolecular folded G-quadruplex (antiparallel structure), **(D)** tetramolecular folded G-quadruplex (parallel structure).

to bind hemin (14). Hemin binds with external guanines in a G4, which indicates that parallel structure is more favorable for the binding of hemin through end-stacking. Therefore, the highest activity was observed for parallel or mixed intramolecular quadruplexes (14, 15). Lower activity of antiparallel quadruplexes is likely attributed to the steric hindrance caused by loops, which makes hemin binding difficult (16). The sequence of loops in a G4 affects the stability, conformation, and activity of DNAzymes. It has been observed that longer loops generate antiparallel quadruplexes and exhibit lower activity (17). Shorter loops stabilize parallel quadruplexes, producing higher enzymatic activity.

ABTS (2,2'-azinobis(3-ethylbenzothiazoline)-6-sulfonic acid), TMB (3,3',5,5'-tetramethylbenzidine), and luminol are commonly used as substrates to observe the catalytic activity of G4-hemin DNAzymes. The oxidation of ABTS or TMB catalyzed by G4-hemin DNAzymes generates colored products, and the concomitant changes in the absorption spectra can be used to monitor the catalyzed reaction. The reaction of luminol with hydrogen peroxide ($H_2O_2$) catalyzed by G4-hemin DNAzymes produces chemiluminescence, for which the luminescence intensity serves as the analytical signal. Cations are necessary for G4 formation. Early studies indicated that the potassium ion ($K^+$) was crucial for G4 formation and the catalytic activity of G4-hemin DNAzymes. However, recent reports showed that other ions could also be used and that, in some cases, replacing $K^+$ with ammonium ($NH_4^+$) ions positively influenced enzymatic activity. Sintim et al. also discovered that the presence of $NH_4^+$ reduced the oxidative degradation of oligonucleotides (17). Nie et al. discovered a unique intramolecular enhancement effect of the adjacent A at 3' ends of G4 structures, which remarkably boost the activity of G4-hemin DNAzymes by just adding an adenine nucleotide at 3' terminals of G-rich sequences (8). Enzymes that exhibit catalytic activity in a wide temperature range are urgently needed. Though G4-hemin DNAzymes are less susceptible to temperature variations and preserve their activity, most G4-hemin DNAzymes work only at modest temperatures. However, Ju et al. reported a thermophilic DNAzyme with efficient POD activity (18). This thermophilic DNAzyme was capable of oxidizing substrates at high temperatures (up to 95 °C) and long reaction times at high temperatures (up to 18 h at 75 °C).

## 13.2 HEAVY METAL IONS DETECTION

Heavy metal contaminations in the environment and foods have attracted intensive attention from the public since they pose serious threats to the ecological system and human health. Traditional detection methods for heavy metals, such as atomic absorption spectroscopy, are sensitive, but these methods have to be implemented in professional laboratories. Therefore, it is of significance to develop convenient and cost-effective technologies for rapid and on-site detection of heavy metals. G4 formation is a metal-ion-dependent process, which has inspired the detection of metal ions based on DNAzymes. In most cases, the $K^+$ is used for quadruplex formation. Wang et al. (19) reported that DNAzyme catalytic activity is selectively induced by the $K^+$ ion because G-rich DNA strands should form G4 before binding with hemin. They proved the $K^+$ selectivity by performing comparative tests with other ions, including NH$^{4+}$, sodium (Na$^+$), lithium (Li$^+$), cesium (Cs$^+$), magnesium (Mg$^{2+}$), and calcium (Ca$^{2+}$) using TMB as a DNAzyme activity indicator. The heavy metal lead (Pb$^{2+}$) is a toxic pollutant with a substantial influence on human health. An assay to detect Pb$^{2+}$ with POD-mimicking DNAzymes as an indicator label was presented by the Dong group (20). They found that Pb$^{2+}$ caused a rearrangement of the K$^+$-stabilized G4 structure and that the resulting G4 did not enhance the catalytic activity of hemin (**Figure 13.2A**). This observation was explained as a weak binding affinity of the G4 structure stabilized by Pb$^{2+}$ toward hemin and, thus, poor catalytic activity in the POD-mimicking reaction. This G4 structure shows allosteric regulation by Pb$^{2+}$, which behaves like an inhibitor and switches the catalytic activity of G4-hemin between active and inactive forms. The catalytic activity of DNAzymes decreased proportionally as the concentration of Pb$^{2+}$ increased. The lowest Pb$^{2+}$ concentration that could be determined colorimetrically was 32 nM (20). In another investigation, Ju et al. found that the activity of parallel G4-hemin DNAzymes was deactivated by Pb$^{2+}$ (21). The K$^+$ ions in the parallel G4 were replaced by Pb$^{2+}$ and consequently decreased the affinity between the topology and hemin, this led to a decrease in DNAzyme activity for catalyzing the oxidation of ABTS by H$_2$O$_2$ to form a green dye with an absorption maximum at 420 nm. The assay did not use any amplification and had a linear response in the 0.01 to 10 μM Pb$^{2+}$ concentration range and a limit of detection (LOD) of 7.1 nM. Also, the method was successfully applied to the analysis of spiked water samples.

Mercury (Hg$^{2+}$) is another dangerous pollutant detrimental to the environment and human health. For the rapid and effective monitoring of Hg$^{2+}$, many sensors have been developed, including those based on POD-mimicking DNAzymes. Hg$^{2+}$ can bind with two thymines to form a T-Hg$^{2+}$-T complex (22, 23). This binding can be used to strengthen DNA duplexes for activating DNAzymes. Kong et al. developed a sensitive and selective Hg$^{2+}$ detection method based on the Hg$^{2+}$-mediated formation of split G-quadruplex-hemin DNAzymes (22). In their strategy, two label-free oligonucleotides are used. In the presence of Hg$^{2+}$, the two oligonucleotides hybridize each other to form a duplex, in which T-T mismatches are stabilized by the T-Hg$^{2+}$-T base pair. As a result, the G-rich sequences of the two oligonucleotides can associate to form a split G-quadruplex, which can bind hemin to form catalytically active G4-hemin DNAzymes (**Figure 13.2B**). The results can be monitored by an

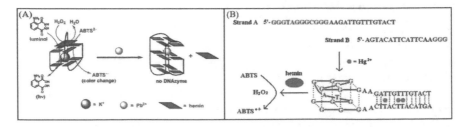

**FIGURE 13.2** (A) Utilizing Pb$^{2+}$-induced allosteric G4 for label-free colorimetric and chemiluminescence detection of Pb$^{2+}$ (Reproduced from (20) with permission from American Chemical Society). (B) Detection of Hg$^{2+}$ ion using a POD-like split G4-hemin DNAzyme. (Reproduced from (22) with permission from Royal Society of Chemistry).

absorbance increase in the $H_2O_2$-ABTS reaction system by using UV-vis absorption spectroscopy. This "turn-on" process allows the detection of aqueous $Hg^{2+}$ at concentrations as low as 19 nM using a simple colorimetric technique. The Wang group utilized the $Hg^{2+}$-mediated T-T base pair to modulate the folding of G-rich DNAs and inhibit the DNAzyme activity, developing a colorimetric approach to sense $Hg^{2+}$ (23). Two G-rich DNAs were adopted, which folded into G4 in low- and high-salt conditions, respectively. These G4 structures were able to bind hemin to form the POD-like DNAzymes in the folded state. Upon addition of $Hg^{2+}$, the folding of G4 was inhibited due to the formation of the T-$Hg^{2+}$-T complex. As a result of $Hg^{2+}$ inhibition, a sharp decrease in the catalytic activity toward the $H_2O_2$-mediated oxidation of ABTS was observed, accompanied by a change in solution color. Through this approach, aqueous $Hg^{2+}$ can be detected down to 50 nM (10 μg/kg) with high selectivity without interference from other metal ions.

Like $Hg^{2+}$, one $Ag^+$ ion can bind with two cytosines to form C-$Ag^+$-C base pair. Based on this phenomenon, Shen et al. mediated POD-mimicking DNAzymes to detect $Ag^+$ (24). In their method, two unlabelled oligonucleotides with different lengths are used. In the absence of $Ag^+$, the two oligonucleotides hybridize each other to form an intermolecular duplex. The addition of $Ag^+$ disrupts the intermolecular duplex and promotes a part of the sequence of the longer oligonucleotide to fold into an intramolecular duplex, in which C-C mismatches are stabilized by C-$Ag^+$-C base pairs. As a result, the G-rich sequence of the same oligonucleotide can fold into a G4, which can bind hemin to form a catalytically active G4-hemin DNAzyme. This can be reflected by an absorbance increase when monitored in the $H_2O_2$-ABTS reaction system by using ultraviolet-visual (UV-vis) absorption spectroscopy. This "turn-on" process allows the detection of aqueous $Ag^+$ at concentrations as low as 20 nM using a simple colorimetric technique.

Zinc ($Zn^{2+}$) is required for the human body, but the deficiency or excessive intake of $Zn^{2+}$ will result in various detrimental effects. Severe neurological diseases, cell viability, and soil microbial activity are related to $Zn^{2+}$. The Xu group has described a method for sensitive colorimetric determination of $Zn^{2+}$ (25). In their design, they used the following: 1) a $Zn^{2+}$-responsive hairpin DNAzyme that assisted target recycling; 2) hybridization chain reaction; and 3) G4-hemin DNAzyme nanoladder. The $Zn^{2+}$-responsive hairpin DNAzyme acted as the recognition and transformation probe. Upon addition of $Zn^{2+}$ and enzyme strand, a duplex was formed in the loop region of the hairpin. The caged initiator sequence was subsequently liberated from the hairpin DNAzyme by the $Zn^{2+}$-selective split of the substrate strand. This cleavage induced an enzyme strand recycling for the next round of cleavage. As a result, the initiator DNA was accumulated and cross-opened hairpins H1 and H2 to start a hybridization chain reaction. The caged G4 was released after the hybridization chain reaction to recruit hemin to form the G4-hemin DNAzyme that was inserted into the DNA nanoladder. Once formed in the DNA nanoladder, these POD-like DNAzyme acted as catalytic labels for the oxidation of $ABTS^{2-}$, resulting in a visual color change. This cascade amplification strategy allowed 10 nM to 100 μM of $Zn^{2+}$ to be linearly quantified by colorimetry at 415 nm with a LOD of 3.5 nM. They tested this in lake water and obtained recoveries ranging from 97.7 to 108.3%, which confirms the high reliability of the method for real-sample analysis.

## 13.3 PESTICIDES DETECTION

Pesticides play an important role in agriculture as approximately one-third of the global agricultural production is dependent on the use of pesticides. However, the increased pesticide application also increased the risk of excessive pesticide residues in food and the environment. For efficient monitoring and control of pesticides and their adverse effects, fast and reliable quantification of pesticide residues is crucial. Malathion, a broad-spectrum insecticide, is widely used for the control of various outdoor insects in agriculture and home maintenance. However, the abuse of malathion leads to serious contamination, posing a threat to the ecological environment and human health. Zou et al. demonstrated a label-free chemiluminescent aptasensor for the sensitive detection of malathion based on exonuclease (Exo)-assisted dual signal amplification and G4-hemin DNAzyme (26). Upon the addition of malathion, the aptamer probe specifically binds to the target, and after Exo I- and III-assisted signal amplification, large numbers of G4-hemin DNAzymes were generated to produce and amplify the detection signal (**Figure 13.3A**). Under the optimal experimental conditions, the proposed aptasensor showed an excellent linear response to malathion with a LOD of 0.47 pM. Li et al. reported a novel photoelectrochemical sensing platform for malathion detection based on the biocatalysis-induced formation of bismuth oxybromide/bismuth sulfide ($BiOBr/Bi_2S_3$) semiconductor heterostructures and HRP-mimicking DNAzyme (27).

Tang et al. fabricated a label-free electrochemical biosensor for the detection of nereistoxin-related insecticides based on nereistoxin binding-triggered conformational switching of DNAzyme and micropipette tip-based miniaturized electrochemical device (28). The model target bensultap, a broad-spectrum carbamate insecticide, led to the formation of catalytically-active G4-hemin DNAzyme. The activity of the G4-hemin DNAzyme was followed by catalyzing the oxidation

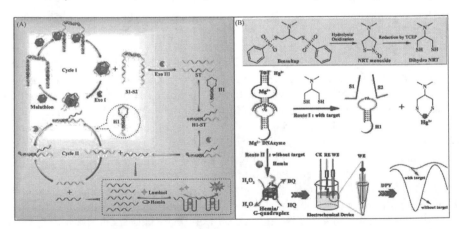

**FIGURE 13.3** (**A**) Sensitive and label-free chemiluminescence detection of malathion using Exo-assisted dual signal amplification and G4-hemin DNAzyme (Reproduced from (26) with permission from Elsevier). (**B**) Target-induced conformational switch of DNAzyme for homogeneous electrochemical detection of nereistoxin-related insecticide (Reproduced from (28) with permission from Elsevier).

of hydroquinone to benzoquinone in the presence of $H_2O_2$ to generate enhanced current output (**Figure 13.3B**). They achieved a low LOD (6.9 ng/L) and a wide linear range (0.01-2000 μg/L), and the strategy was also applied to detect bensultap in agricultural products.

Acetamiprid is widely used as a replacement for organophosphorus and other traditional insecticides owing to its low mammalian toxicity. However, its extensive use may cause adverse effects on food and the environment. Li et al. utilized G4-hemin DNAzyme and functionalized graphene quantum dot to construct a fluorometric biosensor for acetamiprid assay (29). In their strategy, G4-hemin DNAzyme catalyzed the oxidation of o-phenylenediamine by $H_2O_2$ to produce a yellow fluorescent product. This oxidation product interacts with D-penicillamine and histidine-functionalized graphene quantum dot to achieve a rapid energy transfer, forming a fluorometric sensor. As the formation of the G4-hemin DNAzyme was only triggered by acetamiprid, the sensor worked in the 1.0 fM to 1.0 nM acetamiprid concentration range with a LOD of 0.38 fM. This sensor was successfully applied to determine acetamiprid content in tea.

## 13.4 ANTIBIOTICS DETECTION

Antibiotics are biologically active compounds that can act on the metabolism of bacteria, fungi, and protozoa to inhibit or eliminate microbial growth. They have been extensively applied in preventing and treating human bacterial infections and animal infectious diseases. However, due to their overuse and inappropriate applications in the last few decades, as well as discharge from industrial effluents, they have been widely distributed to the environment. This causes severe environmental pollution and serious potential harm to human health, especially the potential risk of proliferation of antibiotic resistance genes, which will make disease treatment less efficient, more costly, and often impossible. Hence, the rapid analysis of antibiotics is of considerable importance and urgent. The Gan group explored a fluorescence "switch-on" assay for the detection of the ultra-trace level of antibiotics based on magnetic aptamer-platinum (Pt)-luminal labeled with G4-hemin DNAzyme (30). Using chloramphenicol (CAP) as a model target, they demonstrated G4-hemin DNAzyme and Pt NPs could be assembled as a nano tracer to catalyze the luminol-$H_2O_2$ system to emit fluorescence (**Figure 13.4A**). Such a dual-amplified "switch-on" signal strategy significantly improved the detection performance affording a wide linear range (0.001–100 ng mL$^{-1}$) and a low LOD (0.0005 ng mL$^{-1}$).

In another system, by combining colorimetric signal transduction of G4-hemin DNAzyme with a competitive biorecognition reaction at aptamer-conjugated magnetic beads, a biosensing method was developed for the rapid and sensitive detection of CAP (32). The one-step competitive reaction between the aptamer-CAP target biorecognition and the hybridization of aptamer and CAP-aptamer allows the capture of Au nanoprobes onto the surface of magnetic beads. The colorimetric signal generation was due to the enzymatic catalytic reaction of the POD-mimicking G4-hemin DNAzyme, which provided LOD down to 0.13 pg/mL of CAP. When tested with milk samples, satisfactory results were obtained, which point to its potential practical applications.

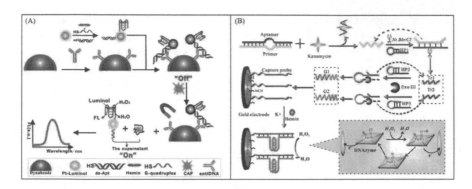

**FIGURE 13.4** (**A**) Switch-on fluorescent detection of CAP based on a magnetic composite probe with aptamer and G4-hemin co-immobilized Pt NPs-luminol as a signal tracer (Reproduced from (30) with permission from Elsevier). (**B**) Label-free detection of kanamycin based on cascade enzymatic amplification coupled with a split G4 DNAzyme (Reproduced from (31) with permission from Royal Society of Chemistry).

Ou et al. developed an aptasensor for colorimetric tobramycin assay based on the catalytic activity of G4-hemin DNAzyme (33). In this study, dual-strand displacement and DNA three-way junction structure were combined to produce a large number of G4-forming sequences. Finally, the G4-hemin DNAzyme catalyzed the $ABTS^{2-}/H_2O_2$ reaction system to generate a colorimetric signal. After multiple signal amplification, highly sensitive detection was achieved with a LOD down to the nanomolar level. In another example, Zhang et al. integrated a split G4 DNAzyme as the signal reporter with an electrochemical sensing platform for kanamycin detection with specificity and sensitivity (31). To enhance the signal-to-noise ratio, two G-rich oligonucleotide sequences (G1 and G2) were blocked into two different hairpin probes, preventing the two segments from assembling into a split G4 structure (**Figure 13.4B**). Furthermore, a two-step enzymatic signal amplification was designed to generate abundant G1 and G2 to improve sensitivity. This biosensor showed excellent performance for sensing kanamycin with a LOD of 83 fM for kanamycin concentrations ranging from 100 fM to 1 nM.

For ultrasensitive detection, cascade enzymatic recycling coupled to G4-hemin DNAzyme amplification was used for antibiotic detection (34). The assay involves two sequential reactions: the first is a λ Exo-assisted cyclic digestion reaction triggered by target-aptamer binding. The second is an endonuclease-aided cyclic nicking reaction, which produces a large amount of G-rich nucleic acid segments. These segments form G4-hemin DNAzymes in the presence of $K^+$ and hemin. Because the G4-hemin DNAzyme acted as an HRP-mimicking DNAzyme with excellent redox activity, the electrochemical signal transduction was accomplished due to the electroreduction of $H_2O_2$. The aptasensor was applied to the quantitation of kanamycin and gave a linear response in the 1 pM to 10 nM kanamycin concentration range, with a LOD of 0.5 pM. To analyze multiple antibiotics simultaneously and intelligently, Qin et al. reported a potentiometric aptasensing platform based on a G4-hemin DNAzyme and logic gate operations for the determination of two antibiotics using a single membrane electrode (35). A bifunctional probe with two aptamer units and a signal reporter oligonucleotide with a DNAzyme sequence are assembled on the magnetic beads to form a DNA hybrid structure. The "OR" and "INHIBIT" logic functions can be performed by using the two aptamers and antibiotics as inputs and using the chronopotentiometry response based on the G4-hemin DNAzyme-$H_2O_2$-mediated oxidation of TMB as output. The commonly used antibiotics, kanamycin, and oxytetracycline were employed as models and were successfully measured.

## 13.5 MYCOTOXINS DETECTION

Mycotoxins are the toxic secondary products of fungi that frequently contaminate foods, grains, vegetable oils, feeds, as well as related products. Mycotoxins can pose a severe threat to human health because some of them present carcinogenic, mutagenic, and genotoxic activities, showing harmful effects even at low concentrations. For safeguarding human health from the toxic effects of mycotoxins, strict regulatory guidelines and maximum residue levels (MRL) have been set for most of the prevalent and toxic mycotoxins in certain commodities. To monitor mycotoxins contamination, effective and reliable analytical techniques for the sensitive determination of mycotoxins in diverse matrices are highly demanded. An ultrasensitive, colorimetric and homogeneous strategy for aflatoxin B1 (AFB1) detection, which used a DNA aptamer and two split G4-forming segments, was developed by Kim et al. (36) In the absence of AFB1, the two split G4-forming segments was able to combine with the free aptamer of AFB1 to generate an intact G4, facilitating the formation of POD-mimicking DNAzyme. However, in the presence of AFB1, the specific recognition of AFB1 by the aptamer led to structural deformation of the aptamer-DNAzyme complex, which caused the destruction of the G4 and a reduction in POD-mimicking activity. Therefore, a gradual decrease of the colorimetric signal was observed as the concentration of AFB1 increased. This strategy was simple, rapid, and low-cost for the detection of AFB1 with a wide linear range ($0.1$-$1.0 \times 10^4$ ng/mL) and low LOD (0.1 ng/mL). It also displayed high selectivity for AFB1 over other mycotoxins and could be employed to assay AFB1 in ground corn samples. A wash-free and label-free colorimetric biosensor for the amplified detection of AFB1 was also constructed based on the integration of an ingenious hairpin DNA probe with Exo III-assisted signal amplification by Chen et al. (37) The presence of AFB1 activated the continuous cleavage reactions by Exo III toward a hairpin probe, leading to the autonomous production of numerous free G4-forming sequences, which catalyzed the oxidation of TMB by $H_2O_2$ to generate a colorimetric signal. The presence of AFB1 triggered numerous G4-hemin DNAzyme made this naked-eye biosensor ultrasensitive, enabling the visual detection of trace amounts of AFB1 as low as 1 pM without any readout device (**Figure 13.5A**). The authors proved that the sensor was robust and could be used with complex food matrices, such as peanut samples. With the advantages of being simple to use and label-free and the generation of visible and intuitive output, the G4-hemin DNAzyme-based colorimetric biosensor is potentially suitable for in-field detection of AFB1.

An ultrasensitive electrochemical aptasensor with DNA tetrahedral nanostructures (DTNs) for the detection of ochratoxin A (OTA) was developed based on G4-hemin DNAzyme-catalyzed polyaniline (PANI) deposition in the presence of

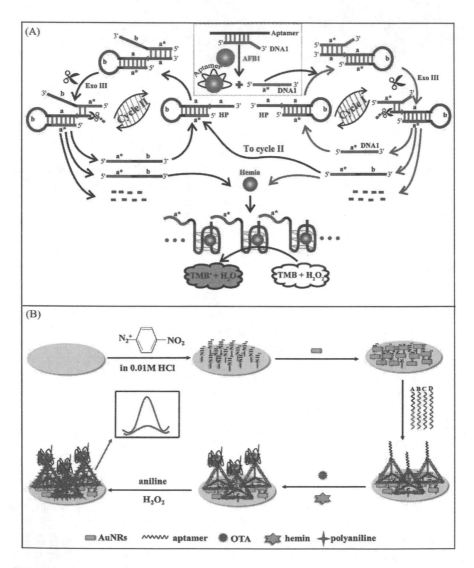

**FIGURE 13.5** (A) Wash-free and label-free colorimetric biosensor for naked-eye detection of AFB1 using G4 as the signal reporter (Reproduced from (37) with permission from Elsevier). (B) Ultrasensitive aptasensor with DNA tetrahedral nanostructure for OTA detection based on G4-hemin catalyzed polyaniline deposition (Reproduced from (38) with permission from Elsevier).

$H_2O_2$ (38). First, the electrode surface was modified with Au nanorods (NRs), which worked as a carrier to immobilize DTNs and promote electron transfer. Then, DTNs were immobilized for PANI deposition owing to their numerous negative charges. In the presence of OTA, the OTA-specific aptamer formed G4 structure and then bound with hemin. Thus, the OTA-induced G4-hemin DNAzyme catalyzed the PANI deposition in the presence of $H_2O_2$ and amplified the electrochemical signal

(**Figure 13.5B**). The amount of generated PANI was dependent on the number of G4-hemin induced by OTA. Therefore, the current signal was related to the concentration of OTA. The fabricated aptasensor exhibited a good linear response toward OTA over a wide range of concentrations from 0.001 ng/mL to 0.5 ng/mL with a LOD of 0.26 pg/mL.

In another study, Yu et al. developed an Exo-assisted multicolor aptasensor for the visual detection of OTA based on the etching of Au NRs mediated by a G4-hemin DNAzyme (39). In this strategy, a DNA probe (AG4-OTA) was designed that comprised an OTA aptamer and G4-forming sequence. OTA binds to AG4-OTA to form an antiparallel G4, which prevents its digestion by Exo I from the 3′ end of the AG4-OTA. Thus, the retained G4-forming sequence can bind to hemin to form G4-hemin DNAzyme. The DNAzyme catalyzes the oxidation of TMB by $H_2O_2$ to produce its diimine derivative ($TMB^{2+}$) in an acidic solution. Then the $TMB^{2+}$ etch the Au NRs by oxidizing Au(0) into Au(I). This results in the generation of rainbow-like colors and provides a multicolor platform for the visual detection of OTA. This strategy utilized only a single DNA probe and output multicolor visual signals for convenient and sensitive detection. It was also successfully applied to the determination of OTA in spiked beer with satisfactory recovery.

## 13.6  SUMMARY AND FUTURE PERSPECTIVES

In this chapter fundamentals concerning the design and engineering of POD-mimicking DNAzymes are reviewed, their properties are described, and how DNAzymes can be applied to contaminants detection in food and the environment are discussed. Due to the unique interactions between metal ions and bases in DNA, several biosensors have been developed to specifically detect toxic metal ions, including $Pb^{2+}$, $Hg^{2+}$, and $Ag^+$. Besides, G4-forming sequences were combined with DNA aptamers for detecting other contaminants, such as pesticides, antibiotics, and mycotoxins. All these biosensors utilized the POD-like catalytic activity of G4-hemin to generate and amplify detection signals, such as colorimetric, fluorescent, or electrochemical signals. To further enhance the detection sensitivity, various DNA amplification or cycling strategies were introduced into the design of the biosensor; these ingenious schemes have been very efficient.

Future work can focus on solving a few key challenges. First, realizing selective metal ion detection is still challenging using G4-hemin DNAzymes as the same binding pocket can accommodate different metal ions with a limited difference. In food and environmental sample matrices, a high background salt may exist and sensing of a small change of target metal ions concentration requires both high sensitivity and excellent specificity. This may be solved by fully understanding the interactions between metal ions and G4 structures as well as the conformational change of G4 structures. Second, ABTS and TMB were frequently used as substrates to generate colored products for visual signal output in most of these studies. Colorimetric methods are convenient and received well, attracting intensive research interests. However, the sensitivity of colorimetric methods is relatively low compared with that of fluorescent or electrochemical strategies. Therefore, new signal transduction strategies are needed to improve the design flexibility of DNAzyme-based sensors.

Also, the background color of ABTS$^{2-}$ and activity of hemin need to be reduced to achieve a high signal-to-background ratio. This might be realized by developing inhibitors that can suppress the activity of free hemin and novel chromogenic strategies. Third, the catalytic activity of G4-hemin DNAzymes is relatively low compared with that of protein enzyme HRP. Though there are already some efficient strategies to improve the catalytic activity and thermal stability of G4-hemin DNAzymes have been reported, further studies for enhancing the catalytic activity are needed. Fourth, most reported strategies have been developed and tested on model analytes in ideal buffer solutions under well-equipped laboratory settings. For rapid analysis of food and environmental samples, matrix effects and interferences should be rigorously tested. Therefore, more investigations for real-sample assays are required to optimize sensing systems for future applications.

## REFERENCES

1. Cech TR. 1988. *JAMA* 260: 3030–4
2. Travascio P, Li Y, Sen D. 1998. *Chemistry & Biology* 5: 505–17
3. Xi H, Juhas M, Zhang Y. 2020. *Biosensors and Bioelectronics* 167: 112494
4. Zhang R, Lu N, Zhang J, Yan R, Li J, et al. 2020. *Biosensors and Bioelectronics* 150: 111881
5. He K, Li W, Nie Z, Huang Y, Liu Z, et al. 2012. *Chemistry – A European Journal* 18: 3992–9
6. Hoang M, Huang P-JJ, Liu J. 2016. *ACS Sensors* 1: 137–43
7. Du Y, Dong S. 2017. *Analytical Chemistry* 89: 189–215
8. Li W, Li Y, Liu Z, Lin B, Yi H, et al. 2016. *Nucleic Acids Research* 44: 7373–84
9. Wu C, Gao G, Zhai K, Xu L, Zhang D. 2020. *Food Chemistry* 331: 127208
10. Zhang C, Zhang H, Wu P, Zhang X, Liu J. 2020. *Biosensors and Bioelectronics* 169: 112603
11. Yang H, Zhou Y, Liu J. 2020. *TrAC Trends in Analytical Chemistry* 132: 116060
12. Huppert JL. 2010. *The FEBS Journal* 277: 3452–8
13. Kong D-M, Cai L-L, Guo J-H, Wu J, Shen H-X. 2009. *Biopolymers* 91: 331–9
14. Cheng X, Liu X, Bing T, Cao Z, Shangguan D. 2009. *Biochemistry* 48: 7817–23
15. Kong D-M, Yang W, Wu J, Li C-X, Shen H-X. 2010. *Analyst* 135: 321–6
16. Travascio P, Witting PK, Mauk AG, Sen D. 2001. *Journal of the American Chemical Society* 123: 1337–48
17. Nakayama S, Sintim HO. 2009. *Journal of the American Chemical Society* 131: 10320–33
18. Guo Y, Chen J, Cheng M, Monchaud D, Zhou J, Ju H. 2017. *Angewandte Chemie International Edition* 56: 16636–40
19. Yang X, Li T, Li B, Wang E. 2010. *Analyst* 135: 71–5
20. Li T, Wang E, Dong S. 2010. *Analytical Chemistry* 82: 1515–20
21. Chen J, Zhang Y, Cheng M, Mergny J-L, Lin Q, et al. 2019. *Microchimica Acta* 186: 786
22. Kong D-M, Wang N, Guo X-X, Shen H-X. 2010. *Analyst* 135: 545–9
23. Li T, Dong S, Wang E. 2009. *Analytical Chemistry* 81: 2144–9
24. Kong D-M, Cai L-L, Shen H-X. 2010. *Analyst* 135: 1253–8
25. Zhu L, Li G, Shao X, Huang K, Luo Y, Xu W. 2019. *Microchimica Acta 187*: 26
26. Wu H, Wu J, Wang H, Liu Y, Han G, Zou P. 2021. *Journal of Hazardous Materials* 411: 124784

27. Li J, Xiong P, Tang J, Liu L, Gao S, et al. 2021. *Sensors and Actuators B: Chemical* 331: 129451

28. Xie S, Yuan W, Wang P, Tang Y, Teng L, Peng Q. 2019. *Sensors and Actuators B: Chemical* 292: 64–9

29. Nana L, Ruiyi L, Xiulan S, Yongqiang Y, Zaijun L. 2020. *Microchimica Acta* 187: 158

30. Miao Y-B, Gan N, Ren H-X, Li T, Cao Y, et al. 2016. *Talanta* 147: 296–301

31. Zhang R, Wang Y, Qu X, Li S, Zhao Y, et al. 2019. *Analyst* 144: 4995–5002

32. Huang W, Zhang H, Lai G, Liu S, Li B, Yu A. 2019. *Food Chemistry* 270: 287–92

33. Ou Y, Jin X, Fang J, Tian Y, Zhou N. 2020. *Microchemical Journal* 156: 104823

34. Han C, Li R, Li H, Liu S, Xu C, et al. 2017. *Microchimica Acta* 184: 2941–8

35. Liu S, Ding J, Qin W. 2019. *Analytical Chemistry* 91: 3170–6

36. Seok Y, Byun J-Y, Shim W-B, Kim M-G. 2015. *Analytica Chimica Acta* 886: 182–7

37. Wu J, Wang X, Wang Q, Lou Z, Li S, et al. 2019. *Chemical Society Reviews* 48: 1004–76

38. Wei M, Zhang W. 2018. *Sensors and Actuators B: Chemical* 276: 1–7

39. Yu X, Lin Y, Wang X, Xu L, Wang Z, Fu F. 2018. *Microchimica Acta* 185: 259

# 14 Nanozymes in Food Contaminants Analysis

*Long Wu*
Key Laboratory of Food Nutrition and Functional
Food of Hainan Province, College of Food
Science and Engineering, Hainan University,
Haikou, Hainan, China
College of Food Science and Engineering,
Hainan University, Haikou City, Hainan Prov.,
PR China

## CONTENTS

DOI: 10.1201/9781003109228-14

## 14.1  INTRODUCTION

Food contaminants, kind of toxic substances that are harmful to humans, have increasingly grown in complexity and followed up on new public health issues, novel safety emergencies, and emerging consumer demands (1). The complexity of the pollutants and food matrices brings great challenges to the analytical methods. For instance, fungi *Alternaria* can generate several toxic secondary metabolites, like alternariol, alternariol monomethyl ether, altenuene, tentoxin, and tenuazonic acid, which are widely found in sorghum, sunflower seeds, cereals, tomatoes, wine, beers, apple juices, and beverages (2). Various analytical strategies have been developed to monitor their occurrence in foods or food production chains. Those wet-chemistry-based analytical methods have been gradually replaced by powerful techniques that enable high enhancements in accuracy, precision, and detection limits. The new technologies can overcome the difficulties of conventional methods, such as time-consuming analysis, laborious procedures, and high cost. The development of novel "rapid" detection methods has decreased detection time dramatically, thus could solve the main concerns of most of the analytical methods. Hence, a new frontier of nanozymes in food contaminants detection gives a glimpse of insight into this concept.

Being different from natural enzymes, nanozymes behave relatively low catalytic activity and specificity and can only mimic limited types of enzymes, which place a big limit on the applications. The advantages and disadvantages of natural enzymes and nanozymes are listed and compared in **Table 14.1**. To resolve the disadvantages of nanozymes, great efforts have been made to develop new nanozymes with

---

## TABLE 14.1
## Comparison Between Natural Enzymes and Nanozymes

|  | Natural enzymes | Nanozymes |
|---|---|---|
| Advantages | High catalytic activity | Controllable catalytic activity |
|  | Good substrate selectivity | Multienzyme mimetic activity |
|  | Excellent biocompatibility | Low cost |
|  | Wide range of applications | Easy to mass-produce |
|  | Mild reaction conditions | Long-term storage |
|  | Stable structure | Robust to harsh environments |
|  | Controllable synthesis via gene | Unique physicochemical properties |
| Disadvantages | High cost | Limited types of nanozymes |
|  | Hard to be separated and purified | Limited substrate selectivity |
|  | Hard to store long term | Limited biocompatibility |
|  | Hard to mass-produce | Limited stability |
|  | Limited application conditions | Potential toxicity |
|  | Easy denaturation | Lack of standards |

superior performance. Up to now, iron-based, noniron metallic, and nonmetallic nanozymes (carbon-, porphyrin-, etc.) have been studied and constructed for different applications. The research direction mainly includes regulating the substrate selectivity, enhance their catalytic activity, and develop their mimetic activity. We introduced different kinds of nanozymes and a series of work on how to construct those nanozymes.

## 14.2 FOOD CONTAMINANTS DETECTION APPLICATIONS

The development of cost-effective, rapid, highly sensitive, and selective detection methods for food contaminants has significant market prospects and huge social benefits. Considering their physiochemical properties, nanozymes have a great potential in improving the performance of contaminants detection methods. In this section, we discuss the application of nanozymes in the detection of different classes of food contaminants, including toxins, pesticide residues, food additives abuse, and microorganism (**Figure 14.1**).

### 14.2.1 Toxins

#### 14.2.1.1 Detection of Mycotoxins

Mycotoxins are secondary metabolites produced by some fungi (mainly *Aspergillus, Penicillium,* and *Fusarium*) during the growth process, which can easily cause

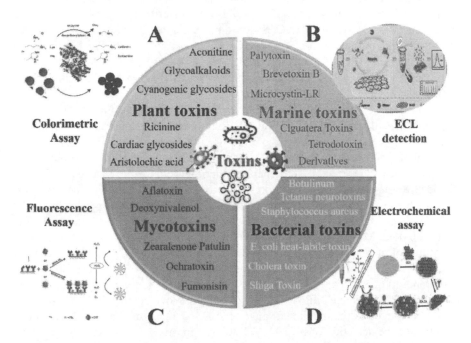

**FIGURE 14.1** Representative illustration of a nanozyme-based method for the detection of all kinds of toxins in food samples [A: (3); B: (4); C: (5); D: (6)].

physiological abnormalities in humans and animals (7). The mycotoxins can enter the food chain through contaminated grains or the products of animals (e.g., milk, meat, and eggs) that are fed with mycotoxin-contaminated feed. The most common mycotoxins are aflatoxin, ochratoxin, fumonisin, zearalenone patulin, and deoxynivalenol. Due to their toxicological effects, the presence of mycotoxins in foods has severe implications on human and animal health even at very low concentration levels (8). If ingested, they may cause acute or chronic disease. The majority of mycotoxins currently known are grouped according to their toxicity (under chronic conditions) as mutagenic, carcinogenic, and teratogenic. For example, aflatoxin is a kind of chemical compound with similar structures and toxicity. In the aflatoxin family, aflatoxin B1 (AFB1) is the most toxic with strong carcinogenicity, immunotoxicity, neurotoxicity, and genotoxicity.

Xu et al. established an indirect competitive metal-organic framework (MOF)-linked immunosorbent assay (MOFLISA) for high throughput and highly sensitive detection of AFB1, which replaces the natural enzyme with functional MOFs to catalyze a chromogenic system (9). The MOFLISA method provided a linear detection range from 0.01 to 20 ng mL$^{-1}$ with a limit of detection (LOD) of 0.009 ng mL$^{-1}$; this LOD is 20-fold lower compared with the results from conventional enzyme-linked immunosorbent assay (ELISA). Based on mesoporous $SiO_2$/Au–Pt (m-SAP), an aptamer and $Fe_3O_4$ magnetic nanoparticles (MNP), a nanozyme, and aptamer-based immunosorbent assay (NAISA) were constructed for AFB1 detection (10). The m-SAP was prepared to act as signal labels, aptamer was adopted to recognize AFB1, and MNP facilitated magnetic separation. The NAISA method showed an LOD of 5 pg mL$^{-1}$, which is 600-fold lower than that of the traditional ELISA method. Based on CdTe/CdS/ZnS quantum dots (QDs), luminol, and HRP-modified Au nanorods (NRs), Wu et al. designed a ratiometric ECL aptasensor for AFB1 detection (11). This sensor exhibited accurate and sensitive analytical performance for AFB1 with a good linear range from 5.0 pM to 10 nM with an LOD of 0.12 pM.

Colorimetric assays have been widely developed for the detection of ochratoxin A (OTA). Tian et al. developed a cascade reaction-based colorimetric aptasensor for the achievement of the high sensitivity of OTA (12). With OTA binding to its aptamer, the alkaline phosphatase-labeled DNA was released and catalyzed ascorbic acid-2-phosphate into ascorbic acid. The generated ascorbic acid further reduces manganese dioxide ($MnO_2$) nanosheets to $Mn^{2+}$ ions, destroying the OXD-mimicking activity of $MnO_2$. Thus, with the increasing amount of OTA, a color change occurs from blue to colorless due to the loss of catalytic activity of $MnO_2$. This method provided an LOD of 0.069 nM for OTA. Furthermore, based on the CAT-regulated fluorescence quenching of mercaptopropionic acid(MPA)-modified CdTe QDs, Lu et al. proposed a competitive fluorescence ELISA for detection of fumonisin B1 (FB1) (5). A system was proposed by using an $FB_1$-labeled CAT as competing antigens $H_2O_2$ decomposition, and $H_2O_2$-sensitive MPA-QDs were adopted provided the signal output. The method exhibited a dynamic linear range of 0.39–12.50 ng mL$^{-1}$ and an LOD of 0.33 ng mL$^{-1}$ for the detection of $FB_1$. This CAT used in this method can be extended to other nanomaterials with the same CAT activity, providing a universal detection platform.

## 14.2.1.2 Detection of Bacterial Toxins

Many foodborne diseases are caused by pathogenic bacteria. Moreover, it has been reported that various bacterial toxins may also act as very dangerous food poisoning substances (13). Emerging bacterial pathogens synthesize toxins that serve as primary virulence factors, including *Staphylococcus aureus (S. aureus)* alpha-toxin, *Shiga* toxin, cytotoxic necrotizing factor type 1, *Escherichia coli (E. coli)* heat-stable toxin, botulinum and tetanus neurotoxins, and *S. aureus* toxic-shock syndrome toxin (14). In some food processes, the elimination of pathogenic microorganisms from foods is an indispensable operation. However, it may suffer from limitations in practical processes due to the complex procedures in food processing. Thus, microbial and product monitoring are important in ensuring food safety. It is expected that feasible analytical techniques can be constructed to monitor pathogenic microorganisms or their products in the food matrix.

Ching et al. described the use of Au NPs in a single lateral flow device for the detection of botulinum neurotoxins A and B (15). If the toxin is present, it binds with the Au-conjugated Ab and together flows to the test capture line, resulting in the resolution of a red line. This is a typical lateral flow immunoassay that can be extended to nanozymes-based analytical techniques. Shlyapnikov et al. reported a new microarray-based immunoassay for the simultaneous detection of five bacterial toxins, including cholera toxin, *E. coli* heat-labile toxin, enterotoxins A and B, and the toxic shock syndrome toxin (16). The assay can be completed in less than 10 min with a low LOD of $0.1-1$ pg mL$^{-1}$ for water and 1 pg mL$^{-1}$ for food samples. Few nanozymes-based analytical techniques have been fabricated for the detection of bacterial toxins. However, nearly all of the immunoassays involve the reaction of enzyme and $H_2O_2$, so it can be a creative way to apply nanozymes in the previously reported immunoassay by replacing the enzyme-conjugated Ab.

## 14.2.1.3 Detection of Marine Toxins

Marine biotoxins are a kind of highly active special metabolic component in marine organisms, which generally has severe toxicity. Marine biotoxins are mainly produced by algae or phytoplankton (17). During the algal blooms, this small subset of algal species produces a large number of toxins, which are a major source of seafood contamination worldwide, thus severely affecting human health, economy, wildlife, and ultimately the ecosystem (18). These are involved in the production of toxins that get accumulated in seafood and transferred to the food chain, such as shellfish, coral reef fish, mollusks, crabs, prawns, mussels, and crustaceans. Therefore, it is crucial to develop rapid and efficient methods for the screening of marine toxins in food products, especially in seafood.

By immobilizing brevetoxin B (BTX-2)–bovine serum albumin (BSA) conjugate on Au NPs-decorated poly(amidoamine) dendrimers, Tang et al. developed an electrochemical assay for the fast screening of BTX-2 in food samples (19). The application of Au NPs can improve the conductivity of dendrimers on the electrode. The BTX-2 assay was conducted with a competitive immunoassay using an HRP-labeled *anti*-BTX-2 Abs and $H_2O_2$–*o*-phenylenediamine (OPD) reaction system. The result was linear over a wide range of $0.03-8$ ng mL$^{-1}$ and the LOD was 0.01 ng mL$^{-1}$ BTX-2. Using a streptavidin-biotin recognition model, Kawatsu et al. developed a direct competitive ELISA for monitoring paralytic shellfish poisoning toxins in shellfish (20). They used a decarbamoyl saxitoxin-POD conjugate as an enzyme label to catalyze the $TMB/H_2O_2$ chromogenic substrate solution. The method showed a specificity of 89.7% (52 of 58 samples) and six false positives (10.3%, 6 of 58) in real samples. Because of the function of POD in the assay, nanozymes with CAT activity can be an alternative to replace POD.

By coupling copper hydroxide ($CuOH_2$) nanozyme and G-quadruplex (G4)/hemin DNAzyme to form a double-integrated mimic enzyme, Liu et al. established a visual, sensitive, and selective immunosensor for detection of microcystin-LR (21). In this strategy, $Cu(OH)_2$ nanozyme acted as the label to capture the secondary Ab for immunoreaction and loading substrate for DNAzymes. The double-integrated mimic enzyme method showed good activity for the chromogenic reaction of ABTS, which realized the visual detection of microcystin-LR in the range from 0.007 to 75 μg $L^{-1}$ with an LOD of 6 ng $mL^{-1}$. Such double-integrated artificial enzyme showed a stable and catalytic ability to $H_2O_2$ and ABTS, further revealing the superiority of functional nanozymes.

### 14.2.1.4 Detection of Plant Toxins

Plant toxins, also known as phytotoxins, are secondary plant metabolites that have acute or chronic toxicity or pose anti-nutritional effects on people. However, as a kind of chemical defense, these toxins may protect the plant from herbivores, bacteria, and fungi. Fortunately, we can distinguish inherent plant toxins in edible crops from plant toxins entering the food and feed chains due to contamination with nonedible plants (22). For example, glycoalkaloids and cyanogenic glycosides are inherent plant toxins in potatoes and cassava. The commonly detected plant toxins include pyrrolizidine alkaloids, grayanotoxins, opium alkaloids, strychnine, ricinine, aconitine, aristolochic acid, and cardiac glycosides (e.g., digitoxin and digoxin).

Hu et al. proposed a sensitive colorimetric aptasensor for the quantitative detection of abrin using Au NPs nanozyme (23). Au NPs possess the POD-like activity that can catalyze TMB in the presence of $H_2O_2$ with color variations. The catalytic activity can be further improved by modifying target-specific aptamer on the surface of Au NPs. However, in the presence of the target molecule, the aptamers will be desorbed from the surface of Au NPs, which causes a decrease in the catalytic abilities of Au NPs. They reported a detection linear range from 0.2 to 17.5 nM and an LOD of 0.05 nM for abrin. Velmurugan et al. reported the fabrication of cobalt hydroxide ($Co(OH)_2$)-enfolded copper(I) oxide ($Cu_2O$) nanocubes on reduced graphene oxide (rGO) to develop an electrochemical caffeine sensor (24). The nanozymes exhibited good electrocatalytic activity toward caffeine in beverage samples and the sensor output was linear from 0.83 to 1200 μM with an LOD of 0.4 μM.

Using chitosan functionalized magnetic graphene oxide ($Fe_3O_4@SiO_2@CS/GO$), Tang et al. developed a method for efficient extraction and determination of alkaloids in hotpot (25). Based on π–π electron interaction, cation–π interaction, and hydrogen bonding, alkaloids were adsorbed from the food matrix, which exhibited great potential for efficacious extraction and separation performance of alkaloids. After separation, the analysis was achieved by ultraperformance liquid chromatography-tandem mass spectrometry (UPLC-MS/MS). The study was conducted by the adsorption properties of nanomaterials, and the detection was carried out without using nanozymes. However, it demonstrated that the detection can be successfully conducted by the pretreatment of nanocomposites, which pose a good guiding sense toward the nanozyme-based analytical techniques. Overall, nanozymes mainly play four key roles in the detection of plant toxins as analyte enricher, sensor structure mediator, target recognizer or reactant, and signaling agent (26).

## 14.2.2 Detection of Pesticide Residues

Pesticides are one of the major inputs used in agriculture to protect crops and seeds before and after harvesting (27). Though they have contributed huge economic benefits to society, the pesticide residues left in the food materials can have a deleterious effect on human health (28). Moreover, the widespread use of pesticides has caused serious concerns in food safety, because the residues are easily exposed to primary and derived agricultural products. Thus, to ensure food safety for consumers, many countries and organizations around the world have established maximum residue limits (MRL) for pesticides in foods (29).

On the other hand, due to the large amounts of pesticides currently being used, an increasing interest has been attracted for developing rapid screening systems to monitor their level in the food products (30). In this section, three kinds of pesticides include organophosphates (OPs), neonicotinoids (NNOs), and triazines (TAs), are introduced as analytes (**Figure 14.2**). To achieve robust detection of pesticides, several analytical techniques based on nanozymes are developed and highlighted.

### 14.2.2.1 Organophosphate Pesticides

Among the toxic pesticides, OPs are the major contaminants in water, fruit, or medicinal plants (32). Residues of Ops, such as chlorpyrifos-methyl, thiometon, and phorate, were found in several food samples at concentrations exceeding their MRL. For example, Wei et al. explored a dual-mode method with nanoceria ($CeO_2$) as a nanozyme for the detection of methyl-paraoxon (MP) in real samples

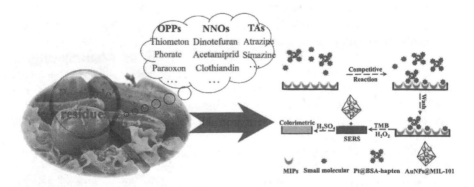

**FIGURE 14.2** Illustration of a nanozyme-based method for the detection of different pesticide residues in food samples (31).

(33). Based on the enzyme-like activity of nanoceria, MP could be hydrolyzed to para-nitrophenol (p-NP) with bright yellow color and characteristic absorption peak, which can be easily analyzed by the colorimetric and spectroscopic techniques. Both strategies showed an LOD of 0.42 μM. Furthermore, Wei et al. established a novel fluorescent method based on Samarium (Sm)-doped nanozyme (Sm-CeO$_2$) and cerium (Ce)-based fluorescent polymer (CFP) for the detection of MP (34). As a new doped nanozyme, Sm-CeO$_2$ exhibits OP hydrolase-like activity to hydrolyze MP. Meanwhile, the product of MP (p-NP) can interrupt the assemble of CFP and quench their fluorescence. This method can afford the fluorescence detection of MP with an LOD of 1.0 μM.

To detect omethoate and dichlorvos, and at the same time evaluate the activity of acetylcholinesterase (AChE), Huang et al. proposed a colorimetric paper sensor using γ-MnOOH nanowires (NWs) as nanozyme and TMB as a chromogenic indicator (35). In the reaction system of AChE and acetylthiocholine iodide (ATCh), thiocholine (TCh) can be produced, which can react with γ-MnOOH selectively and then trigger an activity loss of MnOOH nanozymes toward TMB oxidation. Thus, the concentration of pesticides and AChE activity can be measured by the changes in absorbance at 652 nm or the blue color of oxidized TMB products. The LODs of this system were 0.1 mU mL$^{-1}$ for AChE, 10 ng mL$^{-1}$ for omethoate, and 3 ng mL$^{-1}$ for dichlorvos. Based on Pt nanozyme for signal amplification, Chen et al. described a competitive bio-barcode immunoassay for the detection of trace parathion (LOD = 2.04 ng L$^{-1}$) in food samples (36).

By using Pt NPs as POD catalyzing the oxidation of TMB into an ideal SERS marker, Yan et al. proposed a biomimetic nanozyme-linked immunosorbent assay based on molecularly imprinted polymers (MIPs) and nanozyme labels for detection of triazophos (31). Wherein, MIPs act as a biomimetic Ab, Pt@BSA-hapten as a competitive probe to recognize the MIPs binding site, and Au NPs as the SERS enhanced substrate. Both colorimetric and SERS methods exhibited an LOD of 1 ng mL$^{-1}$, which is promising for the rapid detection of pesticide residues and other small molecules. By combining nanozyme with TMB indicator, SERS may bring about a new prospect for other compound analyses.

### 14.2.2.2  Neonicotinoid Pesticides

Neonicotinoid (NNO) pesticides are a relatively new group of active ingredients with broad-spectrum systemic action, low toxicity, and high insecticidal efficiency to mammals (37). The application of NNOs over large areas of agricultural land could give rise to serious risks in mutagenicity, carcinogenesis, and teratogenicity. Depending on the imidacloprid, acetamiprid pesticides, European Union (EU) has set MRL for pesticide residues in tea in the range 0.05–0.1 mg kg$^{-1}$. Thus, it is crucial to develop reliable analytical methods for proper assessment of human exposure to pesticides through foods.

Weerathunge et al. reported a colorimetric assay for rapid detection of acetamiprid with an acetamiprid-specific aptamer and Au NPs nanozyme (38). The Au NPs nanozyme activity can be inhibited by its surface passivation with target-specific aptamer molecules. In the presence of acetamiprid, the aptamer will be released on Au NPs surface in a target concentration-dependent manner, thus reactivate Au NPs nanozyme activity. This approach can realize the detection of 0.1 ppm acetamiprid within an assay time of 10 min. Based on the fact that aptamer can specifically bind with acetamiprid, an electrochemical aptasensor was also reported to selectively detect acetamiprid residues (39). A hybrid of graphene QD and Au nanostar was prepared and modified on the electrode to enhance electrocatalytic activity. Using differential pulse voltammetry (DPV), the measured signal decreased linearly with an acetamiprid concentration in the range of 1.0 fM–$10^2$ pM with an LOD of 0.37 fM. The ultra-high sensitivity of this sensor was ascribed to the unique catalytic properties of graphene QD and Au nanostars.

Based on an aptamer against acetamiprid, multiple complementary strands (CSs), and Au NPs, a fluorometric aptamer-based assay was developed for the selective detection of acetamiprid (40). In the presence of acetamiprid, they will bind to the aptamer and form CS1-fluorescein (FAM)-labeled CS2 (as a dsDNA), so the FAM-labeled dsDNA does not bind to Au NPs and remains free with strong fluorescence intensity. In reverse, CS3-modified Au NPs will quench the fluorescence of FAM-labeled CS2 without acetamiprid. Therefore, the fluorescence intensity is positively related to the concentration of acetamiprid. The method can realize the detection of acetamiprid in a range of 5–50 nM with an LOD of 2.8 nM. In this work, apart from the nanozyme activity of Au NPs, their quenching effect toward specific fluorescent materials was applied.

### 14.2.2.3 Triazine and Other Pesticides

It was reported that about 50% of pesticides applied in agriculture are related to herbicides (41) and among them, TA pesticides are the most used. Once introduced into the crops, TA pesticides can cause long-term negative effects due to their persistence. Another issue is their easy distribution into other parts of the environment, especially from the soil into groundwater, one of the main sources of drinking water. Thus, it is a vital subject to develop analytical techniques of TA pesticides by easy and cost-effective techniques in environmental chemistry.

By adopting polydopamine functionalized graphene sheets decorated with magnetic metal oxide NPs (FDGs) as efficient nanozyme, Boruah et al. described a study for the detection and degradation of harmful simazine pesticides (42). The detection was based on the hydrogen bonding interactions between pesticide molecules and TMB, which can cause inhibition of the catalytic activity of the FDGs toward TMB oxidation. In this system, the presence of simazine pesticides was detected with an LOD of 2.24 μM. Also, the photocatalytic degradation of simazine is achieved by the excellent photocatalytic activity of FDGs under irradiation of natural sunlight. Similarly, Boruah and Das successfully prepared $Fe_3O_4$-titanium dioxide ($TiO_2$)/rGO nanocomposite with $H_2O_2$ activity and photocatalytic efficiency (43). The colorimetric detection technique is applied for the sensing of atrazine using TMB as substrate molecules, which showed an LOD of 2.98 μg $L^{-1}$ and a linear range of 2–20 μg $L^{-1}$. Further, atrazine molecules can be fully degraded (100%) by $Fe_3O_4$–$TiO_2$/rGO nanozyme under irradiation of natural sunlight. Based on a competitive ELISA, Kwon et al. developed POD-like mesoporous core-shell palladium@platinum (Pd@Pt) NPs-conjugated primary Ab as enzyme labels to detect atrazine (44). The method leads to a high sensitivity with an LOD of 0.5 ng $mL^{-1}$ and recoveries of

99%–115%, demonstrating that atrazine and other low molecular weight herbicides and pesticides can be detected using this immunoassay.

Besides, with the help of heteroatom-doped grapheme, Zhu et al. fabricated a colorimetric nanozyme sensor array for the detection of aromatic pesticides (45). This work takes advantage of nanozyme by differentially masking their active sites, thus different pesticides can be adsorbed on the graphene. As a result, their POD-like activities will decrease. Based on the nanozyme catalyzed TMB/$H_2O_2$ system, five pesticides including fluoroxypyr-meptyl, lactofen, diafenthiuron, bensulfuron-methyl, and fomesafen were successfully detected by the sensor arrays from 5 to 500 μM. The inhibition effect of pesticides toward natural enzymes is suitable for nanozyme, which can be effectively used to indicate the amount of pesticides combining with the TMB/$H_2O_2$ coloring system.

### 14.2.3  VETERINARY DRUG RESIDUES

Veterinary drugs, including pharmaceutical feed additives, are often used to prevent, treat, and diagnose animal diseases or to purposely regulate animal physiological functions (46, 47). However, the abuse of veterinary drugs can easily cause residues of harmful substances in animal-derived foods, which not only cause direct harm to human health but also cause great harm to the development of animal husbandry and the ecological environment (48). Based on their functions, veterinary drugs also include many different groups, such as antibiotics, anthelmintics, growth promoters, antiprotozoal drugs, trypanosomiasis drugs, sedatives, β-adrenergic receptors blockers, etc. (49). The residues very commonly found in animal-derived foods are from antibiotics, sulfonamides, furans, antiparasitic, and hormone drugs. The lack of scientific knowledge and blinding pursuit of economic benefits by farmers cause widespread abuse of veterinary drugs in the animal husbandry industry. Therefore, the detection and analysis of veterinary drug residues in food samples are very necessary. It is fact that has been developed plenty of nanozymes successfully for food safety assay foods (50, 51).

#### 14.2.3.1  Antibiotics

Antibiotics are used to prevent and treat animal diseases and improve the performance of modern animal husbandry (52). Commonly used antibiotics include tetracycline (TCs), penicillin, cephalosporins, macrolides, etc. Nanozymes have certain similarities with natural enzymes in terms of size, shape, and surface charge. Compared with natural enzymes, nanozymes have the advantages of acid resistance, alkali resistance, high-temperature resistance, etc. Many methods for detecting and analyzing antibiotics have been developed. In this section, we will introduce two main nanozyme-based antibiotic analysis methods. The first one is a colorimetric technique, which uses a variety of testing solutions or color developers to determine the color of the solution, or uses an instrument to measure the concentration of the tested substance. The second is electrochemical technology, which is used to catalyze the $H_2O_2$ in the solution using nanozymes modified on the electrode; the

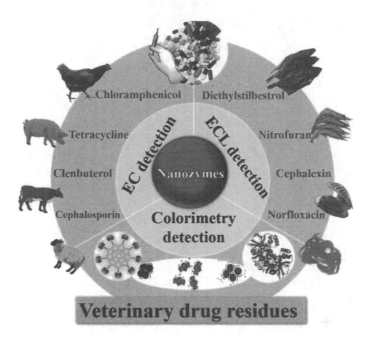

**FIGURE 14.3** Illustration of nanozymes in the design of detection platforms for veterinary drug residues as multifunctional sensing elements.

generated $O_2$ oxidizes specific substances to generate characteristic electrical signals. Different antibiotics drugs of interest in foods and the nanymes-based detection methods are depicted in **Figure 14.3**.

Based on the POD-like activity of Au NCs, Zhang et al. used TCs-specific aptamers to improve the catalysis ability of glutathione (GSH)-stabilized Au NCs to oxidize TMB by $H_2O_2$ and established a colorimetric sensing platform (53). In the presence of $H_2O_2$, the chromogenic substrate TMB is oxidized into a blue product (oxTMB). After adding the aptamer to the system, the POD activity of Au NCs increases with a deep blue color of oxTMB. The electrostatic interaction between the aptamers-modified Au NCs and the substrate TMB promotes the adsorption of TMB, thereby increasing the catalytic activity. However, when Au NCs-aptamers are exposed to TCs, TCs induce conformational changes of the aptamer due to their high affinity, which in turn regulates the surface of Au NCs, thereby inhibiting POD-like activity. In this case, TMB can only be oxidized to blue. Also, Sharma et al. used tyrosine-reduced Au NPs as PODe nanozymes and Ky2 aptamers to construct a colorimetric sensing platform to detect kanamycin (54). Au NPs possess POD activity, which can oxidize the colorless TMB into a blue substance of oxTMB. However, when the ssDNA Ky2 aptamer is modified on its surface, this POD activity will be inhibited. The color of the solution does not change in the absence of kanamycin. On the contrary, the ky2 aptamer exhibits high affinity and specificity in the presence of kanamycin, causing the ky2 molecule to dissociate from the surface of Au

NPs. And then, they will turn on the nanozyme activity of Au NPs again to indicate oxTMB color.

Tian et al. used a composite material of vanadium disulfide ($VS_2$) and Au NPs with perfect electrical conductivity and high specific surface area as carrier materials, using methylene blue labeled hDNA (MB-hDNA) and excellent POD catalytic activity cobalt ferrite ($CoFe_2O_4$) nanozymes as signal amplification components, and a ratio electrochemical biosensor for quantitative detection of kanamycin has been established (55). After the sulfhydryl MB-hDNA was modified with $VS_2$/Au NPs/GCE, the kanamycin-aptamer complex formed a double-stranded structure through the hybridization of the Au–S bond. Subsequently, the obtained $CoFe_2O_4$ nanozyme can be used as a POD mimic to catalyze and accelerate the conversion of $H_2O_2$ into $H_2O$. The presence of kanamycin will cause the decrease of the electrochemical signal of $CoFe_2O_4$ and the increase of the MB signal. This may be due to the $CoFe_2O_4$ nanozyme being dissociated from the electrode surface by the more affinity kanamycin, and the hDNA rebends and folds the MB closer to the electrode surface. Similarly, Khan et al. successfully synthesized a core-shell structure of Au-PDA@$SiO_2$ nanospheres by a one-pot method and used it on a GO electrode for the electrochemical detection of cefotaxime (56).

### 14.2.3.2   Antibacterials

Antibacterial drugs are a class of drugs that can inhibit or kill pathogenic bacteria and are widely used to treat or prevent infectious diseases in animals, such as livestock and poultry. In animal husbandry; some antibacterial drugs also have the effect of stimulating animal growth, increasing feed returns, reducing mortality, and even used as feed additives (57). However, long-term illegal addition of excessive drugs has brought harm to human health and the environment. Therefore, there are strict regulations and dosage control on the use of antibacterial drugs.

The colorimetric analysis method that relies on nanozymes is still the primary detection method for antibacterial drugs. A simple reduction method was used to synthesize Au NCs with 1-methyl-D-tryptophan as the reducing agent and capping agent. In the presence of $H_2O_2$, the obtained Au NCs exhibited POD mimicking properties, which turned TMB redox to blue. Due to the electron transfer regulation of surface charge control, the addition of norfloxacin increases the catalytic efficiency of nanozymes by ten times. The colorimetric sensor system has high selectivity for norfloxacin (58). He et al. used Au@$SiO_2$ NPs as a marker to establish a rapid bionic nano-enzyme-linked immunosorbent assay to detect sulfadiazine. Relying on POD-like activity of Au NPs and molecularly imprinted membranes as biomimetic Abs for recognition, Au@$SiO_2$ nanozymes replaced HRP to complete the sensitive detection of sulfadiazine in beef, pork, and chicken samples. Under the best conditions, the LOD of the immunosorbent test is 0.2 mg $L^{-1}$, which is not significantly different from the results obtained by high-performance liquid chromatography (HPLC) (59).

In recent years, ECL has attracted great interest due to its high sensitivity and selectivity (60). It mainly produces some special substances through electrochemical methods, which can degrade with the substances in the system or by itself, thereby producing the phenomenon of luminescence. Using MIPs and Cu(II) anchored unzipped covalent triazine framework (UnZ-CCTF), Ma et al. described detecting sulfa quinoxaline by ECL. Cu (II) has good dispersibility, conductivity, and POD activity, therefore UnZ-CCTF has a catalytic enhancement effect on the luminol/ $H_2O_2$ system. The detection range of sulfa quinoxaline in milk is 1–20 pM and the LOD is 0.76 pM (61).

### 14.2.3.3 Other Drugs

There are other types of veterinary drugs that contaminate animal foods, such as antiviral drugs and hormones. Antiviral drugs on the market mainly include amantadine, rimantadine, ribavirin, and other drugs represented by the symmetric tricyclic amine structure (62). It is worth noting that excessive use of antiviral drugs will also inevitably lead to excessive drug residues in animals, and eventually enter the human body through the food chain, leading to human anxiety, insomnia, and other adverse reactions (63–65). Among the few detection methods, colorimetry is still the main development and research method. For example, Ma et al. developed a colorimetric immunoassay to detect amantadine by introducing Pt nanocube as a nanozyme and covering the surface with polyvinylpyrrolidone (66). According to this protocol, the sensitivity is 0.195 and 0.134 ng $mL^{-1}$ for the naked-eye and instrumental detection of amantadine, respectively. This system is a significant improvement over the traditional immunoassay. Therefore, it is very meaningful to accelerate the development of rapid detection of veterinary drug residues.

### 14.2.4 Pathogens

The frequent occurrence of food safety incidents is a major worldwide concern. The World Health Organization (WHO) has determined that more than 80% of foodborne diseases occur due to biologically related factors, including microorganisms, parasites, and pests. The ultimate goal of food safety control is to avoid foodborne diseases originating from harmful microorganisms. Many analytical methods have been reported for the detection of bacteria or viruses. However, traditional techniques suffer from the limitation of low sensitivity, complex procedures, and time-consuming operations. Emerging analytical methods based on nanozymes are being developed. In this section, various nanozyme-based assays for harmful microorganisms are described, mainly involving colorimetric assay, lateral flow immunoassay, electrochemical assay, etc. (**Figure 14.4**).

### 14.2.4.1 Bacteria

Bacteria are the main category of foodborne pathogens, including *E.* coli, *Salmonella, Listeria, S. aureus, Shigella, Streptococcus haemolyticus, Vibrio parahaemolyticus,* etc. Among them, *E. coli O157:H7* is a highly infectious pathogen that spreads widely in food and water and poses a major challenge to public health. The Centers for Disease Control and Prevention (CDC) report that millions of people suffer from sickness each year because of *E. coli* infection.

Fu et al. proposed a two-step cascade signal amplification strategy for the detection of *E. coli*, which combines *in-situ* Au growth with nanozyme-catalyzed deposition and greatly improves the sensitivity of conventional Au NPs lateral flow assay (LFA) (67). Based on the principle of the conventional LFA platform,

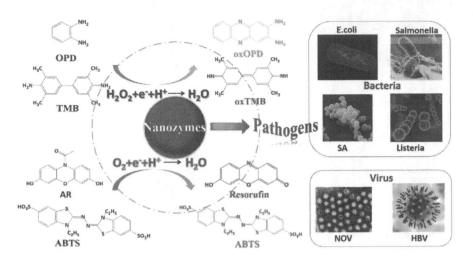

**FIGURE 14.4** Schematic of nanozymes-based colorimetric assays for the detection of food-borne pathogens.

monoclonal antibodies (mAbs)-modified Au NPs were first anchored on test and control lines on the strip, then the *in-situ* growth of Au NPs utilized to amplify the detection signal. After that, the Au NPs nanozyme-mediated catalytic deposition was executed to trigger the deposition of oxidized 3-amino-9-ethylcarbazole on the surface of Au NPs. The *in-situ* engineering of the nanozyme method achieved an ultrahigh LOD of 12.5 CFU mL$^{-1}$, a 400-fold enhancement compared with that of traditional Au NPs- immuno chromatographic assay (ICA). Also, Han et al. adopted concave Pd–Pt NPs as enzyme probes to establish a sensitive LFA for the detection of *E. coli* (68). Pd–Pt NPs were applied as a nanozyme probe to replace Au NPs and generated a nanozyme-based LFA. By using TMB substrate onto the test line, the assay exhibited an enhanced sensitivity of $9.0 \times 10^2$ CFU mL$^{-1}$ in milk, which was 111-fold higher than that of traditional Au NPs-ICA. To get rid of the shackles of traditional LFA and build a more flexible model, increasing studies have been carried out to develop a label-free and low-cost LFA, in which functional nanozymes are widely adopted to replace enzyme-labeled Abs and act as effective recognition agents to generate signals (69, 70).

For the specific and sensitive detection of *S. aureus*, Liu et al. reported a colorimetric assay based on BSA-templated cobalt tetraoxide (Co$_3$O$_4$) magnetic nanozyme conjugated with *S. aureus*-specific fusion-pVIII (71). In this, the functional Co$_3$O$_4$@fusion-pVIII particles could capture *S. aureus* in milk, and then they were isolated from milk by magnetophoretic chromatography. After transferring the complex to a 96-well plate, ABTS and H$_2$O$_2$ were introduced to generate the colorimetric reaction. The method showed a wide detection range of 10–10000 CFU mL$^{-1}$ in milk and an LOD of 8 CFU mL$^{-1}$. Based on Ag NCs nanozyme and aptamer, Liu et al. described a rapid colorimetric assay for *S. aureus* (72). In the study, the Ag NCs can oxidize OPD to the oxidized OPD with color variations. The final detection range of this colorimetric method is from 10 to 10$^6$ cfu·mL$^{-1}$ with an LOD of 10 cfu·mL$^{-1}$. This type of colorimetric assays can become a versatile strategy for the rapid detection of a wide variety of bacteria and pathogens.

### 14.2.4.2 Viruses

Viruses are also foodborne pathogenic microorganisms that can contaminate foods. However, there is a general lack of knowledge about viruses in food safety. At present, the common foodborne viruses are hepatitis A and hepatitis E viruses, rotavirus, astrovirus, enterovirus, and norovirus. Human norovirus (NoV) is one of the most common viruses that cause foodborne outbreaks worldwide (73, 74). It is estimated that 267 million people are infected with NoV each year and more than 200,000 people die, especially the young, the elderly, and people with immunosuppression (75). The present detection technique for NoV is based on gene amplification techniques, such as reverse-transcription quantitative polymerase chain reaction (RtqPCR), but the detection of NoV in food requires matrix-specific virus concentration and the removal of the inhibitory compounds. The RtqPCR method is not amenable to the rapid detection of food samples.

Based on the POD activity of Ag ion-incorporated Au NPs (Au/Ag NP), Khoris et al. developed a colorimetric bioassay for detection of NoV (76). Simply, NoV was captured by anti-NoV genogroup II Abs and formed a sandwich structure with Ab-modified Au NPs. The *in-situ* growth of Au/Ag was controlled by introducing Ag+/hydroquinone solution. When TMB/$H_2O_2$ was added to the wells, Ag ions were released from the surface of Au/Ag NPs and enhanced the oxidation of TMB with intense blue color. The method showed an LOD of 13.2 c132 copies/g feces in the range of $10^2$–$10^6$ copies of viral RNA/mL. Weerathunge et al. proposed a new colorimetric nanozyme aptasensor strategy for rapid (10 min) and sensitive detection of the infective murine norovirus, a readily cultivable surrogate for NoV (77). The strategy involves the noncovalent adsorption of the murine norovirus-specific aptamer molecules onto Au NPs, leading to the loss of its inherent nanozyme activity. In the presence of NoV, the aptamers will be released from Au NPs surface and result in the recovery of the nanozyme activity, producing a blue color. The strategy offers an alternative for practical deployment of norovirus detection with simple pretreatment in contaminated food.

### 14.2.5 Food Additives

Food additives are a kind of raw material added in food or the process of food production, which aim to improve food edibility as well as the taste and aesthetic feeling of food. Although certain levels of food additives are required in the food industry, there is still considerable debate on whether foods or supplements with additives have positive effects on human health. However, what is certain is that the excessive use of additives or illegal use of nonfood additives will cause a series of food safety problems.

Based on their functions, food additives can also be divided into different groups, such as antioxidants, sweeteners, preservatives, colorants, thickeners, flavor enhancers, etc. At present, more than 25,000 food additives are being used around the world. However, high doses of food additives may have harmful long-term effects on animals, such as cancer proliferation (78). Therefore, the analysis of these unavoidable additives in food samples is important. On the other hand, nanozymes are known for their enzyme-like properties. They have many functions beyond catalysis due to the intrinsic nanostructured nature, with which many robust methods are constructed for the detection of food additives.

### 14.2.5.1 Antioxidants

Antioxidants can prevent or delay food oxidation deterioration by reducing oxygen or free radical level around food, and thus improve stability and storage resistance. Commonly used food antioxidants involve butylated hydroxyanisole (BHA), butylated hydroxytoluene (BHT), tert-butyl hydroquinone (TBHQ), and propyl gallate (PG), which possess an aromatic ring and at least one phenol hydroxyl group. The structure indicates that they are favorable to eliminate reactive species, such as reactive oxygen species (ROS). Meanwhile, it has been demonstrated that nanozymes help to simultaneously convert both $O_2$ and $H_2O_2$ to free radicals, which can build a link with antioxidants via the $O_2$- or $H_2O_2$- mediated reactions. Thus, nanozymes with POD activity can be applied in the analysis of antioxidants.

Several analytical procedures have been developed for the detection of antioxidants. In this part, we will introduce two main nanozymes-based analytical methods for the analysis of antioxidants. The first one is an electrochemical technique using nanozymes as a CAT-like modification on electrodes, which act as catalysts toward $H_2O_2$ to obtain $O_2$, then oxidize antioxidants to produce a characteristic signal peak. When combined with specific enzymes (e.g., tyrosinase), the nanozymes-based electrochemical method can achieve a synergistic effect for antioxidants detection. The second one is the traditional chromogenic reaction of TMB producing varied colors in the presence of antioxidants, which can be initiated by nanozymes in the TMB/ $H_2O_2$ reaction system. This method is simple and shows good sensitivity when measured optically.

Wu et al. proposed an electrochemical biosensor for the simultaneous determination of BHA and PG by modifying spiny Au–Pt nanotubes and HRP onto the electrode (79). In the electrochemical process, Au–Pt nanotubes showed synergetic CAT-like activity for BHA and PG with well-defined oxidation peaks at 624 and 655 mV, respectively. The method showed a wide linear range of 0.3–50 mg $L^{-1}$ and 0.1–100 mg $L^{-1}$ for BHA and PG with LODs of 0.046 and 0.024 mg $L^{-1}$. Moreover, BHA and PG were demonstrated by a simple visual detection method, which involved Au–Pt nanotubes, a kind of nanozymes, as catalysts, and TMB as an indicator. By mixing TMB and nanozymes, which is similar to the TMB/$H_2O_2$ coloring system, the mixture showed a characteristic blue color of oxidized TMB. When antioxidants exist, TMB could be less oxidized due to their strong oxidation resistance, which decreased the optical density. Though simple to perform, the detection specificity of the visual detection method was limited. Thus, a combination of visual and electrochemical methods can enhance detection accuracy.

It has been reported that Pd–Au NPs, N-doped carbon, and metalloporphyrin-based hydrophilic porous organic polymer owned POD activity, which can be adopted as nanozymes in colorimetric assays (80, 81). Besides, the electrocatalytic activity of nanozymes is widely used in the construction of electrochemical sensors.

Yue et al. reported an electrochemical sensor for sensitive and selective detection of TBHQ by integrating MIPs, Pd–Au NPs, and electrochemically reduced GO (ERGO) (82). Wherein, MIPs realized the specific recognition with TBHQ, EGRO accelerated the electron transfer and bimetallic Pd–Au NPs acted as a promising catalyst. Pd–Au NPs were demonstrated to be electrocatalytically active, making the method have a favorable accuracy and satisfactory precision for the analysis of TBHQ. Lou et al. successfully prepared N-doped carbon nanozymes for the determination of total antioxidant capacity in real food samples (83). Cui et al. designed and prepared a novel porphyrin-based porous organic polymer, which was adopted in the TMB/$H_2O_2$ reaction system for the evaluation of antioxidants, such as ascorbic acid, gallic acid, and tannic acid (84). The distinguishing inhibitory behavior of these acids implies their different antioxidative mechanisms, further providing a new idea in understanding the biochemical interactions between natural enzymes and antioxidants.

### 14.2.5.2 Food Colorants

Food colorants are any dyes or pigment that imparts color added to food, drink, or any nonfood applications. Synthetic food colors are manufactured chemically, which behave advantages involving high stability to light, air, temperature, pH and storage conditions, color uniformity, relative lower production costs, and so on (85). Thus, synthetic food colors, such as tartrazine, Allura red, sunset yellow FCF, amaranth, ponceau 4R, and indigo carmine are widely applied in the food industry. However, continuous intake of synthetic colorants may impart certain toxicity to the human body (86). Experiments demonstrated that a high dosage of dye like amaranth might increase the incidence of malignant tumors in rats (87). So, the synthetic pigments allowed are regulated in some countries with strictly limited dosage.

A glimpse of structure to analytical methods for food colorants analysis appears to be receiving more attention. One principal reason is that synthetic pigments show a structure–activity relationship concerning groups like hydroxyl (–OH), amine (–$NH_2$), or benzene ring (–$C_6H_5$), which are usually electrochemically active. In this sense, the detection of colorants is more favored with electrochemical methods. Besides, in the oxidation process, catalysts mediated reactions can help colorants form electrocatalytically active species that correspond to distinctive electrochemical responses. In the presence of dissolved oxygen, $H_2O_2$ can be electrochemically produced, which then induces the oxidation of analytes (88). Thus, nanozymes are popular in detecting colorants using electrochemical sensors.

Based on $TiO_2$/ERGO nanocomposites ($TiO_2$/ERGO), Qin et al. described a voltammetric sensor for simultaneous detection of ponceau 4R and tartrazine (89). $TiO_2$ NPs were uniformly supported on ERGO nanoflakes, providing a favorable interface for the adsorption and oxidation of target analytes. The method achieved LODs of 4.0 and 6.0 nM for ponceau 4R and tartrazine, respectively. The good analytical properties are primarily attributed to the synergistic enhancement effect from ERGO nanoflakes and $TiO_2$ NPs. Similarly, Li et al. reported $TiO_2$/ERGO nanohybrids for the electrochemical detection of Allura red with enhanced electrocatalytic activity and voltammetric response, and the LOD is 0.05 μM (90). In another study, nanosized CuS is demonstrated to be an efficient nanozyme with high

POD-mimicking catalytic activity at neutral pH (91). Later, CuS with different morphologies was studied and then applied in tartrazine and sunset yellow detection by voltammetric techniques (92). The CuS nanoflowers constructed electrode realized the detection limits of 12 nM for tartrazine and 6 nM for sunset yellow, which revealed the unique electrocatalytic activities of CuS crystals.

### 14.2.5.3 Other Food Additives

Other additives are commonly detected include preservatives, sweeteners, flavor enhancers, etc. Based on the differences in the structure and property of these food additives, they are often analyzed by the fitting technique or their coupled ones to achieve the best results. In this part, we mainly focus on electrochemical methods with the application of nanozymes.

For example, based on the POD-like catalytic activity of nanozymes, Xi et al. designed Cu/carbon hybrid as potential enzyme mimetics to generate ROS for antibacterial therapy (93). For the electrochemical detection of sweetener, Cu NPs/MWCNTs composite was prepared and modified on the electrode for neotame detection, which exhibited catalytic activity toward the oxidation of neotame at a potential of 1.3 V (94). By employing ZnO NPs/MWCNTs modified glassy carbon electrodes, Balgobind et al. developed a DPV technique for aspartame detection, which promoted the electron transfer and enhanced the performance for aspartame sensing (95). Because the hybrids behave synergistic effects, such as the enhanced electron transfer and electrocatalytic activity, metallic nanozymes hybridized with MWCNTs have stimulated increasing interest in the application of electrochemical sensors.

For the detection of preservatives, Rather et al. proposed a novel electrochemical detection of parabens by depositing polyaniline film (PANI) and Au NPs on a glassy carbon electrode. The square wave voltammetric (SWV) response of ethylparaben (EP) shows a wide linear range from 0.1 to 5.10 nM with an LOD of 0.1 nM. The PANI/Au NPs interface offered a large active surface area, fast electron transfer kinetics, and higher catalytic activity toward EP detection. Pei et al. synthesized the polynaphthylamine/graphene composites by an *in situ* polymerization of naphthylamine monomers and graphene (96). The composites modified electrode exhibits an oxidation cyclic voltammogram (CV) peak located at +0.29 V for benzoic acid, with a linear range of 0.001~2 mM and an LOD of 0.34 $\mu$M. Besides, using Au NPs decorated on a molybdenum disulfide/chitosan (Au@MoS$_2$/CS) as a conductive matrix, Devi et al. constructed an electrochemical immunosensor for the detection of monosodium glutamate, a kind of flavor enhancers (97). A linear detection range was perceived from 0.05 to 200 $\mu$M, with an LOD of 0.03 $\mu$M.

With the participation of nanozymes, the electrochemical oxidation process can be improved by accelerating the electron transfer rate and reducing the reaction potential. The mechanism study showed that the hydroxyl radical could be the key intermediate involved in the POD-like catalysis. We believe that nanozymes will be applied to more new analytical fields with a deep understanding and precise regulation of their catalytic properties.

## 14.2.6  HEAVY METAL IONS

Due to their potential threat to public health, heavy metal ions ($Hg^{2+}$, $Pb^{2+}$, and $Cd^{2+}$) in food have been of increasing concern (98). Long-term intake of these heavy metal ions, even trace amounts in food will cause some severe diseases, such as cognitive deficits, kidney failure, cardiovascular, and neurological disorders (99). Also, $Cu^{2+}$ is an essential element at the trace level in the human body. For example, $Cu^{2+}$ can play a catalytic action in heme synthesis, but the intake of large quantities can be toxic. It is therefore essential to monitor heavy metals in the food or drinking water. Currently, a nanozyme-based analytical method is one of the frontiers in the detection of toxic heavy metal ions.

Huang et al. reported new CS-functionalized molybdenum(IV) selenide nanosheets (CS-$MoSe_2$ NS) for the colorimetric sensing of $Hg^{2+}$ (35). With the principle of $Hg^{2+}$ activated CS-$MoSe_2$ NS nanozyme activities and the indicator of TMB, $Hg^{2+}$ ions could be quantitatively and selectively monitored with an LOD of 3.5 nM. Similarly, Liu et al. developed a new type of $Hg^{2+}$-triggered nanozyme of AuNPs coupled carbon dots (Au NPs@CDs), which can catalyze the oxidation of colorless TMB into blue color. What interesting is that Au NPs@CDs showed almost no POD-like activity, and it was only triggered by $Hg^{2+}$. Based on the regulation of the catalytically triggered activity, the colorimetric method results were linear in the detection range of 7–150 nM and the LOD was 3.7 nM for $Hg^{2+}$ (100). These methods are based on the surface modification of nanozymes, and the catalytic activity can be selectively triggered by the specific target, which could be an example for designing other specific nanozymes.

For the determination of $Pb^{2+}$ ions, Xie et al. proposed Au@Pt NPs nanozyme as a colorimetric probe, which is based on the surface leaching of Au@Pt NPs nanozyme by lead-thiosulfate ($Pb^{2+}$-$S_2O_3^{2-}$) ions, inducing a decreased catalytic activity of the metallic nanozyme (101). As the $Pb^{2+}$ concentration increased, the nanozyme catalytic activity gradually decreased. By using TMB/$H_2O_2$ coloring system as an indicator, an LOD of 3.0 nM with a linear range from 20 to 800 nM was achieved. Liu et al. presented a facile strategy for selective detection of $Cu^{2+}$ by combining the POD-like nanozyme activity of Au NCs with amino acid's ambidentate nature (102). The nanozyme activity of histidine-Au nanoclusters can be inhibited by $Cu^{2+}$, which was developed to a "turn-off" mode that can sensitivity and selectivity recognize $Cu^{2+}$. The nanozyme probe showed a linear range of 1–100 nM and an LOD of 0.1 nM using the TMB/$H_2O_2$ system. Also, Xue et al. proposed an assay for the determination of $Cr^{6+}$ by employing polyethylenimine (PEI)-stabilized Ag NCs as an oxidoreductase mimic (103). Based on the finding that PEI-Ag NCs act as an oxidoreductase-like nanozyme to promote the TMB/chromium ($Cr^{6+}$) reaction, toxic $Cr^{6+}$ can be rapidly detected with an LOD of 1.1 μM. The proposed method was highly selective without the interference of other ions, including $Cr^{3+}$.

Based on the catalytic activity of nanozymes, the constructed methods are adopting the inhibition principle of heavy metal ions. Studies have shown that the addition of metal ions can control nanozyme POD-like activity. Some are based on metallophilic interactions, such as Au–Ag or Au–Hg, with the easy reduction nature of $Ag^+$ and $Hg^{2+}$ being readily modified on the Au NPs to enhance the POD-like activity

(104, 105). Others are using the surface ligands of nanozymes, as described above, to provide binding sites for metal ions, thus reducing the affinity of nanozymes with a substrate like TMB (102). The two strategies can both affect the nanozyme catalytic activity, and the detection can be revealed by the $TMB/H_2O_2$ system. These studies demonstrated that it is of great importance to engineer nanozymes and modify their surfaces.

## 14.3 SUMMARY AND FUTURE PERSPECTIVE

The nanozymes have attracted much attention worldwide. Along with their remarkable properties, nanozymes-based analytical techniques have been booming. In particular, their applications have been widely explored in food safety. As the food contaminants can cause a huge threat to human health and serious economic loss in the food industry, much research is being pursued to develop robust detection strategies. To drive the development of nanozyme research in food safety, it is essential to open a new avenue that can solve the limitations of certain analytical methods. Fortunately, most of the nanozymes are applied in constructing rapid detection methods like fluorescence, colorimetry, electrochemistry, and biosensors, which has provided some potential opportunities to respond to the demands of analytical science. Although nanozymes can enhance the detection performance, they are new artificial enzymes that are full of challenges that remained to be addressed.

 i. Exploring principles and mechanisms of nanozymes. Although a large number of papers have been reported on nanozymes, few experimental studies focused on the theoretical work and mechanism clarification. It is important to explore the fundamental principles and mechanisms of nanozymes, which can reveal the structure–activity relationship and guide the precise design of nanozymes with desirable applications.

 ii. Developing uniform systems and standards. Nanozymes are built up from the concept of an enzyme; however, their properties differ a lot from natural enzymes. So, it is difficult to characterize the nanozyme performance traditionally. For example, the Michaelis–Menten mechanism is popular in discussing natural enzymes, but it is clear that natural enzymes catalyze a reaction through a homogeneous medium, which is different from nanozymes that occur in a heterogeneous mechanism on the surface of nanomaterials. Thus, uniform systems and standards should be constructed to better characterize nanozyme performance.

 iii. Engineering controllable and functional nanozymes. Since size, morphology, and surface groups pose effects on nanozyme activity and functions, it is favorable to achieve nanozymes with high performance. How to controllably engineer nanozymes and extend their functions by surface modification is an important direction.

 iv. Evaluating high-performance nanozymes. In developing improved analytical techniques, various nanozymes are reported for signal production and amplification. However, when applied to real applications, the catalytic

activity of nanozymes is still relatively low. Compared to natural enzymes, the types of nanozymes are limited and nanozymes can hardly catalyze one specific substrate. Therefore, nanozymes with high catalytic activity, various enzymatic activity, and good substrate selectivity are in great need.
v. Integrating distinct techniques. It is encouraging that nanozyme-based detection techniques are narrowing the gap to practical-oriented food analytical methods. But it is almost impossible to achieve all the advances in a single detection technique. Thus, it is an alternative to develop nanozymes-based techniques with multimodes for the rapid, accurate, sensitive, and selective detection of food contaminants. For instance, it can greatly improve the specificity and selectivity of nanozymes by coupling with the molecular imprinting technique.

In general, nanozymes are in the early stages of the development of second-generation artificial enzymes. The powerful functions of nanozymes make them popular from *in vitro* detection to *in vivo* monitoring, and we believe that they will have great potential in the analysis of food contaminants in the near future. The above challenges will be the next frontier for further nanozyme research.

## ACKNOWLEDGMENT

This work was supported by the National Natural Science Foundation of China (31801638) and the Fund of Key Laboratory of Fermentation Engineering (Ministry of Education) (202105FE09). We acknowledge Shuhong Zhou from the Hubei University of Technology for collecting the materials.

## REFERENCES

1. Huang L, Sun D-W, Pu H, Wei Q. 2019. *Comprehensive Reviews in Food Science and Food Safety* 18: 1496–513
2. Pinto VEF, Patriarca A. 2017. *Alternaria Species and Their Associated Mycotoxins*
3. Nilam M, Hennig A, Nau WM, Assaf KI. 2017. *Analytical Methods* 9: 2784–7
4. Yang W, Zhang G, Ni J, Wang Q, Lin Z. 2021. *Sensors and Actuators B-Chemical* 327
5. Lu T, Zhan S, Zhou Y, Chen X, Huang X, et al. 2018. *Analytical Methods* 10: 5797–802
6. Savas S, Altintas Z. 2019. *Materials* 12
7. Zain ME. 2011. *Journal of Saudi Chemical Society* 15: 129–44
8. Cimbalo A, Alonso-Garrido M, Font G, Manyes L. 2020. *Food and Chemical Toxicology* 137
9. Xu Z, Long L-l, Chen Y-Q, Chen M-L, Cheng Y-H. 2021. *Food Chemistry* 338
10. Wu L, Zhou M, Wang Y, Liu J. 2020. *Journal of Hazardous Materials* 399
11. Wu S, Zhu F, Hu L, Xi J, Xu G, et al. 2017. *Food Chemistry* 232: 770–6
12. Tian F, Zho J, Jiao B, He Y. 2019. *Nanoscale* 11: 9547–55
13. Bielecki J. 2003. *Acta Microbiologica Polonica* 52 Suppl: 17
14. Clark GC, Casewell NR, Elliott CT, Harvey AL, Jamieson AG, et al. 2019. *Trends in Biochemical Sciences* 44: 365–79
15. Ching KH, Lin A, McGarvey JA, Stanker LH, Hnasko R. 2012. *Journal of Immunological Methods* 380: 23–9

16. Shlyapnikov YM, Shlyapnikova EA, Simonova MA, Shepelyakovskaya AO, Brovko FA, et al. 2012. *Analytical Chemistry* 84: 5596–603
17. Daly JW. 2004. *Journal of Natural Products* 67: 1211–5
18. Bano K, Khan WS, Cao C, Khan RFH, Webster TJ. 2020. *Biosensors for Detection of Marine Toxins*: John Wiley & Sons, Ltd
19. Tang D, Tang J, Su B, Chen G. 2011. *Biosensors & Bioelectronics* 26: 2090–6
20. Kawatsu K, Kanki M, Harada T, Kumeda Y. 2014. *Food Chemistry* 162: 94–8
21. Liu W, Gan C, Chang W, Qileng A, Lei H, Liu Y. 2019. *Analytica Chimica Acta* 1054: 128–36
22. Mol HGJ, Van Dam RCJ, Zomer P, Mulder PPJ. 2011. *Food Additives and Contaminants Part a-Chemistry Analysis Control Exposure & Risk Assessment* 28: 1405–23
23. Hu J, Ni P, Dai H, Sun Y, Wang Y, et al. 2015. *Analyst* 140: 3581–6
24. Velmurugan M, Karikalan N, Chen S-M, Karuppiah C. 2016. *Microchimica Acta* 183: 2713–21
25. Tang T, Cao S, Xi C, Li X, Zhang L, et al. 2020. *International Journal of Biological Macromolecules* 146: 343–52
26. Chen Q, Zhu L, Chen J, Jiang T, Ye H, et al. 2019. *Food Chemistry* 277: 162–78
27. Bajwa U, Sandhu KS. 2014. *Journal of Food Science and Technology-Mysore* 51: 201–20
28. Jiang X, Li D, Xu X, Ying Y, Li Y, et al. 2008. *Biosensors & Bioelectronics* 23: 1577–87
29. Jallow MFA, Awadh DG, Albaho MS, Devi VY, Ahmad N. 2017. *International Journal of Environmental Research and Public Health* 14
30. Liu T, Tian J, Cui L, Liu Q, Wu L, Zhang X. 2019. *Colloids and Surfaces B-Biointerfaces* 178: 137–45
31. Yan M, Chen G, She Y, Ma J, Hong S, et al. 2019. *Journal of Agricultural and Food Chemistry* 67: 9658–66
32. Yang Q, Wang J, Chen X, Yang W, Pei H, et al. 2018. *Journal of Materials Chemistry A* 6: 2184–92
33. Wei J, Yang L, Luo M, Wang Y, Li P. 2019. *Ecotoxicology and environmental safety* 179: 17–23
34. Wei J, Xue Y, Dong J, Wang S, Hu H, et al. 2020. *Chinese Medicine* 15
35. Huang L, Sun D-W, Pu H, Wei Q, Luo L, Wang J. 2019. *Sensors and Actuators B-Chemical* 290: 573–80
36. Chen G, Jin M, Yan M, Cui X, Wang Y, et al. 2019. *Microchimica Acta* 186
37. Wu L, Zhu L, Ma J, Li J, Liu J, Chen Y. 2020. *Microchimica Acta* 187
38. Weerathunge P, Ramanathan R, Shukla R, Sharma TK, Bansal V. 2014. *Analytical Chemistry* 86: 11937–41
39. Chu H, Hu J, Li Z, Li R, Yang Y, Sun X. 2019. *Sensors and Actuators B-Chemical* 298
40. Bahreyni A, Yazdian-Robati R, Ramezani M, Abnous K, Taghdisi SM. 2018. *Microchimica Acta* 185
41. Gilberto, Abate, Jorge, Cesar, Masini. 2005. *Journal of Agricultural and Food Chemistry* 53: 1612–9
42. Boruah PK, Darabdhara G, Das MR. 2020. *Chemosphere*
43. Boruah PK, Das MR. 2020. *Journal of Hazardous Materials* 385
44. Kwon EY, Ruan X, Wang L, Lin Y, Du D, Van Wie BJ. 2020. *Analytica Chimica Acta* 1116: 36–44
45. Zhu Y, Wu J, Han L, Wang X, Li W, et al. 2020. *Analytical Chemistry* 92: 7444–52
46. Stolker AAM, Brinkman UAT. 2005. *Journal of Chromatography A* 1067: 15–53
47. Rocca LM, Gentili A, Perez-Fernandez V, Tomai P. 2017. *Food Additives and Contaminants Part a-Chemistry Analysis Control Exposure & Risk Assessment* 34: 766–84

48. Masia A, Morales Suarez-Varela M, Llopis-Gonzalez A, Pico Y. 2016. *Analytica Chimica Acta* 936: 40–61
49. Winckler C, Grafe A. 2001. *Journal of Soils and Sediments* 1: 66
50. Wang W, Gunasekaran S. 2020. *Trac-Trends in Analytical Chemistry* 126
51. Zhang X, Wu D, Zhou X, Yu Y, Liu J, et al. 2019. *Trac-Trends in Analytical Chemistry* 121
52. English BK, Gaur AH. 2010. In *Hot Topics in Infection and Immunity in Children Vi*, ed. A Finn, N Curtis, AJ Pollard, pp. 73–82
53. Zhang Z, Tian Y, Huang P, Wu F-Y. 2020. *Talanta* 208
54. Sharma TK, Ramanathan R, Weerathunge P, Mohammadtaheri M, Daima HK, et al. 2014. *Chemical Communications* 50: 15856–9
55. Tian L, Zhang Y, Wang L, Geng Q, Cui J. 2020. *ACS Applied Materials & Interfaces* 12: 52713–20
56. Khan MZH, Daizy M, Tarafder C, Liu X. 2019. *Scientific Reports* 9
57. Devasahayam G, Scheld WM, Hoffman PS. 2010. *Expert Opinion on Investigational Drugs* 19: 215–34
58. Song Y, Qiao J, Liu W, Qi L. 2020. *Analytical and Bioanalytical Chemistry*
59. He J, Liu G, Jiang M, Xu L, Kong F, Xu Z. 2020. *Food and Agricultural Immunology* 31: 341–51
60. Hao N, Wang K. 2016. *Analytical and Bioanalytical Chemistry* 408: 7035–48
61. Ma X, Li S, Pang C, Xiong Y, Li J. 2018. *Microchimica Acta* 185
62. Clercq ED. 2001. *Journal of Clinical Virology* 22: 73–89
63. Chan D, Tarbin J, Sharman M, Carson M, Smith M, Smith S. 2011. *Analytica Chimica Acta* 700: 194–200
64. Wu L, Ding F, Yin W, Ma J, Wang B, et al. 2017. *Analytical Chemistry* 89: 7578–85
65. Mahmoud AM, El Wekil MM, Mahnashi MH, Ali MFB, Alkahtani SA. 2019. *Microchimica Acta* 186
66. Ma X, He S, Zhang Y, Xu J, Zhang H, et al. 2020. *Sensors and Actuators B-Chemical* 311
67. Fu J, Zhou Y, Huang X, Zhang W, Wu Y, et al. 2020. *Journal of Agricultural and Food Chemistry* 68: 1118–25
68. Han J, Zhang L, Hu L, Xing K, Lu X, et al. 2018. *Journal of Dairy Science* 101: 5770–9
69. Cheng N, Song Y, Zeinhom MMA, Chang Y-C, Sheng L, et al. 2017. *Acs Applied Materials & Interfaces* 9: 40671–80
70. Zhang X, Zhang F, Lu Z, Xu Q, Hou C, Wang Z. 2020. *ACS Applied Materials & Interfaces* 12: 25565–71
71. Liu P, Wang Y, Han L, Cai Y, Ren H, et al. 2020. *ACS Applied Materials & Interfaces* 12: 9090–7
72. Liu Y, Wang J, Song X, Xu K, Chen H, et al. 2018. *Microchimica Acta* 185
73. Patel MM, Hall AJ, Vinjé J, Parashar UD. 2009. *Journal of Clinical Virology* 44: 1–8
74. Giamberardino A, Labib M, Hassan EM, Tetro JA, Springthorpe S, et al. 2013. *PLoS ONE* 8
75. Lopman BA, Steele D, Kirkwood CD, Parashar UD. 2016. *PLoS Medicine* 13
76. Khoris IM, Takemura K, Lee J, Hara T, Abe F, et al. 2019. *Biosensors & Bioelectronics* 126: 425–32
77. Weerathunge P, Ramanathan R, Torok VA, Hodgson K, Xu Y, et al. 2019. *Analytical Chemistry* 91: 3270–6
78. Dolatabadi JEN, Kashanian S. 2010. *Food Research International* 43: 1223–30
79. Wu L, Yin W, Tang K, Li D, Shao K, et al. 2016. *Analytica Chimica Acta* 933: 89–96
80. Wang H, Lu Q, Liu Y, Li H, Zhang Y, Yao S. 2017. *Sensors and Actuators B-Chemical* 250: 429–35

81. Liu M, Khan A, Wang Z, Liu Y, Yang G, et al. 2019. *Biosensors & Bioelectronics* 130: 174–84
82. Yue X, Luo X, Zhou Z, Bai Y. 2019. *Food Chemistry* 289: 84–94
83. Lou Z, Zhao S, Wang Q, Wei H. 2019. *Analytical Chemistry* 91: 15267–74
84. Cui C, Wang Q, Liu Q, Deng X, Liu T, et al. 2018. *Sensors and Actuators B-Chemical* 277: 86–94
85. Corradini MG. 2018.
86. Khera KS, Munro IC, Radomski JL. 1979. *Crc Crit Rev Toxicol* 6: 81–133
87. El-Wahab HMFA, Moram ED. 2013. *Toxicology & Industrial Health* 29: 224
88. Wu L, Yan H, Wang J, Liu G, Xie W. 2019. *Journal of the Electrochemical Society* 166: B562–B8
89. Qin Z, Zhang J, Liu Y, Wu J, Li G, et al. 2020. *Chemosensors* 8
90. Gao L, Fan K, Yan X. 2020. *Nanozymology*: 105–40
91. Niu X, Xu X, Li X, Pan J, Qiu F, et al. 2018. *Chemical Communications* 54: 13443–6
92. Li J, Liu M, Jiang J, Liu B, Tong H, et al. 2019. *Sensors and Actuators B-Chemical* 288: 552–63
93. Xi J, Wei G, An L, Xu Z, Xu Z, et al. 2020. *Nano Letters* 20: 800-
94. Bathinapatla A, Kanchi S, Singh P, Sabela MI, Bisetty K. 2015. *Biosensors & Bioelectronics* 67: 200–7
95. Balgobind K, Kanchi S, Sharma D, Bisetty K, Sabela MI. 2016. *Journal of Electroanalytical Chemistry* 774: 51–7
96. Pei LZ, Ma Y, Qiu FL, Lin FF, Fan CG, Ling XZ. 2019. *Materials Research Express* 6
97. Devi R, Gogoi S, Barua S, Dutta HS, Bordoloi M, Khan R. 2019. *Food Chemistry* 276: 350–7
98. Wu L, Zhou M, Liu C, Chen X, Chen Y. 2021. *Journal of Hazardous Materials* 403
99. Zhang X, Wu D, Zhou X, Yu Y, Wu Y. 2019. *TrAC Trends in Analytical Chemistry* 121: 115668–
100. Liu W, Tian L, Du J, Wu J, Lu X. 2020. *The Analyst* 145
101. Xie Z-J, Shi M-R, Wang L-Y, Peng C-F, Wei X-L. 2020. *Microchimica Acta* 187
102. Lu N, Zhang M, Ding L, Zheng J, Zeng C, et al. 2017. *Nanoscale* 9: 4508–15
103. Xue Q, Li X, Peng Y, Liu P, Peng H, Niu X. 2020. *Microchimica Acta* 187
104. Lien C-W, Chen Y-C, Chang H-T, Huang C-C. 2013. *Nanoscale* 5: 8227–34
105. Long YJ, Li YF, Liu Y, Zheng JJ, Tang J, Huang CZ. 2011. *Chemical Communications* 47: 11939–41

# 15 Nanozymes in Food Science and Technology

*Lunjie Huang*[a,b,c] *and Da-Wen Sun*[a,b,c,d,*]

[a]School of Food Science and Engineering, South China University of Technology, Guangzhou, China
[b]Academy of Contemporary Food Engineering, Guangzhou Higher Education Mega Center, South China University of Technology, Guangzhou, China
[c]Engineering and Technological Research Centre of Guangdong Province on Intelligent Sensing and Process Control of Cold Chain Foods, & Guangdong Province Engineering Laboratory for Intelligent Cold Chain Logistics Equipment for Agricultural Products, Guangzhou Higher Education Mega Centre, Guangzhou, China
[d]Food Refrigeration and Computerized Food Technology (FRCFT), Agriculture and Food Science Centre, University College Dublin, National University of Ireland, Belfield, Ireland

## CONTENTS

* Corresponding author: Da-Wen Sun; URLs: www.ucd.ie/refrig, www.ucd.ie/sun.

DOI: 10.1201/9781003109228-15

## 15.1  INTRODUCTION

With high catalytic activity, substrate specificity, and biocompatible properties, enzymes can efficiently catalyze a variety of biochemical reactions. Natural
enzymes, such as protease, carbohydrase, lipase, glycosidase, oxidoreductase, etc.,
played active roles in the modern food industry for food production, processing,
analysis, and safety. Due to these vital roles of enzymes, food enzymology has been
developed as an important branch in food science and technology that has greatly
contributed to the assurance of food safety and quality.

Although natural enzymes are highly effective and specific, many intrinsic
drawbacks have limited their further progress in enzymatic food technologies. For
instance, the production and purification of enzymes are usually laborious and time
consuming so that many enzymes are not easily available or expensive. Meanwhile,
enzymes, due to their biomacromolecular nature, are vulnerable to extreme environmental factors (such as harsh temperature or pH). Thus, strict conditions are required
during the storage and utilization of enzymes to avoid the obvious denaturation of
enzymatic activities. Therefore, the development of reliable and cheap enzyme mimics (artificial enzymes) to replace natural enzymes is valuable to the food industry (1).

Nanozymes have emerged as robust candidates for enzyme mimicry (2—5). In
the food field, increasing effort is made in studying the usability of nanozymes,
which are generally involved in food quality and safety detection techniques (6, 7).

## 15.2  PRINCIPLES OF NANOZYME FOR FOOD QUALITY AND SAFETY DETECTION

### 15.2.1  Nanozyme as a Recognition Receptor

Natural enzymes are intrinsically equipped with various regulatory mechanisms
to adapt their catalytic activities to dynamic biological systems, which mainly rely
on adjusting the concentrations of substrates and bioactive modulator molecules.
Similarly, nanozyme catalysis is responsive to the existence and concentration of
typical substrates or simulative modulators. Based on the mechanism of correlat-
ing catalytic behavior of nanozymes to the analyte concentration, many types of
nanozymes with peroxidase (POD)-, catalase (CAT)-, oxidase (OXD)-, or phospho-
hydrolase (PPH)-like activities have been developed as recognition receptors for
various food analytes, such as ions (8, 9), hydrogen peroxide ($H_2O_2$) (10), antioxidants
(11), glucose (12), pesticides (13), etc. Food detection with these receptor-functioning
nanozymes can be categorized into substrate-dependent or activity-modulating recognition patterns (**Figure 15.1**, top section).

Substrate-dependent recognition relies on the signal changes from nanozyme substrates or substrate-produced products. Typically, POD mimics, which are the most

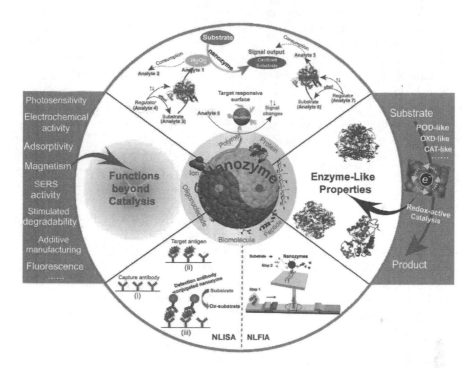

**FIGURE 15.1** The principles of nanozyme-enabled food detection techniques. Right: catalytic paths of nanozymes, Left: multifunctionality of nanozymes, Top and Bottom: roles of nanozymes as a recognition receptor and as a signal tag in the detection strategies, respectively. The diagram of NLFIA was adapted from (14).

important nanozymes in detection applications, catalyze a substrate (colorimetric 2, 2'-azino-bis(3-ethylbenzothiazoline-6-sulfonic acid) (ABTS), 3,3',5,5'-tetramethyl-benzidine (TMB), and o-phenylenediamine (OPD), fluorescent Ampliflu™ Red, or chemiluminescent luminol) into an oxidized product in the presence of $H_2O_2$ as co-substrate (11). Therefore, both typical substrates and $H_2O_2$ co-substrate can function as a variable to affect the catalytic kinetics of POD-like nanozymes within a suitable concentration range. Currently, many analytical methods have been developed based on POD mimics for the quantification of $H_2O_2$ residues in foods (**Figure 15.1**, analyte 1). Besides, food contaminants that can selectively react with $H_2O_2$ (such as melamine) will indirectly influence the signal generation via nanozyme catalysis and, thus, these substances can be measured as a function of $H_2O_2$ consumption (**Figure 15.1**, analyte 2). Similar to the function of $H_2O_2$ for POD-like nanozymes, a few analytes (e.g., glucose, organophosphorus pesticides (OPs), and phenols) can be utilized as a catalytic substrate by enzyme mimics such as nanozymes with glucose oxidase (GOx)-, PPH-, or laccase-like activities to produce detectable oxidation products (**Figure 15.1**, analyte 1). Moreover, inspired by natural domino reactions by the synergistic action of cooperating enzymes, researchers have integrated $H_2O_2$-generating enzymes (or nanozymes) with POD nanozymes to construct artificial cascade reactions for food detection applications (10, 15), achieving detection of these enzymatic substrates (**Figure 15.1**, analyte 3) and associated enzymatic regulators (**Figure 15.1**, analyte 4). Instead, food analytes can be determined by the consumption of the catalytic oxidation products (ox-substrate) via POD-mimicking or OXD-mimicking nanozyme reactions. In this manner, analyte molecules (**Figure 15.1**, analyte 5), such as food antioxidants, can directly decrease the amount of ox-substrates and, thus, can be detected. Particularly, OXD mimics have drawn more attention than POD mimics because OXD mimics can accomplish reactions with no need for unstable $H_2O_2$. Additionally, in contrast to $H_2O_2$-generating enzymes, natural enzymes that generate reductive products, such as alkaline phosphatase (ALP) and acetylcholinesterase (AChE) (16), can be employed to construct multi-enzyme biosensors for food analytes (**Figure 15.1**, analytes 6 and 7).

Enlightened by regulatory mechanisms of natural enzymes, great efforts have been made to develop detection methods relying on the artificial modulation of nanozyme activity. In addition to the structural optimizations (particle size, morphology, defects, and dominant facets) of nanozymes against activity modulation, rational surface engineering strategies (modification, functionalization, and loading) (17) are needed to create stimuli-responsive nanozymes for target recognition and target-dependent catalytic activities (**Figure 15.1**, analyte 8). On the one hand, it is desirable to tailor the nanozyme surface and activity through an assembly of ready-made recognition elements, such as antibodies (Abs), aptamer (Apt) strands, and molecularly imprinted polymers (MIPs), etc. In this manner, the active sites or dispersity of nanozymes can be manipulated by the reversible pairing between these recognizers and homologous target analytes on the nanozyme surface, accomplishing the activity-dependent quantification of food analytes. On the other hand, the rapid advancement in nanobiotechnology has motivated the discovery of several effective nanozyme modulators, comprising ions, small molecules, biomolecules, macromolecules and biomacromolecules, etc. (**Figure 15.1**, central section), which function as artificial enzymatic stimulators/inhibitors to regulate nanozyme activities. Thereby, in such a case, nanozymes with tunable surface chemistry can achieve sensitive recognition and quantification of these modulator-functional or modulator-targeted analytes.

## 15.2.2 Nanozyme Tagging Mechanisms

Different from transforming analyte concentration into changes in nanozyme activity, the nanozyme-labeled strategy is to utilize nanozymes as signal tags, which aims to establish a proportional quantitative relationship between the analyte and nanozyme. As such, nanozyme tags will be advantageous to substitute enzyme tags or amplify signals in immunoassays, aptasensors, and other enzyme-labeled biosensors, owing to their extraordinary and reliable catalytic behaviors.

Due to the simple, rapid, and highly specific immunoreaction between Abs and antigens (analytes), the enzyme-linked immunosorbent assay (ELISA) has been widely used in food safety analyses. In a typical sandwich ELISA assay, the detection procedures include: 1) a specific reaction of antigen (analyte) and the capture Abs immobilized in an ELISA plate; 2) sandwich-type conjugation of the capture Abs, the captured analytes, and horseradish peroxidase (HRP)-labeled detection Abs;3) signal-generating reaction catalyzed by the sandwich complexes; and 4) signal detection by naked eyes, spectrophotometer, or microplate reader. By simply replacing HRP with POD-like or OXD-like nanozymes (**Figure 15.1**, bottom section), the nanozyme-linked immunosorbent assay (NLISA) could gain many superiorities that conventional ELISA cannot reach (18). The advantages of NLISA are: 1) higher reproducibility because nanozymes could either evade activity loss that is often faced by HRP during labeling or washing steps in the assay, or get rid of unstable $H_2O_2$ as co-substrate when exhibiting OXD-like activities; 2) higher sensitivity due to the superior catalytic ability of nanozyme tags when loaded with an equal amount of detection Abs; 3) wider applicability due to the durable robustness of nanozymes in harsh environments where HRP cannot work; and 4) the possibility to create new modes of ELISA-like assays with multifunctional nanozymes.

Lateral flow immunoassay (LFIA) is a lab-on-paper immunodetection technique commonly used in the on-site inspection of food safety. Typically, an LFIA strip is constructed by a sample pad for adsorbing the sample solution, a conjugation pad loaded with detection Abs labeled dark-colored nanoparticles (Abs-NPs), a test pad composed of test line (T-line) and control line (C-line), and an absorbent pad (**Figure 15.1**, bottom section). Particularly, target analytes in the solution will flow with the sample liquid via the capillary force and subsequently be trapped on the T-line of the test pad, where the colored analyte–Abs-NPs–capture Abs complexes are formed. Consequently, the results of LFIA strips can be visually inspected with a drop of the sample within a short time. However, the visual signal of LFIA originates from the gathering effect of intrinsically colored NPs such as gold (Au) NPs, which will be insensitive if the color rendering of NPs is too weak to be visible. In this regard, nanozymes are an important probe material to enhance the detection efficiency and sensitivity of LFIA (14). Besides the above procedures of LFIA, the nanozyme-based LFIA assay involves subsequent catalysis of typical chromogenic/luminescent substrates onto the T-line, where the nanozyme is accumulated in the presence of analytes. As a result, a significant promotion of signal intensity on the T-line can be achieved with the aid of nanozyme catalysis.

Nanozyme tags are also often integrated with food biosensors based on other recognizers, such as Apts (19-21), peptides (22), antibiotics (23), etc. Similar to Abs labeling, these recognizers-modified nanozyme probes show highly selective binding ability to target analytes in food matrices. Meanwhile, under particular circumstances, nanozyme tags sometimes can create a linkage with other functional nanomaterials to trigger a secondary signal amplification of food detection assays, including nanozyme-catalyzed formation/decomposition, luminescence/quenching, or plasmonic effect of functional nanomaterials. More importantly, many nanozymes are multifunctional labeling elements, which can simultaneously exert enzyme-like properties and other sensory features for enhancing food detection, such as photosensitivity (24), electrochemical activity (25), absorptivity (26), magnetism (24, 27), surface-enhanced Raman scattering (SERS) activity (28), degradability (16, 29, 30), manufacturing additivity (31), fluorescence (32, 33), etc. (**Figure 15.1**, left section). The above mechanisms demonstrate that functional nanozyme tags are flexibly available to a variety of food detection methods.

## 15.3   FOOD QUALITY ANALYSIS

### 15.3.1   Antioxidants

Food antioxidants are a group of reductive molecules that often participate in critical biological functions to maintain oxidative stress levels in human bodies (34). Many antioxidants from plant metabolites, including ascorbic acid (AA), thiols, and polyphenols, have been extensively used as conventional additives in food products, and the dietary dosage of which is generally guided by their antioxidative capabilities and mechanisms. Therefore, rapid screening techniques for evaluating antioxidants are needed to guide their usage in different products. Based on the inhibitory effect of common antioxidants on POD or OXD nanozyme activities, many detection methods for food antioxidants have been developed. For example, Wei's group (35) has successfully developed a facile assay to determine the total antioxidant capacity in real samples including four commercial beverages, fresh orange juice, and three kinds of vitamin C tablets by using a POD-like nitrogen-doped carbon nanozyme, which has the potential for evaluation of antioxidant food quality. Jia and coworkers (36) employed the POD-like cobalt tetraoxide ($Co_3O_4$) NPs to compare the antioxidant activity of three food antioxidants (gallic acid, tannic acid, and AA), which showed different levels of antioxidant activity in the following order: tannic acid > gallic acid > AA.

The quantification of antioxidants is important for developing food storage and nutriment recommendation guidelines. Luo et al. (11) reported a colorimetric detection method for reductive AA based on the POD-like and OXD-like activity of mixed-valence cerium (Ce)-based metal-organic framework (MOF) and TMB substrate, which can detect in a linear range of 1—20 µM and a limit of detection (LOD) of 0.28 µM of AA. The applicability of this method was also validated by the reliable results (recoveries between 96.2% and 101.7%) in the analysis of orange and grape juices. Wang et al. (37) synthesized protein-conjugated Au nanoclusters (Au NCs-p-h) for the detection of tea polyphenols in real tea samples, because the POD-like activity of Au NCs-p-h can be restrained due to the tea polyphenols-induced aggregation. Compared to the traditional tartaric acid colorimetric approach, this new method showed identical experimental results but with much higher sensitivity and LOD of 10 nM. Wang's group (38) proposed the ultrasonic synthesis of nano-$PrO_{1.8}$ as a POD nanozyme for the determination of trans-resveratrol in white wine and champagne samples, reaching a LOD of 0.29 µM within a linear range from 0.3 to 16 µM. These studies revealed the potential application of nanozymes for the sensitive and reliable evaluation of antioxidant agents in foods.

### 15.3.2   Proteins

Protein-based dietary ingredients fulfill many technological roles in formulated foods and contribute to nutrient, texture, color, flavor, and other properties of foods (39). For example, food proteins can be as beneficial as being digested into amino acids for the synthesis of bioactive peptides. Besides the digestible food proteins, protein enzymes are especially important for food processing and food function, such as protease, lipase, amylase, cellulose, POD, GOx, etc. Thus, it is significant to detect the existence of food proteins in food matrices. Nandu and Yigit (40) discovered that protein lipase can tune the POD-like activity of two-dimensional (2D) molybdenum disulfide (MoS$_2$) NPs, while other proteins, namely, bovine serum albumin (BSA), alkaline phosphatase (ALP), β-galactosidase, protease, and streptavidin, did not display such behavior. This unique response offered low-nanomolar (5 nM), label-free detection of lipase in samples with unknown identity by using qualitative visual inspection and quantitative statistical analysis.

In certain individuals, some food proteins can cause allergenic reactions, which have become a serious and prevalent food safety and public healthcare concern that affects 5% of adults and 8% of children. Thus, reliable identification of allergenic proteins in foods is vital to the health of people prone to allergies (41). For instance, cow's milk allergy is one of the most frequent and severe immunoglobulin E (IgE)-induced food allergies in children, where β-lactoglobulin (BLG) can serve as an important biomarker for the detection of milk protein. He et al. (42) reported a highly sensitive sandwich NLISA for the detection of BLG based on a specific polyclonal Ab (pAb) against human IgE linear epitopes of BLG and an anti-BLG pAb-platinum (Pt) NPs (POD nanozyme) probe. This NLISA method exhibited a broad linear range of 0.49—1.6 × 10$^4$ ng/mL and a low LOD of 0.12 ng/mL, which was 16 folds lower than that using traditional sandwich ELISA. Furthermore, the proposed approach showed high recovery (93.5%—112.0%) and a low coefficient of variation (1.59%—12.5%) after the analysis of partially hydrolyzed infant formula samples fortified with BLG. To improve its reliability, Li's group (43) proposed a ratiometric SERS NLISA of allergenic BLG via a covalent-organic framework (COF) composite material-based nanozyme tag triggered Raman signal "turn-on" and amplification (**Figure 15.2**).

In the assay, the substrate 4-nitrothiophenol was capable of functioning as a powerful bridge to connect the Au nanostars (with excellent SERS performance) by

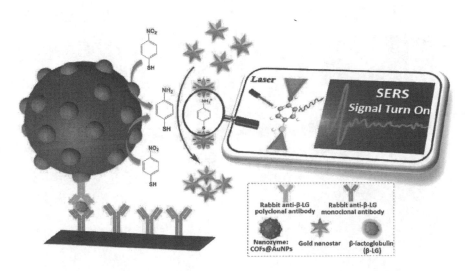

**FIGURE 15.2**  Schematic illustration of the AuNPs doped COF nanozyme-based SERS-NLISA for the detection of allergenic proteins in milk (43).

both the Au-S bond and electrostatic force to further produce a Raman "hot spot." Meanwhile, the Raman signal of 4-nitrothiophenol at 1573 cm$^{-1}$ was weakened, and a new signal at 1591 cm$^{-1}$ generated by 4-aminothiophenol was turned on, leading to the generation of a ratiometric SERS signal. By monitoring the ratiometric SERS signal of $I_{1591}/I_{1573}$, a LOD of 0.01 ng/mL was achieved. The same group also reported a smartphone-integrated portable NLISA of allergenic proteins (α-lactalbumin) by using copper (Cu)-based laccase mimics for signal generation (44). Based on the oxidative coupling reaction between 2,4-dichlorophenol and 4-aminoantipyrine catalyzed by Cu nano-laccase, the NLISA strategy achieved a LOD of 0.056 ng/mL of α-lactalbumin with high specificity and excellent applicability in food sample analysis. These applications indicate that nanozyme probes are advantageous for the detection of food proteins.

### 15.3.3 GLUCOSE, CHOLESTEROL, CHOLINE, ETHANOL, AND OTHERS

Glucose is a sugar and a form of carbohydrate, which is an essential energy source for our bodies. Unfortunately, excessive and prolonged consumption of sugars, such as glucose can drive insulin resistance and hence can increase the risk of diabetes. Accurate quantification of glucose in foods can guide dietary recommendations for diabetic patients. Among the detection methods for glucose, colorimetric assays using nanozymes are attractive because of their simple operation, low cost, and fast visual signal readout by the bare eyes. For instance, Huang et al. (10) reported a colorimetric glucose assay based on the domino reaction of natural GOx with a new type of POD-like mimics such as vanadium disulfide (VS$_2$) nanosheets (NSs) (**Figure 15.3**). Under the optimal conditions, the assay covered a broad glucose concentration range (5 to 250 μM) with a relatively low LOD of 1.5 μM, which could be well applied in fruit juice samples. To achieve higher stability and reusability of the nanozyme

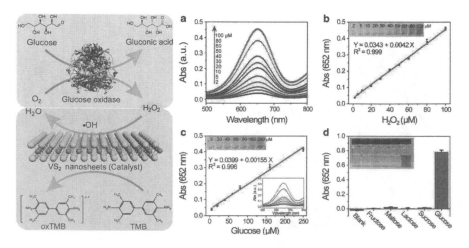

**FIGURE 15.3** Glucose detection based on the cascade reaction of GOx and POD-like VS$_2$ NSs (10).

probe, Xu et al. (45) constructed GOx-immobilized MOF bio-nano-hybrids as a bio-mimetic GOx-POD cascade nanozyme for ultrasensitive glucose biosensing. The stable GOx@MOF detection platform surpassed the free iron (Fe)-MOF/GOx detection system, with a wide linear range (1–500 µM) and a low LOD (0.487 µM).

Cholesterol, a natural organic steroid and alcohol compound, is an essential structural component of mammalian cell membranes to establish proper membrane permeability and fluidity. It is an important building block in the body's hormonal systems for the synthesis of bile acids, steroid hormones, and several fat-soluble vitamins. Further, cholesterol plays an important role in the brain synapses and the immune system including protection against cancer. Although cholesterol is important and necessary for human health, abnormalities of cholesterol levels are symptoms of several diseases, such as hypolipoproteinemia, anemia, septicemia, malnutrition hypertension, coronary heart disease, arteriosclerosis, brain thrombosis, lipid metabolism dysfunction, and myocardial infarction. Thus, estimation of cholesterol levels in foods has attracted extensive attention. Hong et al. (46) proposed a chemiluminescent cholesterol sensor with good selectivity and enhanced sensitivity. This sensor was based on the POD-like activity of cupric oxide (CuO) NPs, where CuO NPs can catalyze the oxidation of luminol by $H_2O_2$, which was produced by the catalysis of cholesterol by cholesterol oxidase. Under the optimal conditions, the chemiluminescence intensity was proportional to the cholesterol concentration over the range of 0.625—12.5 mM, with a LOD of 0.17 mM. The applicability of this method was validated by determining cholesterol in milk powder with satisfactory recovery (95.3—101.9%).

Choline (Cho) is an important precursor for the synthesis of the neurotransmitter acetylcholine (ACh); it is categorized as Vitamin B, an essential nutrient. Cho deficiency in humans leads to some complications, such as liver disease, fatty liver, and hemorrhagic kidney necrosis, atherosclerosis, and possibly neurological disorders. Therefore, Cho determination is essential to food analysis and dietary recommendations. Valekar et al. (47) developed a novel fluorescent assay of Cho and ACh by using amine-grafted MOFs as a promising POD alternative. Based on the excellent POD-like activity of N,N,N′,N′-tetramethyl-1,4-butanediamine-functionalized MIL-100(Fe) nanozyme, AChE, and choline oxidase, Cho and ACh were reliably determined down to 0.027 and 0.036 µM, respectively. Furthermore, the practical applicability of this strategy was successfully demonstrated by detecting Cho in spiked milk samples. Similarly, Nirala et al. (15) reported a quick colorimetric method for the analysis of Cho in milk based on the collaborative utilization of POD-mimicking $MoS_2$ NSs and choline oxidase, which works in the 1—180 µM Cho concentration range with a LOD of 0.4 µM.

Determining ethanol content in alcoholic beverages is important as these beverages are popular but can cause chronic damage to our health. Smutok et al. (48) employed hemin and Au NPs co-modified carbon microfibers as a POD nanozyme for cascade catalysis with ethanol oxidase for amperometric biosensing of ethanol in the grape must and wine samples. The results of ethanol content in the tested samples were 0.13 ± 0.05 mM for grape must and 2280 ± 35 mM for wine, which were in good agreement with the results obtained using an enzymatic kit as a reference approach.

Besides detecting these components in food, the identification of ion species and concentration is also demanded. For example, calcium (Ca) ion is indispensable for various physiological activities of the body, including the maintenance of the biological potential on both sides of the cell membrane, the normal nerve conduction function, and bone development. Wang's group (49) established an amperometric biosensor for Ca ion based on the stimulation effect of Ca ion on CAT-like activity of $Co_3O_4$ nanozymes. The sensor response was linear against Ca concentration of 0.1 and 1 mM with a LOD of 4 µM; the sensor also exhibited good reproducibility and high selectivity against other metal ions ($Na^+$, $K^+$, $Mg^{2+}$, $Mn^{2+}$, $Fe^{3+}$, and $Fe^{2+}$). This method was successfully applied to determine Ca in milk samples.

## 15.4  FOOD SAFETY DETECTION

### 15.4.1  HARMFUL IONS

Harmful cations and anions are commonly found in food products, which result from environmental pollution or improper agronomic and food processing practices. These toxic ions of heavy metals, such as copper ($Cu^{2+}$), mercury ($Hg^{2+}$), chromium ($Cr^{4+}$), arsenite ($As^{3+}$), sulfite ($O_3S^{-2}$), phosphite ($O_3P^{-3}$), nitrite ($NO_2^-$), etc., can accumulate and cause harm to vital biological functions in human bodies. Therefore, rapid and sensitive detection methods for harmful ions are required for food safety detection. Luo et al. (50) found that the $Cu^{2+}$ could selectively and sensitively enhance the POD-like activity of flower-like transition-metal-based material $MMoO_4$ (where, M = Co, Ni), which inspired a simple, sensitive, and selective colorimetric strategy for detecting $Cu^{2+}$. The obvious color signal can be discerned by the naked eye or detected by absorption spectroscopy, achieving a LOD of 0.024 µM in the $Cu^{2+}$ concentration range of 0.1—24 µM. Huang et al. (8) proposed a portable colorimetric detection of mercury(II) ($Hg^{2+}$) based on a green-fabricated 2D material, i.e., chitosan-functionalized molybdenum (IV) selenide ($MoSe_2$) NSs (**Figure 15.4**). The sensing strategy was established on the activating effect of $Hg^{2+}$ on dual POD-like and OXD-like activities of chitosan-$MoSe_2$ NSs, enabled by the *in situ* reduction of chitosan-immobilized $Hg^{2+}$ ions on the $MoSe_2$ NS surface. With TMB substrate as the signal indicator, the assay could quantitatively and selectively monitor as low as 3.5 nM of $Hg^{2+}$ ions by a UV-vis spectrophotometer, with good selectivity against other ions. Furthermore, the smartphone-integrated sensor could detect trace $Hg^{2+}$ (low to 8.4 nM) in drinking water samples in a short time (15 min). Mao et al. (51) utilized a single-atom Fe nanozyme for the fast and highly sensitive colorimetric detection of hexavalent chromium ions (Cr(VI)). With TMB as a colorimetric probe and 8-hydroxyquinoline (8-HQ) as an inhibitor for the oxidation of TMB, the detection of Cr(VI) was realized through a specific interaction between Cr(VI) and 8-HQ, which led to the recovery of blue-colored oxTMB. This method showed superior sensitivity (LOD=3 nM), linear range (30 nM to 3 µM), and specificity; it was successfully applied to detect Cr(VI) in tap water and tuna samples. Additionally, Qiu's group (52) established a method to detect Cr(VI) based on the discovery that the OXD-mimicking activity of ceria nanorods ($CeO_2$ NRs)-templated MOFs could be boosted by Cr ions. It can detect 20 nM of Cr(VI) over a range of 0.03—5 µM with

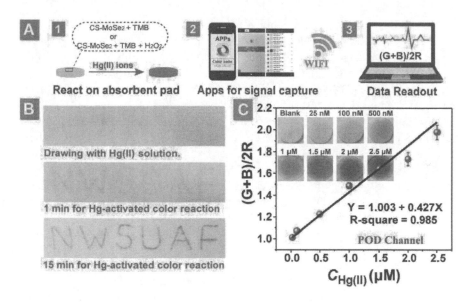

**FIGURE 15.4** The chitosan (CS)-MoSe$_2$ NS/smartphone-based paper chip for the detection of Hg$^{2+}$ ions (8). (A) Principle of the detection assay with a smartphone. (B) chitosan-MoSe$_2$ NS-based test strip for Hg$^{2+}$ visualization. (C) The plot of the (G + B)/2R value vs Hg$^{2+}$ concentration in the POD channel. The images show the color of the test strip varied with the concentration of Hg$^{2+}$.

high selectivity and is workable in different water environment samples with recovery efficiencies within ±5%.

Sulfite is one of the oldest and most ubiquitous food additives; it has been widely used for blanching and preservation of various foodstuffs (dried fruit, vermicelli, preserves, etc.) (53). However, the ingestion of foods containing large amounts of sulfite can cause asthmatic attacks and allergic reactions in sensitive individuals. Hence, sulfite determination in food products is essential for food assurance. Based on the inhibitory effect of sulfite on OXD-like Co$_3$O$_4$ nanozyme, Qin et al. (54) employed a TMB–O$_2$–Co$_3$O$_4$ nanozyme system for colorimetric detection of sulfite in foods, in which a good linear relationship (0.2 × 10$^{-6}$ to 1.6 × 10$^{-5}$ M), a low LOD of 53 nM, and good recovery (93.8% to 100.5%) were obtained. Besides, similar methods have been also developed using OXD-like CoFe$_2$O$_4$ nanozyme and POD-like MoS$_2$/g-C$_3$N$_4$ heterojunctioned 2D nanozymes (55).

Arsenic (As) contamination has drawn great concern across the world due to its hypertoxicity and carcinogenicity. Niu's group (56) reported a novel colorimetric assay of As$^{3+}$ based on the reassembly-induced OXD-like activity inhibition of dithiothreitol-capped palladium (Pd) NPs. Based on this principle, highly sensitive detection of As$^{3+}$ was achieved, providing a wide linear range (33 ng/L to 333.3 μg/L) and an ultralow LOD (35 ng/L). The accurate measurement of As$^{3+}$ in spiked drinking and river water revealed the great promise of this method in food and environmental analysis applications.

Phosphite is widely used in commercial products, such as biostimulants, fungicides, and OPs, and its residue is often found in food products. Liu's group (32) presented a fluorescent "turn-on" sensor for quantitative and highly selective analysis of phosphite based on the different coordination strengths of N and P lone-pair electrons toward OXD-like nickel oxide (NiO) NPs. The mechanism is based on both the effective inhibition of resorufin (the oxidation product of Amplex red) formation by HEPES and the unique ability of phosphite (among various phosphorus-, As-, Se-, and S-containing species) for restoring the activity of NiO nanozyme. The sensor detected P(III) up to 1 mM with a LOD of 1.46 μM under the optimal condition.

Nitrite has been classified as a Group 2A (i.e., probable) carcinogen to humans by the International Agency for Research on Cancer (IARC). Sodium nitrite ($NaNO_2$) and potassium nitrite ($KNO_2$) are used to preserve meat from spoilage as a curing mixture. The extended ingestion of $NO_2^-$ can cause stomach cancer, hypertension, thermo-globinemia, congenital disabilities, and spontaneous abortions. Thus, the detection of $NO_2^-$ residues in foods is significant. Adegoke et al. (26) proposed a rapid and highly selective colorimetric detection of $NO_2^-$ based on the catalytic-enhanced reaction of POD mimetic Au NP-$CeO_2$ NPs-graphene oxide (GO) hybrid nanozyme. Taking $NO_2^-$ as a suitable oxidant within the Au NPs-$CeO_2$ NPs@GO-TMB redox cycle, a unique green color reaction was utilized for the selective detection of $NO_2^-$ within the concentration range of 100—5000 μM with a LOD of 0.3 μg/mL. The colorimetric probe can be successfully applied for $NO_2^-$ detection in tap water.

### 15.4.2 AGROCHEMICAL RESIDUES

Agrochemicals, including biocides (pesticides, herbicides, insecticides, fungicides, etc.), plant growth regulators, fertilizers, veterinary drugs, and feed supplements, are an indispensable component of modern crop management practices as they elevate agricultural productivity of food, fibers, feeds, and fuels. However, their residue in the agri-food products has greatly increased the risks in agri-food safety (57). Therefore, increasing detection strategies using nanozymes have been studied for the sensitive determination of agrochemical residues.

Pesticide detection is among the most common topics of food safety due to its extensive use in agriculture globally and severe toxicity to human bodies (57). Nanozymes are useful in the detection of pesticide molecules. For instance, Weerathunge et al. (20) proposed a highly rapid, specific, and sensitive method for detecting acetamiprid pesticide by combining the inherent POD-like nanozyme activity of Au NPs with the high affinity and specificity of an acetamiprid-specific S-18 Apt. It is shown that the nanozyme activity of Au NPs can be inhibited by its surface passivation with Apt molecules, and can be reactivated in the presence of a cognate acetamiprid in a target concentration-dependent manner. This reversible inhibition of the Au NPs nanozyme activity can either be directly visualized in the form of the color change of the POD reaction product or can be quantified using UV-vis absorbance spectroscopy, allowing detection of 0.1 ppm acetamiprid within an assay time of 10 min. Instead of in solution, detection of pesticide residues in solid matrices is more performable and practical. Huang et al. (29) proposed a portable colorimetric paper sensor based on degradable γ-MnOOH nanowires OXD mimic and chromogenic TMB indicator for rapid and sensitive screening of OPs. The sensing mechanism was established on the induced disintegration of the OXD-like γ-MnOOH NWs into inactive $Mn^{2+}$ ions by the selective reaction with thiocholine (TCh) produced by acetylcholinesterase (AChE) and acetylthiocholine (ATCh) iodide, triggering a remarkable activity loss of MnOOH nanozymes toward TMB oxidation. The concentration of OPs, as an AChE inhibitor, was measured by the color changes of oxTMB product on the portably assembled test papers, achieving relatively low LODs for omethoate (10 ng/mL) and dichlorvos (3 ng/mL). Meanwhile, this sensing system showed great selectivity and anti-interfering capacity, working well in real serum and vegetable samples. Jin et al. (16) proposed a multi-enzyme hydrogel sensor with a smartphone detector for on-site monitoring of OPs. The cascade-reaction sensor, constructed by embedding OXD-mimicking $MnO_2$ nanoflakes, choline oxidase, and AChE into sodium alginate hydrogel, was capable of screening paraoxon within 65 min in a sensitive manner (LOD=0.5 ng/mL). Alternatively, given the promising prospect of POD-like nanozymes in colorimetric detection, it is helpful to eliminate their OXD-like activities and color interference. Taking advantage of the POD-specific activity of white germanium oxide ($GeO_2$) nanozymes its degradability induced by thiocholine, Han's group (58) reported an ultrasensitive colorimetric OPs assay based on the irreversible inhibition of AChE, freeing the corresponding nanozymes-based colorimetric pesticide assay from oxygen (OXD catalysis cosubstrate) and color interferences. This method was capable of detecting OPs in environmental waters (tap water and river water) and food juices (apple juice and cucumber juice) with a linear range of 0.1—50 pM and LOD of 14 fM. Considering that methods to analyze single pesticide residue are not practical for real samples contaminated by multiple pesticides, Zhu et al. (59) fabricated colorimetric nanozyme sensor arrays based on heteroatom-doped graphene for detection of aromatic pesticides (**Figure 15.5**). In the sensor arrays, the presence of different pesticides will inhibit the active sites of this POD nanozyme differentially, resulting in successful discrimination and quantification of five pesticides (i.e., lactofen, fluoroxypyr-meptyl, bensulfuron-methyl, fomesafen, and diafenthiuron) from 5 to 500 μM. The practicality of the sensor arrays enabled successful discrimination of the pesticides in soil samples.

Although the above colorimetric methods are simple and rapid, the sensitivity is not as ideal as required. Thus, nanozyme sensors with more sensitive signal outputs, such as SERS (60) and electrochemical (61), have been explored.

Veterinary drug residues including antibiotic or growth regulators can be found in food of animal origin due to their application for preventive and curative purposes to treat cultivated animals. The control of veterinary drug residues in food is necessary to ensure consumer safety. Because of the advantages of simplicity, cost effectiveness, and visibility, LFIAs have been widely used in the detection of antibiotics, while low sensitivity is still an issue to be solved. Thereby, Wei et al. (62) reported a novel NLFIA based on POD-like Au@Pt nanozymes as a visual tag and a chromogenic substrate 3-amino-9-ethyl-carbazole. The qualitative LOD was 0.1 ng/mL for the Au@Pt nanozyme-based NLFIA, in comparison to 8 ng/mL for conventional LFIA based on Au NPs. Furthermore, the streptomycin residues in milk samples from a local farm were successfully evaluated by the novel LFIA based on Au@Pt nanozyme. Nanozyme tags are abundant but most of them are POD-like

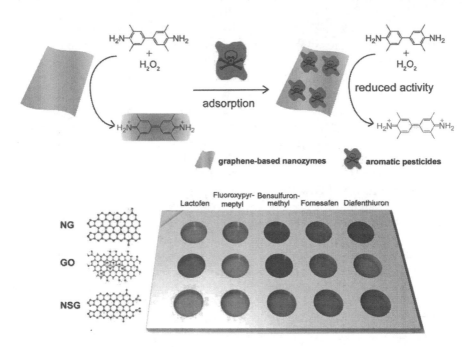

**FIGURE 15.5** Schematic of nanozyme sensor arrays based on heteroatom-doped graphene for detecting pesticides (59).

or OXD-like species, other enzyme nanomimics are rarely utilized in food detection. In particular, Tang's group (63) designed an innovative gas pressure-based aptasensing platform for the electrochemical detection of kanamycin using polyaniline (PANI) nanowire-functionalized reduced graphene oxide (rGO) framework and a CAT-like Pt nanozyme. Under optimum conditions, the compressible PANI/rGO sponge allowed for a pressure-dependent current signal to probe the increase in kanamycin concentration, which covered a dynamic range of 0.2—50 pM with a LOD of 0.063 pM. The assay was highly reproducible, specific, and precise for kanamycin analysis. Moreover, the evaluation results of real milk samples acquired by this method matched well with those obtained by a commercial kanamycin ELISA kit. Except for antibiotic residues, growth-regulating drugs can accumulate in human bodies via meat consumption and adverse biological metabolisms. For example, common β-adrenoceptor agonists, including ractopamine (RAC) and clenbuterol (CLE) could increase the percentage of lean meat and promote the growth of livestock by affecting the flow direction and redistribution of nutrients. Given the accumulation of β-adrenoceptor agonist residues in the edible tissues might cause serious adverse effects, such as dizziness, muscle tremors, and heart palpitations, CLE has been prohibited as a feed additive but RAC is still approved in the USA and some other countries. Liu et al. (64) established a magnetic Prussian blue (PB) nanozyme-mediated dual-readout on-demand multiplex lateral flow immunoassay (MLFIA) for simultaneous detection of ractopamine and clenbuterol in meat samples (**Figure 15.6**). Benefiting from the MPBN tag's intrinsic color and catalysis-enhanced

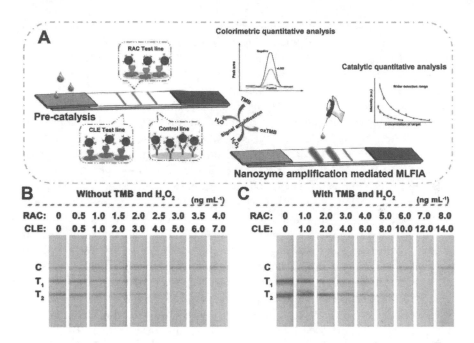

**FIGURE 15.6** The principle (A) and performances (B and C) of the dual-readout NLFIA for simultaneous detection of RAC and CLE (64).

colorimetric signal via POD nanozyme reaction, a dual-readout strategy with improved precision and broadened detection range was achieved, reaching a twofold increase in the detection range that could fulfill different regulatory requirements in various regions.

## 15.4.3 MICROBIAL CONTAMINANTS

Microorganisms, including bacteria, fungi, and viruses, can directly infect human bodies by colonization or indirectly damage human health via producing biotoxins in contaminated foods. Therefore, it is urgent to rapidly and sensitively inspect the microbial safety of foods. With the outbreak of the COVID-19 epidemic, ever-increasing attention has been drawn to microbial food safety as food can be suitable carriers for spreading pathogenic microorganisms (65).

Foodborne bacteria have been a heavy burden for food safety control because they are various species that proliferate rapidly, requiring sensitive and rapid detection techniques. The familiar pathogenic bacteria in the food industry include *Campylobacter jejuni* (*C. jejuni*), *Enterobacter sakazakii* (*E. sakazakii*), *Escherichia coli* O157:H7 (*E. coli* O157:H7), *Listeria monocytogenes* (*L. monocytogenes*), *Salmonella*, *Staphylococcus aureus* (*S. aureus*), *Vibrio parahaemolyticus* (*V. parahaemolyticus*), etc. Nanozyme biosensors are highly available for the detection of these pathogens. Li et al. (66) established a dual-mode immunochromatographic assay for *C. jejuni* detection based on the POD-mimicking and SERS enhancement properties of Pt-coated Au NRs. Under color mode and SERS mode, the proposed assay showed a good linear response in the range of $10^2$–$10^6$ colony-forming units/mL (CFU/mL) and $10^2$–$5 \times 10^6$ CFU/mL with LODs of 75 and 50 CFU/mL, respectively. Additionally, the application of this dual-signal sensor in milk samples obtained good recoveries ranged from 89.33% to 107.62%.

Recent outbreaks of life-threatening neonatal infections caused by *E. sakazakii* call for the urgent development of rapid and ultrasensitive detection approaches. Zhang et al. (67) reported a continual cascade nanozyme biosensor for the detection of viable *E. sakazakii* based on propidium monoazide staining, loop-mediated isothermal amplification (LAMP), and nanozyme catalytic strip. The target analyte, ompA gene of *E. sakazakii*, was recognized by fluorescein isothiocyanate (FITC)-modified primers in the LAMP process, following a magnetic $Fe_3O_4$ nanozyme-linked immunochromatographic reaction, and a nanozyme-amplified colorimetric reaction. As such, the nanozyme biosensor was able to detect 10 CFU/mL viable *E. sakazakii* bacteria within one hour under optimal conditions. *E. coli* O157:H7 is a highly infectious pathogen spreading extensively in food and water, and has led to severe public health accidents. By using concave Pd-Pt NPs as a POD nanozyme probe, Han et al. (68) reported an NLFIA for the sensitive detection of *E. coli* O157: H7 in milk and its sensitivity in milk ($9.0 \times 10^2$ CFU/mL) was 111 folds higher than that of traditional colloidal Au-based LFIA. Similarly, a mannose modified PB nanozyme based NLFIA reported by Wang et al. (69) can detect down to $10^2$ CFU/mL of *E. coli* O157:H7 in potable water and milk, and $10^3$ CFU/mL in watermelon juice and purple cabbage. Using vancomycin as a capture probe and Apt-modified $Fe_3O_4$ NPs cluster as detection probe, Zhang and co-workers (23) developed a rapid and visual amplification aptasensor for *L. monocytogenes* based on POD-mimicking $Fe_3O_4$ NPs, where a visual LOD of $5.4 \times 10^3$ CFU/mL of *L. monocytogenes* and a linear detection range of $5.4 \times 10^3$–$10^8$ CFU/mL could be obtained. *Salmonella* is responsible for many food contamination outbreaks and related human salmonellosis disease. Farka et al. (70) employed PB NPs as a catalytic tag in a sandwich NLISA for the contamination of *Salmonella* typhimurium in powdered milk, with a LOD of $6 \times 10^3$ CFU/mL. In combination with LAMP, Dehghani et al. (71) utilized Pt-Pd NPs/Apt modified magnetic beads as an enzyme-like nano-bioprobe for the on-site detection of *Salmonella* typhimurium in food samples. This approach was possible to detect low-concentration *Salmonella* typhimurium in chicken meat sample (10–15 CFU/mL) and in whole egg sample (3–10 CFU/mL) within less than three hours, obtaining a relative accuracy of 90% with an intra- and inter-assay precision of 8.4% and 9.9%, respectively. Wang's group (72) constructed a colorimetric aptasensor for the detection of *Salmonella* typhimurium using $ZnFe_2O_4$-rGO nanostructures as effective POD mimetics, reaching a linear range from 11 to $1.10 \times 10^5$ CFU/mL and a LOD of 11 CFU/mL. *V. parahaemolyticus* usually contaminates seafood and thus induces foodborne gastroenteritis or even death. Liu et al. (22) proposed a sensitive colorimetric immunoassay of *V. parahaemolyticus* based on specific nonapeptide probe screening from a phage display library conjugated with POD-mimicking $MnO_2$ NSs, demonstrating a wide detection range (20–$10^4$ CFU/mL), low LOD (15 CFU/mL), excellent selectivity, and high reliability for real marine samples. Furthermore, nanozyme tags can be used for multiplexed quantitative analysis of pathogenic bacteria (73).

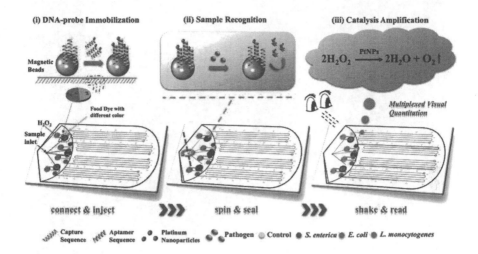

**FIGURE 15.7** Schematic of the assay procedure of nanozyme-generated pressure-based SpinChip for multiple pathogen detection (74).

Wei et al. (74) established a pressure-based SpinChip for multiple pathogen detection using the Apt-modified CAT-like Pt NPs as a signal tag. The biosensor specifically quantified three major foodborne pathogens (*Salmonella enterica*, *E. coli*, and *L. monocytogenes*) simultaneously in apple juice with LODs of about 10 CFU/mL (**Figure 15.7**).

Virus contamination in food, such as human norovirus (21), porcine circovirus (75), Zika virus (76), influenza virus A (77), Ebola virus (78), SARS-CoV-2 (79), etc. often accounts for spreading zoonotic infectious diseases. Combining the enzyme-mimic catalytic activity of Au NPs with the high target specificity of a specific Apt, Weerathunge et al. (21) reported a nanozyme aptasensor for the ultrasensitive colorimetric detection of murine norovirus. The aptasensor achieved fast (10 min) and ultrasensitive (LOD of 3 viruses per assay equivalent to 30 viruses/mL of sample and experimentally demonstrated LOD of 20 viruses per assay equivalent to 200 viruses/mL) detection of murine norovirus in the shellfish sample. We et al. (75) proposed an NLISA method for detecting porcine circovirus type 2 Ab, using Au-Pt/SiO$_2$ nanozyme tag and HAuCl$_4$/H$_2$O$_2$ coloring system. Compared with the conventional ELISA (19.8 ng mL), such an NLISA system yielded 396-fold enhancement (50 pg/mL) in sensitivity for the detection of porcine circovirus type 2 Ab. Hsu et al. (76) proposed a serological point-of-care test for Zika virus detection and infection surveillance using an enzyme-free vial immunosensor with a smartphone. The adoption of core-shell Pt@Au NPs as a nanozyme probe enabled a high sensitivity (1 pg/mL) and desirable specificity for Zika virus detection. Lee's group (77) reported a magnetic NLISA for ultrasensitive influenza A virus detection, in which silica-shelled magnetic nanobeads and enzyme-like AuNPs were combined to monitor influenza A virus (New Caledonia/20/1999) (H1N1) up to fg/mL concentration in the linearity range of $5.0 \times 10^{-15}$–$5.0 \times 10^{-6}$ g/mL. Yan's group (79) presented a nanozyme chemiluminescence paper test for rapid and sensitive detection of SARS-CoV-2

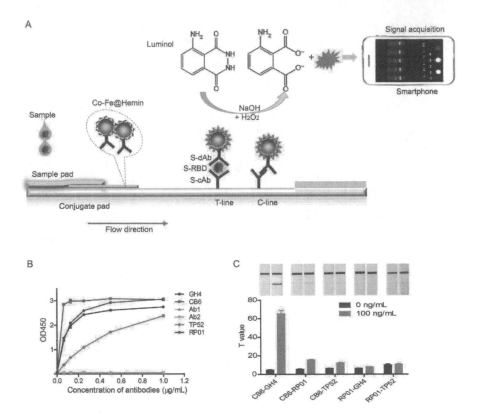

**FIGURE 15.8** Nanozyme chemiluminescent paper test for the detection of SARS-CoV-2 antigen (79). (**A**) Schematic illustration of the nanozyme chemiluminescence paper test for SARS-CoV-2 S-RBD antigen. (**B**) ELISA analysis of Abs binding activity for S-RBD protein. (**C**) Screening of paired Abs using nanozyme colorimetric strip.

antigen (**Figure 15.8**). The Co–Fe@hemin POD nanozyme immobilized on the T-line catalyzes chemiluminescence comparable with natural HRP and thus amplifies immune reaction signal, reaching a LOD of 0.1 ng/mL for recombinant spike antigen of SARS-CoV-2 within a linear range of 0.2—100 ng/mL. Moreover, the strip recognized SARS-CoV-2 antigen specifically, ensuring no cross-reaction with other coronaviruses or influenza A subtypes.

In addition to the detection of microorganisms and their biomarkers, it is equally important to inspect the contamination of biotoxins derived from microorganism activities in food matrices. Among the microbial biotoxins, mycotoxins produced by fungi are of hypertoxicity to humans. They include aflatoxin B1 (AFB1) (30, 80, 81), ochratoxin A (OTA) (82, 83), patulin (84), fumonisin B1 (FB1) (83), and zearalenone (ZON) (85), etc. Xu et al. (81) established a novel indirect competitive MOF-linked immunosorbent assay (MOFLISA) method for the high-throughput and sensitive detection of AFB1. By replacing the natural HRP with enzyme-like MOFs to catalyze a chromogenic system, this MOFLISA can detect as low as 9 pg/mL in a detection range from 0.01 to 20 ng/mL, demonstrating a 20-fold improved LOD value compared with conventional ELISA. In the analysis of Nestle peanut milk samples and Silk soy milk samples, the method obtained good recoveries (86.41—99.74%) and low relative standard deviations (RSD, 2.38—9.04%). Besides, nanozyme tags can be used to drive self-propelled Janus microsensors for sensitive monitoring of enterobacterial contamination of food. For instance, Pacheco et al. (86) prepared nanozyme micromotors by a Pickering emulsion approach to simultaneously encapsulate CAT-like Pt NPs for boosted bubble-propulsion and receptor-modified quantum dots for selective binding with the specific site (3-deoxy-D-manno-oct-2-ulosonic acid) in the endotoxin molecule. Upon interaction with the QDs, the target endotoxins, lipopolysaccharides from *Salmonella*, will trigger a rapid quenching of the fluorescent micromotors in a concentration-dependent manner. The micromotor biosensor can readily determine down to 0.07 ng/mL of lipopolysaccharides in food samples in 15 min, far below the level toxic to humans (275 µg/mL). All the applications suggest that nanozyme tags can be a powerful tool for defense against microbial risk in the food industry.

## 15.4.4 ILLEGAL ADDITIVES

Although being forbidden in food production for safety concerns, illegal food additives are still used by many food companies for economic purposes. The usage of illegal food additives clenbuterol will cause harmful residues in food products, such as clenbuterol and $\beta$-estradiol in animal source foods (33, 64), $H_2O_2$ in milk (87), and melamine in milk powder (88), etc. Zhang et al. (87) fabricated a ready-to-use paper-based chemosensor by using mesoporous carbon-dispersed Pd NPs as a promising POD mimic for the visual determination of $H_2O_2$ in milk. Deng et al. (88) established a novel colorimetric sensor based on the POD-like activity of Au NPs and Au NPs-melamine interaction enhanced catalytic oxidation of TMB, detecting as low as 0.02 mg/L of melamine visually (33). designed and developed an artificial MOF-based nanozyme with dual functions of a catalyst and luminescent sensor specifically for the determination and degradation of hormone 17$\beta$-estradiol and its derivatives. Composed of the luminescent $Tb^{3+}$ ion, catalytic coenzyme factor hemin, and light-harvesting ligand, this MOF-based nanozyme biosensor can be used to both sense 17$\beta$-estradiol as low as 50 pM by its luminescence and degrade 17$\beta$-estradiol like the behavior of natural HRP. The development of nanozyme will strengthen the safety control against illegal food additives.

## 15.4.5 FOOD SPOILAGE

Food spoilage has been a public concern worldwide, calling for reliable sensors or monitoring systems to affirm food freshness of various food commodities, especially highly perishable foods, such as aquatic products and animal source food. Food spoilage can be evaluated by several food freshness biomarkers. As a kind of small molecular compound widely existing in many foods, biogenic amines are mainly formed through the catabolism of amino acids by microorganisms, and thus the levels of which have been chosen as the indexes for the freshness evaluation of aquatic products (25, 89, 90). In this regard, methods for detecting biogenic amines can assist to avoid waste from food spoilage. Li et al. (91) conducted colorimetric detection of putrescine and cadaverine in aquatic products based on the enzyme-mimicking activity of Fe, Co-doped carbon dots (C-dots). With the enzymatic hydrolysis by diamine oxidase (EC 1.4.3.6, DAO), biogenic amine analytes were decomposed to produce $H_2O_2$ to activate a catalytic colorimetric reaction of TMB and Fe, Co-doped C-dots, contributing to the detection of putrescine and cadaverine in various fish samples with a LOD of 0.06 mg/kg.

## 15.5 NANOZYMES OF EMERGING FOOD TECHNOLOGIES

Nanozymes hold great promise to outperform natural enzymes in food sciences. Thus, although nanozyme researches are currently linked to food science mainly by analytical applications, nanozyme techniques beyond food detection are worth exploring in food science. The prospective potentials of the utilization of nanozymes as emerging food techniques in the areas of food preservation, food cleaning, food waste processing, etc., are discussed herein (**Figure 15.9**).

### 15.5.1 NANOZYMES FOR FOOD PRESERVATION

For food preservation, food matrices are generally thermally processed under a temperature range from 60 to 100°C for the duration of seconds to a minute to destroy vegetative microorganisms. However, the energy transferred to the food during this process will trigger unwanted reactions, contributing to undesirable organoleptic and nutritional changes. Ensuring food safety and at the same time meeting consumer demands for retention of nutrition and quality attributes has drawn increased interest in nontraditional preservation techniques for inactivating microorganisms and enzymes in foods. This increasing demand has opened new dimensions for the use of non-destructive preservative techniques. On the one hand, biopreservation agents

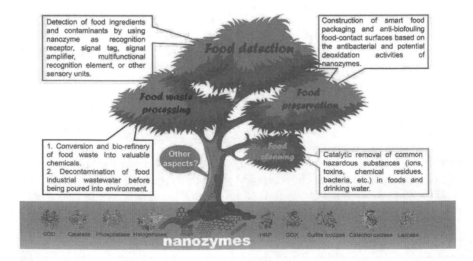

**FIGURE 15.9**  The emerging applications of nanozyme in the field of food science.

have been utilized for extended storage life and enhanced safety of food products (92), such as probiotics, bacteriocins, lactic acid, saponins and flavonoids, chitosan, lactoperoxidase, lysozyme, glucose oxidase, etc. Antimicrobial compounds present in foods can extend the shelf life of unprocessed or processed foods by reducing the microbial growth rate or viability. On the other hand, the rapid development of nanotechnology has transformed many domains of food science, and a wide range of antibacterial nanomaterials, from inorganic metal, metal oxides, and their nanocomposites to nano-organic materials, has been applied for food preservation (93, 94).

As an emerging entity in bionanotechnology, nanozymes are being extensively investigated for combating bacterial and biofilms via durable enzyme mimicry (95). The antibacterial nanozymes consist of POD, OXD, haloperoxidases, and DNase mimics, and the antibacterial activities of which result from, (a) catalyzing the conversion of $H_2O_2$ into mild bactericidal species, (b) catalyzing the conversion of $O_2$ into ROS, (c) catalyzing the decomposition of biofilm components or signal molecules to eliminate biofilm formation. For instance, Dong's group (96) reported a new class of single-atom nanozymes, carbon nanoframe-confined $FeN_5$ active centers ($FeN_5$ SA/CNF), for killing bacteria without the addition of chemical auxiliaries, which catalytically behaved like the axial ligand-coordinated heme of cytochrome P450. The definite active moieties and crucial synergistic effects endow $FeN_5$ SA/CNF with the highest OXD-like activity among other nanozymes (the rate constant is 70 times higher than that of commercial Pt/carbon), which contributed to potent ROS-generation-gifted antibacterial activities against *E. coli* and *S. aureus* pathogens *in vitro* and *in vivo*. Extracellular DNA (eDNA) is an essential structural component during biofilm formation, including initial bacterial adhesion, subsequent development, and final maturation. By confining passivated Au NPs with multiple cerium(IV) complexes on the surface of colloidal magnetic $Fe_3O_4/SiO_2$ core/shell particles, Qu's group (97) constructed a DNase-mimetic artificial enzyme (DMAE) for anti-biofilm applications, which exhibited high cleavage ability towards both model substrates and eDNA. As demonstrated by their anti-biofilm results, the presence of DMAE remarkably potentiated the efficiency of traditional antibiotics to kill biofilm-encased *S. aureus* and eradicate biofilms. Besides, bacterial biofilm formation is closely related to bacterial communication called quorum sensing. Tremel's group mimicked haloperoxidases by $V_2O_5$ nanowires (98) and $CeO_2$-x NRs (99), respectively, to thwart biofilm formation (**Figure 15.10**).

Their results demonstrated that these two haloperoxidases can quench bacterial quorum-sensing behavior by catalytic oxidative bromination of signaling molecules, such as 3-oxo-hexanoylhomoserine lactone. More recently, Qin et al. (100) reported an antiviral strategy using iron oxide nanozymes to target the lipid envelope of the influenza virus, which demonstrated that iron oxide nanozymes functionalized face-mask improves the ability of virus protection against three important subtypes that pose a threat to humans, including H1N1, H5N1, and H7N9 subtype. This evidence proved that nanozymes can be promising bionanocomposites materials capable of tissue engineering, packaging, and surface functionalization techniques. Thus, we believe that the leverage of nanozyme functionalities would provide sustainable, environmentally friendly, and cost-effective strategies for food preservation, food disinfection, anti-biofouling food-contact surface, smart food packaging (**Figure 15.11**), and antibacterial food additives.

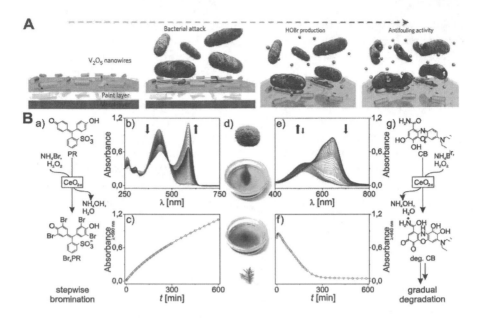

**FIGURE 15.10** Biofilm elimination by haloperoxidase mimicry with (**A**) vanadium pentoxide nanowires (98) and (**B**) CeO₂-x nanorods (99), respectively.

## 15.5.2 Nanozymes for Food Cleaning

Many organic, inorganic, and biological pollutants in the environment, such as pesticides, antibiotics, hormones, toxic ions, mycotoxins, and dyes, will enter the food chain and finally damage human health (57). It is reasonable that the control of hazardous materials in/around the food chain will retard the development of persistent health issues as a result of food contamination. Due to the robust catalytic efficiency and

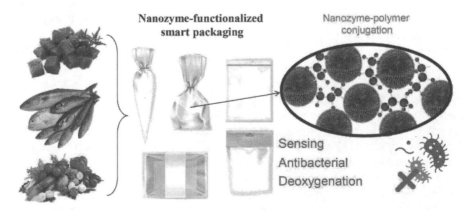

**FIGURE 15.11** Diagram of food preservation techniques by smart food packaging enabled by nanozyme. The nanozyme-engineered packages are possibly smart in sensing, antibacterial, and deoxygenation functionalities.

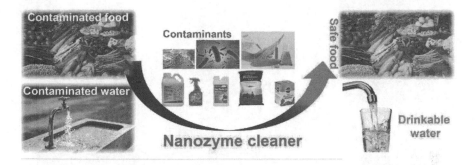

**FIGURE 15.12**   Diagram of food cleaning applications with nanozyme cleaners.

specificity, nanozymes are advantageous for removing hazardous substances from the food industry while avoiding the production of harmful by-products (**Figure 15.12**). For example, Liu' group (101) reported the dehydrogenase-mimicking Au NPs (selected from several nanozymes including nanoceria, $Fe_3O_4$, $Fe_2O_3$, $MnO_2$, and $Mn_2O_3$) could efficiently oxidize estradiol into estrone in the presence of $H_2O_2$ at pH 8, where 5-nm Au NPs catalyzed 4.8 folds faster than 13-nm Au NPs under the same condition. Besides, more literature has validated that functional nanozymes can catalyze the detoxication or degradation of estrogenic endocrine disruptors (33, 101, 102), phenolic compounds (103—106), pesticide residues (13, 24, 107), $H_2O_2$ by-products (108), alcohol (109), organic mercury (28), and dyes (110), etc. These studies pave the way for employing nanozyme to ensure safe food and clean water.

### 15.5.3   NANOZYME FOR FOOD WASTE PROCESSING

During the period of food production and food consumption, considerable food wastes and wastewater can be produced, which may cause resource losses and burden the environmental protection. On the contrary, food waste and food processing wastes, which are abundant in nature and rich in carbon content can also be attractive renewable substrates for sustainable production of biofuel or fine chemicals due to wide economic prospects in industries. However, the selection of catalysts capable of acceptable conversion reaction efficiency and selectivity is usually a challenging issue. In this regard, nanozymes have the potential to surpass traditional catalysts to improve the economy of food waste processing in terms of conversion efficiency, specificity, and cost-effectiveness (111—113). Although no literature reported in this field, the capability of nanozymes for catalyzing natural organic matters potentiates the possibility of processing food wastes with a nanozyme catalysis station (**Figure 15.13**).

## 15.6   SUMMARY AND FUTURE PERSPECTIVES

The current literature has validated that nanozyme will motivate a variety of innovative food technologies in the fields of food analysis, food preservation, food cleaning, food waste processing, etc. However, there are still challenging issues to overcome

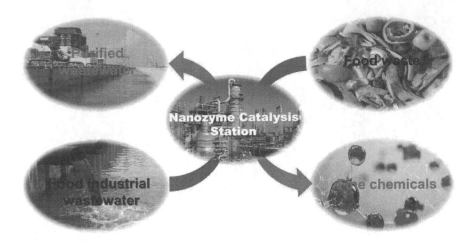

**FIGURE 15.13** Diagram of food waste processing with a nanozyme catalysis station.

to achieve many real successes of nanozymes in food science and technology, as follows:

1. Specificity: The substrate specificity of nanozymes is not as good as that of natural enzymes, which will limit related food applications concerning food processing efficiency and safety. The underlying challenge is the precise design of structure flexibility of nanozymes that feature clear structure-property correlations. The advances in single-atom nanozymes and MOF nanozymes open new avenues to address this issue, which can either manipulate well-defined active sites at the atomic level or reach enzyme-like structural complexity.

2. Target substrate: Current food nanozymology involves mainly oxidoreductase substrates, while the achievements on substrates of other enzymes, such as hydrolases, transferases, lyases, isomerases, or ligases are quite slow. The situation faced by nanozymes is similar to the issue of specificity. Future efforts are encouraged to customize nanozyme design with the inspiration of the characteristic active sites specific to different natural enzymes.

3. Nanotoxicity: The application of nanozymes in the food industry requires a full understanding of nanozyme toxicity, greatly impacting acceptance in the food industry. Currently, the biocompatibility studies of nanozymes *in vitro* and *in vivo* are largely lacking, hindering the future development of nanozyme nanozymology. In this regard, the comprehensive biotoxicity evaluation of promising nanozymes is necessary. Meanwhile, the continuous discovery of naturally sourced or biocompatible (in)organic nanostructures with enzyme-mimicking characteristics is encouraging. Moreover, biocompatible nanozymes with biologically beneficial effects promise to be a nutritive addition for functional foods, which is worthy of further research.

Overall, the solution to the problems in nanozyme specificity, target substrate, nanomaterial toxicity, etc. will require joint efforts from food and nanozyme researchers. Nanozyme that combines nanotechnology and biotechnology is a powerful biomimetic tool to replace the function of natural enzymes in food science and technology.

## REFERENCES

1. Murakami Y, Kikuchi J-i, Hisaeda Y, Hayashida O. 1996. *Chemical Reviews* 96: 721–58
2. Huang Y, Ren J, Qu X. 2019. *Chemical Reviews* 119: 4357–412
3. Jiao L, Yan H, Wu Y, Gu W, Zhu C, et al. 2020. *Angew Chem Int Ed Engl* 59: 2565–76
4. Liang M, Yan X. 2019. *Accounts of Chemical Research* 52: 2190–200
5. Wu J, Wang X, Wang Q, Lou Z, Li S, et al. 2019. *Chemical Society Reviews* 48: 1004–76
6. Huang L, Sun DW, Pu H, Wei Q. 2019. *Comprehensive Reviews in Food Science & Food Safety* 18: 1496–513
7. Wang W, Gunasekaran S. 2020. *TrAC Trends in Analytical Chemistry* 126
8. Huang L, Zhu Q, Zhu J, Luo L, Pu S, et al. 2019. *Inorganic Chemistry* 58: 1638–46
9. Huang L, Zhang W, Chen K, Zhu W, Liu X, et al. 2017. 330: 746–52
10. Huang L, Zhu W, Zhang W, Chen K, Wang J, et al. 2017. *Mikrochim Acta* 185: 7
11. Luo L, Huang L, Liu X, Zhang W, Yao X, et al. 2019. *Inorganic Chemistry* 58: 11382–8
12. Song Y, Qu K, Zhao C, Ren J, Qu X. 2010. *Advanced Materials* 22: 2206–10
13. Wang T, Wang J, Yang Y, Su P, Yang Y. 2017. *Industrial & Engineering Chemistry Research* 56: 9762–9
14. Kim M, Kim MS, Kweon SH, Jeong S, Kang MH, et al. 2015. *Advanced Healthcare Materials* 4: 1311–6
15. Nirala NR, Vinita, Prakash R. 2018. *Mikrochim Acta* 185: 224
16. Jin R, Wang F, Li Q, Yan X, Liu M, et al. 2021. *Sensors and Actuators B: Chemical* 327
17. Liu B, Liu J. 2017. *Nano Research* 10: 1125–48
18. Mulvaney SP, Kidwell DA, Lanese JN, Lopez RP, Sumera ME, Wei E. 2020. *Sensing and Bio-Sensing Research* 30
19. Hu J, Ni P, Dai H, Sun Y, Wang Y, et al. 2015. *Analyst* 140: 3581–6
20. Weerathunge P, Ramanathan R, Shukla R, Sharma TK, Bansal V. 2014. *Analytical Chemistry* 86: 11937–41
21. Weerathunge P, Ramanathan R, Torok VA, Hodgson K, Xu Y, et al. 2019. *Analytical Chemistry* 91: 3270–6
22. Liu P, Han L, Wang F, Li X, Petrenko VA, Liu A. 2018. *Nanoscale* 10: 2825–33
23. Zhang L, Huang R, Liu W, Liu H, Zhou X, Xing D. 2016. *Biosensors & Bioelectronics* 86: 1–7
24. Boruah PK, Das MR. 2020. *Journal of Hazardous Materials* 385: 121516
25. Stasyuk N, Gayda G, Zakalskiy A, Zakalska O, Serkiz R, Gonchar M. 2019. *Food Chemistry* 285: 213–20
26. Adegoke O, Zolotovskaya S, Abdolvand A, Daeid NN. 2021. *Talanta* 224: 121875
27. Gao L, Zhuang J, Nie L, Zhang J, Zhang Y, et al. 2007. *Nature Nanotechnology* 2: 577–83
28. Liu H, Guo Y, Wang Y, Zhang H, Ma X, et al. 2021. *Journal of Hazardous Materials* 405: 124642
29. Huang L, Sun D-W, Pu H, Wei Q, Luo L, Wang J. 2019. *Sensors and Actuators B: Chemical* 290: 573–80
30. Lai W, Wei Q, Xu M, Zhuang J, Tang D. 2017. *Biosensors & Bioelectronics* 89: 645–51
31. Su C-K, Chen J-C. 2017. *Sensors and Actuators B: Chemical* 247: 641–7

32. Chang Y, Liu M, Liu J. 2020. *Analytical Chemistry* 92: 3118–24
33. Wang L, Chen Y. 2020. *ACS Applied Materials & Interfaces* 12: 8351–8
34. Galano A, Mazzone G, Alvarez-Diduk R, Marino T, Alvarez-Idaboy JR, Russo N. 2016. *Annual Review of Food Science and Technology* 7: 335–52
35. Lou Z, Zhao S, Wang Q, Wei H. 2019. *Analytical Chemistry* 91: 15267–74
36. Jia H, Yang D, Han X, Cai J, Liu H, He W. 2016. *Nanoscale* 8: 5938–45
37. Wang S, Liu P, Qin Y, Chen Z, Shen J. 2016. *Sensors and Actuators B: Chemical* 223: 178–85
38. Wang L, Liu Y, Lu C, Yang Z, Liu Y, et al. 2020. *Scientific Reports 10*: 4432
39. Loveday SM. 2019. *Annual Review of Food Science and Technology* 10: 311–39
40. Nidhi Nandu MSH, Neil M. Roberston, Birol Ozturk, and, Yigit MV. 2018. *ChemBioChem*: 1861–7
41. Chafen JJS, Newberry SJ, Riedl MA, Bravata DM, Maglione M, et al. 2010. *JAMA- The Journal of the American Medical Association* 303: 1848–56
42. He S, Li X, Wu Y, Wu S, Wu Z, et al. 2018. *Journal of Agricultural and Food Chemistry* 66: 11830–8
43. Su Y, Wu D, Chen J, Chen G, Hu N, et al. 2019. *Analytical Chemistry* 91: 11687–95
44. Zhang X, Wu D, Wu Y, Li G. 2021. *Biosensors & Bioelectronics* 172: 112776
45. Xu W, Jiao L, Yan H, Wu Y, Chen L, et al. 2019. *ACS Applied Materials & Interfaces* 11: 22096–101
46. Hong L, Liu AL, Li GW, Chen W, Lin XH. 2013. *Biosensors & Bioelectronics* 43: 1–5
47. Valekar AH, Batule BS, Kim MI, Cho KH, Hong DY, et al. 2018. *Biosensors & Bioelectronics* 100: 161–8
48. Smutok O, Kavetskyy T, Prokopiv T, Serkiz R, Wojnarowska-Nowak R, et al. 2021. *Analytica Chimica Acta* 1143: 201–9
49. Mu J, Zhang L, Zhao M, Wang Y. 2014. *ACS Applied Materials & Interfaces* 6: 7090–8
50. Luo L, Su Z, Zhuo J, Huang L, Nian Y, et al. 2020. *ACS Sustainable Chemistry & Engineering* 8: 12568–76
51. Mao Y, Gao S, Yao L, Wang L, Qu H, et al. 2020. *Journal of Hazardous Materials* 408: 124898
52. Wang Y, Liang RP, Qiu JD. 2020. *Analytical Chemistry* 92: 2339–46
53. Zhang X, He S, Chen Z, Huang Y. 2013. *Journal of Agricultural and Food Chemistry* 61: 840–7
54. Qin W, Su L, Yang C, Ma Y, Zhang H, Chen X. 2014. *Journal of Agricultural and Food Chemistry* 62: 5827–34
55. Liu X, Huang L, Wang Y, Sun J, Yue T, et al. 2020. *Sensors and Actuators B: Chemical* 306
56. Xu X, Wang L, Zou X, Wu S, Pan J, et al. 2019. *Sensors and Actuators B: Chemical* 298
57. Sun DW, Huang L, Pu H, Ma J. 2021. *Chemical Society Reviews* 50: 1070–110
58. Liang X, Han L. 2020. *Advanced Functional Materials* 30
59. Zhu Y, Wu J, Han L, Wang X, Li W, et al. 2020. *Analytical Chemistry* 92: 7444–52
60. Yan M, Chen G, She Y, Ma J, Hong S, et al. 2019. *Journal of Agricultural and Food Chemistry* 67: 9658–66
61. Khairy M, Ayoub HA, Banks CE. 2018. *Food Chemistry* 255: 104–11
62. Wei D, Zhang X, Chen B, Zeng K. 2020. *Analytica Chimica Acta* 1126: 106–13
63. Zeng R, Luo Z, Zhang L, Tang D. 2018. *Analytical Chemistry* 90: 12299–306
64. Liu S, Dou L, Yao X, Zhang W, Zhao M, et al. 2020. *Biosensors & Bioelectronics* 169: 112610
65. Laborde D, Martin W, Swinnen J, Vos R. 2020. *Science* 369: 500–2
66. He D, Wu Z, Cui B, Xu E, Jin Z. 2019. *Food Chemistry* 289: 708–13
67. Zhang L, Chen Y, Cheng N, Xu Y, Huang K, et al. 2017. *Analytical Chemistry* 89: 10194–200

68. Han J, Zhang L, Hu L, Xing K, Lu X, et al. 2018. *Journal of Dairy Science* 101: 5770–9
69. Wang Z, Yao X, Zhang Y, Wang R, Ji Y, et al. 2020. *Food Chemistry* 329: 127224
70. Farka Z, Cunderlova V, Horackova V, Pastucha M, Mikusova Z, et al. 2018. *Analytical Chemistry* 90: 2348–54
71. Dehghani Z, Nguyen T, Golabi M, Hosseini M, Rezayan AH, et al. 2021. *Food Control* 121
72. Wu S, Duan N, Qiu Y, Li J, Wang Z. 2017. *International Journal of Food Microbiology* 261: 42–8
73. Cheng N, Song Y, Zeinhom MMA, Chang YC, Sheng L, et al. 2017. *ACS Applied Materials & Interfaces* 9: 40671–80
74. Wei X, Zhou W, Sanjay ST, Zhang J, Jin Q, et al. 2018. *Analytical Chemistry* 90: 9888–96
75. Wu L, Zhang M, Zhu L, Li J, Li Z, Xie W. 2020. *Microchemical Journal* 157
76. Hsu YP, Li NS, Chen YT, Pang HH, Wei KC, Yang HW. 2020. *Biosensors & Bioelectronics* 151: 111960
77. Oh S, Kim J, Tran VT, Lee DK, Ahmed SR, et al. 2018. *ACS Applied Materials & Interfaces* 10: 12534–43
78. Duan D, Fan K, Zhang D, Tan S, Liang M, et al. 2015. *Biosensors & Bioelectronics* 74: 134–41
79. Liu D, Ju C, Han C, Shi R, Chen X, et al. 2020. *Biosensors & Bioelectronics* 173: 112817
80. Shu J, Qiu Z, Wei Q, Zhuang J, Tang D. 2015. *Scientific Reports* 5: 15113
81. Xu Z, Long LL, Chen YQ, Chen ML, Cheng YH. 2021. *Food Chemistry* 338: 128039
82. Huang L, Chen K, Zhang W, Zhu W, Liu X, et al. 2018. *Sensors and Actuators B: Chemical* 269: 79–87
83. Molinero-Fernandez A, Moreno-Guzman M, Lopez MA, Escarpa A. 2017. *Analytical Chemistry* 89: 10850–7
84. Bagheri N, Khataee A, Habibi B, Hassanzadeh J. 2018. *Talanta* 179: 710–8
85. Sun S, Zhao R, Feng S, Xie Y. 2018. *Mikrochim Acta* 185: 535
86. Pacheco M, Jurado-Sanchez B, Escarpa A. 2018. *Analytical Chemistry* 90: 2912–7
87. Zhang W, Niu X, Li X, He Y, Song H, et al. 2018. *Sensors and Actuators B: Chemical* 265: 412–20
88. Deng HH, Li GW, Hong L, Liu AL, Chen W, et al. 2014. *Food Chemistry* 147: 257–61
89. Swaidan A, Barras A, Addad A, Tahon JF, Toufaily J, et al. 2021. *Journal of Colloid and Interface Science* 582: 732–40
90. Wang X, Song X, Si L, Xu L, Xu Z. 2020. *Food and Agricultural Immunology* 31: 1036–50
91. Li Y-F, Lin Z-Z, Hong C-Y, Huang Z-Y. 2021. *Journal of Food Measurement and Characterization*
92. Tiwari BK, Valdramidis VP, O' Donnell CP, Muthukumarappan K, Bourke P, Cullen PJ. 2009. *Journal of Agricultural and Food Chemistry* 57: 5987–6000
93. Bumbudsanpharoke N, Ko S. 2015. *Journal of Food Science* 80: R910–23
94. Youssef AM, El-Sayed SM. 2018. *Carbohydrate Polymer* 193: 19–27
95. Chen Z, Wang Z, Ren J, Qu X. 2018. *Accounts of Chemical Research* 51: 789–99
96. Huang L, Chen J, Gan L, Wang J, Dong S. 2019. *Science Advances* 5: eaav5490
97. Chen Z, Ji H, Liu C, Bing W, Wang Z, Qu X. 2016. *Angewandte Chemie International Edition* 55: 10732–6
98. Natalio F, Andre R, Hartog AF, Stoll B, Jochum KP, et al. 2012. *Nature Nanotechnology* 7: 530–5
99. Herget K, Hubach P, Pusch S, Deglmann P, Gotz H, et al. 2017. *Advanced Materials* 29
100. Qin T, Ma R, Yin Y, Miao X, Chen S, et al. 2019. *Theranostics* 9: 6920–35
101. Zhang Z, Bragg LM, Servos MR, Liu J. 2019. *Chinese Chemical Letters* 30: 1655–8

102. Sun K, Liu Q, Li S, Qi Y, Si Y. 2020. *Journal of Hazardous Materials* 393: 122393
103. Li S, Hou Y, Chen Q, Zhang X, Cao H, Huang Y. 2020. *ACS Applied Materials & Interfaces* 12: 2581–90
104. Huang H, Lei L, Bai J, Zhang L, Song D, et al. 2020. *Chinese Journal of Chemical Engineering*
105. Jiang J, He C, Wang S, Jiang H, Li J, Li L. 2018. *Carbohydrate Polymer* 198: 348–53
106. Li M, Chen J, Wu W, Fang Y, Dong S. 2020. *Journal of the American Chemical Society* 142: 15569–74
107. Efremenko EN, Lyagin IV, Klyachko NL, Bronich T, Zavyalova NV, et al. 2017. *Journal of Controlled Release* 247: 175–81
108. Jiao M, Li Z, Li X, Zhang Z, Yuan Q, et al. 2020. *Chemical Engineering Journal* 388
109. Sun A, Mu L, Hu X. 2017. *ACS Applied Materials & Interfaces* 9: 12241–52
110. Chen Q, Zhang X, Li S, Tan J, Xu C, Huang Y. 2020. *Chemical Engineering Journal* 395
111. Wang F, Zhang Y, Liu Z, Ren J, Qu X. 2020. *Nanoscale* 12: 14465–71
112. Wang J, Huang R, Qi W, Su R, Binks BP, He Z. 2019. *Applied Catalysis B: Environmental* 254: 452–62
113. Yang H, Wu X, Su L, Ma Y, Graham NJD, Yu W. 2020. *Water Research* 171: 115491

# 16 Rational Design of Peroxidase-like Nanozymes

*Xiaoyu Wang[1,*] and Hui Wei[1,2,*]*
[1]Department of Biomedical Engineering, College of Engineering and Applied Sciences, Nanjing National Laboratory of Microstructures, Jiangsu Key Laboratory of Artificial Functional Materials, Nanjing University, Nanjing, Jiangsu, China
[2]State Key Laboratory of Analytical Chemistry for Life Science, School of Chemistry and Chemical Engineering, Chemistry and Biomedicine Innovation Center (ChemBIC), Nanjing University, Nanjing, Jiangsu, China

## CONTENTS

---

* Corresponding authors: Xiaoyu Wang and Hui Wei

DOI: 10.1201/9781003109228-16

**341**

## 16.1   INTRODUCTION

Among different natural enzymes, peroxidase (POD) is a widespread oxidoreductase, which can catalyze the oxidation of some reducing substrates in the presence of peroxides (*e.g.*, hydrogen peroxide, $H_2O_2$). On the one hand, $H_2O_2$ is an intermediate product, which plays an important role in food, environment, pharmaceuticals, and other fields; on the other hand, $H_2O_2$ may generate hydroxyl free radicals ($^{\cdot}OH$) when it is decomposed, and $^{\cdot}OH$ has widespread use in biomedicine. Therefore, tremendous efforts have been devoted to developing nanomaterials with POD-like activities due to their promising applications in sensing, bioimaging, and nanomedicine (1–16).

While great breakthroughs have been made, there remain some bottlenecks in the field of POD-like nanozymes, which greatly limit the further development of POD-like nanozymes. One of these bottlenecks is that the design and preparation of POD-like nanozymes are mainly achieved by using "trial-and-error" strategies (2). The prevalence of "trial-and-error" methods is because the catalytic mechanisms of POD mimics are missing and the structure–catalytic activity relationship remains largely unknown. To tackle these bottlenecks, great efforts have been made to better understand the catalytic process of nanozymes. Some seminal studies have tried to elucidate the catalytic mechanisms of POD-like nanozymes by first-principle calculation (16–25). Besides, the structure–activity relationship was also explored by combining experimental results with computational studies (20, 26). More importantly, several studies have identified predictive descriptors for the rational design of POD mimics (21, 24, 27). Benefitting from the rational design of highly active nanozymes, *in vitro* detection and live bioassays have been developed by using POD mimics (4). In this chapter, we first highlight the recent progress of rational design of POD-like nanozymes and then introduce the representative examples for bioanalytical applications. Finally, the challenges and future perspectives toward POD-like nanozymes are discussed to further advance the field.

## 16.2   CATALYTIC MECHANISM OF POD-LIKE NANOZYMES

Understanding the catalytic mechanism in POD-like catalytic reaction is critical to allow researchers to know why one material is a better POD mimic than another. In terms of nanozyme catalysis, it belongs to heterogeneous catalysis, in which the catalysts and the reactants are present in two phases (28–30). The POD-like catalytic reaction takes place at the surface of solid catalysts, while the reactants (*i.e.*, peroxides and POD substrates) are present in a liquid phase. Therefore, the fundamental concepts of heterogeneous catalysis can be used to elucidate the catalytic mechanisms of POD mimics. Based on fundamental concepts of heterogeneous catalysis, several seminal studies of molecular-level understanding of the catalytic mechanisms in POD-like catalytic reactions have been performed using the first-principle calculation (16–18, 20–25).

## 16.2.1 TMB OXIDATION BY OH GROUP

Shen *et al.* studied the catalytic mechanism of POD mimics by using density functional theory (DFT) calculations (24). Eight $Fe_3O_4$ slabs with different crystal structures, exposed facets, and chemical modifications, were selected to determine the POD-like reaction pathways and possible intermediate and transition-state structures. The POD-like catalytic process of $Fe_3O_4$ slabs involves three reaction steps (**Figure 16.1A**). As shown in equation 16.1 (eq 16.1), the $H_2O_2$ is first adsorbed on the slab surface, which is then dissociated to generate a dual OH adsorbed structure. Subsequently, TMB (3,3′,5,5′-tetramethylbenzidine dihydrochloride) is oxidized by two OH groups in steps 2 and 3 (eqs 16.2–3). For step 1, the slab surface with high reducibility would contribute to the dissociation of $H_2O_2$ because this step is involved in the $H_2O_2$ reduction reaction, while steps 2 and 3 are a protonation-coupled transfer of a hydrogen atom from TMB to the OH groups. In addition to $Fe_3O_4$, the catalytic mechanisms proposed here are also applicable to noble metals and perovskite oxides (17, 21)

$$H_2O_2 \xrightarrow{E_{b,1}} 2OH^*, E_{r,1} \tag{16.1}$$

$$OH_1^* + TMB + H^+ \xrightarrow{E_{b,2}} oxTMB + H_2O, E_{r,2} \tag{16.2}$$

$$OH_2^* + TMB + H^+ \xrightarrow{E_{b,3}} oxTMB + H_2O, E_{r,3}. \tag{16.3}$$

The asterisk in eqs 16.1–3 indicates the adsorption species on the slab surfaces; $OH_1$ and $OH_2$ indicate the hydroxyl absorbates in steps 2 and 3, respectively; and $E_b$ and $E_r$ are the activation energy barrier and reaction energy, respectively.

According to the Arrhenius equation, the reaction rate depends on the activation energy barrier (29). Also, the rate-determining step (RDS), the slowest elementary step of a chemical reaction, determines the rate of the overall reaction process. Therefore, the POD-like activities of nanozymes are generally governed by the energy barrier of RDS. Calculating the energy profiles involved in adsorption energy ($E_{ads}$), activation energy barriers, and reaction energy are critical to obtain the RDS and study the catalytic kinetics. For the POD-like catalytic reaction in **Figure 16.1A**, the calculated energies of the intermediates and transition states on three typical $Fe_3O_4$ slabs are shown in **Figure 16.1B**. For the three steps mentioned above (eqs 16.1–3), step 2 could not be an RDS because structure **iii** is more oxidized than structure **v**. Therefore, steps 1 and 3 were the potential RDS. As shown in **Figure 16.1B**, for slab 14, the $E_{b,1}$ is higher than $E_{b,3}$, suggesting its RDS was step 1. However, the RDSs of slabs 3 and 7 were determined to be step 3 because $E_{b,3}$ was higher than $E_{b,1}$ in these slabs. The different RDSs and energy profiles on different slabs were essentially attributed to the intrinsic structure dependence of the $E_{ads}$, activation energy barrier, and reaction energy. The $H_2O_2$ was easily dissociated on slab 3

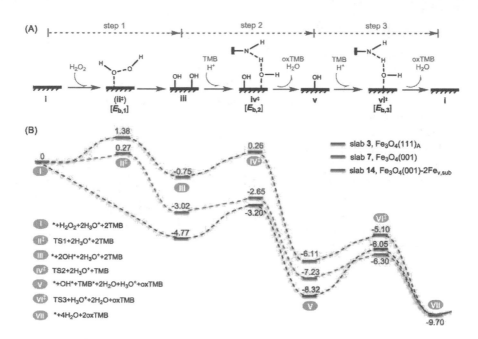

**FIGURE 16.1** Mechanism and kinetics of POD-like reactions catalyzed by iron oxides as determined from DFT calculations. **(A)** Proposed mechanism of POD-like catalysis of iron-oxide slabs, where $[E_{b,1}]$, $[E_{b,2}]$, and $[E_{b,3}]$ are energy barriers for steps 1–3, respectively. **(B)** Relative energy values (in eV) for key intermediates and transition states involved in the catalytic cycles of slabs **3, 7,** and **14**. Reprinted from (24), Copyright 2020, with permission from American Chemical Society.

with high reducibility to generate strongly adsorbed OH groups. However, the OH groups were difficult to remove from the slab 3 surface, so step 3 was the RDS. For slab 14, its low chemical reducibility hindered $H_2O_2$ dissociation, so step 1 was the RDS (24).

### 16.2.2 TMB Oxidation by Hydroxyl Radical ($^\bullet$OH)

Recently, single-atom nanozymes have received extensive attention because their well-defined coordination structure provides an ideal experimental model for catalytic mechanism research (23, 25, 31–40). Several mechanistic studies based on single-atom nanozymes have revealed similar mechanisms (23, 25, 31). As shown in **Figure 16.2**, the catalytic mechanisms of single-atom nanozymes are slightly different from the ones mentioned above (23, 24). The $H_2O_2$ was first adsorbed on the surface of a single-atom nanozyme and followed the homolytic path to form a dual OH adsorbed structure. Subsequently, an OH group desorbed from the surface of nanozyme, resulting in the generation of $^\bullet$OH. Experimentally, the reaction intermediate of $^\bullet$OH was demonstrated by electron spin resonance (ESR) spectra (23).

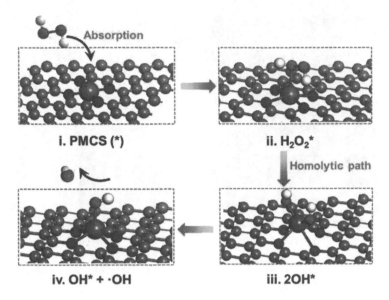

i. PMCS (*)

ii. H₂O₂*

iii. 2OH*

iv. OH* + ·OH

**FIGURE 16.2** Proposed catalytic mechanism of the zinc (Zn)-centered porphyrin-like structure. The pale blue, blue, gray, red, and white balls represent the Zn, N, C, O, and H atoms, respectively. Reprinted from (23), Copyright 2019, with permission from John Wiley and Sons.

## 16.3 FACTORS AFFECTING POD-LIKE ACTIVITY

### 16.3.1 COMPOSITION

Regulating the POD-like activity by changing composition could be roughly classified into two types: type I—by coating or growing material with high POD-like activity on a less active surface and type II—by doping another element into the lattice of nanomaterials to form a solid solution. Some noble metal NPs [*e.g.*, iridium (Ir), ruthenium (Ru), and platinum (Pt)] have been demonstrated to possess excellent POD-like activities (41–46). By coating or growing highly active noble metal NPs on less active material, one would not only enhance the POD-like activity but also improve the atomic utilization efficiency of noble metals (46–48). For example, Xia *et al.* obtained palladium (Pd)-Ir core-shell cubes by depositing a few atomic Ir layers on Pd nanocubes. The POD-like activities of Pd-Ir nanocubes were significantly enhanced by at least 20-fold and 400-fold when compared with the initial Pd cubes and horseradish peroxidase (HRP), respectively (**Figure 16.3**) (48). Also, noble metal NPs were used to regulate the POD-like activity of carbon-based or metal oxide-based nanomaterials, which could not only enhance the POD-like activity of less active carbon or metal oxide-based nanomaterials but improve the cycle stability of metal NPs (49–51). Moreover, numerous studies have shown that there is a synergy between nanomaterials in a hybrid composite (50, 52, 53). For example, the Pt/cube-cerium oxide (CeO₂) was prepared by *in situ* depositing Pt NPs on the surface of cube-CeO₂. Benefiting from the strong metal-support interaction, the

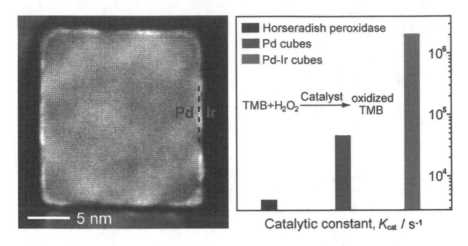

**FIGURE 16.3** Depositing Ir atoms as ultrathin skins on Pd cubes (*i.e.*, Pd-Ir cubes) as enhanced POD mimics. Reprinted from (48), Copyright 2015, with permission from American Chemical Society.

as-hybridized $Pt/cube-CeO_2$ exhibited higher catalytic activity than the mixture of Pt and $cube-CeO_2$ with equivalent quality (50).

Doping other elements into the lattice of nanomaterials was another effective method to enhance the POD-like activity (16, 20, 39, 54–61). The enhanced POD-like activity may be attributed to the modification of the electronic structure by doping another element. Hu *et al.* demonstrated that heteroatom nitrogen (N)-doping into reduced graphene oxide (rGO) and mesoporous carbon could specifically improve their POD-like activities by over 100-fold and 60-fold, respectively (**Figure 16.4**) (20). To further improve the POD-like activities of carbon nanomaterials, sulfur (S)/N co-doped or N/boron (B) co-doped carbon nanomaterials were synthesized, which have shown enhanced POD-like activity when compared with doping with N alone (54, 56, 59). Besides, the POD-like activities of metal oxides could also be improved by doping another metal element. For instance, the first row of transition metals was doped into the lattice of $CeO_2$ to form $M_xCe_{1-x}O_{2-\delta}$ solid solution. Among these doped nanoceria ($CeO_2$), manganese (Mn)-doped Ce solid solution exhibited significantly enhanced POD-like activity (57).

## 16.3.2 STRUCTURE

### 16.3.2.1 Size

In terms of nanozyme catalysis, the chemical reactions take place at the surface of materials. On the other hand, nanomaterials with a smaller size have a higher surface-area-to-volume ratio, which exposes more catalytically active sites on the surface. Therefore, the POD-like activities of nanomaterials are related to their sizes (6, 62–64). Various studies demonstrated that the smaller the size, the higher the POD-like activity. Gao *et al.* first discovered the unexpected POD-like activity of $Fe_3O_4$ NPs and demonstrated their size-dependent catalytic activity (6). The

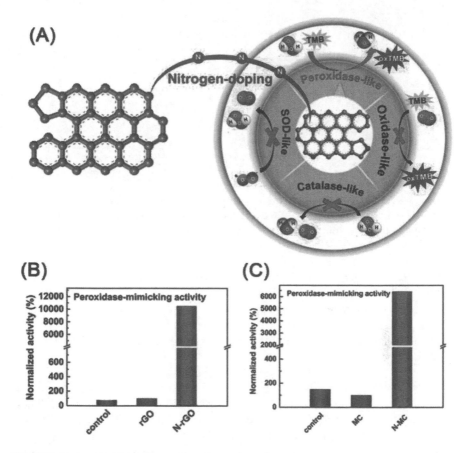

**FIGURE 16.4** (**A**) Illustration of N-doped carbon nanomaterials as efficient POD mimics. (**B**) Normalized POD-like activities of rGO and N-doped rGO (N-rGO). (**C**) Enhancement of the POD-like activities of N-doped mesoporous carbon (N-MC) relative to those of mesoporous carbon (MC). Adapted from (20), Copyright 2018, with permission from American Chemical Society.

POD-like activities decreased with increasing size (30 nm, 150 nm, and 300 nm) of $Fe_3O_4$ NPs (**Figure 16.5A**) (6). They attributed this result to the greater surface-area-to-volume ratio, of smaller NPs, to react with the substrate. However, some studies found that the POD-like activity did not show a consistent trend with decreasing size. He *et al.* investigated the catalytic activities of Au NPs with different sizes by ESR (62). They demonstrated that the ESR signal increased with size from 10 to 50 nm, and then decreased with size from 50 to 100 nm, suggesting that Au NPs with the size of 50 nm possessed the highest catalytic activity (**Figure 16.5B**) (62). Therefore, in addition to changing the surface area-to-volume ratio, other factors, such as the electronic structure of nanomaterials may be tuned by changing their sizes (63, 65, 66). For example, cytosine-rich oligonucleotide stabilized 2.9-nm Pt nanozymes exhibited better POD-like activity than guanine-rich oligonucleotide stabilized 1.8-nm Pt nanozymes. More metallic $Pt^0$ on the surface of 2.9-nm Pt nanozymes enabled

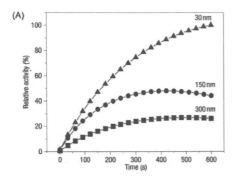
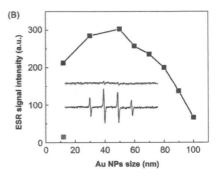

**FIGURE 16.5** **(A)** POD-like activities of $Fe_3O_4$ MNPs with different sizes. **(B)** Effect of Au NPs size on the generation of ˙OH induced by Au NPs. (A) Reprinted from (6), Copyright 2007, with permission from Nature Publishing Group. (B) Reprinted from (62), Copyright 2013, with permission from Elsevier.

the high POD-like activity, while more $Pt^{2+}$ but less $Pt^0$ was present on the surface of 1.8-nm Pt nanozymes (63). Recently, to maximize the atom utilization, single-atom nanozymes with isolated metal atoms dispersed on solid support have been extensively studied (23, 25, 31–35, 38–40). Benefitting from their unique geometric and electronic structures, single-atom nanozymes exhibited excellent POD-like activity (23, 25, 31, 35, 38, 40).

### 16.3.2.2 Morphology and Facet

There are usually several different facets on the surface of a nanomaterial. These facets with different atom arrangements and undercoordinated sites exhibit different $E_{ads}$, reaction energy, and activation energy barriers for the same substrate, determining their different catalytic activities. Since different morphologies have different facets, the morphology could be used to regulate the POD-like activity of nanozymes. Liu *et al.* obtained three kinds of $Fe_3O_4$ nanocrystals with cluster spheres, octahedral, and triangular by a hydrothermal method (67). Their studies suggested that the cluster spheres with exposed {311} facets showed the highest POD-like activity, while triangular plates with {200} facets exhibited moderate POD-like activity, but higher than that of octahedral $Fe_3O_4$ with {111} facets (**Figure 16.6A**). Recently, numerous studies suggested that metal NPs with high-index facets are generally more reactive than low-index ones due to the high density of uncoordinated atomic steps, ledges, and kinks on these facets (68–71). High-index {730} faceted Pt concave nanocubes had superior POD-like activity, which the $K_{cat}$ value of Pt concave nanocubes is about 1500-fold and 4-fold higher than HRP and Pt nanospheres, respectively (71). Wu *et al.* prepared Pd-Pt core-frame nanodendrites by growing a dense array of Pt branches on a Pd core (**Figure 16.6B**) (68). As shown in **Figure 16.6B**, to further enhance the catalytic activity, the less active core (*i.e.*, Pd) was selectively etched, forming the Pt hollow nanodendrites with more exposed active sites and high-index facets (*i.e.*, {110} and {311} facets) (68). Li *et al.* investigated the effect of facet on the POD-like activity of Au nanocrystals by DFT calculations (17). They found that the Au with {111}, {110}, and {211} facets followed the same catalytic mechanism

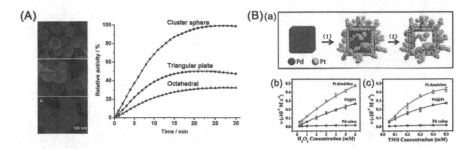

**FIGURE 16.6** (**A**) Time-dependent catalytic activity of cluster sphere, triangular plate, and octahedral $Fe_3O_4$ nanostructures with TMB and $H_2O_2$ as the substrates. (**B**) Schematic showing the two major steps involved in the synthesis of Pt hollow nanodendrites and the reaction velocity of Pt hollow dendrites, Pd@Pt, Pd cubes. (A) Adapted from (67), Copyright 2010, with permission from John Wiley and Sons. (B) Adapted from (68), Copyright 2018, with permission from John Wiley and Sons.

and RDS. According to the activation energy barriers of RDS, the Au {111} with the highest energy barrier was the least reactive, while the Au with {211} facets exhibited the highest activity (17).

## 16.4    ACTIVITY DESCRIPTORS

Composition, size, morphology, and facet could affect the POD-like activity of nanozymes by changing both their geometric and electronic structures. However, the relationship between these aspects and POD-like activity was ambiguous, resulting in the design and synthesis of POD-like nanozymes were mainly achieved by "trial-and-error" strategies. Predictive descriptors are structural parameters of nanomaterials that can act as proxies for their catalytic activities (72). Identifying predictive descriptors can significantly facilitate the search for highly active POD mimics. In this section, we introduce several seminal studies on identifying predictive descriptors for the rational design of POD mimics.

### 16.4.1    $e_g$ Occupancy

For electrocatalysis and photocatalysis, various studies demonstrated that the electronic structure (*e.g.*, the *d*-band center of metals, O 2*p*-band center, and $e_g$ occupancy) could serve as predictive activity descriptors for the rational design of electro-catalysts and photo-catalysts. However, the effect of electronic structure on the POD-like nanozymes remains largely unknown. To demonstrate the structure–activity relationship and identify a predictive descriptor, $ABO_3$-type perovskite transition metal oxide (TMO) with $BO_6$ octahedral subunits (where A is a rare earth or alkaline-earth metal and B is a transition metal) were used as a model system due to their flexible structures, adjustable components, and catalytic properties (**Figure 16.7A**) (21). Ten perovskite oxides were prepared and their POD-like activities were studied (**Figure 16.7B**). A volcano relationship between the $e_g$ occupancy (*i.e.*, the *d*-electron population of the $e_g$ ($\sigma^*$) antibonding orbitals

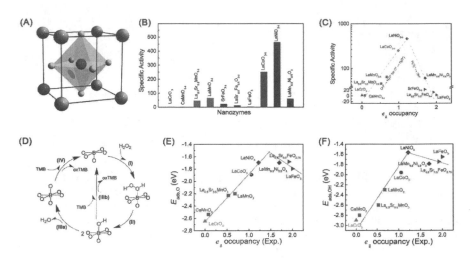

**FIGURE 16.7** (A) Schematic of the $ABO_3$ perovskite structure. (B) Specific POD-like activities of perovskite TMOs. (C) Specific POD-like activities of perovskite TMOs plotted as a function of $e_g$ occupancy, in which equations shown in gray are the rate-limiting reaction steps. (D) The proposed subprocesses responsible for the oxidation of TMB to TMBox with the (001) facet of $ABO_3$ as POD mimics. Adsorption energies of (E) O ($E_{ads,O}$) and (F) OH ($E_{ads,OH}$) plotted as a function of $e_g$ occupancy, where $E_{ads}$ and $e_g$ occupancy were obtained by calculations and experiments, respectively. Adapted from (21), Copyright 2019, with permission from Nature Publishing Group.

associated with the transition metal sites) of B cations and the specific POD-like activities of perovskite oxide-based POD mimics could be obtained (**Figure 16.7C**). Perovskite oxides with $e_g$ occupancy of about 1.2 had the highest POD-like activity, while perovskite oxides with $e_g$ occupancy of 0 or 2 exhibited negligible POD-like activity (**Figure 16.7C**). Therefore, the $e_g$ occupancy can act as a predictive descriptor of perovskite oxide-based POD mimics. Moreover, research has demonstrated the $e_g$ occupancy can also serve as a descriptor for five binary metal oxide NPs with octahedral coordination. Other electronic structure characteristics, such as the oxidation state of a transition metal, $3d$ electron number of B-site ions exhibited no apparent relationship with the catalytic activity of nanozyme. The O $2p$-band center and B-O covalency may serve as secondary descriptors when the occupancy of B cation is close to 1. DFT calculations were performed to theoretically explain the effect of $e_g$ occupancy on the catalytic activity (**Figures 16.7D-7F**). These results suggested that the $e_g$ occupancy could influence the adsorption energies and RDSs, which in turn changed the POD-like activities of perovskite oxides. When $e_g$ was higher than 1.2, the RDS was the dissociation of $H_2O_2$. When $e_g$ was lower than 1.2, the RDS was the oxidation of the substrate. Perovskite oxides with $e_g$ of about 1.2 had optimal energy barrier and can facilitate the RDS efficiently, resulting in an excellent POD-like activity.

## 16.4.2 REDOX POTENTIAL

The catalytic mechanism discussed earlier requires electron transfer from POD-like nanozyme to $H_2O_2$, in which subsequently the electron was transferred from TMB to nanozyme to realize the catalytic cycle. Two half-reactions were involved in the catalytic cycle (*i.e.*, $H_2O_2$ reduction reaction and TMB oxidation reaction). The redox potentials of $H_2O_2$ dissociation and TMB oxidation are 1.566 and 1.13 V, respectively (27, 73). Therefore, from thermodynamic aspects, the ideal redox potential of POD-like nanozyme should lie in between the two half-reactions. Dong *et al.* tried to explain why cobalt tetraoxide ($Co_3O_4$) NPs could serve as excellent POD mimics by redox potential (27). The redox potential of $Co^{3+}/Co^{2+}$ in the $Co_3O_4$ NPs is about 1.30 V, while the redox potentials of $H_2O_2$ dissociation and TMB oxidation are 1.566 and 1.13 V, respectively (**Figure 16.8A**) (27, 73, 74). Therefore, the order of $H_2O_2$, TMB, and $Co_3O_4$ redox potential made the electron transfer process effective. As shown in **Figure 16.8B**, electron transfer occurred first between the $Co^{3+}$ and TMB, in which $Co^{3+}$ was reduced into $Co^{2+}$ and TMB was oxidized into a blue derivative (27). Subsequently, $Co^{2+}$ was reoxidized to $Co^{3+}$ by $H_2O_2$ to accomplish the catalytic cycle. In addition to $Co_3O_4$, the redox potential theory can also be used to explain why Prussian blue (PB) can mimic POD (75). Prussian blue could be oxidized by $H_2O_2$ to form Berlin green (BG) or Prussian yellow (PY) and subsequently BG/PY could be reduced by TMB (75). From thermodynamic aspects, the overall processes were easily achieved because the redox potential of PB is in between TMB and $H_2O_2$. Therefore, for POD-like nanozyme with the catalytic mechanism of TMB oxidation by nanozyme directly, redox potential may be a possible descriptor for the rational design of highly active POD mimics.

## 16.4.3 ADSORPTION ENERGY OF OH GROUP ($E_{ADS,OH}$)

According to principles of chemical reactions and Brønsted–Evans–Polanyi (BEP) relationship, it has been demonstrated that the $E_{ads,OH}$ could be a universal descriptor

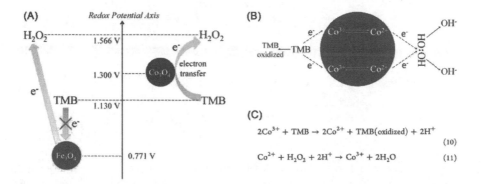

**FIGURE 16.8** (**A**) Theoretical analysis of the NPs as POD mimics. (**B**) Potential mechanism of $Co_3O_4$ NPs as POD mimics. (**C**) The whole reaction process of $Co_3O_4$ NPs as POD mimics. Adapted from (27), Copyright 2014, with permission from American Chemical Society.

for POD mimics (24, 76). The overall reaction for POD mimics could be written as follows:

$$H_2O_2 + 2TMB + 2H^+ \rightarrow (2oxTMB+)2H_2O, \ C \tag{16.4}$$

where $C$ is the reaction energy of POD-like catalytic reaction.

As discussed earlier, this overall reaction (eq 16.4) could be divided into three steps (eqs 16.1-3). The reaction energies ($E_r$) of three elementary reactions were $E_{r,1}$, $E_{r,2}$, and $E_{r,3}$. Therefore, $C$ could be expressed as:

$$C = E_{r,1} + E_{r,2} + E_{r,3}. \tag{16.5}$$

Because both steps 2 and 3 are involved in the protonation-coupled transfer of a hydrogen atom from TMB to the OH groups, the $E_r$ of these two steps followed a linear relationship. Therefore, we can write

$$E_{r,2} = cE_{r,3}. \tag{16.6}$$

Therefore,

$$C = E_{r,1} + cE_{r,3} + E_{r,3} \tag{16.7}$$

$$E_{r,3} = \frac{C - E_{r,1}}{1+c}. \tag{16.8}$$

The catalytic activities of POD mimics were governed by the energy barrier of RDS. As discussed earlier, steps 1 and 3 are potential RDSs in the POD-like catalytic process. According to BEP linear scaling relationships in heterogeneous catalysis, the energy barrier and reaction energy for the same reactions have a positive relationship. Therefore, the energy barriers ($E_b$) of steps 1 and 3 are as follows:

$$E_{b,1} = a_1E_{r,1} + b_1 \tag{16.9}$$

$$E_{b,3} = a_3E_{r,3} + b_3. \tag{16.10}$$

Substituting eq 16.8 into eq 16.10, we obtain the following:

$$E_{b,3} = \frac{-a_3}{1+c}E_{r,1} + \frac{a_3c}{1+c} + b_3. \tag{16.11}$$

Therefore, according to the above deduction (eq 16.9 and eq 16.11), whether it is step 1 or step 3, their $E_b$ were linearly related to $E_{r,1}$. Moreover, $Fe_3O_4$ was taken as an example to demonstrate the linear relationship between $E_{b,1}$ (or $E_{b,3}$) and $E_{r,1}$ (**Figure 16.9**) (24). By plotting the $E_{b,1}$ or $E_{b,3}$ as a function of the corresponding $E_{r,1}$, an inverse volcano curve could be obtained. The lines of $E_{b,1}$ or $E_{b,3}$ intersect where

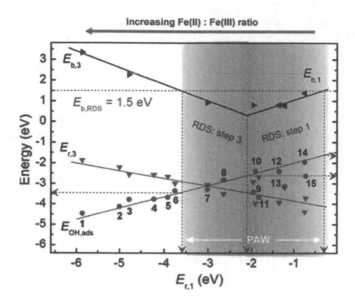

**FIGURE 16.9** Volcano-shaped activity curve. The volcano-shaped plot of POD activity (black lines) as a function of $H_2O_2$ chemisorption energy ($E_{r,1}$) for $Fe_3O_4$ slabs 1–15. $E_{r,3}$, and $E_{ads,OH}$ are also plotted in the figure as linear functions of $E_{r,1}$ (gray lines). The blue zone is the POD activity window (PAW) defined by $E_{r,1}$. The color change from blue to white represents the gradual reduction in the activity from a high value to zero. The vertical and horizontal dashed lines with arrows illustrate how PAWs are defined by $E_{r,1}$ and $E_{ads,OH}$, respectively. Labels ●, ▼, ◄, and ► designate $E_{ads,OH}$, $E_{r,3}$, $E_{b,1}$, and $E_{b,3}$, respectively. Adapted from (24), Copyright 2020, with permission from American Chemical Society.

$E_{r,1}$ = -2.1 eV. When $E_{r,1}$ is lower than -2.1 eV, the $E_{b,3}$ was higher than $E_{b,1}$, thus the RDS is step 3. When $E_{r,1}$ is higher than -2.1 eV, the RDS is step 1. Therefore, $E_{r,1}$ could be an activity descriptor for POD mimics. Further, they found that the $E_{ads,OH}$ exhibited a linear relationship with $E_{r,1}$ (**Figure 16.9**). In addition, the calculation of $E_{ads,OH}$ is easier than $E_{r,1}$. Therefore, $E_{ads,OH}$ could replace $E_{r,1}$ to be a more effective and simpler descriptor for POD mimics. To demonstrate the general applicability of the $E_{ads,OH}$ descriptor, 57 additional nanomaterials, including metals, metal oxides, and carbon were also investigated. The calculated $E_{ads,OH}$ values exhibited great power for predicting the highly active POD mimics.

## 16.5   BIOANALYTICAL APPLICATIONS

### 16.5.1   *IN VITRO* DETECTION

#### 16.5.1.1   Bioactive Small Molecules

POD mimics could catalyze $H_2O_2$ to oxidize the substrate (*e.g.*, TMB), forming an oxidized product. Based on this reaction, the detection principles for bioactive small molecules are mainly classified into three types: 1) $H_2O_2$ (or some targets which could be oxidized by their corresponding oxidase to produce $H_2O_2$) could be detected by oxidizing the POD substrates to generate a signal in the presence of POD mimics; 2) some reductive targets could be detected by reducing the oxidized products (and/or by consuming $H_2O_2$), which subsequently result in decreased signals; and 3) targets could be detected by interacting with POD-like nanomaterials, which could enhance or inhibit the nanozyme activity.

For the first type, $H_2O_2$ detection based on POD mimics has been extensively studied ever since the discovery of unexpected POD-like activity of $Fe_3O_4$ MNPs (1, 2, 7, 39, 52, 77–98). The general principle is based on the $H_2O_2$ mediated oxidation of a substrate to generate an oxidized product for signal transduction with the assistance of POD mimics (**Figure 16.10**) (91). By changing different types of substrates, colorimetric, fluorescent, chemiluminescent, and Raman signals could be used for signaling (7, 93, 98–101). The seminal study of Wei and Wang reported a colorimetric method for $H_2O_2$ detection by using $Fe_3O_4$ MNPs as POD mimics and ABTS [2,2'-azino-bis(3-ethylbenzothiazoline-6-sulfonic acid)] as a substrate (7). By catalyzing $H_2O_2$ to oxidize ABTS with the assistance of $Fe_3O_4$ MNPs, a green-colored product (*i.e.*, ABTS$^{\bullet+}$) could be obtained, enabling $H_2O_2$ detection by the naked eye or absorption spectra (7). By replacing the ABTS with Amplex Red, the fluorescent method could be constructed for $H_2O_2$ detection (102). Leucomalachite green or TMB could be oxidized into Raman-active reporters (*i.e.*, malachite or TMBox) in the presence of $H_2O_2$ with the assistance of POD mimics, which could be used for signaling by surface-enhanced Raman scattering (SERS) spectroscopy (86, 89, 93, 95). Besides, by using electrochemical methods, $H_2O_2$ could be detected in the absence of a POD substrate (81, 87, 103, 104). For example, electrochemical sensing of $H_2O_2$ was achieved by the POD-like $Fe_3O_4$/rGO nanocomposites modified glassy carbon electrode (GCE) (87). The $H_2O_2$ could be reduced by the POD-like $Fe_3O_4$/rGO nanocomposites, which subsequently generate cathodic current for signaling. Moreover, extracellular $H_2O_2$ released from HeLa cells simulated by cadmium telluride (CdTe) quantum dots could be monitored by this as-developed electrochemical method (87). Recently, to enhance the robustness of $H_2O_2$ detection, a ratiometric sensing platform based on fluorescent carbon nitride ($C_3N_4$)-based nanozymes was constructed by Wang *et al.* (98). In the presence of $H_2O_2$, *o*-phenylenediamine (OPD) could be oxidized into OPDox with the assistance of $C_3N_4$-based nanozymes. The OPDox could not only emit fluorescence at 564 nm when excited at 385 nm but quench the fluorescence of $C_3N_4$-based nanozymes at 438 nm. Therefore, the ratio of the fluorescent intensity at 564 nm and 438 nm could be employed as the signal output for ratiometric $H_2O_2$ detection, which showed enhanced robustness (98). By coupling the oxidation of the substrate by their corresponding oxidases, some oxidase substrates can be detected by the aforementioned $H_2O_2$ detection method (91). Until now, various oxidase substrates, including glucose, lactate, cholesterol, choline, sarcosine, and xanthine have been successfully detected when combining their corresponding oxidases (or oxidase mimics) with POD mimics (7, 8, 44, 82, 84, 92, 93, 100, 105–127).

For the second type, targets with reducibility (*e.g.*, ascorbic acid, dopamine, cysteine, homocysteine, and glutathione) could be detected by inhibiting the POD-like catalytic reaction (51, 85, 88, 128–145). Based on the inhibitory effect on TMB oxidation, colorimetric detection of glutathione (GSH) was established by using

POD-like gold (Au) nanoclusters (137). Benefiting from the excellent property of this colorimetric method, GSH in cell lysates could be successfully detected. Moreover, cancer cells could be discriminated from normal cells due to the higher GSH levels in cancer cells than normal cells (137). Lou *et al.* developed N-doped carbon nanozymes with high and specific POD-like activity for ascorbic acid detection (146). The absorbance at 652 nm decreased with the increasing concentration of ascorbic acid. This colorimetric sensing platform could be also used for total antioxidant capacity (TAC) evaluation. TAC of four commercial beverages, fresh orange juice, as well as three kinds of vitamin C tablets was successfully determined by this colorimetric method (146). To perform multiplex detection for biothiols, Wang *et al.* constructed cross-reactive nanozyme sensor arrays (45). Six biothilos, including GSH, cysteine (Cys), mercaptoacetic acid (MA), mercaptosuccinic acid (MS), dithiothreitol (DTT), and mercaptoethanol (ME) could be successfully discriminated by the as-developed nanozyme sensor arrays (**Figures 16.10A, B**) (45). Moreover, biothiols in serum could be also discriminated, demonstrating the practical application of nanozyme sensor arrays (**Figure 16.10C**) (45).

For the third type, some bioactive small molecules (*e.g.*, phosphates, amino acids, and melamine) could be detected by interacting with nanozymes (147–151). By interacting with nanomaterials, some targets could change the structure and surface charge of nanomaterials, which in turn could regulate their catalytic activity. For example, Ni *et al.* found that Au NPs-melamine aggregates could be formed by adding the melamine into bare Au NPs (147). The POD-like activities of bare Au NPs increased with the increasing melamine concentration, enabling the colorimetric detection of melamine (147). Copper ions ($Cu^{2+}$) were found to inhibit the POD-like activity of histidine (His)-Au nanoclusters (AuNCs) (148). The catalytic activities of His-AuNCs could be recovered by coordinating $Cu^{2+}$ with free His. In addition, phosphates could be detected by regulating the POD-like activity of the two-dimensional (2D)-metal-organic framework (MOF) (149). The detection principle was that the structure of 2D-MOF could be destroyed by phosphates and subsequently, the phosphates could interact with TCPP(Fe) (Fe(III) meso-tetra(4-carboxyphenyl)

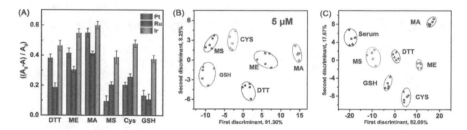

**FIGURE 16.10** Nanozyme sensor arrays for detection of biothiols. (**A**) Colorimetric response patterns of nanozyme sensor arrays toward biothiols. 2-D canonical score plots for the first two factors of response patterns obtained against 5 μM of biothiols (**B**) and 10 μM of biothiols in the presence of 1% FBS (C). Adapted from (45), Copyright 2018, with permission from American Chemical Society.

porphine chloride) monomer, resulting in the inhibition of nanozyme catalytic activity, thus a turn-off colorimetric sensor could be constructed for phosphates detection.

### 16.5.1.2   Biomacromolecules

#### 16.5.1.2.a   Nucleic Acids

The methods for nucleic acid detection based on POD-like nanozymes could be mainly classified into two types: 1) using nanozymes as signaling nanoprobes and 2) regulating nanozyme activities. For the first type, numerous studies have demonstrated that nanozymes could act as tags to label nucleic acids for signaling (59, 152–157). As shown in **Figure 16.11A**, zirconium hexacyanoferrate (ZrHCF) MNPs could act as an artificial POD for electrochemical detection of target DNA (tDNA)

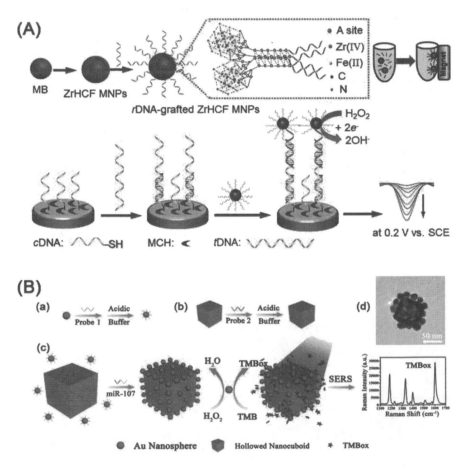

**FIGURE 16.11**   (A) Preparation of rDNA-grafted ZrHCF MNPs and illustration of the stepwise DNA assay. (B) Illustration of triggered self-assembly of plasmonic nanostructures for miR-107 detection. (A) Reprinted from (153), Copyright 2015, with permission from American Chemical Society. (B) Reprinted from (155), Copyright 2019, with permission from John Wiley and Sons.

(153). The reporter DNA (rDNA) was first conjugated with ZrHCF MNPs by the interaction between the Zr (IV) in the ZrHCF MNPs and phosphate groups in the rDNA. The tDNA could not only be brought on the electrode surface by the interaction with preabsorbed capture DNA (cDNA) but can bind with the rDNA-grafted ZrHCF nanozymes by the hybridization reaction between tDNA and rDNA. Then, the rDNA-grafted ZrHCF nanozymes could catalyze the reduction of $H_2O_2$, which in turn produced electrochemical signals for quantification of tDNA concentration (153). In addition to DNA, microRNA could be also detected by using nanozymes as signal tags (155–157). Li et al. developed an SERS detection platform based on targets triggering self-assembly of Au nanosphere on the hollowed Au/silver (Ag) alloy nanocuboids (155). As shown in **Figure 16.11B**, Au nanospheres and hollowed Au/Ag alloy nanocuboids were first modified by probe 1 and probe 2, respectively (155). In the presence of microRNA-107 (miR-107), Au nanospheres and hollowed Au/Ag alloy nanocuboids were self-assembled into plasmonic nanostructures because probe 1 and probe 2 could be complementary to the entire miR-107. The Au nanospheres in the self-assembled nanostructure could catalyze the TMB to TMBox in the presence of $H_2O_2$, and subsequently, TMBox could generate an enhanced SERS signal due to the plasmonic hot spots in the self-assembled nanostructure. With this SERS detection platform, as low as fM-level miR-107 could be detected, which could meet the clinical requirement.

For the second type, the sensing platforms were constructed by regulating the catalytic activity of nanozymes by nucleic acids (158–167). For instance, Liu et al. demonstrated a label-free colorimetric method for tDNA detection by using POD-like Au@Fe-MIL-88 (162). They found that single-stranded DNA (ssDNA) could be easily absorbed on the surface of Au@Fe-MIL-88, resulting in the decreased POD-like activity of Au@Fe-MIL-88 because the absorbed ssDNA could prevent the POD substrates from binding to the catalytic sites. In the presence of tDNA, the ssDNA was removed from the surface of Au@Fe-MIL-88 due to the hybridization reaction between ssDNA and target DNA, enabling that the POD-like activity was recovered. With this method, the linear range for target DNA was 30–150 nM, with a limit of detection (LOD) of 11.4 nM (162). In addition to influencing the interaction between nanozymes and POD substrates, the adsorbed nucleic acids could also prevent the nanomaterials from aggregating in the presence of high concentration salt (NaCl) (158, 159, 164). Guo et al. found ssDNA could be stably absorbed on the surface of hemin-graphene hybrid nanosheets (H-GNs) by π-π interaction, which could prevent the H-GNs from aggregating in NaCl electrolyte since negatively charged ssDNA backbone increased the electrostatic repulsion interaction between H-GNs (159). However, the double-stranded DNA (dsDNA) exhibited very weak adsorption affinity to H-GNs, resulting in the aggregation of H-GNs. Upon centrifugation, the ssDNA-modified H-GNs were not precipitated and the supernatant exhibited excellent POD-like activity. The H-GNs with dsDNA were precipitated after centrifuging, enabling that the supernatant possessed low POD-like activity. By exploiting the distinctly different affinity of ssDNA and dsDNA to H-GNs and the POD-like activity of H-GNs, colorimetric detection of 29-mer hepatitis B virus (HBV) DNA was demonstrated. Moreover, the single-nucleotide polymorphisms (SNPs) could be determined by this method (**Figure 16.12**) (159).

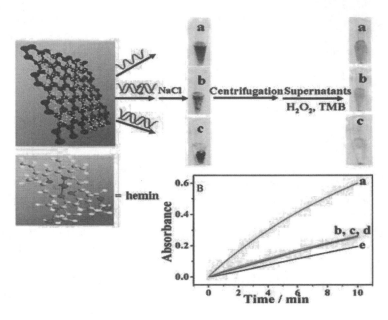

**FIGURE 16.12**   Illustration of the protocols for the detection of SNPs. Reprinted from (159), Copyright 2011, with permission from American Chemical Society.

### 16.5.1.2.b   Proteins

Protein detection based on POD mimics has been extensively studied (48, 61, 168–175). Gao *et al.* reported two interesting immunoassays for HBV antigen and cardiac troponin I detections using POD-like $Fe_3O_4$ MNPs as tags (6). In the subsequent study, they developed an $Fe_3O_4$ MNPs-based immunochromatographic strip (nanozyme strip) for the detection of glycoprotein (GP) of the Ebola virus (EBOV) (171). Because of the catalytically amplified ability of POD-like $Fe_3O_4$ MNPs, the sensitivity of the nanozyme strip exhibited 100-fold higher than the colloidal Au strip, with LOD of 1 ng/mL (**Figure 16.13A**). In addition to $Fe_3O_4$ MNPs, other POD-like nanozymes with higher catalytic activities were also developed as immunoassay tags for signaling. For example, Pd-Ir cubes were obtained by depositing Ir with a few atom layers on Pd cubes, which were subsequently exploited for immunoassays of human prostate surface antigen (PSA) (48). Benefitting from their excellent POD-like activity, the LOD of Pd-Ir cubes-based immunoassays was 110-fold lower than those of HRP-based immunoassays (**Figure 16.13B**). Liu *et al.* developed a nanozyme chemiluminescence paper test for detection of SARS-CoV-2 spike antigen by using POD-like Co-Fe@hemin as catalytic tags (**Figure 16.13C**) (175). The sensitivity of the nanozyme chemiluminescence strip was comparable with that of enzyme-linked immunosorbent assay (ELISA). Moreover, the diagnosis could be completed within 16 min, which was shorter than nucleic acid tests (**Figure 16.13C**). In addition to immunoassays, based on the interaction between nanozymes and proteins, nanozyme sensor arrays could be also constructed for the detection and discrimination of proteins (45, 169, 176).

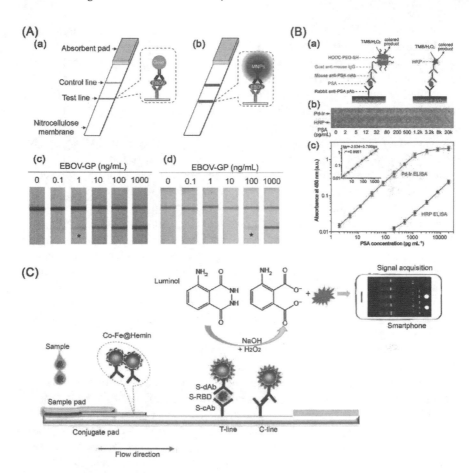

**FIGURE 16.13** (**A**) Standard colloidal Au strip and nanozyme-strip employing $Fe_3O_4$ MNPs in place of Au NPs for EBOV-GP detection. (**B**) Detection of PSA with Pd-Ir cubes-based ELISA (Pd-Ir ELISA) and conventional HRP-based ELISA (HRP ELISA). (**C**) Illustration of the nanozyme chemiluminescence paper test for SARS-CoV-2 S-RBD antigen. Recognition, separation, and catalytic amplification by nanozyme probes. (**A**) Adapted from (171), Copyright 2015, with permission from Elsevier. (**B**) Reprinted from (48), Copyright 2015, with permission from American Chemical Society. (**C**) Reprinted from (175), Copyright 2021, with permission from Elsevier.

### 16.5.1.2.c Enzymes

Some molecules or ions, which could regulate the POD-like activity of nanomaterials, could be generated by catalyzing some substrates in the presence of corresponding enzymes or be consumed as enzyme substrates. Based on this, some enzymes (*e.g.*, urease, acetylcholinesterase (AChE), and phosphatase) could be detected by coupling the POD-like reaction with enzyme-catalyzed reactions (149, 177–190). For instance, Su *et al.* developed a bioassay for urease detection based on the pH-dependent POD activity of Ni/Co layered double hydroxides (LDHs) (177). They found the proton-consuming urease-catalyzed reaction could modulate the catalytic activity of nickel (Ni)/Co LDHs, which formed the basis of determining urease activity. Urease activity over the range of 3.3–270 mU/mL could be detected by monitoring the POD-like activity of Ni/Co LDHs (177). Chen *et al.* constructed a colorimetric detection platform for determining AChE activity by using $Co_3O_4$@Co-Fe oxide double-shelled nanocages (DSNCs) as POD mimics (178). Acetylcholinesterase could catalyze the hydrolysis of acetylthiocholine to generate thiocholine. The thiocholine with –SH group could not only coordinate with the metal centers of $Co_3O_4$@Co-Fe oxide DSNCs to block access to catalytic sites but also reduce the TMBox to TMB, enabling the competitive effect on the POD-like catalytic reaction of $Co_3O_4$@Co-Fe oxide DSNCs. Based on this, a colorimetric platform for AChE activity screening in the linear range over 0.0008–1 mU/mL, was successfully constructed (178). Qin *et al.* fabricated nanozyme-based sensor arrays by using three POD-like 2D-MOF (**Figure 16.14**) (149). Five phosphates, including adenosine monophosphate (AMP), adenosine diphosphate (ADP), adenosine triphosphate (ATP), inorganic pyrophosphate (PPi), and inorganic phosphate (Pi), were successfully discriminated by using the as-prepared 2D-MOF nanozyme sensor array because they could differentially modulate the POD-like activity of 2D-MOF nanozymes. Moreover, as shown in **Figure 16.14**, the sensor arrays were successfully applied to probing two enzymatic hydrolysis processes (*i.e.*, apyrase-catalyzed and pyrophosphatase (PPase)-catalyzed hydrolytic reactions).

### 16.5.1.2.d   Saccharides

Numerous heparin sensing platforms were constructed by using POD mimics (191–195). Hu *et al.* found that heparin could boost the POD-like activity of Au NCs at neutral pH (191). Based on this phenomenon, colorimetric detection of heparin was developed with a linear ranging from 0.5 to 25 μg/mL. Cheng *et al.* developed a series of 2D-MOF nanosheets with excellent POD-like activity (192). Heparin-specific AG73 peptides could block the access of active sites after absorbing onto the 2D-MOF nanosheets, which in turn decreased their catalytic activities. When interacted with heparin, AG73 peptides could be removed from the surface of 2D-MOF, enabling that the POD-like activity of 2D-MOF could be restored Therefore, the 2D-MOF nanosheets were used to detect heparin (**Figure 16.15**). Moreover, by coupling this sensing platform with microdialysis technology, monitoring the heparin's elimination process in living rats was successfully achieved (192).

### 16.5.1.3   Exosomes and Cells

Some characteristic receptors (usually proteins) are over-expressed on the surface of exosomes and cells. These receptors could be specifically recognized by their corresponding antibodies or ligands. Detection probes for exosomes and cells could be constructed by combining an antibody or a ligand with nanozymes. Antibodies or ligands in probes could specifically bind with exosomes or cells, while POD-like nanozymes could be used for signal transduction.

### 16.5.1.3.a   Exosomes

Several studies demonstrate exosomes could be detected by combining an antibody or a ligand with nanozymes (196–200). Wang *et al.* demonstrated that the POD-like

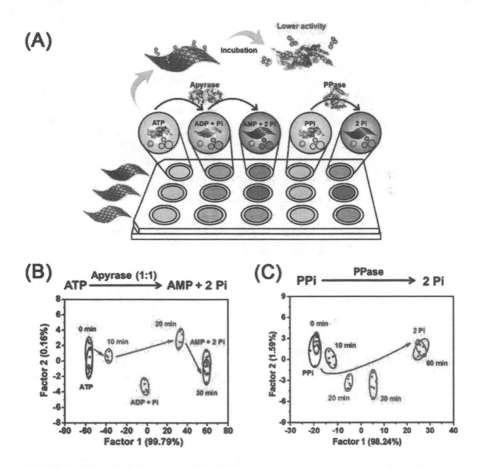

**FIGURE 16.14** (**A**) Schematic of 2D-MOF-nanozyme sensor arrays probing phosphates and their related hydrolytic process. (**B**) 2-D canonical score plot for the first two factors of response patterns obtained against ATP, ADP + Pi, AMP + 2Pi, and assay samples from different time points in the ATP-hydrolysis process catalyzed by apyrase (1:1). (**C**) 2-D canonical score plot for the first two factors of response patterns obtained against PPi, 2Pi, and assay samples from different time points in the PPi-hydrolysis process catalyzed by PPase. Adapted from (149), Copyright 2018, with permission from American Chemical Society.

activity of g-C$_3$N$_4$ nanosheets could be significantly improved by adsorbing CD63-specific aptamer, which was attributed to the enhanced adsorption of TMB-mediated by aptamer. The aptamer could be released from the surface of g-C$_3$N$_4$ nanosheets in the presence of CD63 (a surface marker of an exosome), which subsequently results in decreasing the catalytic activity of g-C$_3$N$_4$ nanosheets. Based on this, colorimetric quantification of exosomes could be achieved by monitoring the catalytic oxidation of TMB (196). Moreover, based on the differential expression of CD63, exosomes produced by a breast cancer line (MCF-7) and a control cell line (MCF-10A) could be discriminated by this colorimetric platform (196). As shown in **Figure 16.16**, Au-loaded Fe$_2$O$_3$ nanocubes (Au-NPFe$_2$O$_3$NC) with magnetic property and POD-like activity were used to construct an ELISA for the detection of exosomes (198).

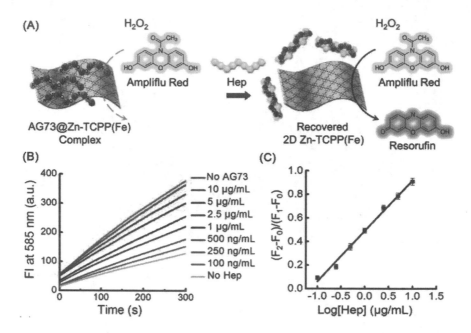

**FIGURE 16.15** **(A)** Illustration of AG73-inhibited POD-like activity of 2-D Zn-TCPP(Fe) nanosheets with Ampliflu Red as the POD substrate. **(B)** Kinetic curves plotting the time-dependent fluorescence emission intensity at 585 nm for Ampliflu Red oxidation reactions catalyzed by Zn-TCPP(Fe) in different AG73 concentrations. **(C)** The normalized catalytic activity of 2-D Zn-TCPP(Fe) nanosheets in different AG73 concentrations. Reprinted from (192), Copyright 2017, with permission from American Chemical Society.

The CD-63 specific antibody was first conjugated with Au-NPFe$_2$O$_3$NC to capture a pool of exosomes in cell culture media, and subsequently, the Au-NPFe$_2$O$_3$NC/CD63/exosomes conjugates were isolated and purified by using a magnetic washing procedure. Then, the screen-printed electrode with antibody modification was used to bind with Au-NPFe$_2$O$_3$NC/CD63/exosome conjugates for the construction of sandwich immunoassays. The POD-like Au-NPFe$_2$O$_3$NC could generate a colorimetric signal or an electrochemical signal for the quantification of exosomes (198).

*16.5.1.3.b   Cells*

Cells (usually cancer cells) could be also detected by an antibody or ligand-modified nanozymes (10, 201–215). As shown in **Figure 16.17A**, Zhang *et al.* constructed a cancer cell detection platform by using folate-modified Pt NPs/graphene oxide (Pt/GO) nanocomposites (201). Folate on the surface of nanocomposites can act as a recognition element by targeting folate receptors on the cell membrane, while the POD-like Pt/GO nanocomposites could act as a signal transducer. This colorimetric detection platform exhibited high sensitivity, which 125 cancer cells could be detected by naked-eye observation (201). Instead of Pt/GO, Au NPs on mesoporous silica (Si)-coated nanosized rGO, AgX, Fe$_2$SiW$_{10}$, Fe-aminoclay, and Cu$_{2-x}$Se/rGO with POD-like activities could be also modified by folate for cancer cells detection

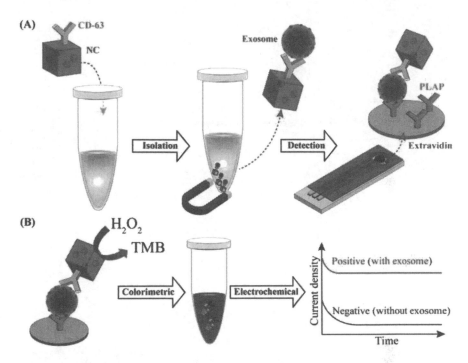

**FIGURE 16.16** (**A**) Schematic representation of Au-NPFe$_2$O$_3$NC with a generic antibody (CD63) functionalization for direct exosome isolation and detection from cell culture media. (**B**) Naked-eye detection along with UV–visible and electrochemical quantification of placenta alkaline phosphatase (PLAP)-specific exosomes present in the cell culture media were achieved by using POD-like Au-NPFe$_2$O$_3$NC. Reprinted from (198), Copyright 2019, with permission from American Chemical Society.

(202–206). In addition to folate, antibodies were also used for specific recognition of cancer cells. For example, Li *et al.* developed a circulating tumor cell (CTC) detection platform by using anti-melanoma-associated chondroitin sulfate proteoglycan (MCSP) antibodies modified Fe$_3$O$_4$ MNPs (**Figure 16.17B**) (211). The MCSP antibodies could specifically recognize the over-expressed MCSP on the surface of melanoma CTCs, while the POD-like Fe$_3$O$_4$ MNPs could be used for CTCs isolation and signal transduction. With this detection platform, as low as 13 melanoma CTCs per mL could be successfully detected within 50 min (211).

## 16.5.2 *In vivo* Detection

### 16.5.2.1 Living Brains

POD mimics have been used for the detection of neurochemical substances in living brains (93, 102, 141, 216–218). Lin *et al.* demonstrated that Prussian blue (PB) could act as an "artificial POD" to replace "natural POD" for simultaneous and selective online detection of glucose and lactate by an electrochemical method (**Figure 16.18**) (216). The glucose or lactate could be oxidized by their corresponding

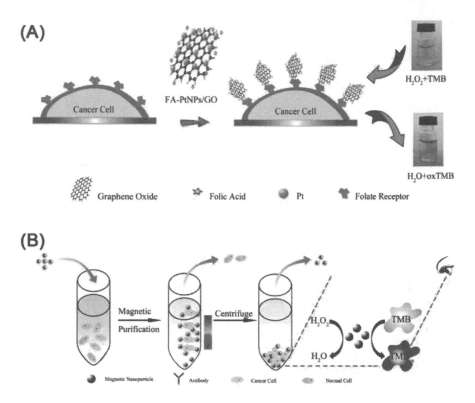

**FIGURE 16.17** **(A)** The colorimetric direction of cancer cells by using folic acid functionalized Pt NPs/GO. **(B)** MNPs for rapid separation and detection of melanoma CTCs. (A) Reprinted from (201), Copyright 2014, with permission from American Chemical Society. (B) Reprinted from (211), Copyright 2017, with permission from Royal Society of Chemistry.

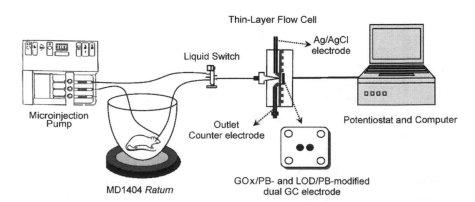

**FIGURE 16.18** Illustration of the online electrochemical method with oxidase/PB-based biosensors for simultaneous and continuous monitoring of glucose and lactate in the brain of freely moving rats. Reprinted from (216), Copyright 2007, with permission from American Chemical Society.

oxidase to generate $H_2O_2$, and then PB could catalyze the reduction of $H_2O_2$ to generate cathodic current for signaling. Based on the cascade reaction, by using a continuous-flow electrochemical cell with glucose oxidase (GOx)/PB and lactate oxidase (LOx)/PB-modified dual GCE, the simultaneous measurements of glucose and lactate in the rat microdialysate from the striatum were achieved (216).

To further enable the efficient mass transfer and minimize $H_2O_2$ decomposition to enhance the catalytic efficiency of the cascade reaction, recently, integrated nanozymes (INAzymes) for *in vivo* sensing were developed by Cheng *et al.* (**Figure 16.19A**) (102). They first developed INAzymes by encapsulating molecule catalyst hemin and GOx into ZIF-8. The INAzymes exhibited enhanced catalytic activity in the cascade reactions due to the nanoscale proximity effect. Encouragingly, the offline detection of cerebral glucose changes in living rats was achieved by *in vivo* microdialysis technology. Moreover, the INAzymes were also successfully used for online monitoring of the live brain glucose level by combining with microfluidic technology (**Figure 16.19B**). The dynamic changes of striatum glucose during ischemic/reperfusion processes were monitored by the online detection platform, demonstrating its practical applications for *in vivo* sensing (**Figure 16.19C**).

In the following study, they developed integrated nanozymes for analytes detection by Raman signals (93). They prepared Au NPs@MIL-101 by *in situ* embedding Au NPs inside MIL-101. The Au NPs can not only exhibit POD-like activity for catalyzing the oxidation of Raman inactive receptor into Raman active one but possess SERS activities to enhance the Raman signals. When decorating Au NPs@MIL-101 with GOx or LOx, glucose and lactate could be detected by the integrative nanozyme platform. The potential applications were further demonstrated by monitoring the dynamic change of glucose and lactate in live rat brains during ischemia/reperfusion

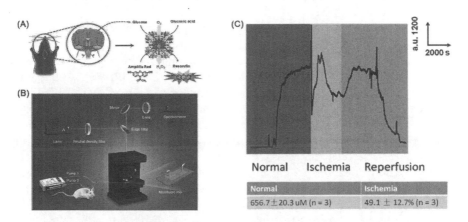

**FIGURE 16.19** (**A**) Illustration of measuring glucose in the brain of living rats by the INAzyme-catalyzed cascade reactions, which produced fluorescent resorufin for signaling. (**B**) The fluorescence sensing optical platform for continuous *in vivo* measurement of neurochemicals in living rats. (**C**) Continuously monitoring the dynamic changes of glucose level in the striatum of a living rat brain following global ischemia/reperfusion with the fluorescence sensing optical platform. Adapted from (102), Copyright 2016, with permission from American Chemical Society.

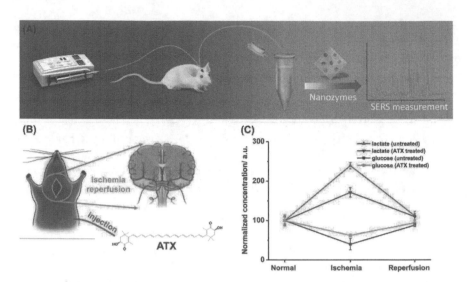

**FIGURE 16.20** Integrative nanozymes for monitoring cerebral glucose and lactate and evaluating the efficacy of ATX. **(A)** Monitoring glucose and lactate in live rats' brains with integrative nanozymes sensing platform. **(B)** ATX pretreatment before global ischemia/reperfusion. **(C)** Dynamic changes of glucose and lactate following global ischemia/reperfusion in the ATX treated or untreated group. Reprinted from (93), Copyright 2017, with permission from American Chemical Society.

processes. More encouragingly, the sensing platform could also be used for evaluating the therapeutic efficacy of anti-oxidant drugs candidate astaxanthin (ATX) for stroke (**Figure 16.20**) (93).

Ascorbic acid, another neurochemical substance, has been demonstrated to play important roles in various physiological and pathological processes. As discussed previously, ascorbic acid could be detected by inhibiting the catalytic process of POD-like nanozymes due to the reducibility of ascorbic acid. Based on this principle, carbon-shielded 3-D Co–Mn nanowire array on Ni foam (CoMn NW/NF@C) with excellent POD-like activity was used to construct the colorimetric sensing platform for ascorbic acid, and linear ranges of 0.1–1 µM and 1–30 µM with an LOD of 42.8 nM were obtained (141). Further, ascorbic acid in brain microdialysate during the cerebral calm/ischemia process was determined by using this as-developed colorimetric method.

### 16.5.2.2 Tumor

Metabolic proteases (*e.g.*, matrix metalloproteinase 9, MMP9) are often upregulated in cancerous cells (219). Therefore, monitoring the protease activity could enable the early diagnosis of cancer. To enable *in vivo* tumor monitoring, nanosensors were engineered by coupling four POD-like Au NCs to a large carrier (*i.e.*, neutravidin, NAv) by using an MMP9-specific peptide sequence (**Figure 16.21A**) (220). The overall nanosensors were too large to excrete with urine. However, in the tumor-bearing rat, the nanosensors would be disassembled by overexpressed MMP9 to release individual Au NCs (**Figure 16.21B**).These Au NCs with ultrasmall size

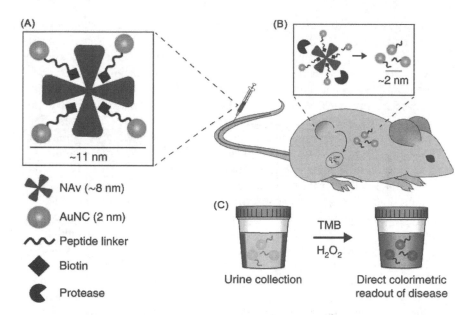

**FIGURE 16.21** Design of a nanocatalyst signal-amplification sensing system. **(A)** Catalytic Au NCs were conjugated to an NAv protein scaffold through a biotinylated protease-cleavable peptide linker. **(B)** The protease-sensitive Au NC/NAv complex (~11 nm) designed to specifically disassemble when exposed to the activity of the relevant dysregulated proteases at the site of disease was injected intravenously. After protease cleavage (top), the liberated Au NCs (~2 nm) were filtered through the kidneys and into the urine. **(C)** The Au NCs were detected in the cleared urine by measuring their ability to oxidize a chromogenic POD substrate (*e.g.*, TMB) in the presence of $H_2O_2$ and generate a visually detectable colored signal. Reprinted from (220), Copyright 2019, with permission from Nature Publishing Group.

(~2 nm) could be efficiently cleared via the renal pathway, accumulating in the collected urine. Therefore, tumor diagnosis could be achieved by monitoring the POD-like activity of Au NCs (**Figure 16.21C**).

## 16.6 SUMMARY AND FUTURE PERSPECTIVES

In this chapter, we highlighted the recent advances in deepening the understanding of catalytic mechanisms, modulating the activities of nanozymes by composition and structure, and identified the predictive activity descriptors for the rational design of highly active POD-like nanozymes. Benefitting from these as-developed excellent POD mimics, great progress for *in vitro* and *in vivo* bioanalytical applications have been pursued. Representative examples in bioanalytical applications have been highlighted. Despite the substantial progress, several challenges remain to further advance this field.

1. *Introduction of Fundamental Concepts of Heterogeneous Catalysis Into Nanozymes.* Until now, hundreds of nanomaterials have been found with POD-like activity. Although a few descriptors have been developed for their rational design, most nanozymes are being prepared via "trial-and-error"

strategies due to the lack of structure–catalytic activity relationship. Further efforts are needed to deepen the understanding of catalytic mechanisms of nanozymes, which essentially belong to the category of heterogeneous catalysis. Therefore, the fundamental concepts of heterogeneous catalysis, such as microkinetic modeling, scaling relations, Sabatier analysis, and activity and selectivity maps, should be introduced into nanozyme catalysis to build a complete theoretical catalytic system, which would benefit understanding the catalytic mechanisms and elucidating the structure–activity relationship.

2. *Machine Learning and High-Throughput Experimentation.* Combining machine learning with high-throughput experimentation provides opportunities to accelerate nanozyme discovery. By statistical learning to analyze nanozyme experiment data, machine learning could help identify activity descriptors to rationalize and predict POD-like activity. In addition, machine learning can decrease the computational costs of DFT calculation. For example, accelerating the search for transition states in DFT calculations could be achieved with the assistance of machine learning. A series of candidate nanozyme could be obtained by combining machine learning with DFT calculations. Subsequently, high-throughput experimentation should be developed to validate the catalytic activity of candidate nanozyme. If the initial machine learning fails to anticipate nanozyme activity satisfactorily, the high-throughput experimentation data should be used to refine the model and tune parameters for the next cycle of machine learning. Therefore, a closed-loop machine learning-driven high-throughput experimentation method could be constructed to fast-track nanozyme discovery.

3. *Selectivity.* As-developed nanozymes generally have multi-enzymatic activities, which significantly limit their extensive applications for bioanalysis. For example, when nanozymes with both POD- and oxidase-like activities are used for $H_2O_2$ detection, a strong background will be generated even in the absence of $H_2O_2$, which greatly affects the detection sensitivity. Also, biological samples (especially for *in vivo* analysis) are extremely complex, so nanozymes with highly specific POD-like activity are needed for highly selective detection. Therefore, further efforts are necessary to develop various methods to effectively control the nanomaterials to specifically mimic POD.

4. *High-Impact Applications.* Till now, quite limited studies were involved in the *in vivo* applications of nanozymes in bioanalytical fields. To demonstrate the unique advantages of nanozymes, developing live assays with POD-like nanozymes is encouraged. We also expect to see more practical bioanalytical applications. For instance, Liu *et al.* developed immunoassays for the detection of SARS-CoV-2 (175).

## ACKNOWLEDGMENT

The work from the Wei lab described in this chapter was supported by the China Postdoctoral Science Foundation (2019TQ0144 and 2019M661786), the National Key R&D Program of China (2019YFA0709200), National Natural

Science Foundation of China (21722503 and 21874067), PAPD Program, Open Funds of Key Laboratory of Analytical Chemistry for Biology and Medicine (Wuhan University), Ministry of Education (ACBM2019001), and Fundamental Research Funds for the Central Universities (021314380145).

## REFERENCES

1. Wei H, Wang E. 2013. *Chemical Society Reviews* 42: 6060–93
2. Wu J, Wang X, Wang Q, Lou Z, Li S, et al. 2019. *Chemical Society Reviews* 48: 1004–76
3. Chen Z, Wang Z, Ren J, Qu X. 2018. *Accounts of Chemical Research* 51: 789–99
4. Si-Rong L, Yen-Chun H, Jia-Rui L, Er-Kang W, Hui W. 2018. *Progress in Biochemistry and Biophysics* 45: 129–47
5. Jiang D, Ni D, Rosenkrans ZT, Huang P, Yan X, Cai W. 2019. *Chemical Society Reviews* 48: 3683–704
6. Gao L, Zhuang J, Nie L, Zhang J, Zhang Y, et al. 2007. *Nature Nanotechnology* 2: 577–83
7. Wei H, Wang E. 2008. *Analytical Chemistry* 80: 2250–4
8. Song Y, Qu K, Zhao C, Ren J, Qu X. 2010. *Advanced Materials* 22: 2206–10
9. Fan K, Cao C, Pan Y, Lu D, Yang D, et al. 2012. *Nature Nanotechnology* 7: 459–64
10. Tao Y, Lin Y, Huang Z, Ren J, Qu X. 2013. *Advanced Materials* 25: 2594–9
11. Ding H, Cai Y, Gao L, Liang M, Miao B, et al. 2018. *Nano Letters* 19: 203–9
12. Cao F, Zhang L, Wang H, You Y, Wang Y, et al. 2019. *Angewandte Chemie International Edition* 58: 16236–42
13. Li S, Shang L, Xu B, Wang S, Gu K, et al. 2019. *Angewandte Chemie International Edition* 58: 12624–31
14. Zhen W, Liu Y, Wang W, Zhang M, Hu W, et al. 2020. *Angewandte Chemie International Edition* 59: 9491–7
15. Wang P, Liu S, Hu M, Zhang H, Duan D, et al. 2020. *Advanced Functional Materials* 30: 2000647
16. Liang Q, Xi J, Gao XJ, Zhang R, Yang Y, et al. 2020. *Nano Today* 35: 100935
17. Li J, Liu W, Wu X, Gao X. 2015. *Biomaterials* 48: 37–44
18. Zhao R, Zhao X, Gao X. 2015. *Chemistry–A European Journal* 21: 960–4
19. Fang G, Li W, Shen X, Perez-Aguilar JM, Chong Y, et al. 2018. *Nature Communications* 9: 129
20. Hu Y, Gao XJ, Zhu Y, Muhammad F, Tan S, et al. 2018. *Chemistry of Materials* 30: 6431–9
21. Wang X, Gao XJ, Qin L, Wang C, Song L, et al. 2019. *Nature Communications* 10: 704
22. Guo S, Guo L. 2019. *The Journal of Physical Chemistry C* 123: 30318–34
23. Xu B, Wang H, Wang W, Gao L, Li S, et al. 2019. *Angewandte Chemie-International Edition* 58: 4911–6
24. Shen X, Wang Z, Gao X, Zhao Y. 2020. *ACS Catalysis* 10: 12657–65
25. Lu X, Gao S, Lin H, Yu L, Han Y, et al. 2020. *Advanced Materials* 32: 2002246
26. Wang Z, Zhang R, Yan X, Fan K. 2020. *Materials Today* 41: 81–119
27. Dong J, Song L, Yin J-J, He W, Wu Y, et al. 2014. *ACS Applied Materials & Interfaces* 6: 1959–70
28. Nørskov JK, Bligaard T, Rossmeisl J, Christensen CH. 2009. *Nature Chemistry* 1: 37–46
29. Nørskov JK, Studt F, Abild-Pedersen F, Bligaard T. 2014. *Fundamental Concepts in Heterogeneous Catalysis*: John Wiley & Sons
30. Schloegl R. 2015. *Angewandte Chemie-International Edition* 54: 3465–520
31. Huo M, Wang L, Wang Y, Chen Y, Shi J. 2019. *ACS Nano* 13: 2643–53

32. Niu X, Shi Q, Zhu W, Liu D, Tian H, et al. 2019. *Biosensors & Bioelectronics* 142: 111495
33. Lin S, Wei H. 2019. *Science China-Life Sciences* 62: 710–2
34. Huang L, Chen J, Gan L, Wang J, Dong S. 2019. *Science Advances* 5: eaav5490
35. Cheng N, Li J-C, Liu D, Lin Y, Du D. 2019. *Small* 15: 1901485
36. Ma W, Mao J, Yang X, Pan C, Chen W, et al. 2019. *Chemical Communications* 55: 159–62
37. Zhao C, Xiong C, Liu X, Qiao M, Li Z, et al. 2019. *Chemical Communications* 55: 2285–8
38. Zhang H, Lu XF, Wu Z-P, Lou XWD. 2020. *ACS Central Science* 6: 1288–301
39. Kim MS, Lee J, Kim HS, Cho A, Shim KH, et al. 2020. *Advanced Functional Materials* 30: 1905410
40. Jiao L, Yan H, Wu Y, Gu W, Zhu C, et al. 2020. *Angewandte Chemie-International Edition* 59: 2565–76
41. Wu G-W, He S-B, Peng H-P, Deng H-H, Liu A-L, et al. 2014. *Analytical Chemistry* 86: 10955–60
42. Li W, Chen B, Zhang H, Sun Y, Wang J, et al. 2015. *Biosensors & Bioelectronics* 66: 251–8
43. Ye H, Mohar J, Wang Q, Catalano M, Kim MJ, Xia X. 2016. *Science Bulletin* 61: 1739–45
44. Jin L, Meng Z, Zhang Y, Cai S, Zhang Z, et al. 2017. *ACS Applied Materials & Interfaces* 9: 10027–33
45. Wang X, Qin L, Zhou M, Lou Z, Wei H. 2018. *Analytical Chemistry* 90: 11696–702
46. Xi Z, Ye H, Xia X. 2018. *Chemistry of Materials* 30: 8391–414
47. He W, Wu X, Liu J, Hu X, Zhang K, et al. 2010. *Chemistry of Materials* 22: 2988–94
48. Xia X, Zhang J, Lu N, Kim MJ, Ghale K, et al. 2015. *ACS Nano* 9: 9994–10004
49. Kim MS, Kweon SH, Cho S, An SSA, Kim MI, et al. 2017. *ACS Applied Materials & Interfaces* 9: 35133–40
50. Li Z, Yang X, Yang Y, Tan Y, He Y, et al. 2018. *Chemistry–A European Journal* 24: 409–15
51. Ivanova MN, Grayfer ED, Plotnikova EE, Kibis LS, Darabdhara G, et al. 2019. *ACS Applied Materials & Interfaces* 11: 22102–12
52. Sun X, Guo S, Chung C-S, Zhu W, Sun S. 2013. *Advanced Materials* 25: 132–6
53. Xie J, Cao H, Jiang H, Chen Y, Shi W, et al. 2013. *Analytica Chimica Acta* 796: 92–100
54. Zhu Y, Wu J, Han L, Wang X, Li W, et al. 2020. *Analytical Chemistry* 92: 7444–52
55. Ahmed A, John P, Nawaz MH, Hayat A, Nasir M. 2019. *ACS Applied Nano Materials* 2: 5156–68
56. Kim MS, Cho S, Joo SH, Lee J, Kwak SK, et al. 2019. *ACS Nano* 13: 4312–21
57. Guo W, Zhang M, Lou Z, Zhou M, Wang P, Wei H. 2019. *ChemCatChem* 11: 737–43
58. Feng L, Zhang L, Zhang S, Chen X, Li P, et al. 2020. *ACS Applied Materials & Interfaces* 12: 17547–56
59. Chen W, Zhang X, Li J, Chen L, Wang N, et al. 2020. *Analytical Chemistry* 92: 2714–21
60. Li S, Zhao X, Gang R, Cao B, Wang H. 2020. *Analytical Chemistry* 92: 5152–7
61. Xi Z, Wei K, Wang Q, Kim MJ, Sun S, et al. 2021. *Journal of the American Chemical Society* 143: 2660–4
62. He W, Zhou Y-T, Warner WG, Hu X, Wu X, et al. 2013. *Biomaterials* 34: 765–73
63. Fu Y, Zhao X, Zhang J, Li W. 2014. *The Journal of Physical Chemistry C* 118: 18116–25
64. Xi Z, Gao W, Xia X. 2020. *ChemBioChem* 21: 2440–4
65. Nilsson A, Pettersson LGM, Hammer B, Bligaard T, Christensen CH, Norskov JK. 2005. *Catalysis Letters* 100: 111–4
66. Xi Z, Cheng X, Gao Z, Wang M, Cai T, et al. 2019. *Nano Letters* 20: 272–7
67. Liu S, Lu F, Xing R, Zhu J-J. 2011. *Chemistry-A European Journal* 17: 620–5

68. Wu R, Chong Y, Fang G, Jiang X, Pan Y, et al. 2018. *Advanced Functional Materials* 28: 1801484
69. Tian N, Zhou Z-Y, Sun S-G, Ding Y, Wang ZL. 2007. *Science* 316: 732–5
70. Yang L, Song X, Qi M, Xia L, Jin M. 2013. *Journal of Materials Chemistry A* 1: 7316–20
71. Gao Z, Lv S, Xu M, Tang D. 2017. *Analyst* 142: 911–7
72. Zhao Z-J, Liu S, Zha S, Cheng D, Studt F, et al. 2019. *Nature Reviews Materials* 4: 792–804
73. Shinde SS, Maroz A, Hay MP, Anderson RF. 2009. *Journal of the American Chemical Society* 131: 5203–7
74. Li WY, Xu LN, Chen J. 2005. *Advanced Functional Materials* 15: 851–7
75. Zhang W, Hu S, Yin J-J, He W, Lu W, et al. 2016. *Journal of the American Chemical Society* 138: 5860–5
76. Bligaard T, Nørskov JK, Dahl S, Matthiesen J, Christensen CH, Sehested J. 2004. *Journal of Catalysis* 224: 206–17
77. Huang Y, Ren J, Qu X. 2019. *Chemical Reviews* 119: 4357–412
78. Zhuang J, Zhang J, Gao L, Zhang Y, Gu N, et al. 2008. *Materials Letters* 62: 3972–4
79. Dai Z, Liu S, Bao J, Jui H. 2009. *Chemistry-A European Journal* 15: 4321–6
80. Jv Y, Li B, Cao R. 2010. *Chemical Communications* 46: 8017–9
81. Kim MI, Ye Y, Won BY, Shin S, Lee J, Park HG. 2011. *Advanced Functional Materials* 21: 2868–75
82. Shi W, Wang Q, Long Y, Cheng Z, Chen S, et al. 2011. *Chemical Communications* 47: 6695–7
83. Shi W, Zhang X, He S, Huang Y. 2011. *Chemical Communications* 47: 10785–7
84. Dong Y, Zhang H, Rahman ZU, Su L, Chen X, et al. 2012. *Nanoscale* 4: 3969–76
85. Ai L, Li L, Zhang C, Fu J, Jiang J. 2013. *Chemistry–A European Journal* 19: 15105–8
86. McKeating KS, Sloan-Dennison S, Graham D, Faulds K. 2013. *Analyst* 138: 6347–53
87. Fang H, Pan Y, Shan W, Guo M, Nie Z, et al. 2014. *Analytical Methods* 6: 6073–81
88. Zhang J-W, Zhang H-T, Du Z-Y, Wang X, Yu S-H, Jiang H-L. 2014. *Chemical Communications* 50: 1092–4
89. Jin J, Zhu S, Song Y, Zhao H, Zhang Z, et al. 2016. *ACS Applied Materials & Interfaces* 8: 27956–65
90. Cai S, Han Q, Qi C, Lian Z, Jia X, et al. 2016. *Nanoscale* 8: 3685–93
91. Wang X, Hu Y, Wei H. 2016. *Inorganic Chemistry Frontiers* 3: 41–60
92. Wang X, Cao W, Qin L, Lin T, Chen W, et al. 2017. *Theranostics* 7: 2277–86
93. Hu Y, Cheng H, Zhao X, Wu J, Muhammad F, et al. 2017. *ACS Nano* 11: 5558–66
94. Ding Y, Yang B, Liu H, Liu Z, Zhang X, et al. 2018. *Sensors and Actuators B: Chemical* 259: 775–83
95. Wu J, Qin K, Yuan D, Tan J, Qin L, et al. 2018. *ACS Applied Materials & Interfaces* 10: 12954–9
96. Cai S, Xiao W, Duan H, Liang X, Wang C, et al. 2018. *Nano Research* 11: 6304–15
97. Jiao L, Xu W, Yan H, Wu Y, Liu C, et al. 2019. *Analytical Chemistry* 91: 11994–9
98. Wang X, Qin L, Lin M, Xing H, Wei H. 2019. *Analytical Chemistry* 91: 10648–56
99. Chen W, Hong L, Liu A-L, Liu J-Q, Lin X-H, Xia X-H. 2012. *Talanta* 99: 643–8
100. Hu A-L, Liu Y-H, Deng H-H, Hong G-L, Liu A-L, et al. 2014. *Biosensors & Bioelectronics* 61: 374–8
101. Luo F, Lin Y, Zheng L, Lin X, Chi Y. 2015. *ACS Applied Materials & Interfaces* 7: 11322–9
102. Cheng H, Zhang L, He J, Guo W, Zhou Z, et al. 2016. *Analytical Chemistry* 88: 5489–97
103. Karyakin AA, Karyakina EE. 1999. *Sensors and Actuators B-Chemical* 57: 268–73
104. Karyakin AA, Puganova EA, Budashov IA, Kurochkin IN, Karyakina EE, et al. 2004. *Analytical Chemistry* 76: 474–8

105. Wang C-I, Chen W-T, Chang H-T. 2012. *Analytical Chemistry* 84: 9706–12
106. Su L, Feng J, Zhou X, Ren C, Li H, Chen X. 2012. *Analytical Chemistry* 84: 5753–8
107. Hong L, Liu A-L, Li G-W, Chen W, Lin X-H. 2013. *Biosensors and Bioelectronics* 43: 1–5
108. Chen Y, Cao H, Shi W, Liu H, Huang Y. 2013. *Chemical Communications* 49: 5013–5
109. Deng L, Chen C, Zhu C, Dong S, Lu H. 2014. *Biosensors & Bioelectronics* 52: 324–9
110. He S-B, Wu G-W, Deng H-H, Liu A-L, Lin X-H, et al. 2014. *Biosensors and Bioelectronics* 62: 331–6
111. Lin T, Zhong L, Song Z, Guo L, Wu H, et al. 2014. *Biosensors and Bioelectronics* 62: 302–7
112. Qu K, Shi P, Ren J, Qu X. 2014. *Chemistry–A European Journal* 20: 7501–6
113. Hayat A, Haider W, Raza Y, Marty JL. 2015. *Talanta* 143: 157–61
114. Qian J, Yang X, Yang Z, Zhu G, Mao H, Wang K. 2015. *Journal of Materials Chemistry B* 3: 1624–32
115. Nirala NR, Pandey S, Bansal A, Singh VK, Mukherjee B, et al. 2015. *Biosensors & Bioelectronics* 74: 207–13
116. Qian F, Wang J, Ai S, Li L. 2015. *Sensors and Actuators B-Chemical* 216: 418–27
117. Jiang X, Sun C, Guo Y, Nie G, Xu L. 2015. *Biosensors and Bioelectronics* 64: 165–70
118. Han L, Li C, Zhang T, Lang Q, Liu A. 2015. *ACS Applied Materials & Interfaces* 7: 14463–70
119. Lu C, Liu X, Li Y, Yu F, Tang L, et al. 2015. *ACS Applied Materials & Interfaces* 7: 15395–402
120. Nirala NR, Abraham S, Kumar V, Bansal A, Srivastava A, Saxena PS. 2015. *Sensors and Actuators B: Chemical* 218: 42–50
121. Huang Y, Zhao M, Han S, Lai Z, Yang J, et al. 2017. *Advanced Materials* 29: 1700102
122. Wang Q, Zhang X, Huang L, Zhang Z, Dong S. 2017. *Angewandte Chemie-International Edition* 56: 16082–5
123. Wang Q, Zhang X, Huang L, Zhang Z, Dong S. 2017. *ACS Applied Materials & Interfaces* 9: 7465–71
124. Hassanzadeh J, Khataee A. 2018. *Talanta* 178: 992–1000
125. Valekar AH, Batule BS, Kim MI, Cho K-H, Hong D-Y, et al. 2018. *Biosensors & Bioelectronics* 100: 161–8
126. Nirala NR, Vinita, Prakash R. 2018. *Microchimica Acta* 185: 224
127. Wu X, Chen T, Wang J, Yang G. 2018. *Journal of Materials Chemistry B* 6: 105–11
128. Ma Y, Zhang Z, Ren C, Liu G, Chen X. 2012. *Analyst* 137: 485–9
129. Zheng A-X, Cong Z-X, Wang J-R, Li J, Yang H-H, Chen G-N. 2013. *Biosensors & Bioelectronics* 49: 519–24
130. Ray C, Dutta S, Sarkar S, Sahoo R, Roy A, Pal T. 2014. *Journal of Materials Chemistry B* 2: 6097–105
131. Tan H, Ma C, Gao L, Li Q, Song Y, et al. 2014. *Chemistry–A European Journal* 20: 16377–83
132. Lin X-Q, Deng H-H, Wu G-W, Peng H-P, Liu A-L, et al. 2015. *Analyst* 140: 5251–6
133. Dutta S, Ray C, Mallick S, Sarkar S, Sahoo R, et al. 2015. *The Journal of Physical Chemistry C* 119: 23790–800
134. Jiang Z, Gao P, Yang L, Huang C, Li Y. 2015. *Analytical Chemistry* 87: 12177–82
135. Nagvenkar AP, Gedanken A. 2016. *ACS Applied Materials & Interfaces* 8: 22301–8
136. Jia H, Yang D, Han X, Cai J, Liu H, He W. 2016. *Nanoscale* 8: 5938–45
137. Feng J, Huang P, Shi S, Deng K-Y, Wu F-Y. 2017. *Analytica Chimica Acta* 967: 64–9
138. Fan S, Zhao M, Ding L, Li H, Chen S. 2017. *Biosensors and Bioelectronics* 89: 846–52
139. Ding Y, Zhao J, Li B, Zhao X, Wang C, et al. 2018. *Microchimica Acta* 185: 131
140. Wang J, Hu Y, Zhou Q, Hu L, Fu W, Wang Y. 2019. *ACS Applied Materials & Interfaces* 11: 44466–73

141. Lu M, Li B, Guan L, Li K, Lin Y. 2019. *ACS Sustainable Chemistry & Engineering* 7: 15471–8
142. Yu R, Wang R, He X, Liu T, Shen J, Dai Z. 2019. *Chemical Communications* 55: 11543–6
143. Huang X, Xia F, Nan Z. 2020. *ACS Applied Materials & Interfaces* 12: 46539–48
144. Lin J, Wang Q, Wang X, Zhu Y, Zhou X, Wei H. 2020. *Analyst* 145: 3916–21
145. Pedone D, Moglianetti M, Lettieri M, Marrazza G, Pompa PP. 2020. *Analytical Chemistry* 92: 8660–4
146. Lou Z, Zhao S, Wang Q, Wei H. 2019. *Analytical Chemistry* 91: 15267–74
147. Ni P, Dai H, Wang Y, Sun Y, Shi Y, et al. 2014. *Biosensors & Bioelectronics* 60: 286–91
148. Liu Y, Ding D, Zhen Y, Guo R. 2017. *Biosensors & Bioelectronics* 92: 140–6
149. Qin L, Wang X, Liu Y, Wei H. 2018. *Analytical Chemistry* 90: 9983–9
150. Xia W, Zhang P, Fu W, Hu L, Wang Y. 2019. *Chemical Communications* 55: 2039–42
151. Lv J, Wang S, Zhang C, Lin Y, Fu Y, Li M. 2020. *Analyst* 145: 5032–40
152. Wang Q, Lei J, Deng S, Zhang L, Ju H. 2013. *Chemical Communications* 49: 916–8
153. Zhang G-Y, Deng S-Y, Cai W-R, Cosnier S, Zhang X-J, Shan D. 2015. *Analytical Chemistry* 87: 9093–100
154. Ling P, Lei J, Zhang L, Ju H. 2015. *Analytical Chemistry* 87: 3957–63
155. Li J, Koo KM, Wang Y, Trau M. 2019. *Small* 15: 1904689
156. Li X, Li X, Li D, Zhao M, Wu H, et al. 2020. *Biosensors & Bioelectronics* 168: 112554
157. Tian L, Qi J, Oderinde O, Yao C, Song W, Wang Y. 2018. *Biosensors & Bioelectronics* 110: 110–7
158. Song Y, Wang X, Zhao C, Qu K, Ren J, Qu X. 2010. *Chemistry–A European Journal* 16: 3617–21
159. Guo Y, Deng L, Li J, Guo S, Wang E, Dong S. 2011. *ACS Nano* 5: 1282–90
160. Park KS, Kim MI, Cho DY, Park HG. 2011. *Small* 7: 1521–5
161. Liu M, Zhao H, Chen S, Yu H, Quan X. 2012. *ACS Nano* 6: 3142–51
162. Liu YL, Fu WL, Li CM, Huang CZ, Li YF. 2015. *Analytica Chimica Acta* 861: 55–61
163. Liu B, Liu J. 2015. *Nanoscale* 7: 13831–5
164. Chau LY, He Q, Qin A, Yip SP, Lee TMH. 2016. *Journal of Materials Chemistry B* 4: 4076–83
165. Hizir MS, Top M, Balcioglu M, Rana M, Robertson NM, et al. 2016. *Analytical Chemistry* 88: 600–5
166. Chen C, Li N, Lan J, Ji X, He Z. 2016. *Analytica Chimica Acta* 902: 154–9
167. Tan B, Zhao H, Wu W, Liu X, Zhang Y, Quan X. 2017. *Nanoscale* 9: 18699–710
168. He W, Liu Y, Yuan J, Yin J-J, Wu X, et al. 2011. *Biomaterials* 32: 1139–47
169. Li X, Wen F, Creran B, Jeong Y, Zhang X, Rotello VM. 2012. *Small* 8: 3589–92
170. Zhu Y-D, Peng J, Jiang L-P, Zhu J-J. 2014. *Analyst* 139: 649–55
171. Duan D, Fan K, Zhang D, Tan S, Liang M, et al. 2015. *Biosensors and Bioelectronics* 74: 134–41
172. Tian Z, Li J, Zhang Z, Gao W, Zhou X, Qu Y. 2015. *Biomaterials* 59: 116–24
173. Loynachan CN, Thomas MR, Gray ER, Richards DA, Kim J, et al. 2018. *ACS Nano* 12: 279–88
174. Su Y, Wu D, Chen J, Chen G, Hu N, et al. 2019. *Analytical Chemistry* 91: 11687–95
175. Liu D, Ju C, Han C, Shi R, Chen X, et al. 2021. *Biosensors and Bioelectronics* 173: 112817
176. Qiu H, Pu F, Ran X, Liu C, Ren J, Qu X. 2018. *Analytical Chemistry* 90: 11775–9
177. Su L, Yu X, Miao Y, Mao G, Dong W, et al. 2019. *Talanta* 197: 181–8
178. Chen Q, Zhang X, Li S, Tan J, Xu C, Huang Y. 2020. *Chemical Engineering Journal* 395: 125130
179. Jin R, Xing Z, Kong D, Yan X, Liu F, et al. 2019. *Journal of Materials Chemistry B* 7: 1230–7

180. Wang M, Liu L, Xie X, Zhou X, Lin Z, Su X. 2020. *Sensors and Actuators B-Chemical* 313: 128023
181. Zhang X, Lu Y, Chen Q, Huang Y. 2020. *Journal of Materials Chemistry B* 8: 6459–68
182. Guo Y, Li X, Dong Y, Wang G-L. 2019. *ACS Sustainable Chemistry & Engineering* 7: 7572–9
183. Song H, Niu X, Ye K, Wang L, Xu Y, Peng Y. 2020. *Analytical and Bioanalytical Chemistry* 412: 5551–61
184. Wang C, Gao J, Cao Y, Tan H. 2018. *Analytica Chimica Acta* 1004: 74–81
185. Wang X, Jiang X, Wei H. 2020. *Journal of Materials Chemistry B* 8: 6905–11
186. Xie X, Wang Y, Zhou X, Chen J, Wang M, Su X. 2021. *Analyst* 146: 896–903
187. Ye K, Wang L, Song H, Li X, Niu X. 2019. *Journal of Materials Chemistry B* 7: 4794–800
188. Zheng S, Gu H, Yin D, Zhang J, Li W, Fu Y. 2020. *Colloids and Surfaces A-Physicochemical and Engineering Aspects* 589: 124444
189. Lien C-W, Huang C-C, Chang H-T. 2012. *Chemical Communications* 48: 7952–4
190. Jiang X, Wang X, Lin A, Wei H. 2021. *Analytical Chemistry*: DOI: 10.1021/acs.analchem.1c00721
191. Hu L, Liao H, Feng L, Wang M, Fu W. 2018. *Analytical Chemistry* 90: 6247–52
192. Cheng H, Liu Y, Hu Y, Ding Y, Lin S, et al. 2017. *Analytical Chemistry* 89: 11552–9
193. You J-G, Wang Y-T, Tseng W-L. 2018. *ACS Applied Materials & Interfaces* 10: 37846–54
194. Ma X, Kou X, Xu Y, Yang D, Miao P. 2019. *Nanoscale Advances* 1: 486–9
195. Gu H, Huang Q, Zhang J, Li W, Fu Y. 2020. *Colloids and Surfaces A-Physicochemical and Engineering Aspects* 606: 125455
196. Wang Y-M, Liu J-W, Adkins GB, Shen W, Trinh MP, et al. 2017. *Analytical Chemistry* 89: 12327–33
197. Xia Y, Liu M, Wang L, Yan A, He W, et al. 2017. *Biosensors & Bioelectronics* 92: 8–15
198. Boriachek K, Masud MK, Palma C, Hoang-Phuong P, Yamauchi Y, et al. 2019. *Analytical Chemistry* 91: 3827–34
199. Di H, Mi Z, Sun Y, Liu X, Liu X, et al. 2020. *Theranostics* 10: 9303–14
200. Wang Q-L, Huang W-X, Zhang P-J, Chen L, Lio C-K, et al. 2020. *Microchimica Acta* 187: 61
201. Zhang L-N, Deng H-H, Lin F-L, Xu X-W, Weng S-H, et al. 2014. *Analytical Chemistry* 86: 2711–8
202. Maji SK, Mandal AK, Kim Truc N, Borah P, Zhao Y. 2015. *ACS Applied Materials & Interfaces* 7: 9807–16
203. Wang G-L, Xu X-F, Qiu L, Dong Y-M, Li Z-J, Zhang C. 2014. *ACS Applied Materials & Interfaces* 6: 6434–42
204. Sun C, Chen X, Xu J, Wei M, Wang J, et al. 2013. *Journal of Materials Chemistry A* 1: 4699–705
205. Lee Y-C, Kim MI, Woo M-A, Park HG, Han J-I. 2013. *Biosensors & Bioelectronics* 42: 373–8
206. Guo QJ, Pan ZY, Men C, Lv WY, Zou HY, Huang CZ. 2019. *Analyst* 144: 716–21
207. Song Y, Chen Y, Feng L, Ren J, Qu X. 2011. *Chemical Communications* 47: 4436–8
208. Kim MI, Kim MS, Woo M-A, Ye Y, Kang KS, et al. 2014. *Nanoscale* 6: 1529–36
209. Ge S, Liu F, Liu W, Yan M, Song X, Yu J. 2014. *Chemical Communications* 50: 475–7
210. Gao L, Liu M, Ma G, Wang Y, Zhao L, et al. 2015. *ACS Nano* 9: 10979–90
211. Li J, Wang J, Wang Y, Trau M. 2017. *Analyst* 142: 4788–93
212. Tian L, Qi J, Qian K, Oderinde O, Cai Y, et al. 2018. *Sensors and Actuators B-Chemical* 260: 676–84
213. Tian L, Qi J, Qian K, Oderinde O, Liu Q, et al. 2018. *Journal of Electroanalytical Chemistry* 812: 1–9

214. Weerathunge P, Pooja D, Singh M, Kulhari H, Mayes ELH, et al. 2019. *Sensors and Actuators B-Chemical* 297: 126737
215. Wang H, Wu T, Li M, Tao Y. 2021. *Journal of Materials Chemistry B* 9: 921–38
216. Lin Y, Liu K, Yu P, Xiang L, Li X, Mao L. 2007. *Analytical Chemistry* 79: 9577–83
217. Sardesai NP, Ganesana M, Karimi A, Leiter JC, Andreescu S. 2015. *Analytical Chemistry* 87: 2996–3003
218. Ding Y, Ren G, Wang G, Lu M, Liu J, et al. 2020. *Analytical Chemistry* 92: 4583–91
219. Zelikin AN. 2020. *Nature Chemistry* 12: 11–2
220. Loynachan CN, Soleimany AP, Dudani JS, Lin Y, Najer A, et al. 2019. *Nature Nanotechnology* 14: 883–90

# 17 Potential Toxicology of Nanozymes

*Weizheng Wang and Sundaram Gunasekaran*[*]
Department of Biological Systems Engineering,
University of Wisconsin–Madison, WI, USA

## CONTENTS

## 17.1 INTRODUCTION

The field of toxicology traditionally deals with the adverse effects of bulk chemical agents, and their diagnosis and treatment, to living organisms and the environment. This concept was initially proposed by Paracelsus, who implied a linear relationship between dose and dose–response (1). Later research has allowed for a comprehensive revision of dose and dose–response relationships, which proved to be more complicated. In the conventional model, the typical feature of the dose–response relationship (also called exposure–response relationship) is "S" -shaped, indicating

---

[*] Corresponding author: Sundaram Gunasekaran

DOI: 10.1201/9781003109228-17

that a nonlinear relationship in high and low dose ranges (2). This model plays an important role in describing the toxicity of chemical substances in bulk, with consideration of substance concentration and exposure time as two key parameters. At the nanoscale, however, the effects of substances vastly differ from their bulk counterparts due to a substantial increase in surface-to-volume ratio or surface functionality alteration (3). These new properties significantly affect their reactivity, for example, their enzymatic properties.

Along with the exploding growth of nanotechnology and its application, concerns began to arise regarding the safety of nanomaterials (NMs). In the late 20th century, several early toxicological and epidemiological experiments were conducted to evaluate the adverse effects of "ultrafine" (<100 nm) particles on the respiratory system (4–6). Such research primarily focused on the potential effect of ultrafine particles on their behaviors while they were in the aerosols and their effect on human health. The data collected have provided strong evidence that the size of nanoparticles (NPs) plays a necessary role in their behavior when they come in contact with the respiratory tract. Later, additional investigations were carried out on the potentially harmful effects of NPs on various other organs and systems, involving an inflammatory response in lungs (7, 8), dermal penetration (9), and even the brain of largemouth bass (10). In 2004, nanotoxicology was first adopted by Donaldson et al. and has quickly begun to draw increasing attention globally, mainly focusing on the toxicological aspect of NMs (11). Over the years, there has been an exponential growth in the published literature on nanotoxicology. For example, just from 2000 to 2007, the peer-review publications on nanotoxicology have increased sixfold (12, 13).

Unfortunately, the risk assessment of NPs is in its early stage, there are still many unknowns in fully assessing their toxicological effects. The biggest problem is to completely know how NMs interact with living systems. Especially, how the binding and interaction with biological entities are altered when the NMs are in different environments. For example, even with the same NM, the size, shape, or surface modification would change how it could affect our health. There is also a lack of accepted or standardized protocols to evaluate the toxic effects of NMs on various biological targets. Furthermore, it is rather complicated to compare the results of toxicity tests *in vitro* with those observed *in vivo*. In this chapter, we mainly review the toxic effect of NMs on living organisms, including the exposure route, biodistribution (BD), mechanisms of nanotoxicity, and toxicity risk in different organs or systems. Some nanotoxicological effects on the environment are also discussed.

## 17.2   POTENTIAL NANOZYME EXPOSURE AND BIODISTRIBUTION

Since iron oxide ($Fe_3O_4$) NPs have been first recognized with peroxidase (POD) behavior in 2007, numerous NMs of metals, metal oxides, carbon, etc. have been used as enzyme mimics (14). Therefore, nanozyme applications, described in previous chapters, have been largely explored and are beneficial to society. With the increasing development of nanozyme applications, it is anticipated that nanozyme products will dominate food, agricultural, medical, environmental, and industrial areas in the future. However, along with increased applications in diverse fields, the risk of passively receiving these nanozymes and releasing them into the environment and in biomedical applications, which may, unsuspectingly, become harmful to the health and wellbeing of living entities and the surrounding environment. In this chapter, we discuss several possible uptake paths of NPs which allow them to get access into human bodies and how those NPs biodistribute and impact our health.

## 17.2.1  Exposure Routes for Nanoparticles

An overview of possible exposure pathways of NPs is presented in **Figure 17.1**. As can be observed, inhalation and dermal penetration are two major exposure routes for humans who work or live with NMs, while ingestion is always associated with food, drink, or drug uptake. People when they get an injection of NPs-based vaccines or medical liquid (15).

The respiration system is the route for NPs from the air to enter the human body. As a major organ in the respiratory system, the lung helps to exchange oxygen ($O_2$) and carbon dioxide ($CO_2$) into or out of the blood vessels. The deposition of NPs onto the respiratory tract is the first step after air containing NPs is inhaled, which is greatly dependent on the size of the NPs, and as the size is reduced, both deposition ratio and retention time on the lung surface could rapidly increase (16). When bulk and nanoscale foreign particles deposit in the respiratory tract, most of them can be removed by mucociliary clearance; however, NPs of size ranging from 1 to10

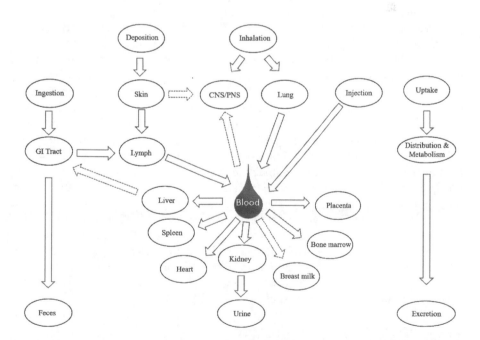

**FIGURE 17.1**  Exposure routes of NPs and their demonstrated (solid arrow) and hypothetical (dashed arrow) translocation routes. CNS, central nervous system, PNS, peripheral nervous system. Redrawn based on and with permission from Environmental Health Perspectives (18).

nm may escape and could reach the alveolar region throughout the lungs based upon Brownian movement (17).

Once NPs reach the alveoli, they cannot be removed since the balloon-shaped air sacs lack the mucociliary clearance mechanism. Instead, NPs so entered are immediately endocytosed and translocated into the bronchial tubes by macrophages (19, 20). This translocation process of various NPs, involving zinc oxide (ZnO) NPs, gold (Au) NPs, multiwalled carbon nanotubes (MWCNT), etc., have been investigated as a function of size and amount of NPs (21–23). Additionally, it has also been reported that a small amount (<0.05% of provided dose) of NPs is capable of crossing the thin air–blood barrier that protects blood from foreign particles, and finally enters the bloodstream (24). Besides the pulmonary-blood pathway, the olfactory bulb-neuronal cell pathway is another approach for transmigration of foreign NPs from the respiratory tract into the brain, where endocytosis plays a key role in the interneuron translocation of the NPs (25). It is computationally simulated that the percentage of inhaled NPs deposited on the olfactory bulb is higher in rats than in humans and the calculated olfactory dose is higher in the human body owing to the larger average amount of air inhaled by humans than by rats (26).

Penetrating through the skin is another most likely route for NPs to enter the body and gain access to various organs. As the largest organ in the human body, with a surface area of 1.4–2 m$^2$, skin consists of three layers: 1) epidermis; 2) dermis; and 3) hypodermis (27). Strongly keratinized stratum corneum layer (SCL), the outermost layer of the epidermis, functions as the main barrier to the exogenetic microscale particles and stimulus to protect the body. However, given their size, NPs can get across the SCL via aqueous pores or apolar intercellular route (28). For example, silver (Ag) NPs and maghemite ($\gamma$-Fe$_2$O$_3$) have been known to penetrate SCL via the follicular pathway; and the NPs so enter are usually stored in hair follicular pores, which also provide the exogenetic NPs the shortest route for entering (29–31). Yet, it has been shown via skin biopsy that without further penetration Au NPs of average core diameter of 15 nm can only accumulate and store in the follicular openings (32).

Besides the above two routes, another potential route for NPs exposure is the gastrointestinal tract (GIT). NPs from foods, drinks, or drugs and those removed by the mucociliary clearance through the respiratory system can reach the GIT and be transported to the inner circulation system (15). Based on previous observations, four translocation pathways allow NPs to enter the bloodstream post oral uptake. The primary and common pathway among these is transcytosis that occurs at the surface of small intestinal lymphoid aggregates (known as Peyer's Patches), which assists to transmigrate NPs to neighboring/interlocking mononuclear cells (33). Even so, NPs post oral uptake has only minor adverse effects, since they are most likely to be excreted out of the body (>97% of dose administration) (18). However, more research is needed to fully evaluate the assimilation of NPs via GIT.

## 17.2.2 BIODISTRIBUTION OF NANOPARTICLES

Biodistribution (BD) is an assessment that tracks the travel sites of small bulk particles in the body. Once bulk particles enter the vascular system, they are carried by body fluids flowing throughout to reach different organs or systems depending on various physicochemical properties of the bulk particle-based products and their ability to penetrate the barriers encountered. Unlike bulk particles, BD of NPs largely depends on characteristics of NPs, such as their size, shape, and chemical functionalities.

Nanoscale size is one of the significant advantages for NPs that enhances their chemical reactivity. A size-dependent BD study carried out in rodents demonstrated that tissue distribution significantly relies on the size of NPs. Larger Au NPs (50–250 nm) are most likely to be distributed and accumulated only in blood, liver, and spleen. On the contrary, smaller particles (~10 nm) are usually present broadly once they get access to the bloodstream, including in blood, liver, spleen, lung, kidney, testis, heart, thymus, and even brain (34, 35). In addition, the time to reach the maximum level in the same organ varies between longer and shorter NPs. In a study, as shown in **Figure 17.2A**, long carbon nanohorns (CNH) reached the maximum level in the liver and spleen in 48 h and then the amount slightly decreased in seven days, while the short CNH took seven days to reach the maximum level (36).

Chemical modification, achieved by altering the biochemical properties and surface charge, is another essential factor for BD of NPs. As shown in **Figure 17.2B**, unmodified NPs are much easier to stimulate and accelerate opsonization and phagocytosis in the liver and spleen as they are capable of binding to various blood proteins including opsonins (37, 38). Polyethylene glycol (PEG)-modified NPs (i.e., PEGylated NPs) can reduce the rate of being phagocytic captured in the liver and spleen, improving their systemic circulation (39). Moreover, NPs covered apolipoprotein E can specifically and effectively overcome the blood–brain barrier (BBB), eventually accumulating in the brain (40). Hirm et al. (41) examined the surface charge of NPs and their distribution in organs using Au NPs. They found that negatively charged NPs accumulate more in the liver and kidney; whereas more positively charged NPs are found in the spleen, heart, kidney, and carcass.

## 17.3   MECHANISM OF NANOTOXICITY

### 17.3.1   Dose Metric for Nanoparticles

Dose and dose–response play essential roles in the toxicology of bulk particles. When using bulk particles, the dose depends only on the mass or concentration of toxins present and is usually defined as mass or moles of toxic substance per unit of body weight (such as mg/kg or moles/kg) (42). This metric is inadequate to comprehensively describe the toxicological effect of NPs due to their unique properties and high chemical reactivity. Many attempts have been made to examine the effect of physicochemical attributes dose–response relationship. However, there is still no consensus on how these factors account for the toxicological effects of NPs (43), including surface area (44), size (45), number (46), and surface chemical functionalization (47).

### 17.3.2   Nanozyme Characterizations

As mentioned earlier, the high-surface-area-to-volume ratio of NPs contributes to their substantially high biochemical reactivity compared to their bulk counterparts.

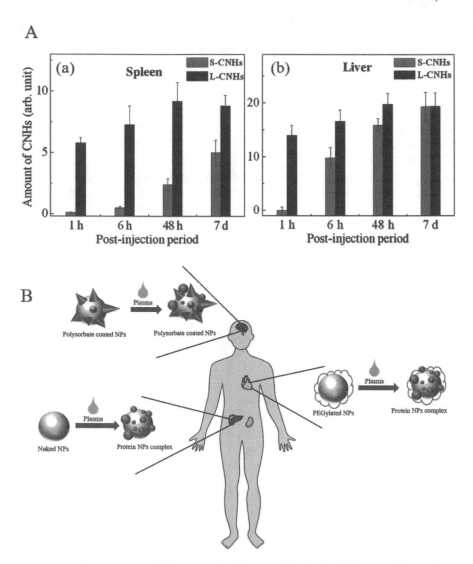

**FIGURE 17.2** (**A**) Amount of long CNH (L-CNHs, length 100 nm) and short CNH (S-CNHs, length 30–50 nm) in the spleen (a) and liver (b) after one week of exposure. Adapted with permission from (36). (**B**) Scheme for the pattern of BD of NPs in the human body in the presence of various surface modifications. Uncoated NPs bind many proteins that mainly present in the liver and spleen. "PEGylated" NPs with few proteins bound flow throughout the body via the bloodstream. "Polysorbate-coated" NPs bind with apolipoprotein E and reach CNS. Redrawn based on (37)

While high reactivity is helpful for enzyme-mimicking properties as nanozymes, there is also a concomitant increase in the potential nanotoxicity of NPs. There are a couple of important and determining factors to the toxicity of NPs in terms of size, shape, length, agglomeration, concentration, biochemical functionalization, and solvent. Agglomeration usually appears in the vast majority of NPs due to Van der Waals' attractive and electrostatic double-layer forces between NPs (48, 49). Upon agglomeration, the large aggregates induce multiple cellular responses in bodies, resulting in unpredictable results. A study conducted by Albanese et al. (50) revealed that toxic responses in different cell lines varied when they were treated by the transferrin-coated Au NPs based on various target receptors, endocytosis mechanisms, and cell phenotypes. The adverse effects of agglomeration are also dependent on surface functionalization, disperse media, concentration, as well as length of NPs (51–53).

For one-dimensional (1-D) NMs, such as MWCNT, length is another important determinant for influencing nanotoxicology. This was initially found with asbestos, where long rigid asbestos fibers (length >20 μm) surrounded the chest surface and abdominal cavities causing mesothelioma (54). Later, Poland et al. (55) intraperitoneally injected saline solutions containing MWCNTs of different lengths into normal mice and found that longer MWCNTs (>20 μm) are the most likely to accumulate in diaphragmatic mesothelium compared to the shorter and tangled nanotube aggregates. Consequently, long MWCNTs significantly increased granulomatous lesion formation. This indicated that inflammation risk increases with the exposure to MWCNTs, probably caused by the long MWCNTs, whose length exceeds the engulfment ability of macrophages (shown in **Figure 17.3**) (56). Another observation is that the pro-inflammatory effect of long, needle-like MWCNTs (~13 μm) on primary macrophages of normal blood cells, suggested that long MWCNTs activate inflammasome by stimulating the pathophysiological mechanism (57).

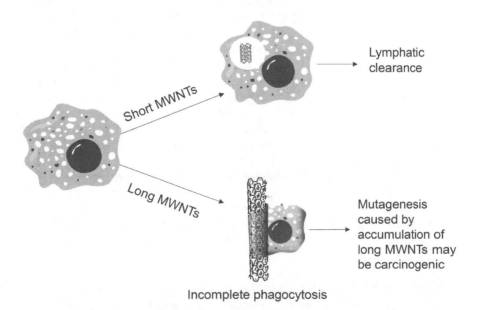

**FIGURE 17.3**   A. Length of MWNTs influences phagocytosis through macrophages and clearing mechanism. Shorter MWNTs can be cleared by macrophages; however, longer MWNTs cannot be cleared and accumulate in tissues [based on (1)].

### 17.3.3  Nanotoxicological Mechanism

#### 17.3.3.1  Molecular Factor

As has been discussed in previous chapters, following the catalysis mechanism of nanozyme in the presence of oxidizing agents (e.g., hydrogen peroxide ($H_2O_2$) and $O_2$) and their substrates [e.g., 3,3′,5,5′ tetramethylbenzidine (TMB) and 2,2-azinobis (3-ethylbenzothizoline-6-sulfonic acid) (ABTS)], nanozymes are classified as various natural enzyme-mimics, such as POD, oxidase (OXD), superoxide dismutase (SOD), catalase (CAT), etc. (58). OXD-mimic helps electron transfer from organic substrates (e.g., TMB) to dissolve $O_2$. Consequently, dissolved $O_2$ is reduced to a highly reactive superoxide anion ($O_2 \cdot^-$), which is rapidly converted to $H_2O_2$ or directly to $H_2O$. While SOD-mimic catalyzes highly reactive $O_2 \cdot^-$ to $H_2O_2$, which can be further reduced to $H_2O$ in the presence of CAT- or POD-mimic. Based on these processes, it is demonstrated that substantial $O_2 \cdot^-$, hydroxyl radicals ($\cdot OH$) and $H_2O_2$ are constantly generated for oxidizing substrates during catalysis. Those three oxygen derivatives are also known as reactive oxygen species (ROS).

An important question is "what might happen when nanozymes are in the cellular environment?" Endogenous generation of ROS in mitochondria is an intrinsic behavior of cells that support multiple physiological processes in the body, including proliferation, signaling, senescence, pathological process, etc. (59) Under normal conditions, the amount of ROS and its oxidative-damaged effects are usually under the regulation of cellular antioxidant cascade constituted in several natural enzymes: SOD, OXD, CAT, glutathione peroxidase (GPx), and some antioxidants, such as glutathione (GSH) (60). Nevertheless, if nanozymes are introduced, excessive byproducts derived from $O_2$ perhaps predominates in the cell, acting as toxicological intermediates. This behavior destroys the delicate balance between ROS production and intrinsic antioxidant defenses of the biological system known as oxidative stress (OS). Increasing OS level has been reported to enhance the inflammation of cells through activation of principle cascades with the involvement of nuclear factor-κB, phosphoinositide 3-kinase pathways, and mitogen-activated protein kinase (61, 62). Apart from ROS directly inducing the OS in cells, excessive ROS released via catalysis of NPs can also initialize lipid peroxidation in the mitochondrial membrane, thus damaging mitochondria (63). In general, there are limited pathological outcomes (e.g., apoptosis, inflammation, and hypertrophy) that appear in biological systems when they are injured or invaded by foreign biochemical substances, due to the ability of integration for multiple injury pathways. Nonetheless, mechanisms of each pathological outcome brought by nanozymes might be different and novel, even if there is no new pathology introduced. Elucidations of these specific mechanisms can be achieved via investigations conducted under controlled conditions *in vitro* and data collected *in vivo* (64).

#### 17.3.3.2  Genotoxic Penitential of Nanozyme

Genotoxicity occurs when genetic information is damaged by chemical substances within a cell, which may lead to cancer. According to the mechanism of genetic damage, genotoxicity can be classified as primary or secondary (65, 66). Primary genotoxicity usually refers to genetic information damaged by particles/NPs through direct or indirect pathways without initializing inflammation; whereas, secondary genotoxicity is associated with inflammation induced by ROS or other intermediates (67). Based on their intrinsic properties, nanozymes can cause either primary or secondary genotoxicity when they are introduced into the bodies. There is evidence that DNA damage can be induced by carbon nanotubes (CNTs) and graphene nanofibers (GNF) (68). *In vitro* experiments with these carbon NMs indicated that they induced a dose-dependent genotoxic effect in human bronchial epithelial cells, which may be due to the fibrous nature of these NMs with a possible contribution by catalyst metals (Co, Mo, and Fe) present in them.

Some NPs may simultaneously induce primary and secondary genotoxicity. For example, when ZnO NPs were used for treating human neuronal cells under various exposure conditions, the results showed that ZnO NPs are responsible for DNA damage both directly and via ROS produced after ZnO NPs exposure, which also resulted in oxidative DNA damage (69). Investigation into the immunological responses of NPs revealed that single-walled carbon nanotubes (SWCNTs) functionalized by peptides form immunogenic complexes that increase antibody response (70, 71). In another study, Ag NPs treatment in rats evidenced increasing chromosome breakage and polyploidy cell growth, which are usually associated with the activation of DNA damage response (72). However, further study is necessary to shed more light on the specific immune response to the antigenicity of NPs and their complexes.

## 17.4 TOXIC RISK OF NANOZYMES TO DIFFERENT ORGANS AND SYSTEMS

As NPs are distributed throughout the biological system, due to their small size and high surface-area-to-volume ratio, they usually participate in several basic cellular processes in many organs, such as proliferation, metabolism, and cellular death. There are different toxic effects and outcomes for cells in different organs. In this section, we discuss pathways of exposure to NPs in the human body, affected organs, and associated diseases from epidemiological, *in vivo* and *in vitro* studies. (**Figure 17.4**) (73) and more information on nanomaterials and dosage pertaining to specific toxic effects are summarized in **Table 17.1**.

### 17.4.1 NANOTOXICITY TO THE RESPIRATORY SYSTEM

As discussed previously, the respiratory system is the most common route for NPs to enter and begin to accumulate upon exposure. Consequently, several lung disorders may be attributed to NPs exposure such as pulmonary fibrosis and exacerbation of asthma in asthmatic individuals (106). Pulmonary fibrosis occurs as NPs accumulate on the lung surface. The formation of thick and stiff fibrosis affects the normal activity of the lung tissues. The extent of fibrosis can cause a variety of respiratory symptoms, including hypoxemia, pulmonary hypertension, bronchiectasis, etc. (107). ROS-initializing oxygen species are considered as the first and important step in pulmonary fibrosis that triggers inflammatory signal by activating sensing toxic mediators that is expressed by macrophages and neutrophils, causing inflammatory response (108). Once this happens, a repair mechanism occurs to respond to this

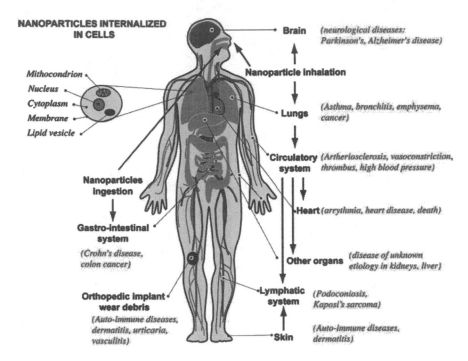

**FIGURE 17.4** Schematic of human body with pathways of exposure to nanoparticles, affected organs, and associated diseases from epidemiological, *in vivo* and *in vitro* studies. Reproduced from Buzea et al. (73) with the permission of the American Vacuum Society.

activity in the lung. Ryman-Rasmussen et al. (74) studied mice exposed to aerosol MWCNTs and found that incidence of fibrosis and number and size of scarring aggregates increased significantly with MWCNTs exposure. Furthermore, Manke et al. (77) reported that the longer the SWCNTs the higher the potential for fibrogenesis in the lung. Cerium dioxide ($CeO_2$) NPs have also been observed to significantly increase the release of two fibrotic toxic mediators, osteopontin (OPN) and transform growth factor (TGF)-β release, that induces lung fibrosis in rats (78, 79). Likewise, several other NPs, e.g., ZnO and CuO, are also deemed responsible to aggravating pulmonary fibrosis in the lung (80, 83).

Asthma is a chronic respiratory disease, characterized by a nonspecific lung hypersensitivity induced by inflammation and vulnerable to nanotoxicity in the lung. In a recent study, it was evidenced that asthmatic individuals are more sensitive than healthy people to CuO and carboxylated CuO NPs aerosols in a dose-dependent manner, and the set of genes responding to mucociliary clearance vary in the asthmatic and healthy population (81). The difference in sensitivity to CuO NPs in an asthmatic and healthy population is possibly due to a combination of lung hyperresponsiveness and insufficient clearance mechanism. Further research, especially with enzyme-mimic NPs, is needed to elucidate any adverse effects of nanozymes on the asthmatic population.

**TABLE 17.1**
**Toxicity of Nanoparticles to Different Organs and Systems in the Abe Human Body**

| Nanomaterial | Size | Dose/Concentration | Result | Ref. |
|---|---|---|---|---|
| | | **Lung** | | |
| MWCNTs | Width (10 ~50 nm), length (less than 100 nm – more than 10 μm) | High dose: 30 mg/m³, low dose: 1 mg/m³ | Number and size of subpleural fibrosis are significantly increases as dose increases | (74) |
| Bacterial lipopolysaccharides (LPS)–MWCNTs | Width(10~30 nm), length (0.3 ~50 μm) | 4 mg/kg | LPS-MWCNT significantly enhances the pulmonary fibrosis formation | (75) |
| MWCNTs | Width (49 + 13.4 nm), length (3.86 +1.94 μm) | 1.86 mg/kg | Acute inflammatory and fibrotic responses, macrophages polarization | (76) |
| SWCNTs | Long: length (12.31~13.4 μm), diameter (11.3 nm); Short: (1.13~0.89 μm), diameter (10.8 nm) | 0.02~0.2 μg/cm² | Longer SWCNTs provide higher ROS response, collagen production and TGF-β release thus higher fibrogenic response | (77) |
| CeO₂ NPs | 6.4~14.8 nm | 0.15~7 mg/kg | TGF-β and OPN releasing increase thus inducing the Pulmonary fibrosis | (78) |
| CeO₂ NPs + diesel exhaust particles (DEPs) | 6.4~14.8 nm | 0.15~7 mg/kg | DEPs +CeO₂ NPs induce lung injury after combined exposure | (79) |
| CuO NPs | 46.5 nm | 2.5, 5 and 10 mg/kg | CuO NPs increasingly deteriorate pulmonary inflammation as dose increases in C57BL/6 mice | (80) |
| nCuO$^{COOH}$ NPs and CuO NPs | 10–20 nm | Low dose: 23 and 32 mg/m³ Mid dose: 120 and 128 mg/m³ High dose 470 and 495 mg/m³ | A set of genes responding to mucociliary clearance mechanism varies among asthmatic and healthy population | (81) |
| ZnO NPs | 10.7+0.7 nm | 50 cm²/rat and 150 cm²/rat | ZnO NPs induces pulmonary fibrosis, goblet cell hyperplasia, eosinophilia, in different pH | (82) |

*(Continued)*

**TABLE 17.1 (Continued)**

**Toxicity of Nanoparticles to Different Organs and Systems in the Abe Human Body**

| Nanomaterial | Size | Dose/Concentration | Result | Ref. |
|---|---|---|---|---|
| ZnO NPs + toluene | 380 + 20 nm | Low dose: 5 mg/m³ ZnO + 200 ppm toluene. High dose: 10 mg/m³ ZnO +200 ppm toluene | ZnO NPs + toluene significantly increases pulmonary mediators' level thus inducing the pulmonary fibrotic response | (83) |
| | | **Liver** | | |
| Ag NPs | 35 ~ 45 nm | 20 and 50 ppm | Red blood cells (RBC), Hb, and Hct level do not change significantly, while significant change occurs in ALT and AST level in hepatocytes of both male and female mice after 2, 7, 14 days exposure. | (84) |
| Ag NPs | 18 ~ 19 nm | Low dose: 0.6×10⁶ particle/cm³, 49 µg/cm³ Middle: 1.4×10⁶ particle/cm³, 133 µg/cm³ High dose: 3.0×10⁶ particle/cm³, 515 µg/cm³ | No significant dose-related differences among blood parameters and several histopathological changes are identified such as bile-duct hyperplasia and hepatocellular necrosis | (85) |
| Ag NPs | 10~30 nm | 500 mg/kg | AST level increased significantly and the amount of ALT decreased but then increased at day 30 in rats. Autophagy and inflammatory reaction are induced. | (86) |
| Ag NPs | 13 ~ 40nm | 4, 10, 20, and 40 mg/kg | Significant change occurs among the blood parameters involving RBC, white blood cells (WBC), Hb, and platelets in high dose groups (20 and 40 mg/kg). Several liver functional enzymes, such as ALT and AST significantly increased after Ag exposure. | (87) |
| Au NPs | 10 and 50 nm | 50 µL | AST and ALP in liver cells are dependent on the small size (10 nm), large size is determinate for GGT and ALT level | (88) |

*(Continued)*

**TABLE 17.1 (Continued)**
**Toxicity of Nanoparticles to Different Organs and Systems in the $_{Abe}$Human Body**

| Nanomaterial | Size | Dose/Concentration | Result | Ref. |
|---|---|---|---|---|
| SWCNTs | Diameter (0.88~1.42 nm for FH-P-SWCNT, 1.27~1.42 nm for SO-SWCNT), Length (5–10 μm for FH-P-SWCNT, 1~5 μm for SO-SWCNT) | 0.1 mg/mL | Enzymatic metabolites of CYP3A4, CYP3A5, and CYP2D6 are significantly reduced in the presence of SO-SWCNT | (89) |
| SWCNTs | Length (7.0 nm), diameter (1.6 50 and 100 μg/mL nm) | | A significant reduction of CYP3A4 enzyme metabolites is observed in the presence of c-SWCNT in a dose-dependent manner, while PEGylated c-SWCNT can mitigate this effect | (90) |
| Ag NPs | 181 +17 nm | 5, 10, 25, 50, 100 μg/mL | No significant change on CYP1A, CYP2C, CYP2D, CYP2E1, and CYP3A enzymatic activities in rat liver *in vivo*, but strong inhibition effect only on CYP2C and CYP2D activities | (91) |
| Ag NPs | 25 ~40 nm Average: 32.8 nm | 480 mcg/day with 32 ppm Ag NPs | No observation on inhibition activity of Ag NPs to CYP1A2, CYP2C9, CYP2C19, CYP2D6, and CYP3A4 *in vivo* | (92) |
| | | **Dermal Toxicity** | | |
| MWCNTs | – | 0.6 and 0.06 μg/mL | The dermal fibroblasts cell cycle is arrested and apoptosis/ necrosis increases | (93) |
| c-MWCNTs | Outer diameter (30 nm) Length (5–20 μm) | 1 μg/cm$^2$ | c-MWCNTs induced keratinocyte toxicity and skin allergic condition is not mediated by ROS generation but in a carboxylation-dependent manner | (94) |
| Ag NPs | – | – | Inhibition to proliferation and morphology affected were found after Ag NPs exposure in human epidermal keratinocytes cells | (95) |
| TiO$_2$ NPs | 4, 10, 25, 60 and 90 nm | 400 μg/cm$^2$ | TiO$_2$ NPs penetrate to skin after chronic dermal exposure (60 days) and translocate to different tissues and organs. And those NPs are responsible for increased OS in the skin cell. | (96) |

*(Continued)*

**TABLE 17.1 (Continued)**
**Toxicity of Nanoparticles to Different Organs and Systems in the $_{Abe}$Human Body**

| Nanomaterial | Size | Dose/Concentration | Result | Ref. |
|---|---|---|---|---|
| | | **Brain** | | |
| TiO$_2$ NPs | 15 ~30 nm | 14, 28, 42 and 56 mg/kg | TiO$_2$ NPs synthesized in aqueous medium generated OS in vivo, and skin cells are damaged and have genetic alteration | (97) |
| TiO$_2$ NPs (GT)$_6$ – SWCNT | 30 nm — | 2.5 ~ 120 ppm 5 μg/mL | Microglia produce ROS in response to TiO$_2$ NPs exposure (GT)$_6$ – SWCNTs induce the inflammatory response in mice SIM-A9 microglial cells, while this could be mitigated by PEGylation | (98) (99) |
| Au NPs | 20 nm | 20 μg/kg | OS generation and antioxidant enzyme decreases, suggesting Au NPs might lead to DNA damage/cell death | (100) |
| Graphene oxide | Thickness (1.02 + 0.15 nm), lateral lengths (0.5 μm) | 0.01 ~ 1 μg/L | Brain cells apoptosis and senescence were triggered in the zebrafish larvae model, and Parkinson's disease-like symptom induced | (101) |
| Ag NPs | 25, 40 and 80mm | Final dose: 10.4 μg/cm$^2$ | The cytotoxic response was induced by smaller Ag NPs (25 and 40 nm) in rat brain microvessel endothelial cells. BBB permeability improved as size increases | (102) |
| SPIONs | 51.88nm | 10~200 μg/mL SPIONs to PC12 cells, 1 μg/μL SPIONs to hippocampus or striatum | A high dose of SPIO NPs induces a cytotoxic response in PC12 cells, decreasing cell viability and tyrosine hydroxylase protein but increasing the cell apoptosis. | (103) |

*(Continued)*

**TABLE 17.1 (Continued)**
**Toxicity of Nanoparticles to Different Organs and Systems in the [Abe]Human Body**

| Nanomaterial | Size | Dose/Concentration | Result | Ref. |
|---|---|---|---|---|
| | | **Cardiovascular System** | | |
| ZnO NPs | ZnO NPs (diameter: 20 nm) and ZnO NPs (diameter: 90~210 nm) | 0, 20, 50, 150 μg/mL | Cell viability decreased and OS generated in human coronary artery endothelial cells after ZnO NPs exposure. And Ca+ signaling pathway, neuroactive ligand-receptor interaction, hypertrophic cardiomyopathy, renin-angiotensin system, and dilated cardiomyopathy are affected by ZnO NPs | (104) |
| $Y_2O_3$, $\gamma$-$Fe_2O_3$, and ZnO NPs | $\gamma$-$Fe_2O_3$ NPs (45 nm and 5 nm) $Y_2O_3$ NPs (20~60 nm) ZnO NPs: (length: 100~200 nm Diameters:20~70 nm) | 0.001 ~ 50μg/mL | $Fe_2O_3$ NPs do not affect inflammation response in human aortic endothelial cells (HAECs), while $Y_2O_3$ and ZnO NPs are responsible to induce the inflammation activity in HAECs at above 10 μg/mL and ZnO NPs are cytotoxic at the highest concentration | (105) |
| | | **Others** | | |
| Ag NPs | 6.2~629 nm (61%: 27.3~106.2%) | 5 mg/kg | Organ damage occurs in the liver, kidney, thymus, and spleen after Ag NPs exposure. Mild irritation was in the thymus and spleen, but chromosome breakage and polyploidy cell rates significantly increased in the liver and kidney. | (72) |

## 17.4.2 NANOTOXICITY TO THE LIVER

The liver is essential to regulate metabolism and detoxify potential toxic xenobiotics, and it is where injected NPs are most likely to store and accumulate. Histopathologic change and hematologic level are recognized to cause liver injury. Mice exposed to Ag NPs showed that serum aspartate aminotransferase (AST) significantly increases during the entire experiment; whereas, the level of serum alanine aminotransferase (ALT) decreases in the first couple of days but increases at day 30 after exposure, indicating membrane rupture within hepatic cells (84, 86). Cytoplasmic granulation, inflammation, and cytoplasmic vacuolation with necrosis of hepatocytes were detected in mice hepatic cells during different time intervals after Ag NPs exposure. Although several publications indicate that there is no significant dose-related impact on serum parameters alteration (e.g., red blood cell, hemoglobin, and hematocrit, etc.), available hematological data are insufficient (85, 87). Moreover, inflammation reaction was also found in mice exposed to Au NPs. An increase in enzyme AST and a decrease in alkaline phosphatase (ALP) levels in mice are associated with smaller Au NPs, while ALT and gamma-glutamyl transferase (GGT) levels depend on larger NPs after three days of exposure (88). However, a discrepancy occurs in the size-related response of histopathological change after exposure to Au NPs that have a similar size range (109).

Another concern is due to the interaction between NPs and hepatocellular enzymes, for example, cytochrome P450 (CYP) that is a supergroup of enzyme consisting of cofactor-heme, functioning for detoxification of xenobiotics. This behavior can influence the enzymatic activity in hepatic cells and affect detoxification. SWCNTs have been identified to significantly reduce the level of metabolites of CYP2D6, CYP3A4, and CYP3A5, which are the three most abundant enzymes associated with drug-metabolizing function in CYP family (89, 90). Essentially, the process of reducing enzymatic metabolites is largely dependent upon several factors such as dose, a metal catalyst for SWCNTs synthesis [Fe (FH-P-SWCNT) versus nanocomposites of nickel and yttrium (SO-SWCNT)], additive proteins [bovine serum albumin (BSA)], and surface chemical modification [carboxylated SWCNT (c-SWCNT) versus PEGylated SWNT (PEG-SWCNT)]. El-Sayed, et al. (90) found that 6β-hydroxy testosterone, a major CYP3A4 enzyme metabolite, was inhibited when CYP3A4 enzyme was exposed to c-SWCNT in a dose-dependent manner. Yet, BSA corona helps to prevent enzyme inhibition activity by c-SWCNT and the efficiency of prevention to enzyme inhibition is positively related to the amount of BSA. Furthermore, PEG-SWCNT can mitigate the inhibition activity of c-SWCNT to the CYP3A4 enzyme in a molecular weight-dependent manner (**Figure 17.5**). This suggests that SWCNTs can inhibit the activity of CYP enzymes via three probable routes (90, 110, 111): 1) active site disruption; 2) competitive binding of enzymatic subtracts; and 3) active site bioactivity of enzyme prohibition. Though, on the contrary, El-Sayed et al. (112) observed pristine and oxidized SWCNTs are biodegraded by CYP3A4 *in vitro*. Besides, recent research found a notable inhibition activity of Ag NPs on CYP enzymes *in vitro*, though not *in vivo* perhaps due to ion formation occurring *in vivo* after Ag NPs exposure, which cannot interact with any key amino acids of CYP inhibition endpoint (91, 92, 113). However, this may suggest

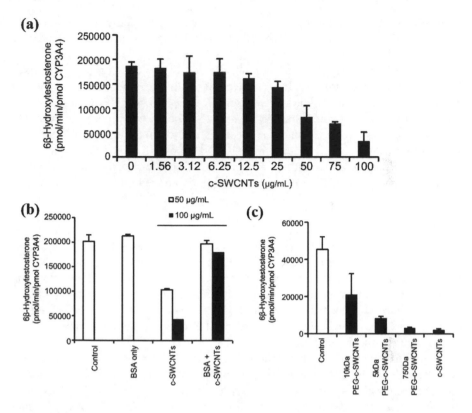

**FIGURE 17.5** Effect of different factors on CYP3A4 activity. (**a**) Inhibition effect of c-SWCNTs concentration on CYP3A4 catalysis activity by measuring the conversion of testosterone to 6 6β-hydroxy testosterones. (**b**) BSA, c-SWCNT, and their mixture. (**c**) c-SWCNT and different molecular weights of PEGylated c-SWCTN. Adapted with permission from (90).

that Ag NPs are potential hepatotoxins if they are present in an insufficient amount in the liver.

## 17.4.3 DERMAL TOXICITY

The absorption and accumulation of toxic NMs on the skin are dependent on their chemical composition and surface chemical modifications. Dermal toxicity occurs when NMs come in contact with the skin and then are transmitted through various inner translocation routes. Health hazards to workers potentially in various manufactural processes arise from exposure to NPs, supported by data of MWCNTs uptake through human epidermal keratinocytes (114). Ding et al. (93) pointed out that MWCNTs cause human dermal fibroblast cell cycle arrest and apoptosis/necrosis increase mediated by an immune and inflammatory response. In their study, strong immune and inflammatory responses were regulated by genes, which are activated by MWCNTs. When c-MWCNTs mixed with 2,4-dinitrofluorobenzene (DNFB) was used to treat mice ear, ear swelling was aggravated significantly in 6 h and 12 h, and high carboxylation level exacerbated the DNFB effect on ear swelling response (**Figure 17.6A**) (94).

Other NPs, including those of titanium dioxide ($TiO_2$) and Ag, have also been implicated for dermal toxicity. In a study by Wu et al. (96), dermal penetration of $TiO_2$ NPs occurred after 60 days of exposure *in vivo*, allowing NPs to get access to different tissues and organs in hairless mice body. The mice's skin then appeared to develop excessive keratinization, thinner dermis, and wrinkled epidermis after eight weeks of exposure to 10-nm and 25-nm $TiO_2$ NPs, possibly due to OS. Ag NPs are responsible for epidermal keratinocytes damage after skin penetration, resulting in significant changes in cell morphology and inhibition of cell proliferation (95).

## 17.4.4 Neurotoxicity

Once NPs have entered the blood vessel or lymph node via exposure pathways, they could gain access to the CNS across the BBB which is one of the most essential parts for brain protection. As the NPs are deposited in the CNS, multiple important regions in the brain are potential storage sites, including the hippocampus, cortex, striatum, olfactory bulb, and cerebellum (115). The accumulation of NPs is found to damage the CNS in different ways based on their physicochemical characteristics and surface chemical modifications.

Neuroinflammation mainly occurs in a type of macrophages-like cells covered throughout the CNS known as microglia, usually induced after NPs access the CNS. Microglia are activated and proliferated immune defense for CNS when brain homeostasis is destroyed or some toxic substances enter (116). As NPs enter the CNS, microglia shift from their quiescent state to an activated state, modifying morphology and further releasing pro-inflammatory factors (117). Long et al. (98) found that $TiO_2$ NPs exposure to mouse BV2 microglia induces ROS to release without photoactivation, which concurred with an earlier report (118). The "efficiency" of NPs exposure is size-dependent, i.e., smaller NPs could rapidly stimulate BV2 microglia to generate ROS. Besides, $(GT)_6$ single-stranded DNA conjugated SWCNTs were examined as neurosensory for mice SIM-A9 microglial cells *in vitro*, which could change the morphology of cells from round and motile to multipolar and ramified cells, and upregulate genes for microglial immune responses to express, but mitigated by PEGylation (99). Apart from occurring in microglial cells, neuroinflammation is also induced by NPs in other regions of the brain, including microvascular endothelial cells (102, 119), and neurons (120). For example, Au NPs were intraperitoneally injected into male rats resulting in significantly increased pro-inflammatory factors, such as malondialdehyde (MDA) (46% increase), 8-hydroxydeoxyguanosine (8OHdG) (57% increase), caspase-3 (38% increase), and heat-shock protein 70 (Hsp70) (45% increase), but decrease (21%) the important antioxidant enzyme GPx in neuron cells (**Figure 17.6B**) (100). This suggests that Au NPs are capable of inducing neuroinflammation in neuron cells and may lead to cell death.

Another concern for the CNS after NPs exposure is their ability to induce multiple types of cell death, such as apoptosis, autophagy, and necrosis. Superparamagnetic iron oxide (SPIO) NPs were found to increase the apoptosis of PC12 cells obtained

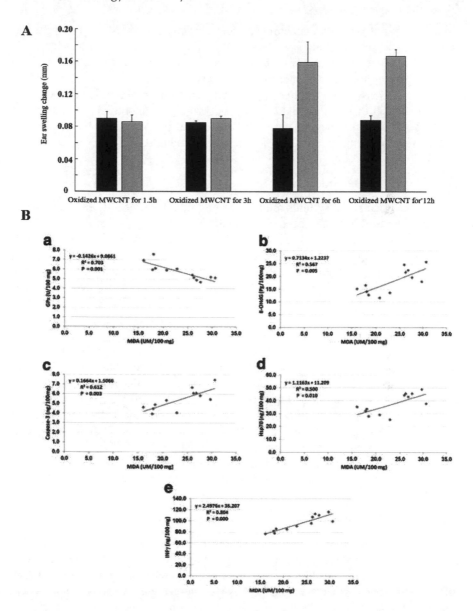

**FIGURE 17.6** (**A**) Effect of oxidized MWCNTs on contact hypersensitivity ear swelling response after exposure in 1.5, 3, 6, and 12 h. On day 0, mice were pretreated by 0.05% DNFB. On day 5, the right ear of mice was treated by 20 μL/ear of 0.2% DNFB (black bar), and the left ear was treated by various carboxylation levels of MWCNTs at 1 μg/ear dose with 0.2% DNFB (gray bar). Adapted with permission from (94). (**B**) Correlation between MDA production that represents lipid peroxidation and GPx (a), 8-OHdG (b), caspase-3 (c), Hsp70 (d), and INFγ (e), after 20 nm Au NPs treatment. Adapted with permission from (100).

from rat adrenal medulla pheochromocytoma region, and cells in the hippocampus and dorsal striatum region *in vivo* (103). This suggested that SPIO NPs could potentially induce neurotoxicity in the CNS. A recent finding on the zebrafish larvae model suggested that a low concentration of graphene oxide could not only induce Parkinson's disease-like symptoms by observation on normal amino acid and fatty acid metabolism disturbance and but also trigger the cell apoptosis and senescence based upon oxygen species generated (101). However, further research is required to shed more light on the mechanism of NPs inducing cell death.

### 17.4.5 OTHER ORGANS

Some other organs and systems are also prone to damage by NPs exposure in the body. Metal-based NPs have been observed to be responsible for cardiovascular toxicity in laboratory animals. For example, when human vascular endothelial cells (HVECs) were exposed *in vitro* to different sizes and concentrations of ZnO NPs, a couple of genes associated with cardiovascular disease were downregulated, while the level of several cardiovascular dysfunctional and inflammatory factors, such as interleukin-6 (IL-6), interleukin-8 (IL-8), were significantly increased (104, 105). Similar effects on the cardiac system were observed when HVECs were exposed to TiO$_2$ NPs both *in vitro* and *in vivo* (121, 122).

Kidney and intestine cells were also reported to have been damaged by NPs. Ag NPs were reported to break down the chromosomes and significantly increase polyploidy cells in rat liver and kidney *in vivo*, demonstrating that Ag NPs potentially have genotoxicity to kidney and liver (72). This corroborated the results of Milic et al., who reported a significant decrease in the ratio of porcine kidney cell viability after exposure to Ag NPs. When exposed to 25–70 mg/L of Ag NPs, there was a corresponding decrease in cell viability 32%–54% in 24 h (123). Additionally, CuO NPs were observed to cause oxidative, cell damage, and death both in liver and intestine cells, which suggests the potential cytotoxicity of CuO NPs (124).

## 17.5 ECOTOXICOLOGY

The adverse effects of NMs on the environment have also been studied. Once NMs are released into the environment, they spread quickly in the air, water, and soil. The NMs enter the atmosphere, biosphere, hydrosphere, and lithosphere through different pathways. Understanding how NMs interact with various elements and the toxicity risks of NMs should be an important consideration in the eco-friendly design of NMs to protect the environment from nanoscale materials pollution. The ecotoxicological effects of several NPs, including those of Ag, ZnO, and CuO, have been reviewed by Ivask et al. (125). Nanotoxicity of CuO NPs to a variety of aquatic organisms, including algae, shrimps, and rotifer, was determined via observation on the kinetics of target cell and mortality as toxicological endpoint (126). The toxicity of ZnO NPs is considerably higher to crustaceans (*Daphnia magna* and *Thamnocephalus platyurus*) than that of CuO NPs (127). Acute toxicity to *Daphnia magna* from ZnO, SWCNTs, MWCNTs, and other NPs over 48 h were compared in a comprehensive study conducted by Zhu et al. (128). Experiments on aquatic lives (daphnies, algae, rotifer, and plants) demonstrated size-dependent cell growth inhibition after TiO$_2$ NPs exposure (129).

## 17.6  SUMMARY AND FUTURE PERSPECTIVES

As an emerging facet of nanotechnology, nanozymes are now at an early stage but will undoubtedly bring many benefits. But, unfortunately, there are some adverse effects that may cause toxicity to the health of the biological system and the ecosystem. With intrinsic properties of NMs, nanozymes toxicity can be referred to as nanotoxicology. Therefore, it is crucial to consider nanotoxicology for the safer and sustainable development of nanozyme technology.

In this chapter, we have presented some critical information on the toxicological effects of NPs on living entities and the environment. Several exposure routes of NPs include skin contact, inhalation, injection, and ingestion. Upon entering the body, the BD of NPs is dependent on their morphology and surface function. There are several putative mechanisms of nanotoxicity to organisms that involve ROS, OS, characteristics of NPs, and genotoxicity. However, the biggest challenge of nanotoxicology is on the mechanism of toxicological damage and disorders that arise in each organ or system after NPs exposure, due to multiple factors involved in the nanotoxicology matrix. These factors are physical properties, such as size, shape, surface-area-to-volume ratio, chemical functions, as well as dosage. Furthermore, the dose matrix is also complicated to be estimated for each type of NPs, requiring considerations of determinants, such as mass, the number of NPs, etc. The ecosystem is also subject to adverse effects of NPs when they are released into the environment, which should be further investigated. In general, compared to the voluminous literature on various aspects of nanotechnology, information available on nanotoxicology is rather limited. Thorough and comprehensive investigations on all aspects of various NMs and the attendant nanotoxicological effects are to be fully considered and carefully documented. This should form a basis for further development of nanozymes and other nanotechnological developments that interact with living systems and the environment. Such a holistic understanding of the properties, functions, and end effects of NMs will help lead to safer and more responsible endues applications—ones that do not endanger the systems that nanozymes interact with.

## REFERENCES

1. Borzelleca JF. 2000. *Toxicological Sciences* 53: 2–4
2. Timbrell J. 2001. *Introduction to toxicology*: CRC Press
3. Elsaesser A, Howard CV. 2012. *Advanced Drug Delivery Reviews* 64: 129–37
4. Pui DYH, Fruin S, McMurry PH. 1988. *Aerosol Science and Technology* 8: 173–87
5. McClellan RO. 1987. *Annual Review of Pharmacology and Toxicology* 27: 279–300
6. Kanapilly GM, Wolff RK, DeNee PB, McClellan RO. 1982. In *Inhaled Particles V*, pp. 77–91: Elsevier
7. Schlesinger RB, Snyder CA, Chen LC, Gorczynski JE, Ménache M. 2000. *Inhalation Toxicology* 12: 927–39
8. Warheit DB, Laurence BR, Reed KL, Roach DH, Reynolds GAM, Webb TR. 2004. *Toxicological Sciences* 77: 117–25

9. Shvedova A, Castranova V, Kisin E, Schwegler-Berry D, Murray A, et al. 2003. *Journal of Toxicology and Environmental Health Part A* 66: 1909–26
10. Oberdörster E. 2004. *Environmental Health Perspectives* 112: 1058–62
11. Donaldson K, Stone V, Tran CL, Kreyling W, Borm PJA. 2004. *Nanotoxicology*. BMJ Publishing Group Ltd
12. Ostrowski AD, Martin T, Conti J, Hurt I, Harthorn BH. 2009. *Journal of Nanoparticle Research* 11: 251–7
13. Santamaria A. 2012. In *Nanotoxicity*, pp. 1–12: Springer
14. Wang W, Gunasekaran S. 2020. *TrAC Trends in Analytical Chemistry* 126: 115841
15. Hagens WI, Oomen AG, de Jong WH, Cassee FR, Sips AJAM. 2007. *Regulatory Toxicology and Pharmacology* 49: 217–29
16. Anderson DS, Patchin ES, Silva RM, Uyeminami DL, Sharmah A, et al. 2015. *Toxicological Sciences* 144: 366–81
17. Singh AK. 2015. *Engineered nanoparticles: structure, properties and mechanisms of toxicity*: Academic Press
18. Oberdörster G, Oberdörster E, Oberdörster J. 2005. *Environmental Health Perspectives* 113: 823–39
19. Sturm R. 2015. *Annals of Translational Medicine* 3
20. Hoet PHM, Brüske-Hohlfeld I, Salata OV. 2004. *Journal of Nanobiotechnology* 2: 12
21. Bengalli R, Gualtieri M, Capasso L, Urani C, Camatini M. 2017. *Toxicology Letters* 279: 22–32
22. Patra HK, Banerjee S, Chaudhuri U, Lahiri P, Dasgupta AK. 2007. *Nanomedicine: Nanotechnology, Biology and Medicine* 3: 111–9
23. Sahu SC, Casciano DA. 2009. *Nanotoxicity: from in vivo and in vitro models to health risks*: John Wiley & Sons
24. Kreyling WG, Semmler M, Möller W. 2004. *Journal of Aerosol Medicine* 17: 140–52
25. Kao Y-Y, Cheng T-J, Yang D-M, Wang C-T, Chiung Y-M, Liu P-S. 2012. *Journal of Molecular Neuroscience* 48: 464–71
26. Garcia GJM, Schroeter JD, Kimbell JS. 2015. *Inhalation Toxicology* 27: 394–403
27. Meyer W, Seegers U. 2012. *Journal of Fish Biology* 80: 1940–67
28. Baroli B. 2010. *Journal of Pharmaceutical Sciences* 99: 21–50
29. Tak YK, Pal S, Naoghare PK, Rangasamy S, Song JM. 2015. *Scientific Reports* 5: 16908
30. Baroli B, Ennas MG, Loffredo F, Isola M, Pinna R, López-Quintela MA. 2007. *Journal of Investigative Dermatology* 127: 1701–12
31. Schneider M, Stracke F, Hansen S, Schaefer UF. 2009. *Dermato-endocrinology* 1: 197–206
32. Sykes EA, Dai Q, Tsoi KM, Hwang DM, Chan WCW. 2014. *Nature Communications* 5: 1–8
33. Powell JJ, Faria N, Thomas-McKay E, Pele LC. 2010. *Journal of Autoimmunity* 34: J226–J33
34. De Jong WH, Hagens WI, Krystek P, Burger MC, Sips AJAM, Geertsma RE. 2008. *Biomaterials* 29: 1912–9
35. Sonavane G, Tomoda K, Makino K. 2008. *Colloids and Surfaces B: Biointerfaces* 66: 274–80
36. Zhang M, Yamaguchi T, Iijima S, Yudasaka M. 2013. *Nanomedicine: Nanotechnology, Biology and Medicine* 9: 657–64
37. Aggarwal P, Hall JB, McLeland CB, Dobrovolskaia MA, McNeil SE. 2009. *Advanced Drug Delivery Reviews* 61: 428–37
38. Alexis F, Pridgen E, Molnar LK, Farokhzad OC. 2008. *Molecular Pharmaceutics* 5: 505–15

39. Larsen EKU, Nielsen T, Wittenborn T, Birkedal H, Vorup-Jensen T, et al. 2009. *ACS Nano* 3: 1947–51
40. Wagner S, Zensi A, Wien SL, Tschickardt SE, Maier W, et al. 2012. *PLoS ONE* 7: e32568
41. Hirn S, Semmler-Behnke M, Schleh C, Wenk A, Lipka J, et al. 2011. *European Journal of Pharmaceutics and Biopharmaceutics* 77: 407–16
42. Hodgson E. 2004. *A textbook of modern toxicology*: John Wiley & Sons
43. Oberdörster G, Oberdörster E, Oberdörster J. 2007. *Environmental Health Perspectives* 115: A290-A
44. Schmid O, Stoeger T. 2016. *Journal of Aerosol Science* 99: 133–43
45. Montes-Burgos I, Walczyk D, Hole P, Smith J, Lynch I, Dawson K. 2010. *Journal of Nanoparticle Research* 12: 47–53
46. Wittmaack K. 2007. *Environmental Health Perspectives* 115: 187–94
47. Grass RN, Limbach LK, Athanassiou EK, Stark WJ. 2010. *Journal of Aerosol Science* 41: 1123–42
48. Stumm W, Morgan JJ. 2012. *Aquatic chemistry: chemical equilibria and rates in natural waters*: John Wiley & Sons
49. Hotze EM, Phenrat T, Lowry GV. 2010. *Journal of Environmental Quality* 39: 1909–24
50. Albanese A, Chan WCW. 2011. *ACS Nano* 5: 5478–89
51. Tripathy N, Hong T-K, Ha K-T, Jeong H-S, Hahn Y-B. 2014. *Journal of Hazardous Materials* 270: 110–7
52. Römer I, White TA, Baalousha M, Chipman K, Viant MR, Lead JR. 2011. *Journal of Chromatography A* 1218: 4226–33
53. Ntim SA, Sae-Khow O, Desai C, Witzmann FA, Mitra S. 2012. *Journal of Environmental Monitoring* 14: 2772–9
54. Davis JM, Addison J, Bolton RE, Donaldson K, Jones AD, Smith T. 1986. *British Journal of Experimental Pathology* 67: 415
55. Poland CA, Duffin R, Kinloch I, Maynard A, Wallace WAH, et al. 2008. *Nature Nanotechnology* 3: 423
56. Kostarelos K. 2008. *Nature Biotechnology* 26: 774–6
57. Palomaki J, Valimaki E, Sund J, Vippola M, Clausen PA, et al. 2011. *ACS Nano* 5: 6861–70
58. Jiang D, Ni D, Rosenkrans ZT, Huang P, Yan X, Cai W. 2019. *Chemical Society Reviews*
59. Kim KS, Lee D, Song CG, Kang PM. 2015. *Nanomedicine* 10: 2709–23
60. Blokhina O, Virolainen E, Fagerstedt KV. 2003. *Annals of Botany* 91: 179–94
61. Khanna P, Ong C, Bay BH, Baeg GH. 2015. *Nanomaterials* 5: 1163–80
62. Nel A, Xia T, Mädler L, Li N. 2006. *Science* 311: 622–7
63. Yu K-N, Yoon T-J, Minai-Tehrani A, Kim J-E, Park SJ, et al. 2013. *Toxicology in Vitro* 27: 1187–95
64. Arora S, Rajwade JM, Paknikar KM. 2012. *Toxicology and Applied Pharmacology* 258: 151–65
65. Modrzynska J, Berthing T, Ravn-Haren G, Jacobsen NR, Weydahl IK, et al. 2018. *Particle and Fibre Toxicology* 15: 2
66. Schins RPF. 2002. *Inhalation Toxicology* 14: 57–78
67. Schins RPF, Knaapen AM. 2007. *Inhalation Toxicology* 19: 189–98
68. Lindberg HK, Falck GCM, Suhonen S, Vippola M, Vanhala E, et al. 2009. *Toxicology Letters* 186: 166–73
69. Valdiglesias V, Costa C, Kiliç G, Costa S, Pásaro E, et al. 2013. *Environment International* 55: 92–100
70. Pantarotto D, Partidos CD, Graff R, Hoebeke J, Briand J-P, et al. 2003. *Journal of the American Chemical Society* 125: 6160–4

71. Pantarotto D, Partidos CD, Hoebeke J, Brown F, Kramer ED, et al. 2003. *Chemistry & Biology* 10: 961–6
72. Wen H, Dan M, Yang Y, Lyu J, Shao A, et al. 2017. *PLoS ONE* 12: e0185554
73. Buzea C, Pacheco II, Robbie K. 2007. *Biointerphases* 2: MR17–MR71
74. Ryman-Rasmussen JP, Cesta MF, Brody AR, Shipley-Phillips JK, Everitt JI, et al. 2009. *Nature Nanotechnology* 4: 747–51
75. Cesta MF, Ryman-Rasmussen JP, Wallace DG, Masinde T, Hurlburt G, et al. 2010. *American Journal of Respiratory Cell and Molecular Biology* 43: 142–51
76. Dong J, Ma Q. 2018. *Nanotoxicology* 12: 153–68
77. Manke A, Luanpitpong S, Dong C, Wang L, He X, et al. 2014. *International Journal of Molecular Sciences* 15: 7444–61
78. Ma JY, Mercer RR, Barger M, Schwegler-Berry D, Scabilloni J, et al. 2012. *Toxicology and Applied Pharmacology* 262: 255–64
79. Ma JYC, Young S-H, Mercer RR, Barger M, Schwegler-Berry D, et al. 2014. *Toxicology and Applied Pharmacology* 278: 135–47
80. Lai X, Zhao H, Zhang Y, Guo K, Xu Y, et al. 2018. *Scientific Reports* 8: 1–12
81. Kooter I, Ilves M, Gröllers-Mulderij M, Duistermaat E, Tromp PC, et al. 2019. *ACS Nano* 13: 6932–46
82. Cho W-S, Duffin R, Howie SEM, Scotton CJ, Wallace WAH, et al. 2011. *Particle and Fibre Toxicology* 8: 1–16
83. Jain S, Rachamalla M, Kulkarni A, Kaur J, Tikoo K. 2013. *Inhalation Toxicology* 25: 703–13
84. Heydrnejad MS, Samani RJ, Aghaeivanda S. 2015. *Biological Trace Element Research* 165: 153–8
85. Sung JH, Ji JH, Park JD, Yoon JU, Kim DS, et al. 2009. *Toxicological Sciences* 108: 452–61
86. Lee T-Y, Liu M-S, Huang L-J, Lue S-I, Lin L-C, et al. 2013. *Particle and Fibre Toxicology* 10: 1–13
87. Tiwari DK, Jin T, Behari J. 2011. *Toxicology Mechanisms and Methods* 21: 13–24
88. Abdelhalim MAK, Moussa SAA. 2013. *Saudi Journal of Biological Sciences* 20: 177–81
89. Asai Y, Sakakibara Y, Inoue R, Inoue R, Nadai M, Katoh M. 2018. *Biopharmaceutics & Drug Disposition* 39: 275–9
90. El-Sayed R, Bhattacharya K, Gu Z, Yang Z, Weber JK, et al. 2016. *Scientific Reports* 6: 1–12
91. Kulthong K, Maniratanachote R, Kobayashi Y, Fukami T, Yokoi T. 2012. *Xenobiotica* 42: 854–62
92. Munger MA, Hadlock G, Stoddard G, Slawson MH, Wilkins DG, et al. 2015. *Nanotoxicology* 9: 474–81
93. Ding L, Stilwell J, Zhang T, Elboudwarej O, Jiang H, et al. 2005. *Nano Letters* 5: 2448–64
94. Palmer BC, Phelan-Dickenson SJ, DeLouise LA. 2019. *Particle and Fibre Toxicology* 16: 1–15
95. Lam PK, Chan ESY, Ho WS, Liew CT. 2004. *British Journal of Biomedical Science* 61: 125–7
96. Wu J, Liu W, Xue C, Zhou S, Lan F, et al. 2009. *Toxicology Letters* 191: 1–8
97. Unnithan J, Rehman MU, Ahmad FJ, Samim M. 2011. *Biological Trace Element Research* 143: 1682–94
98. Long TC, Saleh N, Tilton RD, Lowry GV, Veronesi B. 2006. *Environmental Science & Technology* 40: 4346–52
99. Yang D, Yang SJ, Del Bonis-O'Donnell JT, Pinals RL, Landry MP. 2020. *ACS Nano* 14: 13794–805

100. Siddiqi NJ, Abdelhalim MAK, El-Ansary AK, Alhomida AS, Ong WY. 2012. *Journal of Neuroinflammation* 9: 1–7
101. Ren C, Hu X, Li X, Zhou Q. 2016. *Biomaterials* 93: 83–94
102. Trickler WJ, Lantz SM, Murdock RC, Schrand AM, Robinson BL, et al. 2010. *Toxicological Sciences* 118: 160–70
103. Liu Y, Li J, Xu K, Gu J, Huang L, et al. 2018. *Toxicology Letters* 292: 151–61
104. Chuang K-J, Lee K-Y, Pan C-H, Lai C-H, Lin L-Y, et al. 2016. *Food and Chemical Toxicology* 93: 138–44
105. Gojova A, Guo B, Kota RS, Rutledge JC, Kennedy IM, Barakat AI. 2007. *Environmental Health Perspectives* 115: 403–9
106. Li JJe, Muralikrishnan S, Ng C-T, Yung L-YL, Bay B-H. 2010. *Experimental Biology and Medicine* 235: 1025–33
107. Dheda K, Booth H, Huggett JF, Johnson MA, Zumla A, Rook GAW. 2005. *The Journal of Infectious Diseases* 192: 1201–10
108. Cheresh P, Kim S-J, Tulasiram S, Kamp DW. 2013. *Biochimica et Biophysica Acta (BBA)-Molecular Basis of Disease* 1832: 1028–40
109. Yang L, Kuang H, Zhang W, Aguilar ZP, Wei H, Xu H. 2017. *Scientific Reports* 7: 1–12
110. Zuo G, Huang Q, Wei G, Zhou R, Fang H. 2010. *ACS Nano* 4: 7508–14
111. Zuo G, Gu W, Fang H, Zhou R. 2011. *The Journal of Physical Chemistry C* 115: 12322–8
112. El-Sayed R, Waraky A, Ezzat K, Albabtain R, Elgammal K, et al. 2019. *Biochemical and Biophysical Research Communications* 515: 487–92
113. Wasukan N, Kuno M, Maniratanachote R. 2019. *Journal of Chemical Information and Modeling* 59: 5126–34
114. Monteiro-Riviere NA, Nemanich RJ, Inman AO, Wang YY, Riviere JE. 2005. *Toxicology Letters* 155: 377–84
115. Lin Y, Hu C, Chen A, Feng X, Liang H, et al. 2020. *Archives of Toxicology* 94: 1479–95
116. Bachiller S, Jiménez-Ferrer I, Paulus A, Yang Y, Swanberg M, et al. 2018. *Frontiers in Cellular Neuroscience* 12: 488
117. Ge D, Du Q, Ran B, Liu X, Wang X, et al. 2019. *International Journal of Nanomedicine* 14: 4167
118. Gurr J-R, Wang ASS, Chen C-H, Jan K-Y. 2005. *Toxicology* 213: 66–73
119. Trickler WJ, Lantz-McPeak SM, Robinson BL, Paule MG, Slikker Jr W, et al. 2014. *Drug Metabolism Reviews* 46: 224–31
120. Chibber S, Ansari SA, Satar R. 2013. *Journal of Nanoparticle Research* 15: 1–13
121. Zhang Q, Liu Z, Du J, Qin W, Lu M, et al. 2019. *The Journal of Toxicological Sciences* 44: 35–45
122. Chen Z, Wang Y, Zhuo L, Chen S, Zhao L, et al. 2015. *Toxicology Letters* 239: 123–30
123. Milić M, Leitinger G, Pavičić I, Zebić Avdičević M, Dobrović S, et al. 2015. *Journal of Applied Toxicology* 35: 581–92
124. Abudayyak M, Guzel E, Özhan G. 2020. *Advanced Pharmaceutical Bulletin* 10: 213
125. Ivask A, Juganson K, Bondarenko O, Mortimer M, Aruoja V, et al. 2014. *Nanotoxicology* 8: 57–71
126. Manusadžianas L, Caillet C, Fachetti L, Gylytė B, Grigutytė R, et al. 2012. *Environmental Toxicology and Chemistry* 31: 108–14
127. Blinova I, Ivask A, Heinlaan M, Mortimer M, Kahru A. 2010. *Environmental Pollution* 158: 41–7
128. Zhu X, Zhu L, Chen Y, Tian S. 2009. *Journal of Nanoparticle Research* 11: 67–75
129. Clément L, Hurel C, Marmier N. 2013. *Chemosphere* 90: 1083–90

# Index

9780367623883